Individual Participant Data Meta-Analysis

WILEY SERIES IN STATISTICS IN PRACTICE

Advisory Editor, Marian Scott, University of Glasgow, Scotland, UK

Founding Editor, Vic Barnett, Nottingham Trent University, UK

Statistics in Practice is an important international series of texts which provide detailed coverage of statistical concepts, methods, and worked case studies in specific fields of investigation and study.

With sound motivation and many worked practical examples, the books show in down-to-earth terms how to select and use an appropriate range of statistical techniques in a particular practical field within each title's special topic area.

The books provide statistical support for professionals and research workers across a range of employment fields and research environments. Subject areas covered include medicine and pharmaceutics; industry, finance, and commerce; public services; the earth and environmental sciences, and so on.

The books also provide support to students studying statistical courses applied to the above areas. The demand for graduates to be equipped for the work environment has led to such courses becoming increasingly prevalent at universities and colleges.

It is our aim to present judiciously chosen and well-written workbooks to meet everyday practical needs. Feedback of views from readers will be most valuable to monitor the success of this aim.

A complete list of titles in this series appears at the end of the volume.

Human and Biological Sciences

Brown and Prescott · *Applied Mixed Models in Medicine*
Ellenberg, Fleming, and DeMets · *Data Monitoring Committees in Clinical Trials: A Practical Perspective*
Lawson, Browne, and Vidal Rodeiro · Disease Mapping With WinBUGS and MLwiN
Lui · Statistical Estimation of Epidemiological Risk
Marubini and Valsecchi · Analysing Survival Data from Clinical Trials and Observation Studies
Parmigiani · Modeling in Medical Decision Making: A Bayesian Approach
Senn · Cross-over Trials in Clinical Research, Second Edition
Senn · Statistical Issues in Drug Development
Spiegelhalter, Abrams, and Myles · Bayesian Approaches to Clinical Trials and Health-Care Evaluation
Turner · New Drug Development: Design, Methodology, and Analysis
Whitehead · Design and Analysis of Sequential Clinical Trials, Revised Second Edition
Whitehead · Meta-Analysis of Controlled Clinical Trials
Zhou, Zhou, Liu, and Ding · Applied Missing Data Analysis in the Health Sciences

Earth and Environmental Sciences

Buck, Cavanagh and Litton · *Bayesian Approach to Interpreting Archaeological Data*
Cooke · *Uncertainty Modeling in Dose Response: Bench Testing Environmental Toxicity*
Gibbons, Bhaumik, and Aryal · *Statistical Methods for Groundwater Monitoring, Second Edition*
Glasbey and Horgan · *Image Analysis in the Biological Sciences*
Helsel · *Nondetects and Data Analysis: Statistics for Censored Environmental Data*
Helsel · *Statistics for Censored Environmental Data Using Minitab® and R, Second Edition*
McBride · *Using Statistical Methods for Water Quality Management: Issues, Problems and Solutions*
Ofungwu · *Statistical Applications for Environmental Analysis and Risk Assessment*
Webster and Oliver · *Geostatistics for Environmental Scientists*

Industry, Commerce and Finance

Aitken and Taroni · *Statistics and the Evaluation of Evidence for Forensic Scientists, Second Edition*
Brandimarte · *Numerical Methods in Finance and Economics: A MATLAB-Based Introduction, Second Edition*
Brandimarte and Zotteri · *Introduction to Distribution Logistics*
Chan and Wong · *Simulation Techniques in Financial Risk Management, Second Edition*
Jank · *Statistical Methods in eCommerce Research*
Jank and Shmueli · *Modeling Online Auctions*
Lehtonen and Pahkinen · *Practical Methods for Design and Analysis of Complex Surveys, Second Edition*
Lloyd · *Data Driven Business Decisions*
Ohser and Mücklich · *Statistical Analysis of Microstructures in Materials Science*
Rausand · *Risk Assessment: Theory, Methods, and Applications*

Individual Participant Data Meta-Analysis

A Handbook for Healthcare Research

Edited by

Richard D. Riley
Keele University
Keele, UK

Jayne F. Tierney
MRC Clinical Trials Unit at UCL
London, UK

Lesley A. Stewart
University of York
York, UK

WILEY

This edition first published 2021

Registered Offices

John Wiley & Sons, Inc., 111 River Street, Hoboken, NJ 07030, USA

John Wiley & Sons Ltd, The Atrium, Southern Gate, Chichester, West Sussex PO19 8SQ, UK

Editorial Office

9600 Garsington Road, Oxford, OX4 2DQ, UK

For details of our global editorial offices, customer services, and more information about Wiley products visit us at www.wiley.com.

Wiley also publishes its books in a variety of electronic formats and by print-on-demand. Some content that appears in standard print versions of this book may not be available in other formats.

Library of Congress Cataloging-in-Publication Data

Names: Riley, Richard D., editor. | Tierney, Jayne F., editor. | Stewart, Lesley A., editor.

Title: Individual participant data meta-analysis : a handbook for healthcare research / edited by Richard D. Riley, Jayne F. Tierney, Lesley A. Stewart.
Other titles: Statistics in practice.
Description: Hoboken, NJ : Wiley, 2021. | Series: Wiley series in statistics in practice | Includes bibliographical references and index. | Contents: Individual Participant Data Meta-Analysis for Healthcare Research / Richard D. Riley, Lesley A. Stewart, Jayne F. Tierney – Rationale for Embarking on an IPD Meta-Analysis Project / Jayne F. Tierney, Richard D. Riley, Catrin Tudur Smith, Mike Clarke, and Lesley A. Stewart – Planning and Initiating an IPD Meta-Analysis Project / Lesley A. Stewart, Richard D. Riley, and Jayne F. Tierney – Running an IPD Meta-Analysis Project : From Developing the Protocol to Preparing Data for Metaanalysis / Jayne F. Tierney, Richard D. Riley, Larysa H.M. Rydzewska, and Lesley A. Stewart – The Two-stage Approach to IPD Meta-Analysis / Richard D. Riley, Thomas P.A. Debray, Tim P. Morris, and Dan Jackson – The One-stage Approach to IPD Meta-Analysis / Richard D. Riley and Thomas P.A. Debray – Using IPD Meta-Analysis to Examine Interactions between Treatment Effect and Participant-level Covariates / Richard D. Riley and David J. Fisher – One-stage versus Two-stage Approach to IPD Meta-Analysis : Differences and Recommendations / Richard D. Riley, Danielle L. Burke, and Tim Morris – Examining the Potential for Bias in IPD Meta-Analysis Results / Richard D. Riley, Jayne F. Tierney, and Lesley A. Stewart – Reporting and Dissemination of IPD Meta-Analyses / Lesley A. Stewart, Richard D. Riley, and Jayne F. Tierney – A Tool for the Critical Appraisal of IPD Meta-Analysis Projects (CheckMAP) / Jayne F. Tierney, Lesley A. Stewart, Claire L. Vale, and Richard D. Riley – Power Calculations for Planning an IPD Meta-Analysis / Richard D. Riley and Joie Ensor – Multivariate Meta-Analysis Using IPD / Richard D. Riley, Dan Jackson, and Ian R. White – Network Meta-Analysis Using IPD / Richard D. Riley, David M Phillippo, and Sofia Dias – IPD Meta-Analysis for Test Accuracy Research / Richard D. Riley, Brooke Levis, and Yemisi Takwoingi – IPD Meta-Analysis for Prognostic Factor Research / Richard D. Riley, Karel G.M. Moons, and Thomas P.A. Debray – IPD Meta-Analysis for Clinical Prediction Model Research / Richard D. Riley, Kym I.E. Snell, Laure Wynants, Valentijn M.T. de Jong, Karel G.M. Moons, and Thomas P.A. Debray – Dealing with Missing Data in an IPD Meta-Analysis / Thomas P.A. Debray, Kym I.E. Snell, Matteo Quartagno, Shahab Jolani, Karel G.M. Moons, and Richard D. Riley.

Identifiers: LCCN 2021000638 (print) | LCCN 2021000639 (ebook) | ISBN 9781119333722 (cloth) | ISBN 9781119333760 (adobe pdf) | ISBN 9781119333753 (epub) | ISBN 9781119333784 (oBook)

Subjects: MESH: Meta-Analysis as Topic | Data Interpretation, Statistical | Models, Statistical | Randomized Controlled Trials as Topic

Classification: LCC R853.S7 (print) | LCC R853.S7 (ebook) | NLM WA 950 | DDC 610.72/7–dc23

LC record available at https://lccn.loc.gov/2021000638

LC ebook record available at https://lccn.loc.gov/2021000639

Cover Design: Wiley

Cover Image: © Zaie/Shutterstock

C9781119333722_050521

MIX
Paper from responsible sources
FSC www.fsc.org FSC® C013604

To Lorna, Sebastian and Imogen
To Phil and Ellie
To Simon, Catriona and Kirstin

Contents

Acknowledgements

The Editors would like to acknowledge the support of their colleagues in their host institutions and departments: the School of Medicine, Keele University; the Centre for Reviews and Dissemination, University of York; and the MRC Clinical Trials Unit at University College London. Particular thanks to Lucinda Archer, John Allotey, Sarah Burdett, Thomas Debray, Miriam Hattle, Mel Holden, Carl Moons, Max Parmar, Bob Phillips, Larysa Rydewska, Mark Simmonds, Kym Snell, Shakila Thangaratinam, and Claire Vale, who have worked with us on many of our applied IPD meta-analysis projects, and to Danielle Burke and Joie Ensor for organising the Statistical Methods for IPD Meta-Analysis course at Keele. We are particularly grateful to Mike Clarke who has shared the IPD journey from the start and has contributed so much to the field. We also recognise the contributions by the convenors and other members of the Cochrane IPD Meta-Analysis Methods Group over many years, and acknowledge stimulating discussions with participants at our various workshops and training courses. We thank our colleagues and research collaborators on the various applied and methodological IPD meta-analysis projects we have been involved in, many of which formed motivating examples and case studies in the book chapters. In particular, we are indebted to the participants in the various trials and studies, and the associated investigators, without whom IPD meta-analysis projects would not be possible.

1

Individual Participant Data Meta-Analysis for Healthcare Research

Richard D. Riley, Lesley A. Stewart, and Jayne F. Tierney

1.1 Introduction

Healthcare and clinical decision-making should be guided by the evidence arising from high-quality research studies. Often a single study is insufficient to make firm recommendations, and so multiple studies are conducted to address the same research question. This motivates the need for *evidence synthesis*: the combination of data from multiple studies to provide an overall summary of current knowledge. For example, when multiple randomised trials have examined the effect of a particular treatment, evidence syntheses are needed to combine and summarise the information from these trials, in order to establish whether the treatment is effective or not.

Systematic reviews are the cornerstone of evidence synthesis and evidence-based decision-making in healthcare. They use transparent methods to identify, appraise and combine a body of research evidence, with the goal of producing summary results that guide best practices for stakeholders including patients, clinicians, health professionals, and policy-makers. Systematic review methodology has been championed by organisations such as Cochrane, who publish systematic reviews in the Cochrane Library summarising the effects of interventions,[1] the accuracy of diagnostic tests,[2] the prognostic effect of particular factors,[3] and the performance of risk prediction models.[4] Most systematic reviews include a *meta-analysis*,[5] which is a statistical technique for combining (synthesising) quantitative data obtained from multiple research studies. Traditionally, most meta-analyses have used aggregate data extracted from study publications, but there is growing demand for meta-analyses that utilise individual participant data (IPD).[6–9]

This book is intended as a comprehensive handbook for healthcare researchers undertaking IPD meta-analysis projects. In this introductory chapter, we clarify differences between IPD and aggregate data, and outline why IPD meta-analysis projects are increasingly needed. Then, we detail the scope of our book and its intended audience, and signpost where to find material in subsequent chapters.

1.2 What Is IPD and How Does It Differ from Aggregate Data?

IPD refers to the raw information recorded for each participant in a research study (e.g. a randomised trial), such as baseline characteristics, prognostic factors, treatments received, outcomes and follow-up details, and can be represented by a dataset containing a separate row per participant and columns containing values for each participant-level variable. For example, IPD for a randomised trial of anti-hypertensive treatment will usually include the pre- and post-treatment blood pressure level, a treatment group indicator, important clinical characteristics and prognostic factors

Individual Participant Data Meta-Analysis: A Handbook for Healthcare Research, First Edition.
Edited by Richard D. Riley, Jayne F. Tierney, and Lesley A. Stewart.

recorded at baseline (such as age, sex, BMI and comorbidities), and relevant follow-up information (such as time to cardiovascular disease or death). An IPD meta-analysis project, therefore, involves the collection, checking, harmonisation and synthesis of IPD from multiple studies to answer particular research questions. An excerpt of IPD collected from 10 randomised trials for an IPD meta-analysis project is given in Box 1.1(a), after harmonisation into a single dataset ready for meta-analysis to summarise the effect of anti-hypertensive treatment. This dataset contains a single row *per participant* in every trial.

In contrast, aggregate data refers to information averaged or estimated across all participants in a particular study, such as the treatment effect estimate, the total participants, and the mean age and proportion of males in each treatment group. Such aggregate data are derived from the IPD, and therefore the IPD can be considered the original source material. A conventional meta-analysis uses aggregate data (e.g. as extracted from study publications), rather than IPD. An example of aggregate data obtained from 10 randomised trials of anti-hypertensive treatment is shown in Box 1.1(b), after collation into a single dataset ready for meta-analysis. This dataset contains a single row *per trial.*

1.3 IPD Meta-Analysis: A New Era for Evidence Synthesis

"Data sharing is an important part of ensuring trust in research, and it should be the norm."[10]

IPD meta-analysis projects began to emerge in the late 1980s and early 1990s,[11,12] originating mainly in the cancer and cardiovascular disease fields.[13] Calls to support IPD meta-analysis grew strongly throughout the 1990s alongside the formation of methodology working groups,[8,14] in particular the Cochrane IPD Meta-Analysis Methods Group (https://methods.cochrane.org/ipdma/).[7] In the decades since, the number of IPD meta-analysis projects has risen sharply (Figure 1.1). Early meta-analyses based on IPD were commonly described as *overviews* or *pooled analyses,*[7,11,15,16] until *IPD meta-analysis* emerged as the preferred, and now most widely used, label. The IPD abbreviation initially referred to *individual patient data*, but now *individual participant data* is the more inclusive and accepted term.

The growth of IPD meta-analysis projects reflects their potential to revolutionise healthcare research,[14,17] especially as they align with three major contemporary initiatives: *reducing research waste,*[18] *data sharing,*[19–24] and *personalised healthcare.*[25,26] The sharing of IPD maximises the contribution of existing data from millions of research participants, and so is becoming an increasingly frequent stipulation of research funding. Leading medical journals now require data-sharing statements, with some even enforcing the sharing of IPD on request.[23] This has led to dedicated data-sharing platforms and repositories being established to house IPD from existing studies.[27–31] Furthermore, as the drive for personalised healthcare (also known as stratified or precision medicine) continues,[25,26] researchers have recognised that, compared to using published aggregate data, IPD allows a more reliable evaluation of how participant-level characteristics are associated with outcome risk and response to treatment.[32,33] Thus, IPD meta-analysis projects are now central to modern evidence synthesis in healthcare.

1.4 Scope of This Book and Intended Audience

Meta-Analysis Using Individual Participant Data: A Handbook for Healthcare Research provides a comprehensive introduction to the fundamental principles and methods that healthcare

Box 1.1 Example of individual participant data (IPD) and how it differs from aggregate data

Illustrative example of 10 randomised trials examining the effect of anti-hypertensive treatment

(a) IPD

- The following table shows hypothetical IPD collected, checked and harmonised from 10 randomised trials examining the effect of anti-hypertensive treatment versus control in participants with hypertension.
- Each row provides the information for each participant in each trial, and each column provides participant-level information such as baseline characteristics and outcome values.
- Only a subset of the IPD is shown for brevity, as in reality many more rows and columns will be needed for each trial, to include all available participants and variables.

Trial ID	Participant ID	Treatment group, 1 = treatment 0 = control	Age (years)	SBP before treatment (mmHg)	SBP at 1 year (mmHg)
1	1	1	46	137	111
1	2	1	35	143	133
(other rows for trial 1 omitted for brevity)					
1	1454	0	62	209	219
2	1	0	55	170	155
2	2	1	38	144	139
(other rows for trial 2 omitted for brevity)					
2	337	1	44	153	129
(rows for trials 3 to 9 omitted for brevity)					
10	1	0	71	149	128
10	2	1	59	168	169
(other rows for trial 10 omitted for brevity)					
10	4695	0	63	174	128

- This IPD can be used to produce aggregate data for each trial, as shown in the table on the following page.

(Continued)

Box 1.1 (Continued)

(b) Aggregate data

- Now each row corresponds to a particular trial, and each column is a trial-level variable containing aggregated data values such as the total number of particulars and the mean age in each group.

Trial ID	Number of participants		Mean age (years)		Mean SBP before treatment (mmHg)		Mean SBP at 1 year (mmHg)		Treatment effect on SBP at 1 year adjusted for baseline (treatment minus control)
	Control	Treatment	Control	Treatment	Control	Treatment	Control	Treatment	Estimate (variance)
1	750	704	42.36	42.17	153.05	153.88	139.75	132.54	−6.53 (0.75)
2	199	138	69.57	69.71	191.55	188.30	179.89	164.67	−13.81 (4.95)
(rows for trials 3 to 9 omitted for brevity)									
10	2297	2398	70.21	70.26	173.94	173.75	165.24	154.87	−10.26 (0.20)

Source: Richard Riley.

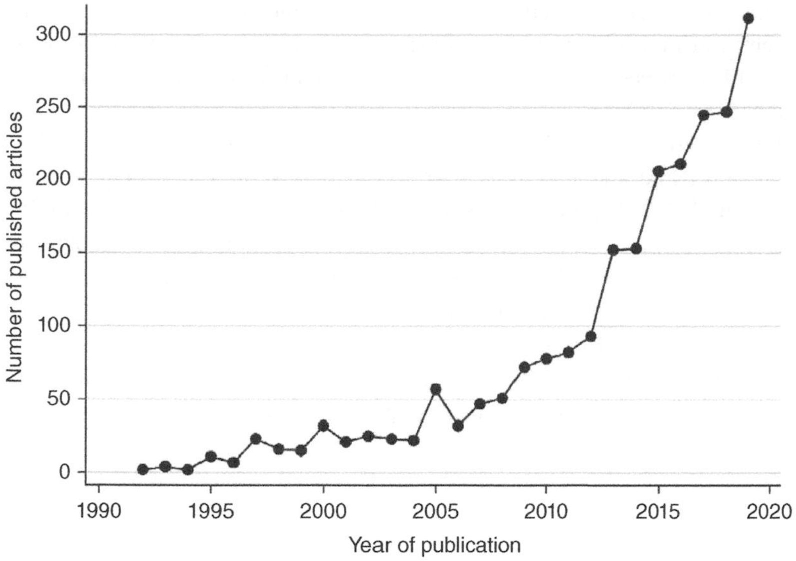

Figure 1.1 Number of published IPD meta-analysis articles over time, based on a crude search* in PubMed
Source: Richard Riley.
*from searching for the following keywords in the Title or Abstract of the article: (meta-analysis AND individual patient data) OR (meta-analysis AND individual participant data) OR (meta-analysis AND IPD).

researchers need when considering, conducting or using IPD meta-analysis projects. Written and edited by researchers with substantial experience in the field, the book details key concepts and practical guidance alongside illustrated examples and summary learning points.

IPD meta-analysis projects require a multi-disciplinary research team, including clinicians and healthcare professionals, statisticians, evidence synthesis experts, search and information specialists, database managers, trialists, and patient and public advisory groups, amongst others. Therefore, this book is aimed at a broad audience, and guides the reader through the journey from initiating and planning IPD projects to obtaining, checking, and meta-analysing IPD, and appraising and reporting findings. Very little prior knowledge is required. We assume readers are aware of the importance of systematic reviews and meta-analysis in general, and are reading this book to help guide their decisions as to whether to take the IPD approach; to learn what an IPD project entails (from start to finish); and to understand appropriate methodology and best practice, for example to inform protocols, data retrieval plans, statistical analyses, bias assessments, reporting standards, and critical appraisal.

Our book is split into five parts. Parts 1 to 3 focus on the synthesis of IPD from randomised trials to examine treatment effects. Parts 4 and 5 branch out to cover special topics and applications, including diagnosis, prognosis and prediction. **Part 1** includes chapters 2 to 4, and covers practical guidance for initiating, planning and conducting IPD meta-analysis projects. **Part 2** includes chapters 5 to 8, and covers fundamental two-stage and one-stage statistical methods for conducting an IPD meta-analysis of randomised trials to examine a treatment effect. These chapters are more technical than others, but should still be broadly accessible, as recommendations and illustrated examples are given throughout to reinforce the key messages. **Part 3** includes Chapters 9 to 11, and focuses on the critical appraisal and dissemination of IPD projects. **Part 4** includes Chapters 12 to 14, and covers special topics in statistics, including calculating power (in advance of IPD collection) and analysing multiple outcomes and multiple treatments. **Part 5** concludes with Chapters 15 to 18, which broaden application of IPD projects to the evaluation of diagnostic tests, prognostic factors, and clinical prediction models.

This book is the first to be devoted entirely to IPD meta-analysis projects, and complements other textbooks on systematic reviews and meta-analysis that focus mainly on the aggregate data approach, such as the following.[1,34–37] A general statistical textbook would also provide complementary reading to Part 2 of this book.[38–41] Relevant methods for IPD meta-analysis of prognosis studies are introduced in *Prognosis Research in Healthcare: Concepts, Methods and Impact*,[32] and Part 5 builds extensively on this work. Detailed information is also available on our companion website for this book: www.ipdma.co.uk. Introductory videos are included, alongside links to relevant publications, talks, training courses, and workshops. Statistical code is also provided for educational purposes, so that readers can replicate various examples given throughout the book and reinforce their learning.

Part I

Rationale, Planning, and Conduct

2

Rationale for Embarking on an IPD Meta-Analysis Project

Jayne F. Tierney, Richard D. Riley, Catrin Tudur Smith, Mike Clarke, and Lesley A. Stewart

Summary Points

- Many of the principles, methods and processes of IPD meta-analysis projects are similar to those of a conventional systematic review and meta-analysis of aggregate data. The most substantial differences relate to the collection, checking and analysis of data at the participant level, and collaboration with the investigators responsible for the existing trials.
- Compared to using aggregate data, IPD projects can potentially provide substantial improvements to the extent and quality of data available, and give greater scope and flexibility in the analyses, for example to examine participant-level associations.
- Important differences can occur between IPD and aggregate data meta-analysis results. This depends on many aspects including the availability of IPD, whether IPD leads to improvements in the completeness and quantity of information, and how analysis methods planned by the IPD researchers compare with those done by original trial investigators.
- Given the additional resource requirements, it is important to consider carefully whether an IPD project is needed instead of a conventional systematic review using aggregate data. The decision will depend on the particular research question, and whether IPD would produce a more reliable and comprehensive answer than using the aggregate data already available for eligible trials.

2.1 Introduction

In this chapter, we overview those elements of an IPD meta-analysis project that differ from a conventional meta-analysis of aggregate data (Section 2.2), describe the advantages (Section 2.3) and challenges of the IPD approach (Section 2.4), and summarise empirical evidence comparing results of IPD and aggregate data meta-analyses (Section 2.5). Although IPD projects almost always provide advantages, sometimes a standard aggregate data meta-analysis may be sufficient to answer a particular research question. Hence, researchers should only embark on an IPD project after careful consideration, especially as it requires additional time, resources and skills. We provide guidance to help researchers decide when the use of IPD is likely to provide more robust conclusions than using available aggregate data alone (Section 2.6). We focus on the synthesis of evidence from randomised

Individual Participant Data Meta-Analysis: A Handbook for Healthcare Research, First Edition.
Edited by Richard D. Riley, Jayne F. Tierney, and Lesley A. Stewart.

trials evaluating treatment effects, but most of what is presented also applies to other study types and to other types of research questions, such as those for diagnosis and prognosis (Part 5).

2.2 How Does the Research Process Differ for IPD and Aggregate Data Meta-Analysis Projects?

IPD meta-analysis projects follow many of the same principles and research processes as conventional systematic reviews and meta-analyses of aggregate data. However, there are also important differences, as now described.

2.2.1 The Research Aims

A first and fundamental step of all research projects is to define their aims. As for systematic reviews and meta-analyses based on aggregate data, the aims of an IPD meta-analysis project should be defined in relation to key components such as the participants, interventions, comparators or controls, outcomes and study designs of interest, aided by a framework such as PICOS (an example is given in Section 3.3).[42] Most reviews based on aggregate data focus on summarising the overall treatment effect, and often IPD meta-analysis projects also have this objective. However, IPD additionally allows participant-level information to be examined and analysed, and so most IPD projects are specifically set up to utilise this. In particular, they may aim to summarise treatment effects conditional on prognostic factors (Chapters 5 and 6); to assess whether the treatment effect varies according to participant-level characteristics (Chapter 7), or to evaluate treatment effects at multiple time-points during follow-up (Chapter 13). Indeed, the potential research questions that can be addressed by an IPD project are broad, and a wide variety of applications are demonstrated throughout this book.

2.2.2 The Process and Methods

Figure 2.1 provides key differences in the process of conducting IPD meta-analysis projects compared to conventional reviews based on aggregate data.[7,43] Best practice is to publish and adhere to a protocol, regardless of whether aggregate data or IPD are being used, although protocols for IPD projects will usually be more detailed (Section 4.2.2). Methods for identifying trials are very similar in the two approaches, but in an IPD project searches may be conducted prior to or in tandem with protocol development, in order to generate a preliminary list of trials (Section 4.2.3), and to identify the associated investigators from whom IPD will be sought (Section 3.2).

Prior to data collection, an IPD project may require ethical approval (Section 3.10) and development of formal data-sharing agreements (Section 3.11), as well as the preparation of a detailed data dictionary (Section 4.2.7). These are rarely required for an aggregate data review. Furthermore, the subsequent data collection, checking and analytical aspects of an IPD project are much more exacting than those for aggregate data reviews. They may include data entry, data re-coding and harmonisation, together with checking, querying and subsequent validation of IPD with original trial investigators (Chapter 4),[7,43,44] as well as advanced statistical methods for meta-analysis (Part 2).

Unlike aggregate data reviews, IPD projects usually involve and benefit from establishing partnerships with trial investigators who, in addition to providing their IPD, play an active role throughout the process, from identifying relevant trials through to helping interpret and disseminate IPD

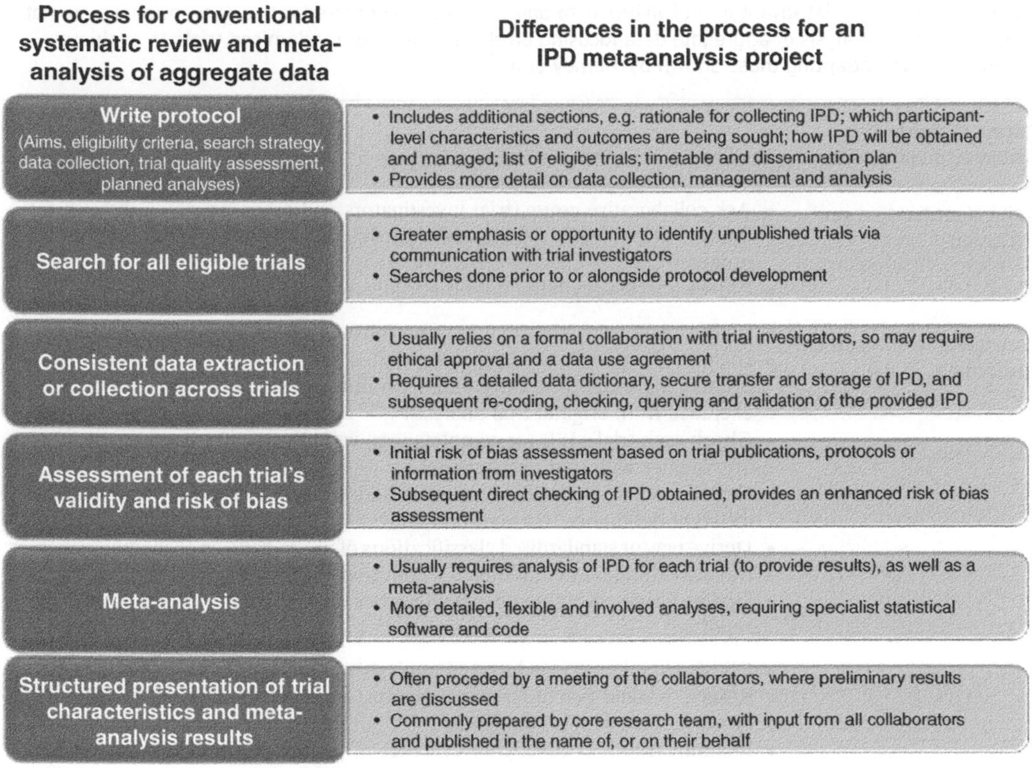
Process for conventional systematic review and meta-analysis of aggregate data
Differences in the process for an IPD meta-analysis project
Write protocol
(Aims, eligibility criteria, search strategy, data collection, trial quality assessment, planned analyses)
• Includes additional sections, e.g. rationale for collecting IPD; which participant-level characteristics and outcomes are being sought; how IPD will be obtained and managed; list of eligibe trials; timetable and dissemination plan
• Provides more detail on data collection, management and analysis
Search for all eligible trials
• Greater emphasis or opportunity to identify unpublished trials via communication with trial investigators
• Searches done prior to or alongside protocol development
Consistent data extraction or collection across trials
• Usually relies on a formal collaboration with trial investigators, so may require ethical approval and a data use agreement
• Requires a detailed data dictionary, secure transfer and storage of IPD, and subsequent re-coding, checking, querying and validation of the provided IPD
Assessment of each trial's validity and risk of bias
• Initial risk of bias assessment based on trial publications, protocols or information from investigators
• Subsequent direct checking of IPD obtained, provides an enhanced risk of bias assessment
Meta-analysis
• Usually requires analysis of IPD for each trial (to provide results), as well as a meta-analysis
• More detailed, flexible and involved analyses, requiring specialist statistical software and code
Structured presentation of trial characteristics and meta-analysis results
• Often proceded by a meeting of the collaborators, where preliminary results are discussed
• Commonly prepared by core research team, with input from all collaborators and published in the name of, or on their behalf

Figure 2.1 Key differences between the process for a IPD meta-analysis project and a conventional systematic review and meta-analysis of aggregate data. *Source:* Jayne Tierney.

meta-analysis results. This may include establishing a collaborative group that authors the main project publication, with all those involved being listed as co-authors, and holding a meeting of this Group where preliminary results are presented and discussed (Section 3.8).[7,43] Recently, a range of clinical study data repositories and platforms have been established, offering another source of IPD from existing trials, but there are both advantages and disadvantages of obtaining for IPD meta-analysis projects in this way (Sections 3.2.2 and 4.4.5).[45]

Given these differences, IPD meta-analysis projects require a greater range of skills (Section 3.5), generally take longer (Section 3.7), and need more resources (Section 3.8) than traditional systematic reviews and meta-analyses based on aggregate data.

2.3 What Are the Potential Advantages of an IPD Meta-Analysis Project?

Provided it is conducted appropriately, an IPD meta-analysis project offers many advantages over the conventional aggregate data approach (Table 2.1).[7,9,43,44] A key benefit is the potential to improve the quantity and quality of data, because there is no need to be limited by what has been published. For example, IPD from unpublished trials can be included (Section 4.2.3), as can any outcomes that were not reported for published trials, or even participants who were

Table 2.1 Key potential advantages of an IPD meta-analysis project compared with a conventional systematic review and meta-analysis of aggregate data focusing on the synthesis of randomised trials to evaluate treatment effects, adapting those shown by Tierney et al.[9]

Aspect of systematic review or meta-analysis	Advantages of an IPD meta-analysis project
Trial identification and inclusion	• Ask collaborative group (trial investigators and other experts in the clinical field) to help identify eligible trials (particularly those that are unpublished or ongoing)* • Clarify a trial's eligibility with the trial's investigators*
Data completeness and uniformity	• Include data from trials that are unpublished or not reported in full* • Include unreported data (e.g. unpublished subgroups, outcomes and time-points), more complete information on outcomes, and data on participants excluded from original trial analyses* • Check each trial's IPD for completeness, validity and consistency, and resolve any queries with trial investigators • Derive new or standardised outcome definitions across trials or translate different definitions to a common scale • Derive new or standardised classifications of participant-level characteristics, or translate different definitions to a common scale • Update follow-up of time-to-event or other time-related outcomes beyond those reported*
Risk of bias assessment	• Clarify trial design, conduct and analysis methods with trial investigators* • Resolve unclear risk of bias assessments (i.e. based on trial reports) through direct contact with investigators* • Examine trial IPD directly for evidence of potential bias in trial design and conduct, and resolve any queries with trial investigators • Obtain extra data where necessary to alleviate or mitigate against potential biases*
Analyses	• Apply a consistent method of analysis for each trial (independent of original trial analyses) • Analyse all important outcomes irrespective of whether published* • Explore validity of analytical assumptions e.g. normality of residuals in a linear regression analysis • Derive outcomes and measures of effect directly from IPD (independent of trial reporting), potentially at multiple time-points of interest • Use a consistent unit of analysis for each trial (e.g. consistently analyse preterm birth events per mother rather a mix of per mother and per baby in trials that include twin pregnancies) • Account for complexities in each trial in the analysis, such as cluster randomised trials or multi-centre trials • Analyse continuous outcomes on their continuous scale and adjust for baseline value • Adjust for a pre-defined set of prognostic factors • Apply consistent definitions for categorised data (e.g. stage of cancer) • Conduct more detailed and appropriate analysis of time-to-event outcomes (e.g. handling of censored observations, generating Kaplan Meier curves, examination of non-proportional hazards) • Achieve greater power for assessing interactions between effects of interventions and participant-level characteristics • Model associations at the participant level, including potential non-linear relationships • Use appropriate but non-standard models (e.g. that account for repeated measurements or correlation between multiple outcomes) or measures of effect • Explain potential heterogeneity and inconsistency in network meta-analysis

	• Address additional important questions over and above efficacy, or not considered by original trials e.g. to explore the natural history of disease, prognostic factors or surrogate outcomes
Interpretation	• Discuss implications for clinical practice and research with a multi-disciplinary group of collaborators including trial investigators who supplied data, and patient research partners*
Dissemination	• Achieve more widespread dissemination though collaborative group networks and patient groups

* These advantages accrue from direct contact with trial investigators (rather than the IPD *per se*), so potentially could be achieved for conventional systematic reviews if more active communication with trial investigators were adopted. This is seldom done in practice.

Source: Adapted from Tierney et al.,[9] with permission, © 2015 Tierney et al. (CC BY 4.0).

inappropriately excluded from the original trial analyses.[7,9,43] As well as helping to circumvent potential reporting biases,[46] this can increase the quantity of information available for analysis and, therefore, boost the statistical power to detect genuine effects.[47] In addition, there is greater ability to standardise outcome and covariate definitions across trials (Section 4.5), which not only facilitates the conduct of meta-analysis, but also aids the interpretation of findings. Detailed data checking helps to ensure the completeness, validity and internal consistency of data items for each trial, further enhancing data quality (Section 4.5.4),[7,9,43,44] as well as providing independent scrutiny of the trial data.

In general, having access to IPD also supports more flexible and sophisticated analyses than are possible with only existing aggregate data. IPD are vital for a thorough investigation of participant-level associations, for example to identify treatment effect modifiers (Chapter 7).[7,9,43] For instance, an IPD meta-analysis project by the Early Breast Cancer Trialists Group, which combined IPD from 37,000 women in 55 randomised trials, established that the drug tamoxifen works better in the subgroup of breast cancer patients who are classed as oestrogen receptor positive.[15]

With IPD, there is no need to rely on, or be restricted by, the original trial methods of analysis. For example, the IPD meta-analysis research team could opt for alternative effect measures (e.g. hazard ratios rather than odds ratios) or assumptions (e.g. non-proportional rather than proportional hazards), as appropriate, and consider a broader set of outcomes than originally reported. Collecting IPD also allows continuous variables to be analysed on their continuous scale; potential non-linear relationships to be examined; and the analysis of outcomes, covariates (e.g. prognostic factors) and time-points that were recorded, but not originally analysed by trial investigators.

As most IPD meta-analysis projects are collaborative endeavours, direct contact with trial investigators can help to identify trials that may not be easily identifiable via other forms of searching,[7,9,43] and to clarify the eligibility of potentially relevant trials. Trial investigators can also provide extra information leading to more reliable risk of bias assessments than are achievable from trial reports (Section 4.6),[48] and if potential biases or errors are identified, they may be able to supply additional data to resolve or minimise these (Section 4.5.4).[7,9,43] Bringing together a group of international and multi-disciplinary collaborators can also facilitate wider discussion and interpretation of results, and aid dissemination of key findings (Chapter 10).

The advantages shown in Table 2.1 focus on the synthesis of randomised trials to evaluate treatment effects, but IPD meta-analyses have further advantages for non-efficacy questions. In particular, they are pivotal in guiding and tailoring diagnostic strategies (Chapter 15), identifying risk and prognostic factors (Chapter 16), and individualising risk prediction (Chapter 17) to guide healthcare policy and practice.[32]

2.4 What Are the Potential Challenges of an IPD Meta-Analysis Project?

The processes for collecting, checking and analysing IPD are more involved and complex than for conventional aggregate data reviews of the same topic, and therefore, more time and resources are required (Chapter 3).[7,9,43] Thus, before embarking on an IPD project, careful consideration about whether it is an appropriate course of action is needed (Section 2.6).[47,49]

As most IPD projects rely on collaboration with the teams responsible for the included trials, negotiating and maintaining relationships with investigators from different countries, settings and disciplines can take considerable time, effort, diplomacy and careful management (Section 3.2.1).[43,44] In an era in which the value of clinical data sharing is more widely appreciated, persuading trial investigators of the value of participating has perhaps become easier. That said, IPD meta-analysis research teams and those providing IPD are now faced with additional tasks, such as seeking ethical or other institutional approval for the exchange of IPD (Section 3.10), as well the development of detailed data-sharing agreements (Section 3.11).

Over the years, advances in database and statistical software and electronic communication have greatly reduced the burden of labour required for the data exchange, management and analysis aspects of IPD projects.[43] Even so, these remain the most time-consuming and resource-intensive phases (Section 3.8), and require skills and expertise beyond those needed for a conventional aggregate data review (Section 3.5). This is emphasised by a growing number of methodological articles relating to IPD meta-analysis projects, covering issues such as data checking and harmonisation,[7,28] statistical methodology,[33,50–57] examining potential biases,[46,58] dealing with unavailable IPD,[59] reporting,[60] and statistical software development,[61] amongst others.

2.5 Empirical Evidence of Differences Between Results of IPD and Aggregate Data Meta-Analysis Projects

There are many empirical comparisons of results produced by IPD meta-analyses with results based on corresponding analyses of published aggregate data. An early example, in advanced ovarian cancer, found that results based on published aggregate data suggest a 7.5% absolute improvement in the percentage of women surviving at 30 months with platinum-based chemotherapy, whereas the IPD meta-analysis suggests a 2.5% improvement in the percentage surviving.[8] This disparity, which could have led to different clinical conclusions, seemed to be driven by the IPD meta-analysis project including more trials, participants and follow-up, as well as including all of the events in a time-to-event analysis, rather than calculating a risk ratio from events observed at a fixed time-point.

In contrast, in a different example, there was no clear evidence of an effect of ovarian ablation on survival of women with early breast cancer, based on the published aggregate data, but a 10% absolute increase in the percentage surviving at 15 years based on IPD.[62] In this case, the IPD for the included trials incorporated much greater follow-up, leading to a near doubling of events. This, and a more appropriate time-to-event analysis, were likely to be the key drivers for the discrepancy with the aggregate data findings. Many other comparisons of results from IPD and aggregate data meta-analysis projects have been carried out, not only in cancer and cardiovascular disease where IPD meta-analysis first gained traction, but also in other healthcare areas such as infectious diseases, neurology, nephrology and critical care. The differences shown between IPD and aggregate data findings are variable and seem context specific (e.g. depending on the research question; Sections 2.2.1 and 2.6.1).[63]

A large systematic review that brought together published comparisons of treatment effects from IPD and aggregate data meta-analyses found that many pairs of IPD and aggregate data analyses agreed in terms of the statistical significance of the overall results for the main outcomes. However, the disagreement observed in 20% of cases could have led to different clinical conclusions.[63] The discrepancies did not seem to be clearly associated with variation in the number of trials, number of participants or length of follow-up.[63] Importantly, discrepancies are likely to be more pronounced when going beyond overall treatment effects, which is often a key aim of an IPD meta-analysis project, such as when examining treatment-covariate interactions at the participant level (Chapter 7).[33]

Evidence from a large cohort of systematic reviews of the effects of cancer therapies on survival showed that, on average, meta-analysis results for the overall treatment effect derived from published aggregate data (based on hazard ratios) were slightly more in favour of the research treatment than those from IPD.[47] Although most results were similar between aggregate data and IPD meta-analyses, those discrepancies that did occur were often substantial.[47] Importantly, results from aggregate data were most likely to agree with those from IPD when the number of participants or events (absolute information size) and the proportion of participants or events available from the aggregate data relative to the IPD (relative information size) were large. This emphasises that assessing the amount of information provided by the available aggregate data, and what the obtainable IPD might add for a particular research question, is an important step in determining when IPD will bring the greatest value (Section 2.6.3).

2.6 Guidance for Deciding When IPD Meta-Analysis Projects Are Needed to Evaluate Treatment Effects from Randomised Trials

Based on practical experience[7,43] and the empirical evidence summarised in Section 2.5,[47,63] any decision about undertaking an IPD meta-analysis project should be based on the nature of the specific research question (Section 2.6.1), the completeness and uniformity of the available aggregate data (Section 2.6.2), the information size (Section 2.6.3), and the data and analyses required to address the research question reliably (Section 2.6.4). A checklist of questions to aid in this decision-making is provided in Table 2.2, and is explained in more detail in the following subsections. The focus is on the evaluation of treatment effects from randomised trials. If the answer to one or more of the questions is "yes", then an IPD project is likely to add considerable value compared to a conventional systematic review and meta-analysis of aggregate data.

2.6.1 Are IPD Needed to Tackle the Research Question?

In certain circumstances, the rationale for obtaining and analysing IPD is immediately very strong, such as when the research question is focused on participant-level relationships to inform more stratified or personalised approaches to treatment. In particular, if the desire is to evaluate whether particular types of participants benefit more or less from an intervention than others (Chapter 7), IPD will almost always be needed to obtain a reliable assessment of treatment-covariate

Table 2.2 Signalling questions to help decide when aggregate data are insufficient for meta-analysis and IPD are needed, focusing on the evaluation of treatment effects from randomised trials.

Why IPD might be required	Signalling questions to help consider whether IPD are needed	Yes/No
To address the specific research question	Is going beyond overall treatment effects an aim of the project? (e.g. to examine treatment effects in relation to particular participant characteristics)	
	Is independent scrutiny of one or more eligible trials required? (e.g. if some trial results are controversial or all trials arise from a single sponsor)	
	Is it reasonable to wait some time for the research question to be addressed? (e.g. if a good-quality aggregate data meta-analysis already exists, but IPD are needed for a more thorough or up-to-date analysis)	
To improve the completeness and uniformity of the information	Are suitable aggregate data lacking for key outcomes of the trials? (e.g. publications do not provide a risk ratio, mean difference or hazard ratio for the overall effect; a treatment-covariate interaction for each participant-level covariate of interest, or the data to calculate these)	
	Are outcome definitions corresponding to the aggregate data unsuitable or do they lack uniformity across trials? (This could make synthesis or interpretation of outcome effects using aggregate data difficult)	
	Are participant-level covariate definitions corresponding to the aggregate data unsuitable or do they lack uniformity across trials? (This could make synthesis or interpretation of treatment-covariate interactions using aggregate data difficult)	
To improve the information size	Is the absolute information size represented by the aggregate data too small to detect realistic effects of treatment on the main outcomes? (i.e. the total number of participants, and total events if applicable)	
	Is the relative information size represented by the aggregate data 'low' or potentially unrepresentative? (i.e. the proportion of all potentially eligible participants or events, if applicable)	
	For time-to-event outcomes, is the duration of follow-up captured by the aggregate data too short?	
To improve the quality of the analyses	Are the statistical analysis methods and assumptions used by the trials to produce the aggregate data inappropriate?	
	Are the statistical analyses used by across the trials to produce the aggregate data incompatible?	
	Are continuous outcomes and variables handled inappropriately in the trial analyses that produced the aggregate data?	
	Answer to key questions "YES" = IPD may add considerable value	

Source: Jayne Tierney, adapting the figure presented by Tudur Smith et al.,[64] with permission.

interactions.[33] This is also true for situations where participant-level diagnosis, prognosis and prediction are of interest (Chapters 15 to 17). Another powerful motivation for seeking IPD is in controversial areas, where independent scrutiny of the trial IPD may improve credibility and increase transparency, which may be sufficient justification in itself.[20,65] On the other hand, if it is clear that a conventional aggregate data meta-analysis could provide reliable (albeit less detailed) results, then an IPD project may be of less value, or may not be considered a priority. For example, if the sole research objective is to investigate the overall effect of a treatment, then it may be reasonable to rely on aggregate data from existing trials (reported or otherwise available) that summarise these effects (Section 2.6.2).

It will not always be possible to complete an IPD meta-analysis project in a suitably timely manner for the question of interest, because, for example, trial investigators are focused on completion of their individual trials, trial data are embargoed for a period, or it will take too long to set up data-sharing agreements. Therefore, if a therapeutic area is moving very quickly, there is an urgent policy need, or results are required to inform an ongoing trial of the same treatment(s), a prospective aggregate data meta-analysis,[66, 67] perhaps as part of a living systematic review,[67, 68] may be more suitable for delivering results in the shortest time frame. However, ultimately the merits of any aggregate data synthesis need to be balanced against the benefits that a good-quality IPD project could bring, and for an important question, the extra time needed for IPD meta-analysis may be justified to better inform decision-making in the longer term. Instead, researchers might choose to complete a conventional aggregate data meta-analysis first, with the intention of conducting an IPD meta-analysis project in a subsequent stage, if more reliable and nuanced results are needed.

2.6.2 Are IPD Needed to Improve the Completeness and Uniformity of Outcomes and Participant-level Covariates?

Before deciding whether to collect IPD for meta-analysis, an important step is to assess the completeness and uniformity of the available aggregate data, either based on a pre-existing systematic review that addresses a similar research question, or by conducting a scoping or systematic review of existing trials of interest. If outcomes and participant-level covariates have been collected in the eligible trials, but are not (adequately) described in the associated trial reports (such as side effects of treatment, multiple time-points or continuous values of prognostic factors), this can be rectified by the collection and analysis of IPD. Even if all the outcomes, participant-level covariates and, if relevant, interactions required for the analyses have been reported, if they are not defined consistently across trials it can be difficult to include or combine their results in aggregate data meta-analysis in a meaningful way. At best, this could lead to findings that are difficult to interpret, and at worst, that are unreliable. If this is a cause for concern, IPD might be sought to allow standardisation of the variables in readiness for analysis (Section 4.5).

2.6.3 Are IPD Needed to Improve the Information Size?

A major motivation for meta-analysis is to increase the statistical power over that for a single trial. However, meta-analysis may still not be sufficient to answer a particular research question reliably, as it depends on the potential *absolute* information size available from all existing trials. Determining this potential absolute information size, and subsequently statistical power (Chapter 12),[69] should be considered in advance, and depends on the nature of the research question. For example, when using meta-analysis to examine the overall effect of a treatment for a binary or time-to-event outcome, the absolute information size depends on the number of trials potentially available for meta-analysis, as well as the number of participants and events in these trials. Between-trial heterogeneity is also important, though it is difficult to gauge in advance. When examining participant-level treatment-covariate interactions, the variability of covariate values in each trial also contributes toward the potential absolute information size (Chapter 12).[70]

If the potential absolute information size based on all trials and their participants is small, and so statistical power is low, any meta-analysis will struggle to detect realistic and clinically meaningful effects of the treatment under investigation, regardless of whether aggregate data or IPD are ultimately used. In this situation, conducting a meta-analysis based on IPD, in particular, may not be the best use of time, effort and resources,[47] unless it is specifically needed to inform the rationale and design (e.g. sample size) of a new trial that is geared to increasing the absolute information size for a subsequent meta-analysis (Chapter 12).[71,72]

The absolute information size of a meta-analysis may differ depending on whether aggregate data or IPD can be obtained, as suitable aggregate data may not be available for all trials, and similarly IPD may not be obtainable for all trials. It has been shown that when the absolute information size represented by an aggregate data meta-analysis is small, the overall results are less likely to agree with those of a corresponding IPD meta-analysis project.[47]

Even when the absolute information size of the available aggregate data is large, and power considered adequate, if these data represent a small proportion of all eligible participants (for example, because aggregate data for particular trials, participants or outcomes are not reported, or the follow-up is limited), then the *relative* information size will be small. Any meta-analysis of such aggregate data would not only suffer from reduced precision, but could be potentially biased or otherwise unrepresentative.[47] In this situation, if the collection of IPD were to bring about a substantial increase in the proportion of eligible trials, participants or events, thereby increasing the relative information size available for meta-analysis, then the approach could add considerable value, and may also give very different results to an equivalent aggregate data meta-analysis. For example, in the earlier example about the effects of ovarian oblation on survival in early breast cancer (Section 2.5), the collection of IPD brought about a substantial increase in the duration of follow-up, and the consequent number of events compared to the aggregate data, increasing both reliability and precision.

In contrast, if the absolute information size of the aggregate data is large (and so power considered sufficient), and the relative information size is also large (i.e. it represents a high proportion of the total eligible participants or events available from all existing trials), a meta-analysis of these aggregate data would be expected to provide a reliable estimate. However, the aggregate data may only be sufficient in some respects, but not others. For example, whilst the absolute and relative information size of aggregate data may be sufficient when focussing on overall (unadjusted) treatment effects,[47] they may be low when considering other measures (estimands) of interest, such as conditional treatment effects (i.e. adjusted for prognostic factors; see Chapters 5 and 6), subgroup results and treatment-covariate interactions (see Chapter 7), and time-dependent treatment effects (e.g. non-constant hazard ratios) and multiple time-points (see Chapter 13). IPD may substantially increase the information size for estimating such nuanced measures, and so researchers need to decide if they are a priority. For example, if an aggregate data meta-analysis has large absolute and relative information sizes, and shows an overall benefit of treatment, this might provide a strong motivation for collecting IPD to examine subgroup effects or time-dependent effects. In contrast, if there is no evidence of an overall effect based on such aggregate data, then there might be less justification for going to the trouble of collecting IPD, unless other reasons might warrant it (Table 2.2).

2.6.4 Are IPD Needed to Improve the Quality of Analysis?

Even if the necessary aggregate data are available for a trial, it may have been obtained using an inappropriate analytic method. For example, a treatment effect measured by an odds ratio derived from a logistic regression analysis may have been reported for a trial, when a hazard ratio based on a

Cox regression would have been more appropriate, due to the time-to-event nature of the data; or a cluster randomised trial may have been analysed without accounting for the clustering. Another issue is that trial analyses may not provide the estimate of interest. For example, when conditional treatment effects are of interest, a trial may have derived treatment effect estimates without adjustment for key prognostic factors (e.g. if continuous outcome values at the end of follow-up were analysed without adjustment for the continuous outcome values at baseline). Analyses may also not be sufficiently comprehensive; for example, a Cox regression model may have been fitted without examining the proportional hazards assumption for the treatment variable, even when non-constant hazard ratios are a concern (e.g. from overlapping Kaplan-Meier curves), or missing data may not have been handled appropriately (Chapter 18).

Analyses may also be inconsistent across trials. For example, even in situations where estimates of treatment-covariate interactions are reported for each trial, they may differ in their definitions of categorical covariates, handling of continuous covariates (e.g. age might be dichotomised in some trials, but not in others) and the assumed relationships (e.g. linear or non-linear trends).

All of these issues give rise to concern that a meta-analysis based on aggregate data would not be robust or adequate for answering the research question of interest, and that an IPD meta-analysis would be more comprehensive and flexible. Again, this can be determined only by first appraising the individual trial analyses, and evaluating which methods trial investigators used and the extent of aggregate data available.

2.7 Concluding Remarks

While there are many similarities between IPD and aggregate data meta-analysis projects, they differ substantially in collaborative, data management and analytical aspects. If done well, the IPD approach can bring substantial improvements to both the quality of the data and the analyses, often increasing statistical power, and leading to more reliable results and more nuanced examinations, for example, those relating to treatment effect modifiers at the participant level (Chapter 7). However, IPD projects incur additional costs in terms of the time, resource and skills required (Chapter 3), and so should not be undertaken lightly. Hence, researchers must give careful consideration to the research question, and whether IPD will add value over existing aggregate data. If IPD are likely to add value, the next phase is to examine the feasibility of obtaining IPD, and to plan and initiate the IPD project, as described in Chapter 3.

3

Planning and Initiating an IPD Meta-Analysis Project

Lesley A. Stewart, Richard D. Riley, and Jayne F. Tierney

Summary Points

- IPD meta-analyses are major research projects that typically take upwards of two years to complete. Specific research funding is usually required, and they cannot be done on a volunteer basis or in spare time. They require broader skills than conventional systematic reviews and meta-analyses of aggregate data, including greater statistical expertise and experience in managing participant-level data.
- Many IPD meta-analysis projects are collaborative, involving partnership with trial investigators who contribute IPD from their trials for re-analysis and whose role is acknowledged through membership of a collaborative group and authorship arrangements. An advisory group may be set up to include wider clinical, topic or methodological expertise and to facilitate patient and public involvement.
- Obtaining IPD from repositories or data-sharing platforms is emerging as a possible alternative or complement to direct collaboration with trial investigators.
- Initiating an IPD meta-analysis requires careful planning and detailed preparation. A clear overview of the entire project is needed at the outset, to give the best chance of success.
- Set-up tasks can include developing a project scope, establishing the central research team and advisory group, seeking in principle agreement to collaborate from trial investigators and/or identifying other sources of IPD, developing data-sharing agreements, applying for research funding, and for ethical approval or exemption.
- A competent central research team should include members with experience of successfully completing an IPD meta-analysis project, advanced statistical knowledge, experience in managing and coding IPD, and strong communication skills. The team should be as independent as possible and should not include members with a vested interest or strongly held views on the particular topic under investigation, such as whether a particular intervention is or is not effective.
- Prospective IPD meta-analysis projects need detailed and specialist planning.

Individual Participant Data Meta-Analysis: A Handbook for Healthcare Research, First Edition.
Edited by Richard D. Riley, Jayne F. Tierney, and Lesley A. Stewart.

3.1 Introduction

As described in Chapters 1 and 2, IPD meta-analysis projects are often regarded as a gold standard approach to evidence synthesis. However, they require a broader skillset than conventional systematic reviews, and generally require more resources and take longer to complete. Decisions to embark on IPD projects should therefore not be made lightly, and careful planning is essential. In this chapter, we cover the preparatory phase of an IPD meta-analysis project and provide guidance for planning and initiation. We outline the importance of carefully refining the research question to be addressed through development of a project scope, building the collaborative framework for the project, and establishing a team equipped with the necessary skills to ensure that it can be delivered successfully. We discuss data-sharing agreements, outline the potential need for ethical approval, and share our experience of typical timescales and of preparing funding applications. Throughout, we assume that the IPD project aims to synthesise IPD from multiple randomised trials to evaluate treatment effects. However, most of our guidance is also appropriate to other types of IPD meta-analysis projects including those focused on diagnostic or prognostic topics (Part 5).

Figure 3.1 (phase 1 section) outlines the main activities that need to be completed during the set-up and initiation phase of an IPD meta-analysis project, illustrating the approvals that may need to be sought and documentation to be prepared. In order to plan and prepare for an IPD project, and in particular to estimate costs for a funding application, it is necessary to think through all steps of the project at the outset (i.e. all elements of Figure 3.1), as these are often inter-dependent. Unlike a conventional systematic review and meta-analysis of existing aggregate data, where if something has been overlooked, syntheses can be unpicked and redone relatively straightforwardly, IPD meta-analysis projects are not well suited to rapid, frequent or last-minute changes, because of the considerable additional time that it can take to obtain and check additional data, and re-run analyses.

3.2 Organisational Approach

3.2.1 Collaborative IPD Meta-Analysis Project

IPD meta-analysis projects are most commonly initiated and carried out by a central research team, who establish a wider collaboration including representatives of the included trials. Partnership with trial investigators brings benefits in terms of detailed understanding of the topic area as well as generating 'buy in' and ultimately supporting provision of IPD. It also gives trial investigators appropriate academic credit through membership of the collaborative group, in whose name the IPD project is often published. However, direct involvement of trial investigators is at odds with some systematic review standards, such as those produced by the Institute of Medicine which recommend that systematic reviews are undertaken by those who are independent of the primary studies and who do not have vested interest in the review outcome.[73] This standard is much easier to comply with when using aggregate data extracted from trial publications. In our view, attempting an IPD meta-analysis project without some degree of involvement from trial investigators (over and above simply providing or allowing access to their IPD) would significantly reduce the chances of successful completion, and could lead to less insightful and nuanced interpretation of findings. Nonetheless, direct involvement (as a member of the central research team or otherwise having a decision-making role) of those whose trial is included in the IPD meta-analysis, or who otherwise hold strong views about the anticipated findings of the research in question, has potential to be both problematic and undermine credibility.

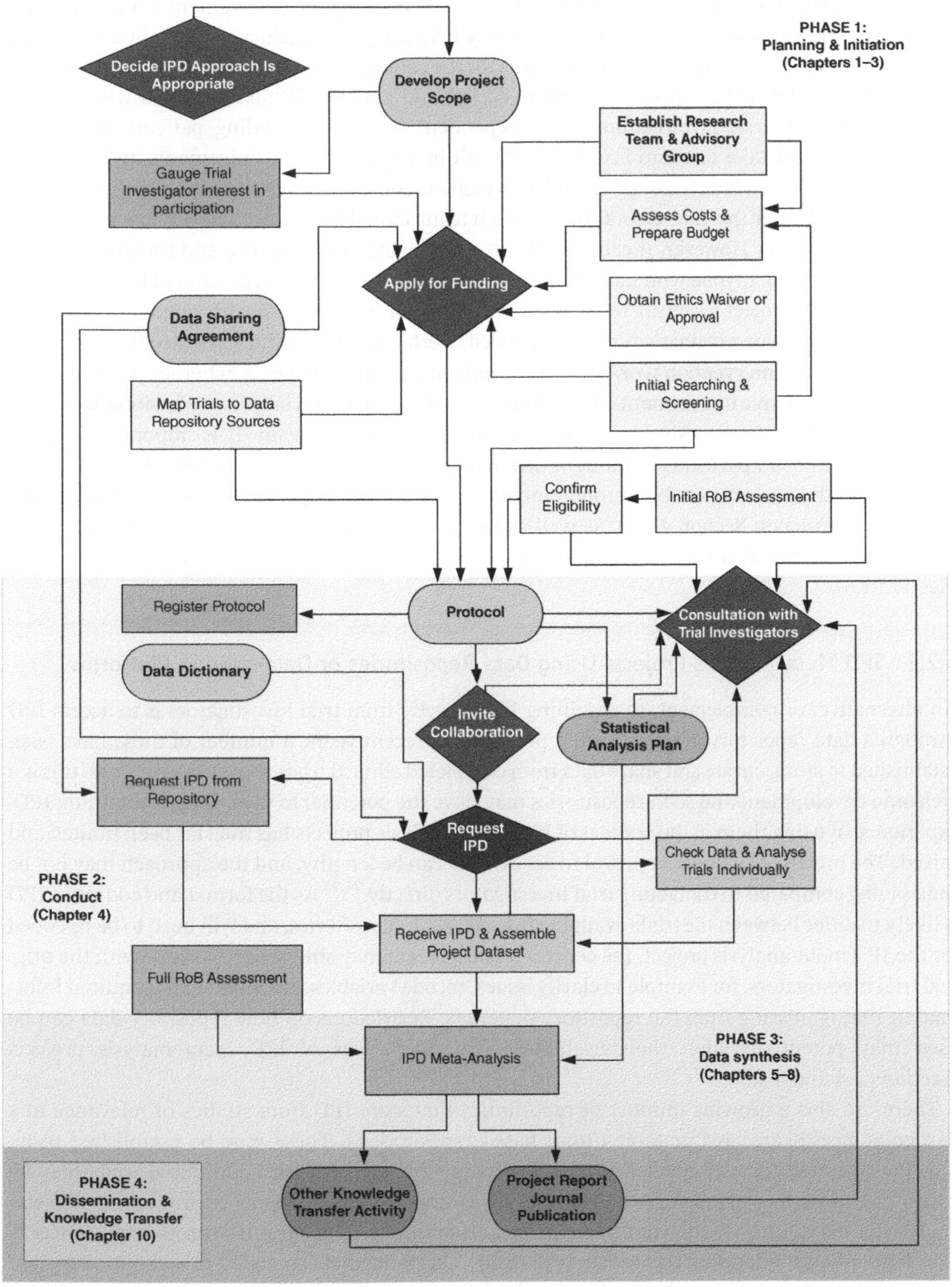

Figure 3.1 Typical phases of an IPD meta-analysis project. *Source:* Lesley Stewart.

Therefore, establishing a mechanism that allows trial investigator involvement without permitting vested interest is vital. One approach that may help safeguard against undue influence, whilst still valuing and benefitting from partnership, is for the central research team to have clearly understood responsibility for all aspects of project design and analysis. Whilst the team will listen to advice from both trial investigators and independent advisors (including patients and public stakeholders), and take this into account, they will be responsible for judgements and decisions made. For example, which trials are included, which outcomes are analysed, and which subgroups are examined. Under this framework, the research team should ideally exclude anyone responsible for an included trial. However, it can be difficult to gain sufficient expertise and understanding of the research topic if anyone who has involvement with an eligible trial is precluded from membership of the IPD project's central research team, particularly for rare health conditions. Thus, a degree of transparent pragmatism may be needed. Certainly, those who have strong beliefs (e.g. about whether an intervention works overall or only in certain individuals, whether particular biomarkers are predictive of treatment effect) or who stand to gain financially or professionally according to the results of synthesis, should not be part of the central team. It is important that the responsibilities of all partners are thought through well in advance, and are made clear to all from the outset of the project, possibly through inclusion in a project scope (Section 3.3) or charter (and later in the protocol; Section 4.2.2), as well as being reflected in the data-sharing agreement. An advisory group can also help ensure that the central research team maintains its independence (Section 3.6).

3.2.2 IPD Meta-Analysis Projects Using Data Repositories or Data-sharing Platforms

An alternative, or complement, to obtaining IPD directly from trial investigators is to access IPD through a data repository or data-sharing platform. In recent years, a number of these have been established to store, curate and share data from completed clinical trials (Box 3.1). Although this is a welcome development and such repositories may have the potential to save time in obtaining IPD, experience of using them in the context of IPD meta-analysis projects has thus far been limited and mixed. The process of gaining approval to access data can be lengthy, and the approach may not be time saving compared to contacting trial investigators directly.[74,75] As the format and coding of IPD is likely to differ between the trials available through such repositories, and will need to be re-coded for the IPD meta-analysis project, the central research team may still need to consult with the original trial investigators, for example to clarify issues, recode variables, and obtain any required information that is missing from the repository materials. Restrictions on how repository data can be used may potentially limit their usefulness for some types of IPD meta-analysis projects (Sections 3.4 and 4.4.5).

There are also a growing number of repositories that store IPD from studies of relevance to a particular healthcare area or topic ('topic-based repositories'). These may be established using the IPD collected for a completed IPD meta-analysis project, to which additional trials may be added over time. For example, ACCENT is a topic-based database developed from an IPD meta-analysis of the efficacy of adjuvant fluorouracil and folinic acid for stage II/III colorectal cancer.[76] Consequently, an important advantage is that IPD have already been coded to a common format and checked prior to their inclusion in the original IPD meta-analysis. Although such repositories are often used as a resource for subsequent research carried out by the initial collaborative group, it may also be possible for others to gain access to the repository data. Clearly, if considering using such data from a repository for an IPD meta-analysis, it is important to establish at the outset whether the repository data will be obtainable.

Box 3.1 Examples of data-sharing platforms and data repositories

Clinical Study Data Request (CDSR) (https://clinicalstudydatarequest.com/)

Includes access to data from a consortium of pharmaceutical companies including Astrellas Pharma, Bayer, Chugai, Esai, Novartis, ONO, Roche, Sanofi, Sunovion, Shiongi, UCB and ViiV; and academic research funders including the Wellcome Trust, the Bill and Melinda Gates Foundation, the UK Medical Research Council and Cancer Research UK. Lists anonymised data from over 3,000 studies (10 from academic funders). Data are provided in a secure analytic environment that includes free and open source analytic packages and software. Access to data is provided for 12 months that can be extended to 24 months. No charge for access is made.

DataSphere (https://www.projectdatasphere.org/)

Provides access to IPD from academic and industry phase III cancer clinical trials. Includes 160 datasets and data from over 10,000 patients. Data are made available within a secure environment that includes SAS analytic tools. Some data may be downloaded. No charge for access is made.

SOAR (https://dcri.org/our-work/analytics-and-data-science/data-sharing/)

Co-located with the Duke Databank for Cardiovascular Disease. Includes clinical study reports and de-identified IPD from Bristol–Myers Squibb clinical trials for drugs licensed for use in the United States and Europe and completed after 2008. Information from terminated programmes to be available two years after discontinuation. Data are released to researchers and no charge is made.

Vivli (http://vivli.org/)

An independent repository and analytic platform providing access to IPD and metadata. Participating commercial partners include AbbVie, Biogen, Boehringer Ingelheim, Celgene, Daiichi-Sanko, GSK, Lilly, Pfizer, Takeda, Tempus and UCB, along with a number of academic and charitable partners. Includes data from almost 5,000 clinical trials and 2.7 million participants. Data are accessed and analysed in a secure analytic environment that includes a number of commercial and open source software and analytic packages; data may also be downloaded with permission. Data access and use is free for a period after which a charge is made, currently $12 or $25 per day depending on whether their standard or premium research environment is being used.

Yale Open Data (http://yoda.yale.edu/)

Includes access to data from Johnson & Johnson and SI-BONE Inc. and from Queen Mary University of London. Depending on the data partner, IPD are either made available in a personalised account on a secure data server or released using a secure electronic data transfer. No charge for access to data is made.

All platforms require submission of a research proposal that is reviewed before data are released, and are subject to data sharing agreements. Some publicly list applications and access decisions as well as publishing project findings. Information is correct as of March 2020. The status of platforms change frequently and up to date and further information should be sought from their websites.

Source: Lesley Stewart.

In the longer term, it may be possible to use trial data–sharing platforms and repositories to assemble complete IPD meta-analysis datasets. However, as many IPD meta-analysis projects will seek to include older or academic/non-industry trials, neither of which are well represented in existing repositories, for the foreseeable future most IPD meta-analyses will continue to be conducted by negotiating provision of IPD directly from and working with trial investigators. This may be supported or supplemented by obtaining IPD from repositories and data sharing platforms.

3.3 Developing a Project Scope

Developing a project scope is a good way of refining and developing the research question to be addressed, and rapidly prototyping key aspects of project design. A scope should be brief, perhaps around two to three pages in length, and capture the key aims and methods of the project including: the proposed inclusion and exclusion criteria, the main and other outcomes, and any important clinical subgroups and participant-level variables of interest, such as those to be examined as potential effect modifiers. Careful specification of proposed inclusion and exclusion criteria in terms of the PICOS (Population, Intervention, Comparator, Outcomes, Study design) framework at the outset, and reference to them throughout the IPD meta-analysis project, should ensure that the final results are clinically relevant and applicable as intended. If a collaborative approach is adopted, it may also be helpful to outline the terms of collaboration such as the publication policy (e.g. whether group or named authorship will be used, and how many group members/authors are allowed per trial), data safeguarding arrangements, and responsibilities of group membership. An example extract from the scope of an IPD meta-analysis project is given in Box 3.2.

Feedback on a draft scope can be sought from a range of relevant stakeholders and experts, who may find it easier and be more inclined to comment on a short document than a full protocol, enabling the scope to be refined rapidly and iteratively. It can also be circulated to potential collaborators at an early stage of project development, perhaps when sounding out potential willingness to collaborate in the project, and may also serve as a basis for developing a funding application and the project protocol.

3.4 Assessing Feasibility and 'In Principle' Support and Collaboration

Having concluded that an IPD meta-analysis is warranted (Section 2.6) and used the development of a project scope to work through design and organisational issues, it is important to assess whether the project is likely to be feasible – in particular, whether sufficient IPD will be available to support credible analysis.

It is worth bearing in mind that it is not always possible or necessary to obtain IPD from *every* eligible trial. IPD from some older trials may have been lost or destroyed, important participant-level outcomes or covariates may not have been collected in some trials, and not all investigators may wish to collaborate. Deciding how many trials are sufficient for the IPD meta-analysis project to proceed is not straightforward, and depends not only on the number of trials likely to be available, but on their size and which outcome and covariate data are available, as these influence the statistical power that the IPD meta-analysis will have (Chapter 12). For example, when examining participant-level covariates, the within-trial variability of covariate values is also influential toward the power of an IPD meta-analysis, in additional to the total number of participants and events.[33]

Box 3.2 Extract of the scope developed for the Evaluating Progestogens for Preventing Preterm birth International Collaborative (EPPPIC) IPD meta-analysis

Main Aims

1) Effectiveness of any progestogen versus no active intervention (co-treatment is permitted)
2) Effectiveness of vaginally administered progesterone versus 17-OHPC (co-treatment is permitted)

Exploring potential differences in effectiveness according to **type of progestogen** and route of administration.

Considering impact on **preterm birth** (<37 weeks, <34 weeks, <28 weeks), **fetal/neonatal death**, serious **neonatal complications**, infant **disability** and important **maternal morbidity**.
In **asymptomatic** women considered at high risk of preterm birth, but **not** at immediate risk of preterm birth, and **not** those for whom progestogen is administered to prevent miscarriage and does not continue beyond 16 weeks of gestation.

Separate evaluation of **singleton and of multi-fetal** pregnancies exploring:
Whether effectiveness differs according to **key risk factors at trial entry** (previous spontaneous preterm birth, multiple gestation pregnancy, cervical length, positive fetal fibronectin test) and additional trial and patient-level characteristics to investigate whether there are particular types of woman or pregnancy that derive greater benefit (or harm) from intervention.

....

Population
Included: Trials including asymptomatic women considered at increased risk of preterm birth
Excluded: Trials of progestogen given to women only before 16 weeks to prevent miscarriage; trials of progestogen administered for immediately threatened preterm labour including PPROM and/or uterine contractions

Intervention
Included: Trials evaluating any form of progestogen (natural progesterone, 17-OHPC and medroxyprogesterone acetate delivered by any route (vaginal gels, capsules, suppositories, intramuscular, intravenous injection, oral)
Excluded: Trials that ceased administration of progestogen prior to 16 weeks of pregnancy

Comparators
Included: Trials of progestogen versus placebo or no intervention; trials of vaginally administered progesterone versus 17-OHPC

Outcomes
Included: All trials that meet the above criteria will be included and contribute to the IPD meta-analysis project's pre-specified outcomes (above) for which they collected data

Study Design
Included: Randomised controlled parallel group trials
Excluded: Quasi randomised trials, cluster randomised trials, cross-over trials

Source: Lesley Stewart.

If many small trials are unavailable, this may have little impact on an IPD meta-analysis project, because they will usually add little information to the analyses (Section 2.6.3). Conversely, if IPD are not available for several large trials, this may raise serious questions about feasibility.

If the available trials are in keeping with current practice, and the unavailable trials are old and less relevant, it may not be necessary to include the older trials, and it may even be better to exclude them (although it is preferable to identify and address this through tighter eligibility criteria when developing the project scope). If unavailable trials are deemed at high risk of bias, their omission could in fact lead to more robust results. There may even be an element of self-selection, if those responsible for low-quality trials, or *in extremis,* fraudulent trials may decline to participate because their data would not stand up to scrutiny.

Determining whether available data will be sufficient for credible analysis requires ascertaining what trials are likely to make data available. This may include gauging whether trial investigators would, in principle, be willing to share their IPD and/or establishing what data are available in repositories, and on what terms.

Before contacting trial investigators to request in principle agreement to partner in the IPD meta-analysis, the team should ascertain whether any clarification about their trial's eligibility is needed, for example, whether the trial population matches the IPD project's inclusion criteria. These enquiries may be particularly important in clarifying trial design factors, such as details of randomisation and allocation concealment, which are often not well reported in trial publications. This information might then be used as part of an initial informal risk of bias assessment for each trial, if, for example, only those trials at low risk of bias are to be included in the IPD meta-analysis. Whilst undertaking full risk of bias assessment (based on trial publications) can be done, it is not generally essential at this stage. It can however be helpful to explore key domains. Section 4.6 discusses risk of bias assessment and its relationship with data retrieval and checking. Initial communications with trial investigators should therefore be clear that their trial is *potentially eligible* for inclusion in the IPD project and request any additional information required to determine eligibility. Subsequently, any trials found to be inappropriate (e.g. due to inclusion criteria, design, or high risk of bias), should be excluded as early as possible and with little inconvenience for trial investigators.

When seeking in principle agreements and trying to establish feasibility, it should be borne in mind that trial investigators may not pledge support until it is certain that the IPD meta-analysis project will go ahead, or until they know that certain other trial investigators are participating. This can make it challenging to provide an early assessment of feasibility, for example, within a funding application. Building collaboration is time consuming and an iterative process such that the decision to go ahead with an IPD meta-analysis project almost always involves a leap of faith, and a judgement that even though not all data are yet pledged, there is a reasonable chance that, with persistence (Section 4.3), additional trials can be brought on board as the project progresses.

If planning to use IPD from a repository, it is important to map out which repository holds data from each trial, and to investigate current repository data release processes and timescales. This should include finding out the duration for which IPD will be made available in the repository, as access may be granted only within a specified time period, which could cause logistical problems if using IPD from different repositories or sources, and any charges involved. It is particularly important to find out whether data can be provided for use outside the confines of the repository, or whether analyses must be done within the repository platform.

Many repositories do not allow IPD to be exported, and so require analyses to be done within a secure space on their site, yet not all trials required for an IPD meta-analysis project will be included within the same, or indeed any, repository. This precludes the central IPD meta-analysis research team from creating a harmonised 'master database' that contains IPD from all trials and housing it locally. Importing IPD from other trials into the repository (to create a master database to be used to perform the IPD meta-analysis within the repository space) may not be acceptable to other trial investigators. A similar issue occurs when a trial agrees to share IPD, but only allows the IPD meta-analysis team to access it via a secure server at the trial's host institution.

If IPD have to be accessed at more than one location, this forces a two-stage meta-analysis (Chapter 5) whereby IPD for each trial are firstly analysed separately within the confines of their host repository or database to generate aggregate data, and then these aggregate data are exported and combined in a meta-analysis in the second stage. Whilst this is often entirely appropriate, there are circumstances where a one-stage approach (Chapter 6), which analyses IPD from all studies simultaneously, is preferable, especially when outcomes are rare (Chapter 8) or when developing risk prediction models (Chapter 17). In future, sharing data across repositories or distributed syntheses (where a central data processor communicates with several data hubs, passing statistical information back and forth, without exposing the raw data at each site) may help get round such problems.[77] But for now, a one-stage approach is rarely feasible if trials' IPD are stored in different databases and locations. Therefore, at the outset, careful consideration must be given as to whether the trial IPD stored in repositories and the conditions of use will support the planned IPD synthesis. If restricted access would preclude or weaken the planned synthesis, repositories can be approached to see whether an exception can be made (with a careful explanation of why analysing within the repository space is not adequate).

3.5 Establishing a Team with the Right Skills

As for any research project, having the right team in place is vital. Before embarking on an IPD meta-analysis project, it is important to think carefully about what skills and resources will be required for successful completion, and to calculate the associated costs if funding will be sought. Given the work involved, necessary skillset and timescale, IPD meta-analysis projects require dedicated resources and would be very difficult to conduct in reviewers' spare time. In particular, they generally require a broader range of skills and greater expertise in certain areas than is needed for a conventional review using aggregate data. A strong team will include researchers with experience in systematic review methods; information specialists; those who are able to manage, check and harmonise participant-level data using data management and statistical software; statisticians able to implement appropriate statistical methods using suitable statistical software; and clinicians and health professionals with expertise in the topic area.

Assuming that a collaborative group approach is to be taken, the importance of skills in establishing and managing collaboration, negotiating provision of data, navigating politics and brokering a group consensus interpretation of findings cannot be overstated. A successful IPD meta-analysis research team will, therefore, include members with strong communication and interpersonal skills who are able to build rapport and exercise tact and diplomacy when needed. Active involvement of senior researchers and topic experts with an appropriate track record can improve the likelihood of success, as they can enhance credibility and may gain or broker easier access to conversations with senior data holders and trial investigators.

The role of the research lead (usually the principal investigator for the IPD project) is particularly important. In addition to being responsible for the overall design and delivery of the project, they will usually be responsible for overseeing project management and the contributions of other team members, and will often undertake much of the negotiation and external communications activity (which can be very time consuming for some projects). Depending on their background, they may be directly responsible for supervising (or undertaking) the analyses, and at least should work with the senior statistician to agree the analyses required and subsequently on interpretation of results. Given the nature of the role, the research lead will be involved at all stages of the projects and more of their time will be required than for a principal investigator role in other types of systematic review. Ideally, they should have previous experience of completing IPD meta-analysis projects, or have considerable support from someone who does.

IPD meta-analysis projects require expertise in handling, coding and checking participant-level data, skills that are perhaps more similar to those used in data management within clinical trials and other primary research studies than those used in a conventional systematic review. As standardisation and data checking require developing code and running analysis, it is important that the person performing this role has strong quantitative skills, although this may be a different person from the team statistician.

As is evident from Parts 2 to 5 of this book, the types of statistical analyses that can be performed with IPD are considerably more complex than those that are usually carried out for conventional meta-analyses of existing aggregate data, and there is a risk of unknowingly introducing analytic errors, for example by accepting default options in statistical packages or when adapting existing code. Therefore, it is vital that the project team includes a statistician with experience of relevant analytic techniques, preferably someone who been part of an IPD meta-analysis project previously, or familiar with appropriate modelling of large data from clustered sources such as healthcare practices or hospitals. They should also be familiar with the importance of building relationships with trial investigators and how this relates to data assembly, and recognise that analysis is not a stand-alone activity. For this reason, 'drafting in' a statistician to focus only on the analysis is not advised; the statistician must be part of the central team, even if during some periods their involvement is less than at others. It can work well to have a highly experienced statistician, with an established track record in IPD meta-analysis, to specify appropriate methods and oversee and guide the day-to-day work of a more hands-on but potentially less experienced statistician.

3.6 Advisory and Governance Functions

It is usually helpful to establish an advisory group during the planning stage, as having a strong advisory group that endorses the IPD meta-analysis project may add to credibility, be helpful in persuading trial investigators to participate, and strengthen funding applications.

As well as providing independent advice, an advisory group can play an important role in garnering wider clinical or topic expertise, and providing additional methodological oversight. It is also a good way to engage patients and the public in a meaningful way, ensuring that the patient voice is heard. Therefore, an advisory group will often include members from different specialties and professions that are relevant to the review topic, representation from patient support groups, individual patients and carers (who will often have a different perspective to support groups), and methodologists. For example, the advisory group for an IPD meta-analysis project (and linked economic evaluation) examining intensive behavioural interventions based on applied behaviour analysis (ABA) for young children with autism included: representation from the National Autistic Society, research study investigators, parents of children with autistic spectrum disorder, adults with autism spectrum disorder, ABA practice specialists, psychiatrists, clinical and educational psychologists, specialists in IPD meta-analysis, and health economists.[78] Having well-respected international members of the advisory group might be particularly helpful when requesting IPD from trial investigators working in different countries to the central research team.

As participant-level data are being used, commissioners may sometimes suggest that an IPD meta-analysis project should establish governance structures similar to those for a clinical trial. However, with the exception of those that are prospective (Section 3.12), IPD meta-analysis projects use participant-level data that have already been collected in existing trials and no new participants are being recruited; therefore, there should usually be no requirement for a steering or data monitoring and ethics committee (as would be needed for a clinical trial).

3.7 Estimating How Long the Project Will Take

Unlike a conventional systematic review, the pace and progress in an IPD meta-analysis project is not entirely under the control of the research team. The time required for some activities can be reasonably estimated, such as producing a protocol, running searches, eligibility screening, and preparation of a data dictionary (Section 4.2). However, the time taken to assemble, code and check the quality and applicability of received IPD is highly dependent on the actions of the data providers (Sections 4.4 to 4.6), and so is often difficult to estimate in advance.

There is inevitably a lag between inviting trial investigators to participate and receiving IPD. After having been persuaded personally of the value of the proposed project (which may itself take some time), some trial investigators will need to obtain institutional or other approval to release data. This can take several months, particularly if granted at institutional review board or committee meetings, which may be scheduled infrequently. Data and documentation may then have to be located in stores and archives, and prepared for release.

After data have been received, the central research team then need to check the trial IPD and send queries to trial investigators and resolve them. Again, this can take considerable time, particularly if the lead trial investigator needs to liaise with others such as the trial data manager or statistician, to determine exactly how data have been coded or which variables were used to define outcomes in the original trial analyses. It is important to remember that whilst the IPD meta-analysis may be a top priority for the research team leading it, the same may not be true for trial investigators, who are likely to have many competing demands for their time.

Another important consideration when estimating timing and resource requirements is whether those responsible for included trials would prefer to prepare and code their IPD in the format required for the IPD meta-analysis project, or whether they prefer to send it in its original format and for the central research team then to do any recoding required. Even when trial investigators prepare data, the central research team still need to spend some time assimilating it. An estimated minimum of around a day should be allowed for processing the data for each trial, and longer if the suggested coding has not been followed as intended. Dealing with data that have not been prepared by the trial investigators can be very time consuming, depending on the complexity of the data and the way that it is structured. For a very large and complex trial dataset, with variables stored across many electronic forms and with, for example, repeated follow-up and measurements, it may take a team member several weeks to fully understand it, write code to extract and transform data to meta-analysis format, and to check thoroughly that this has generated the correct values. It can be difficult to estimate what proportion of trials this will apply to. Our experience is that most trial investigators are willing to prepare and recode data, but that it would be wise to factor in time for the research team to prepare data from at least 20% of trials.

Unless there are very specific assurances that IPD will be released rapidly and that any issues encountered during data checking will be resolved promptly by trial investigators, as a rule of thumb, upwards of a year should be planned for collecting and checking the IPD from the full set of eligible trials. IPD collection, cleaning and harmonisation for large projects involving many trials may take much longer than a year, and typically 18 to 24 months is needed prior to the IPD meta-analysis itself. Much of the elapsed time is taken up by communications and by trial investigators gaining approvals. As older trials may be difficult and time-consuming to trace, and agreement more difficult to reach for controversial topics, these sorts of issues should also be factored into planning project timelines.

Likewise, there will usually be a lag between requesting IPD from a data repository and subsequent provision of that IPD. There will usually be a process for approving project proposals prior to the release of a trial's IPD that may take several months to complete. As noted earlier, experience to date has been mixed; whilst some teams have found that communication with the data providers has become more streamlined and that pre-coded datasets can reduce the time taken to prepare data for analysis,[74] others have found that obtaining permissions when multiple data owners are involved has been difficult.[75] Based on the limited experience so far, it is sensible to still factor in at least a year to obtain the necessary approvals and gain access to IPD from data repositories and data-sharing platforms.

As trial data usually arrive sporadically over a period of time, data checking is usually done concurrently with data collection and coding. Data are checked as soon as possible after receipt, and any issues discussed and resolved with trial investigators, usually with a series of iterations (Section 4.5.4). This often includes analysing each trial individually and comparing with any published analyses, both to understand any differences that may arise as a result of, for example, using different outcome definitions, and to ensure that the central research team has understood the data correctly. The time and resource needed for checking will depend on how clean the data are on arrival and the extent of checking required. Allowing about three or four days per trial for carrying out data checking is a good starting point. It is useful to allow extra time beyond when the last dataset might be received, in order to complete the checking processes.

Sufficient time must also be factored into timelines for the meta-analyses, and it is important that this critical phase does not get squeezed if data collection takes longer than anticipated. There is sometimes a misconception that statistical analyses are straightforward and can be done at the click of a button, but this is never the case. Assuming data are cleaned and ready for analysis, usually at least six months will be required for the statistical phase of an IPD meta-analysis of randomised trials to evaluate treatment effects. Often, multiple analyses will be needed, for example to analyse multiple outcomes, subgroups, and participant-level covariates, as well as sensitivity analyses and production of associated summary tables and graphs. If complex modelling is planned, such as using multiple imputation to deal with missing data (Chapter 18), analysing non-linear relationships (e.g. for treatment-covariate interactions; Chapter 7) or network meta-analysis (Chapter 14), then six to 12 months will be a more sensible time frame. Furthermore, although most problems with data should be identified when checking data, issues may still arise during synthesis that require further communication with the trial investigators.

Generally, IPD meta-analysis projects will take upwards of two years to complete, and sometimes longer depending on how many trials are involved and the complexities of negotiating collaboration, data coding, checking, cleaning and analysis. Delays may be outside the control of the project team. Flexibility in staffing and scheduling is needed to accommodate this, which can make setting and meeting funder milestones challenging. In our experience, extensions to the original timelines agreed with funders may be required, particularly if key trials delay sending their IPD. Work may be most intense at the beginning and end of a project, and this can be borne in mind when planning resourcing and staffing. Nonetheless, it is important that projects are actively managed at all times and that the research team keep on top of projects and moving them forward.

Prospective IPD meta-analysis projects will additionally need to run to timelines that accommodate those of the participating trials (Section 3.12).

3.8 Estimating the Resources Required

IPD meta-analysis projects cannot be done by a small volunteer review team and usually cost more than a standard systematic review. However, they are considerably less expensive than carrying out a new clinical trial, which may be the only reliable alternative to addressing the research question that the IPD meta-analysis aims to resolve.

Box 3.3 lists the main costs involved in an IPD meta-analysis project, and may be useful starting point in preparing a budget and seeking funding. Most items should be self-explanatory. Some costs are similar to conventional systematic reviews such as those involved in acquiring publications (e.g. inter-library loan charges) and some aspects of dissemination activity such as open access publishing fees. Additional costs are more specific to individual projects, and largely correlate with the number of trials, complexity of the IPD obtained, and type and number of analyses required, as these are major drivers the staff effort needed.

Funding staff time is likely to be the largest project cost. Whilst the staff resource needed for some tasks will be similar to a conventional systematic review, such as those associated with searching and screening studies for inclusion, other costs will be highly dependent on the size and scope of the project. As described in Section 3.7, sufficient staff time needs to be allowed for checking and recoding variables within IPD and for performing the analyses.

In addition to the time taken to manage and oversee a major research project, the time needed for managing the wider collaborative process, for negotiating data provision, and for communication and collaboration must also be budgeted for, but is easily overlooked. For example, an IPD meta-analysis project that included IPD from 31 trials involved sending and receiving over 5,000 separate emails.[79] Given that even the simplest of these probably takes a few minutes to handle, it is not difficult to see how the resource spent on this type of activity mounts up. As managing the

Box 3.3 Typical costs incurred in an IPD meta-analysis project

Staff Costs

- Principal investigator (considerable time may be needed for this strategic and diplomatic role)
- Clinical/topic expert members of team (resource depends on level of involvement)
- Experienced statistician (to plan supervise and undertake complex syntheses)
- Statistician(s) (to plan, code and carry out analyses)
- Researcher(s) (to screen, assess risk of bias, re-code, check data)
- Information specialist (likely to be similar to a standard systematic review)
- Administrative support (e.g. to organise results meeting)
- IT support (if there are special requirements or if not provided by host institution)
- Legal input to data-sharing agreements (if not provided by host institution)

General Costs

- Inter-library loans and document acquisition (similar to a standard systematic review)
- Telephone and teleconference calls with trial investigators
- Conference calls for advisory or collaborative group meetings
- Any travel likely to be needed to secure provision of data
- Any specialist software required for data management or statistical analysis

Fees

- Data preparation bursaries or fees to trial investigators for preparing data (if these are used)
- Any fees to data-sharing repositories for access to data
- Any special licenses required to read/handle repository data

Advisory Group Meetings

- Travel and venue costs (can be reduced by holding most meetings virtually)
- Catering for face-to-face meetings

Patient and Public Involvement Costs

- Payment for contributed time, including preparing for and attending meetings
- Travel to meetings and incidental expenses

Collaborative Group Meeting

- Venue and equipment hire
- Catering during meeting
- Other catering costs (customary to include at least a group evening meal)
- Travel costs or bursaries (taking account of geographical location of studies when costing)
- Accommodation (those travelling long distance may require this pre- or post-meeting)

Dissemination Costs

- Costs associated with presenting results at relevant conference
- Open access publishing fees
- Production of plain language summaries
- Production of any web or other audio/visual materials

The above listing covers typical costs, and should be adapted according to the specific requirements of the project.

Source: Lesley Stewart.

collaboration has potential to be sensitive and political, a significant amount of principal investigator time may be needed for communication.

A commonly asked question is whether trial investigators should be paid to participate and prepare their IPD. Whilst this acknowledges contribution and may reimburse or partially reimburse time taken to prepare data, there is no evidence that offering funds provides an incentive to collaborate, particularly if it is a token amount (as shown in a randomised trial[75]). Many IPD meta-analysis projects have been completed successfully without offering payment, and routinely paying for data provision could render many IPD projects unaffordable. Ideally, the ability to provide robust answers to questions that are likely to matter to trial investigators and the academic credit generated through involvement in an IPD meta-analysis (including authorship), will provide sufficient motivation to participate. Moreover, for more recent trials that have been managed and stored following good practice, it should be relatively straightforward for trial personnel to export and potentially even to re-code their IPD. Indeed, many trials are funded by organisations that expect trial data to be made available for other researchers on trial completion (Box 3.4). One option may be to provide some assistance in the form of data preparation bursaries for those who would otherwise have difficulty in securing the staff time needed to prepare the data. For example, bursaries might be warranted if trial personnel have moved institutions but are willing to prepare IPD in their own time; or if IPD are archived and costs are associated with retrieving this or in transposing data from obsolete storage media. However, this is difficult to predict and remains a difficult issue that will require careful assessment in relation to specific IPD meta-analysis circumstances.

If IPD are to be obtained from repositories, any costs associated with this need to be incorporated in the budget, including any hidden costs such as a requirement for specialist software or licences to read original data. For example, an IPD network meta-analysis that wished to use data from pharmaceutical company trials through clinicalstudydatarequest.com was required to have a WHO Drug Dictionary license at an approximate cost of almost £7,000 per sponsor.[75]

Costs for any planned patient and public involvement and engagement (PPIE) should be included. These should capture reimbursement of travel and incidental expenses associated with attending meetings and include payment for time preparing for and attending these meetings. Payment for time may be made at a generally accepted rate, for example those recommended by INVOLVE in the UK (available at www.invo.org.uk/resource-centre/payment-and-recognition-for-public-involvement/).[80] Because payment to individuals may have implications for their tax or welfare payments, a donation to a patient group or charity may be preferred. For costing purposes it is reasonable to assume that these would be the same amount as would be paid to individuals. Costs associated with advisory group meetings should also be accounted for, for all group members.

One aspect of a collaborative IPD meta-analysis that can incur additional cost is hosting an in-person meeting of trial investigators and advisory group members, at which results are first presented and discussed. As well as providing some incentive to participate, this can aid interpretation and help cascade and disseminate results (Chapter 10). Past experience suggests that holding these as physical meetings works well, although they can be costly. Hosting results meetings alongside a major conference that trial investigators are likely to attend can reduce costs, although it may be more difficult to find a venue and keep participants present and engaged. Costing such a meeting will need to include venue and catering costs, and any accommodation and travel that will be supported through the project. Providing accommodation and subsistence for the duration of the IPD meeting is commonly done. Sometimes travel bursaries are offered, for example, to cover costs for those who would not be attending a main conference to which the IPD project meeting may be aligned. For a well-funded project, travel (economy) may be supported for all those attending. Travel should always be reimbursed for PPIE members.

An alternative is to hold a virtual meeting. Although there is not yet a great deal of experience of how successful on-line meetings are for presenting and discussing IPD meta-analysis results, with ever-improving virtual meeting software and with more individuals mindful of environmental sustainability and their carbon footprint, they may ultimately be the best option and help contain the costs of IPD meta-analysis projects. Furthermore, following the 2020 SARS-CoV2 pandemic and widespread use of online meeting software to host meetings and conferences, virtual meetings have become more commonplace.

Box 3.4 Examples of research funder support for sharing clinical trial data

Cancer Research UK

https://www.cancerresearchuk.org/sites/default/files/cruk_data_sharing_policy_2017_final.pdf
Cancer Research UK regards it good research practice for all researchers to consider at the research proposal stage how they will manage and share the data they will generate. Therefore, Cancer Research UK requires that applicants applying for funding provide a data management and sharing plan as part of their application. This plan will be reviewed as part of the funding decision.

European Research Council

https://erc.europa.eu/sites/default/files/document/file/ERC_info_document-Open_Research_Data_and_Data_Management_Plans.pdf
Grantees to provide information on how their data sets can be accessed, including the terms-of-use or the licence under which they can be accessed and re-used, and information on any restrictions that may apply. It is also important to specify and justify the timing of data sharing. This could be, for example, as soon as possible after the data collection, or at the end of the project. For data that underlie publications it could be, for example, at the time of publication or pre-publication.

National Institutes of Health

https://grants.nih.gov/grants/policy/data_sharing/
In NIH's view, all data should be considered for data sharing. ***Data should be made as widely and freely available as possible while safeguarding the privacy of participants, and protecting confidential and proprietary data.*** *To facilitate data sharing, investigators submitting a research application requesting $500,000 or more of direct costs in any single year to NIH on or after October 1, 2003 are expected to include a plan for sharing final research data for research purposes, or state why data sharing is not possible.*

Medical Research Council

https://mrc.ukri.org/research/policies-and-guidance-for-researchers/open-research-data-clinical-trials-and-public-health-interventions/
The MRC expects valuable data arising from MRC-funded research to be made available to the scientific community with as few restrictions as possible to maximise the value for research and for eventual patient and public benefit. Such data must be shared in a timely and responsible manner. The MRC is aware of the risks of fully open access to individual participant data (IPD), in particular the need to comply with participant consent and avoid inadvertent or deliberate identification of participants. The MRC expects researchers to follow the guidance in "Good Practice Principles for Sharing Individual Participant Data from Publicly Funded Clinical Trials" which details good practice principles and practical guidance on sharing IPD in a controlled way. A data sharing policy should be developed for each study.

The Patient-Centered Outcomes Research Institute

https://www.pcori.org/about-us/governance/policy-data-management-and-data-sharing
PCORI is committed to the principles of open science, particularly maximizing the utility and usability of data collected in research projects that PCORI funds. PCORI seeks to encourage scientifically rigorous secondary use of clinical research data to foster scientific advances that will ultimately improve clinical care and patient outcomes. As such, PCORI believes it is important for our research awardees to systematically create and preserve research data and data documentation in order to facilitate data sharing.

Wellcome

https://wellcome.ac.uk/grant-funding/guidance/clinical-trials-policy
When you register you must include a data sharing plan as part of the trial registration, in line with the 2017 International Committee of Medical Journal Editors (ICMJE) requirements on data sharing statements for clinical trials.

Source: Lesley Stewart.

3.9 Obtaining Funding

There are three main funding routes: funding as part of a core research programme, investigator-led applications and commissioned calls from funders. Each of these has its own advantages and challenges.

It can be difficult to predict how much IPD will be available, what condition it will be in when it arrives, or how much time will be needed to negotiate collaboration and receive IPD. It is therefore perhaps most straightforward for IPD meta-analysis projects to be funded as part of a core evidence synthesis research programme (or unit), which allows the research team to work across different IPD meta-analyses (and other projects) running to differing schedules and to exercise flexibility on start and end dates. A similar approach is to embed the IPD project (undertaken by a suitably experienced and qualified team) within a larger long-term programme of research in a particular topic area.

For investigator-led applications for a single IPD meta-analysis project, whilst time can be taken to build the project scope, explore possible collaborations and assess feasibility, a challenge may be in explaining the rationale for why an IPD synthesis is required rather than a standard review of existing aggregate data (Chapter 2). As IPD projects are rare relative to standard systematic reviews, peer reviewers and funders may be unfamiliar with what they entail, and so careful exposition of methods and the benefits that the IPD approach will bring is essential. Detailed costs and their justification will also be needed. A survey of members of the Cochrane IPD Meta-Analysis Methods Group exploring barriers and successes in applying for funding for IPD meta-analysis projects identified six key themes as being important to funding applications and how they were received by funders.[81] These were:

1) Originality, relevance and potential impact of the project
2) Explaining the importance of using IPD
3) Clear articulation of aims and methods
4) Likely availability of IPD from existing trials
5) Justification and supporting evidence for the level of resource requested
6) Experience of the research group undertaking the review

Clearly a number of these points apply to all funding applications, but issues around the rationale for using IPD (and justification of the associated level of resource) and about the likely availability of IPD require specific and detailed consideration and explanation. Providing evidence that key trials (especially the largest, most recent or highest-quality trials) have pledged or already provided their IPD can be a persuasive element of a successful funding application. Power calculations, based on characteristics (such as number of participants, number of outcome events, and variance of participant-level covariates) of those trials promising their IPD, can help persuade funders (and indeed the IPD project team themselves) that the endeavour is worth the investment (Chapter 12).[33,49]

Commissioned calls for IPD meta-analysis projects are relatively rare but seem to be increasing in frequency. Here, the case for the IPD meta-analysis *per se* may not need to be made in as much detail. However, the challenge of preparing a funding bid (which will include performing many of the preparatory steps outlined in this chapter) to a short deadline is substantial. One aspect that can be particularly tricky is the need to convince the funder that the project team will obtain sufficient IPD for credible analysis. For many IPD meta-analysis projects, it is difficult to ascertain willingness to participate in the short period of time between a funding call and grant submission. Although trial investigators can be approached for in principle agreement to collaborate, it can be difficult to make a persuasive case until the project is established. Furthermore, there is potential for considerable confusion if several research teams making competing applications approach the same trial investigators for in principle support. Within a short time frame it is almost impossible to gain detailed knowledge of which IPD will be available, and there is no crude credibility threshold above and below which the project is deemed feasible or infeasible. As mentioned, a statistical power calculation may be helpful, but for commissioned calls this will most likely need to be made conditional on assuming that particular trials do provide their IPD (Chapter 12).[49] This will require careful explanation in the application, and it may help to provide a range of power calculations based on different assumed IPD retrieval rates.

3.10 Obtaining Ethical Approval

During the planning period, it is important to establish what, if any, form of ethical approval is required for the proposed IPD meta-analysis project. This matters not just in ensuring that the project itself is adhering to ethical standards and good research practice, but is also information that those supplying IPD may need in order to gain their own clearance to release data. Host institutions may take different approaches; although some will grant a waiver from requirement for formal ethical review, others may decide that this approval is required. If formal ethical review is needed, this should be factored into the project timelines, especially as it may take some time to complete. Research funders will often require that either a waiver is in place or approval has been granted before they will release funds.

Key points that may be made when applying for exemption or making an application for ethical approval include:

- IPD meta-analyses use existing data and do not involve recruitment of participants (although see Section 3.12 regarding prospective IPD meta-analysis).
- The IPD obtained and used will not contain any direct identifiers for participants, such as names or identifying numbers that are known to anyone outside of the immediate trial management team.
- The IPD will be held securely at the central research team's host institution with access restricted to members of the team.
- The IPD will be held, managed and used according to a binding data-sharing agreement or contract, including commitment that the recipient project team will make no attempt to re-identify trial participants.
- The research questions to be addressed in the IPD meta-analysis project are the same as or close to those to which the trial participants originally consented.

It is also worth highlighting these points in the IPD meta-analysis protocol, and in data-sharing agreements, as they may help IPD providers gain permission to release their data.

Discussions around ethical approval might draw on evidence that patients are generally supportive of their clinical trial data being re-used in further research activity provided that there are appropriate safeguards around confidentiality. A consultation exercise undertaken in 2008 by the National Cancer Research Institute (NCRI) demonstrated that most respondents believed that material and data collected from patients with cancer should be used, without identifiable information, as broadly as possible and that retrospectively seeking consent was inappropriate.[82] A systematic review of quantitative and qualitative research studies found widespread, although conditional, support among patients and the public for data sharing for health research.[83] Although participants recognised actual or potential benefits, they expressed concerns about breaches of confidentiality and potential abuses of the data.

In our experience, trial investigators do not generally require formal ethical approval to share their trial IPD, and sharing may even be a pre-condition of the original funding for their trial. They may, however, need to apply to an institutional review board or a central legal department for formal approval. Requirements will vary internationally, institutionally and according to the design of the study from which they are sought, and are subject to change. Those providing data will need to comply with legal and ethical requirements accordingly. In an IPD meta-analysis project that developed a risk prediction model for infection in children being treated for cancer presenting with febrile neutropenia (a fever indicating possible infection and risk of complications),[84] we collected de-identified IPD from both clinical trials and audit, and ascertained which data providers required ethics, institutional or other approval and authorisation before they could share IPD with the project. Table 3.1 shows those that did and did not require formal approval.

Table 3.1 Consent sought to collaborate in an IPD analysis of predictive factors for infection in children being treated for cancer presenting with febrile neutropenia

Country	Study type(s)	Review body approached	Review body	Answer
Belgium	Prospective	Yes	University Hospital Review Boards	Agreed
Bulgaria	Prospective	No[1]	–	–
Canada	Prospective	No[1]	–	–
Canada			Institutional Review Board	Agreed
Chile	Prospective	No[1]		–
Germany	Prospective	No[1]	–	–
Italy	Prospective	No[1]	–	–
Netherlands	Prospective	No[1]	–	–
Slovenia	Prospective		Medical Ethics Committee	Agreed
Switzerland	Prospective and retrospective		Hospital Review Board	Agreed
Turkey	Audit	No[2]	–	–
UK	Audit		NHS Ethics Committee	Agreed
United States	Retrospective notes review		Institutional Review Board	Agreed
United States	Prospective	No[1]	–	

1) No prior consent to primary study;
2) not required
Source: Adapted from Phillips et al.,[85] with permission from BMJ Publishing Group Ltd.

3.11 Data-sharing Agreement

An important preparatory step is developing or selecting an appropriate data-sharing agreement, as funders may require this to be included as part of a funding application, or require that it be agreed with them before funding is released (as these agreements often set out issues around intellectual property rights, amongst other things). The central research team for the IPD meta-analysis project will almost certainly need to have the data-sharing agreements approved by their institutional legal team, which can be time-consuming, making it wise to start discussions early. In our experience, data-sharing agreements can be unhelpfully obscure, written in legal language with terms worded in a way that may not best serve collaboration or persuade data providers to partner in the IPD project.

In an attempt to make agreements as clear as possible and more readily understood by those who are agreeing to work together (the IPD meta-analysis team and the trial investigators), we have developed a data-sharing agreement written in language as plain as possible. This has been used successfully in several projects. Researchers are free to use and adapt this under a creative commons licence. The agreement can be found in a forthcoming publication by Stewart et al., and will be available at www.ipdma.co.uk.

One aspect of sharing agreements that requires careful consideration is commitment from trial investigators not to withdraw their IPD once provided. Although the ability of either party to withdraw is often a standard component of contractual arrangements (and may be an option recommended by institutional legal teams), this would be problematic for IPD meta-analysis projects. For example, in more than one of our previous IPD projects, certain trial investigators did not like the IPD meta-analysis results produced, and then wanted to withdraw their IPD on that basis. Aside from the practical and resourcing difficulties arising from having to redo the IPD meta-analysis, the subsequently reduced IPD meta-analysis dataset could very well be biased (Chapter 9). For this reason, our model data-sharing agreement restricts the right to withdraw data to instances where there is a breach of the agreement that cannot be resolved. For similar reasons, it is important that the agreement makes full reference to the IPD meta-analysis protocol, including details of the planned analyses, in order that all partners have committed to these in advance (so that, after viewing the IPD meta-analysis results, the way IPD were analysed could not be cited as grounds for withdrawing data).

3.12 Additional Planning for Prospective Meta-Analysis Projects

As introduced in Chapters 1 and 2, prospective meta-analysis projects are a particular type of meta-analysis in which the research questions are specified and collaborations established *before* the results of any of the component trials are known. Although they can be completed using aggregate data once the trials are completed, they are more commonly undertaken using IPD. They can be set up to bring trials that are already underway together, or can be initiated by convening a group of interested parties at the design stage to create a set of trials that will ultimately contribute to a new meta-analysis. The latter may be particularly useful in tackling emergent health problems and new technologies and in addressing research questions in rare conditions or small populations, where any single trial would struggle to build a persuasive case that it could provide robust results. An excellent overview of the role and operations of prospective meta-analysis is given by Seidler et al.[86]

There are many similarities between prospective and IPD meta-analyses of existing trials, particularly in terms of the analytic techniques used (Part 2) and in the collaborative ethos within which they operate. However, prospective IPD meta-analyses additionally require management within each of the partner trials, as well as managing the overarching and inter-trial collaborations, which may last for many years. Even more time, thought and consultation are likely to be required when planning a prospective meta-analysis project, particularly for those started from scratch, given that component trials must each be designed in addition to the overarching IPD meta-analysis project. Inter-dependencies between trials may need to be considered and complex governance mechanisms put in place. It may take considerable time to develop collaborations and agree management structure and responsibilities between collaborators, and to get funding in place.

In addition to funding for the central coordination and research team (which will be similar to those described in Sections 3.5, 3.7 and 3.8), funding is required for each trial. Each trial will need to obtain its own ethical approval according to the requirements of the jurisdiction in which it is carried out. Those designed from the outset as part of the meta-analysis project should be clear about this and careful explanation of statistical power will be needed. Consideration of data and patient confidentiality may need greater explanation, as by design the data from any one trial will be shared beyond the immediate trial team. Prospective meta-analysis projects that are set up to include trials that are already underway may need to support amended ethics approval for included trials.

Issues around establishing and managing collaborations are similar to those already described for retrospective IPD meta-analyses (Section 3.1). However, motivating factors may differ, with opportunity for greater mutual benefit, additional publications and academic reward if the overarching prospective meta-analysis makes it possible to conduct an individual trial that on its own would be difficult to justify and obtain funding for. As for retrospective IPD meta-analysis projects, collaborative terms need to be clear and transparent. For example, an explicit authorship policy should be in place from the outset and agreement reached. Similarly, transparent processes and *a priori* agreements, on the relative timing of publication of individual trials and the overarching prospective meta-analysis, are crucial for building and maintaining trust within a prospective meta-analysis collaboration. As with IPD meta-analysis projects of already completed trials, good communication is essential.

Prospective meta-analyses are necessarily long-term projects. For those designed from scratch, an intensive set-up phase will be followed by a quieter period waiting for individual trials to complete (depending on the nature of the health condition and questions and outcomes addressed, this can take several years), followed by an intensive analysis phase. For example, in NeoPROM (Neonatal Oxygenation Prospective Meta-Analysis) five groups prospectively planned to conduct separate, but similar, trials assessing different target ranges for oxygen saturation in preterm infants. The project was established in 2005.[86] The first trial started in 2005, the last trial results became available in 2016 and the final prospective meta-analysis was published in 2018 (indicating that around two years were required for the final stage of assembling the trial data, performing the IPD meta-analysis and agreeing and reporting project conclusions, which is not dissimilar to the time scale required for a retrospective IPD meta-analysis project; Section 3.7).[87] For those that bring together trials that are already underway, the processes involved will be very similar to those already described in this chapter for retrospective IPD meta-analysis projects, although project timing will need careful consideration (end dates for ongoing trials are often unpredictable, making it difficult to plan when the data assembly and meta-analyses are to be done – which may have knock-on implications for funding). Where there are some existing trials, prospective meta-analyses could be nested within a wider IPD meta-analysis combining the benefits of both approaches. A summary of options is given within the article by Seidler et al.[86]

It would be unwise to attempt to initiate a new prospective meta-analysis without involvement of someone with prior experience of these unique projects.

3.13 Concluding Remarks

In summary, initiating an IPD meta-analysis project requires a great deal of thought, planning and preparation, which can take a considerable length of time. However, this investment is essential to maximising chances of success, and time invested at this stage will pay dividends later. Once the team and funding are in place and necessary approvals granted, the project can move on to developing the full protocol and beginning to collect, assemble and check the IPD that will be needed for analysis, as described in Chapter 4.

4

Running an IPD Meta-Analysis Project

From Developing the Protocol to Preparing Data for Meta-Analysis

Jayne F. Tierney, Richard D. Riley, Larysa H.M. Rydzewska, and Lesley A. Stewart

Summary Points

- Collecting, checking and managing IPD is more involved and complex than extracting or collecting existing aggregate data, but is fundamental for ensuring that subsequent IPD meta-analyses are robust and comprehensive.
- An IPD meta-analysis protocol should be registered or published, and include details of: the objectives, eligibility criteria, outcomes to be evaluated and the particular participant-level covariates to be included or examined; the processes for collecting, coding and checking data and assessing risk of bias, and the statistical methods.
- A separate comprehensive statistical analysis plan may also be necessary.
- The project should aim to maximise the quantity of high-quality IPD collected, in order to limit bias and uncertainty of results, and to complete the planned analyses reliably.
- Negotiating and maintaining collaboration with trial investigators can take considerable time and effort, but is critical to the success of most IPD projects.
- IPD should be transferred and stored securely, and used carefully and appropriately, in order to respect participant confidentiality, whilst also adhering to the data use agreements put in place with the data providers.
- Variables contained in the supplied IPD will often need to be re-coded, re-defined or derived in a format that is common to all trials, to enable subsequent meta-analysis.
- Data checking is essential to help identify and rectify any major errors, inconsistencies or biases in the IPD, as well as promoting better understanding of individual trials. Such scrutiny may also afford credibility, which may be important for controversial or high-profile projects.
- A detailed log of all changes and transformations made to trial IPD should be maintained, to enable transparency and reproducibility.
- Assessment of risk of bias for each trial is initially based on information from trial publications or protocols, supplemented by any information provided by the trial investigator, and is then refined once IPD have been received, checked and cleaned.
- Some risk of bias concerns may be alleviated by having the IPD (e.g. inclusion of participants excluded from trial analyses), and others that may only become apparent from checking the IPD (e.g. an allocation pattern indicative of flawed randomisation).
- Ultimately, all collaborators will have input into the interpretation and dissemination of results.
- It can be helpful to incorporate patient and public involvement and engagement throughout the project, for example, to input into the development of the research questions, and the interpretation and dissemination of results.

Individual Participant Data Meta-Analysis: A Handbook for Healthcare Research, First Edition.
Edited by Richard D. Riley, Jayne F. Tierney, and Lesley A. Stewart.

4.1 Introduction

Once it has been established that an IPD meta-analysis project is both appropriate (Chapter 2) and feasible (Chapter 3), and suitable personnel, governance and funding are in place (Chapter 3), there is a need to set up systems and processes that will ensure it will be conducted well. This chapter provides guidance on the preparations needed just prior to the collection of IPD (Section 4.2), and how to go about establishing and maintaining collaboration with IPD providers. It also outlines the steps (shown in Figure 4.1) needed to obtain, check and manage IPD (Sections 4.4 and 4.5), and to investigate risk of bias (Section 4.6), prior to final verification and merging of data (Sections 4.8 and 4.9) in readiness for analysis (Part 2). This stage is often underappreciated, but is critical to ensuring the success of the project and that subsequent meta-analyses are robust and comprehensive. We focus on projects that aim to collate IPD from multiple randomised trials to examine the effect of a particular treatment, but very similar principles apply when seeking IPD from other study types, such as observational studies for diagnosis or prognosis (Part 5).

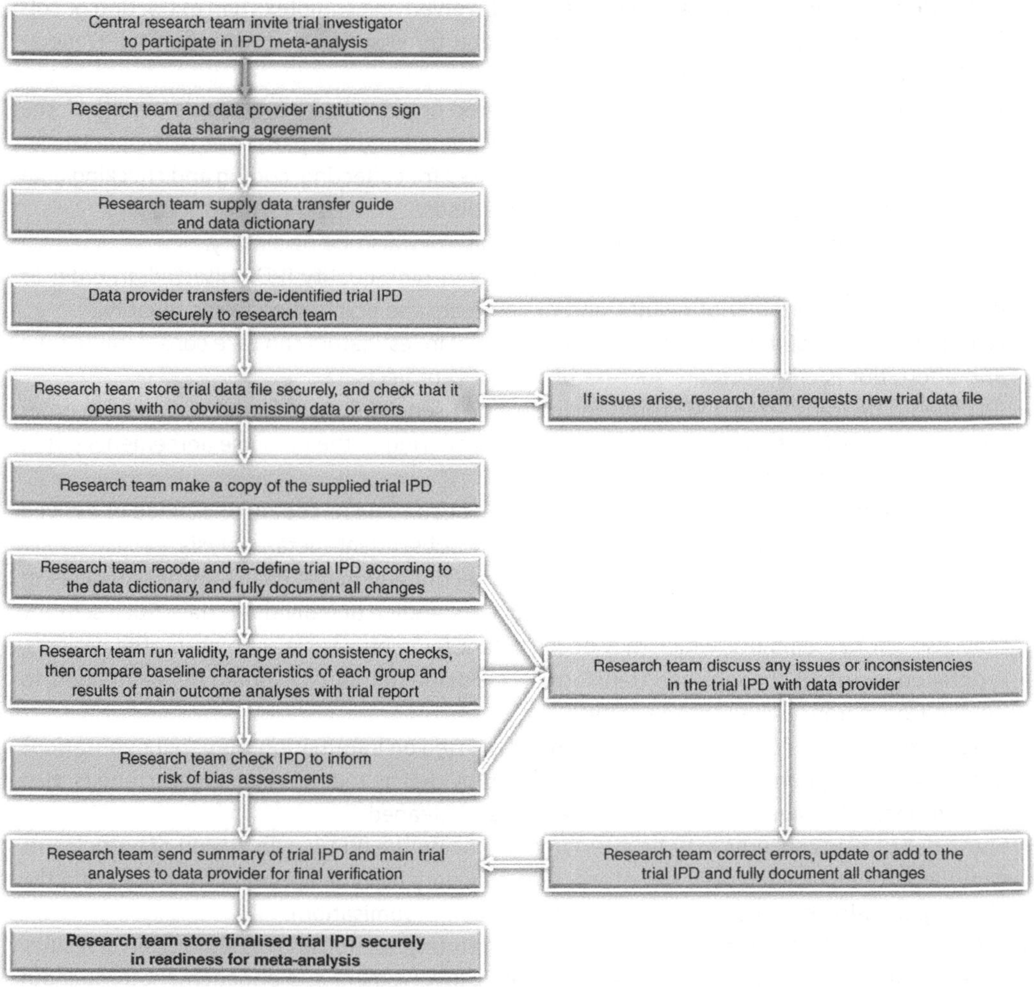

Figure 4.1 Overview of key steps involved in obtaining, managing and checking IPD from a single trial. *Source:* Larysa Rydzewska and Jayne Tierney.

4.2 Preparing to Collect IPD

In this section, we discuss various aspects that should be considered when preparing to collect IPD. This critical set-up stage occurs before formal requests for IPD are sent to trial investigators, but may still involve initial discussions with them, in order to gain clarity on the eligibility of their trials and the IPD they might be able to provide.

4.2.1 Defining the Objectives and Eligibility Criteria

Usually, the objectives and eligibility criteria for trials (and thus their IPD) will have already been defined, either in full or in part, using the PICOS or another similar framework,[42] when developing a project scope (Section 3.3) or funding application (Section 3.9). However, they may still need to be refined at this stage. Figure 4.2 shows the PICOS elements that underlie the objective and eligibility criteria for an IPD meta-analysis of pre-operative chemotherapy for non-small-cell lung cancer.[88]

The type of trials deemed eligible for an IPD meta-analysis project may depend not only on the specifics of the research question and the healthcare area, but also the proportion that are required for reliable synthesis, and are feasible to collect. Such elements should be explicitly considered in formulating the research question, and be built into the inclusion and exclusion criteria, with the rationale for doing so described. In healthcare areas where trials tend to be very large, it may not be worth including IPD from small trials if they would contribute little weight to the evidence base, but take a similar effort to obtain and manage as the larger trials. For example, in an IPD meta-analysis of the efficacy and safety of more intensive lowering of LDL cholesterol, eligibility was restricted to those randomised trials that aimed to recruit 1,000 or more participants with a treatment duration of at least two years.[89] However, depending on the research question, it should be noted that the information size for a trial usually depends on more factors than the total participants (Section 2.6.3), and that statistical power calculations can be used in advance of IPD collection to more appropriately identify which trials provide the most information (Chapter 12), and thereby indicate which should be prioritised for data collection.

Similarly, if older trials are potentially eligible, but might be particularly difficult to track down or are less applicable, then it might be appropriate to exclude them. For example, older trials using long-term alkylating agents were excluded from an IPD meta-analysis of the effects of adjuvant chemotherapy for non-small-cell lung cancer,[90] because previously they had been found to be harmful to patients,[12] and therefore were no longer of relevance to the clinical question.

The central research team might also prioritise seeking IPD from the trials deemed to be of higher quality, based on a formal risk of bias assessment,[91] in order to focus their efforts on trials that would provide the most reliable IPD meta-analysis results (Chapter 9). At the project design stage, necessarily, these judgements would have to be based on information obtained from trial protocols, publications, reports or trial investigators, rather than the IPD itself (Section 4.6).

4.2.2 Developing the Protocol for an IPD Meta-Analysis Project

As for all research studies, a protocol is an invaluable tool for working through the design and guiding the conduct of an IPD meta-analysis project. It serves not only to describe the planned methods in advance of data collection, but is also a main vehicle for communicating the rationale for the project, and convincing potential collaborators of the value of participation – reassuring them that the project is sensible and methodologically sound, and that their IPD will be used appropriately.

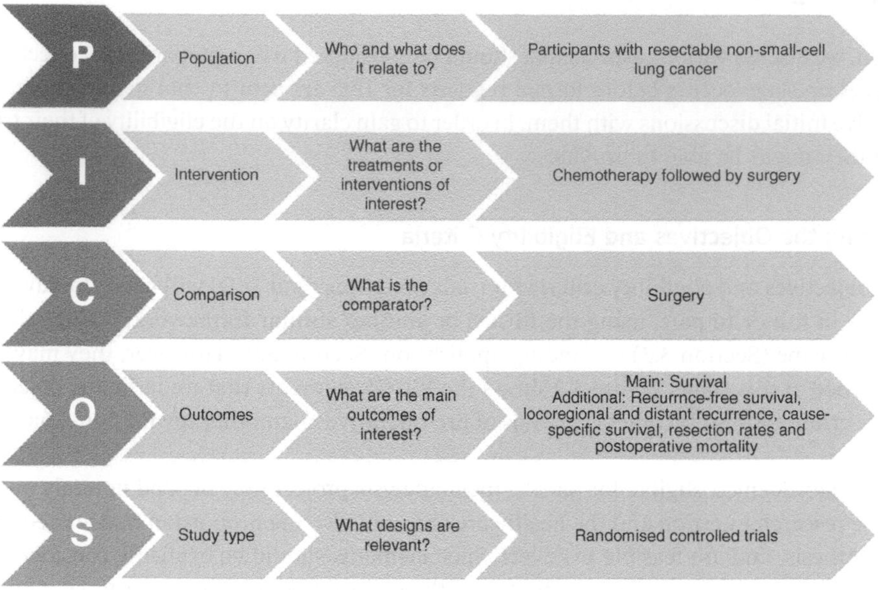

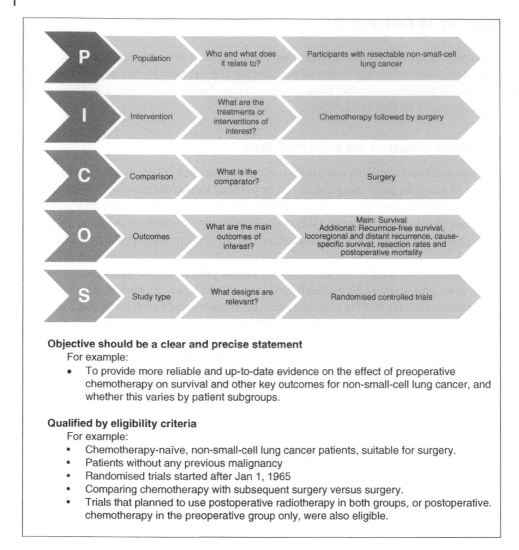

Objective should be a clear and precise statement

For example:

- To provide more reliable and up-to-date evidence on the effect of preoperative chemotherapy on survival and other key outcomes for non-small-cell lung cancer, and whether this varies by patient subgroups.

Qualified by eligibility criteria

For example:

- Chemotherapy-naïve, non-small-cell lung cancer patients, suitable for surgery.
- Patients without any previous malignancy
- Randomised trials started after Jan 1, 1965
- Comparing chemotherapy with subsequent surgery versus surgery.
- Trials that planned to use postoperative radiotherapy in both groups, or postoperative. chemotherapy in the preoperative group only, were also eligible.

Figure 4.2 PICOS example: objective and eligibility criteria for an IPD meta-analysis of pre-operative chemotherapy for non-small-cell lung cancer.[88] *Source:* Based on NSCLC Meta-Analysis Collaborative Group. Preoperative chemotherapy for non-small cell lung cancer: a systematic review and meta-analysis of individual participant data. *Lancet* 2014;383:1561–71.

However, if funders wish to receive or sign off a protocol before releasing project funds, for example, this can pose practical difficulties. A way around this may be to provide funders with a project scope (Section 3.3) or draft version of the protocol, and explain that it will be finalised after collaborators have had the opportunity to comment. This then allows the central research team to modify plans according to the feedback received, and describe which data the included trials have actually collected and will make available.

Key sections to include in the project protocol are shown in Box 4.1. Although the structure is broadly similar to that for a conventional systematic review and meta-analysis of existing aggregate data, greater attention should be paid to explaining the rationale for seeking IPD, describing how data will be checked and used, and, in particular, detailing the analyses that

Box 4.1 Key sections to include in an IPD meta-analysis protocol

- The rationale, including reference to any prior motivating systematic review or meta-analysis, and why IPD are needed
- A description of the research objectives
- The inclusion and exclusion criteria relating to participants, interventions, comparisons, outcomes and study design types (i.e. PICOS), including whether these will be applied at the trial level or participant level, and any other factors such as the qualifying dates for trial completion
- A summary of the methods used for trial identification, including bibliographic search strategies and any additional means of identifying eligible trials, such as communication with trial investigators, along with information about the screening process
- A description of how IPD received will be checked and verified, and how trial quality and the risk of bias will be assessed based on the IPD
- Details of the participant-level variables to be collected
- A list of main and additional outcomes and their definitions
- A summary of the statistical approaches and models to be used, both for analysing trials separately (if applicable) and for IPD meta-analysis, including details of methods for: accounting for clustering of participants within trials, quantifying and exploring heterogeneity, modelling participant-level variables (and any interactions), and any sensitivity analyses. These should be specified in sufficient detail in the protocol or in a separate statistical analysis plan (SAP), in order to permit scrutiny and, if necessary, replication (through access to the same IPD)
- An initial power calculation or sample size justification, conditional on assuming IPD are available from particular trials
- An approximate timetable for the project
- Details of members of the central research team, the project advisory group or steering committee, patient and public involvement representatives and funders
- A dissemination plan
- A provisional table of eligible studies
- Appendices of, for example, search strategies for individual databases and the data dictionary

Source: Jayne Tierney and Lesley Stewart.

will be performed. The latter is particularly important, because IPD offer greater analytical breadth, flexibility and complexity, thereby introducing more potential for inappropriate analyses, and also more opportunity for 'data dredging', data manipulation or the selection of analyses that will generate particular findings, or support prior beliefs. Developing a detailed and publicly accessible protocol prior to receiving IPD helps safeguard against these practices, and at the same time counters any unfounded suspicion or allegations of such manipulation. At a minimum, this would include the main and additional outcomes, and their definitions; methods of individual trial analysis (if relevant) and meta-analysis, including those for exploring potential effect modifiers at the trial or participant level; and methods for quantifying and accounting for heterogeneity.

As for other clinical studies, an additional statistical analysis plan (SAP) may be required, in which case, the protocol should focus on the general methods and a summary of the planned analyses, whilst the SAP would provide more detailed explanation of statistical methods and modelling techniques (see guidance in Part 2). The anticipated scale and complexity of the project will help guide whether the protocol is sufficient, or whether an additional SAP is needed.

Although the protocol and SAP should pre-specify the analyses in some detail, this does not preclude analyses that become necessary to further explore, explain, or add to the main findings. The protocol should make it clear that such analyses may be needed, and will be labelled as post-hoc or exploratory in any report or publication, to distinguish them clearly from planned per-protocol analyses. Furthermore, what is planned at the outset may need to be modified according to, for example, emerging information about data availability (including variables recorded in each trial's IPD), or the identification of new factors that may be prognostic or interact with a treatment effect. Therefore, it can be useful to produce several versions of the protocol and/or SAP, to allow for the incorporation of new proposals and suggestions, either from the project advisory group or trial investigators, or to deal with issues of data availability. Given the inevitable concerns about independence of trial investigators and potential conflicts of interest, it is important to maintain a date-stamped log of such protocol amendments, including who proposed and sanctioned any substantive ones.

For the benefit of potential collaborators, it is useful to include information on how the project will be managed, alongside a timetable and plans for the dissemination of results. Also, as the first full draft of the protocol will usually be completed after the searches for trials and subsequent screening have been completed (Section 4.2.3), this should include a table of the eligible trials identified to date. For this reason, developing the full draft protocol and undertaking searching and screening often occur concurrently.

The IPD meta-analysis protocol should be registered in a publicly accessible registry such as PROSPERO (https://www.crd.york.ac.uk/prospero/) when a comprehensive draft is available (e.g. the version to be circulated to trial investigators for comment). If subsequent amendments are needed, this can be reflected in updates to the registration record, with the reason for changes captured and date-stamped in the associated audit trail held within the registry.

4.2.3 Identifying and Screening Potentially Eligible Trials

Identification of eligible trials should be based on a systematic and comprehensive search of a number of sources, to ensure that all relevant trials are identified, using the same or similar methods to those employed in a conventional systematic review of existing aggregate data.[92] However, IPD meta-analysis projects often have a greater emphasis on searching grey literature sources, such as conference proceedings, as well as trial registers to identify unpublished trials, and any ongoing trials that may complete in time for inclusion in the IPD meta-analysis.[7,9,43] For example, in an IPD meta-analysis project examining the effects of chemoradiation for cervical cancer,[93] about 25% of the included trials were unpublished or published only as an abstract. Although there may be initial concerns about the quality of unpublished trials, this can be formally evaluated (Sections 4.5 and 4.6), and having the accompanying protocol, case report forms and trial IPD enables more detailed quality checking than when relying on aggregate data reported in publications. Indeed, a high standard of reporting does not necessarily correspond to high-quality trial design and conduct, and similarly, some good-quality trials can be quite badly reported.

Trial investigators should be asked whether they can supplement the provisional list of eligible trials, and additional appeals might also be made via project websites, social media or conference presentations. A summary of the sources searched for an IPD meta-analysis of recombinant human bone morphogenetic protein-2 for spinal fusion is given in Box 4.2.

Box 4.2 Summary of the sources searched for an IPD meta-analysis of randomised trials examining recombinant human bone morphogenetic protein-2 for spinal fusion.

- Cochrane Central Register of Controlled Trials
- MEDLINE 1948 to present
- EMBASE 1974 to present
- Science Citation Index 1899 to present
- Automated "current awareness" searches to June 2012
- ClinicalTrials.gov (to identify ongoing or unpublished randomised trials)
- Published a call for evidence

Source: Lesley Stewart, listing the sources used by Simmonds et al.,[65] with permission.

The screening process for deciding which trials are relevant for inclusion is very similar to that for standard systematic reviews.[92] However, with IPD meta-analysis projects, because there is usually greater contact with trial investigators, any doubt as to the eligibility of a particular trial (e.g. in relation to whether particular variables or outcomes are recorded in the trial's IPD) can be clarified through discussion. This process should be well documented, so that it can be used to help populate a PRISMA-IPD flow diagram (Chapter 10).[60]

4.2.4 Deciding Which Information Is Needed to Summarise Trial Characteristics

After relevant trials are identified, it is important to obtain a good understanding of the attributes and characteristics of these trials, for descriptive purposes. This may include contacting trial investigators to request extra information about the trial population and treatment and control interventions. In addition, gathering structured trial-level information about the methods of randomisation, allocation concealment, blinding, planned and actual recruitment, and any stopping rules that were applied can be valuable when assessing risk of bias (Section 4.6), particularly if these aspects are not clearly reported in trial publications.[48] This may be particularly pertinent for older trials with limited documentation.

As there may be a considerable amount of information to collect, it is helpful to use a pre-prepared paper or online data collection form, which may be included as an appendix in the project protocol and accompany the invitation to collaborate. An example is shown in Figure 4.3.

This form is also useful for seeking administrative details for each trial, such as the trial identifier and/or acronym, the International Standard Randomised Controlled Trial Number (ISRCTN) number (if relevant), trial title and up-to-date trial publication information. Also, it is worth including a question about whether the principal trial investigator will be the key contact for the IPD meta-analysis project, or whether another individual, such as the trial statistician or data manager, will be responsible (providing space for their contact details). This would also be the place to ask trial investigators if they are aware of any potentially eligible trials not currently included in the draft protocol.

4.2.5 Deciding How Much IPD Are Needed

The searching and screening process will have produced a set of potentially eligible trials. This may have been refined by seeking early clarifications about trial characteristics, and possibly also by setting an information size threshold (e.g. based on contribution toward power; see Chapter 12),

MRC | Clinical Trials Unit

Smarter Studies
Global Impact
Better Health

UCL

STOPCAP M1

Speeding up the evaluation of therapies for metastatic hormone-sensitive prostate cancer

Trial details:

Trial title: Enter full trial name or title

Trial acronym: Enter trial acronym

Trial registration number: Enter e.g. NCT or ISRCTN number

Name(s) of Principal/Chief Investigator: Enter full name here

Participation in the STOPCAP Programme:

Are you willing to provide data for the STOPCAP programme? Yes ☐ No ☐

Contact details:

Email: Enter PI email **Telephone**: Enter number, with country/area code(s)

Please provide details of <u>most appropriate data contact</u> for this trial, if different from the above:

Name: e.g. data contact name (if not PI)

Email: Enter data contact email **Telephone**: Enter number, with country/area code(s)

Please provide details of <u>most appropriate person to contact about data transfer agreements</u> for this trial:

Name: e.g. data transfer contact name (if not PI)

Email: Enter data transfer contact email **Telephone**: Enter number, with country/area code(s)

Trial design:

Did all men included in this trial have hormone-sensitive prostate cancer? Yes ☐ No ☐

Did some of the men included in this trial have distant metastatic disease? Yes ☐ No ☐

Was informed consent obtained from each patient randomised to the trial? Yes ☐ No ☐

Date trial <u>opened</u> to accrual Day: Pick day **Month**: Pick month **Year**: Pick year

Date trial <u>closed</u> to accrual Day: Pick day **Month**: Pick month **Year**: Pick year

Method of randomisation (sequence generation) Enter full details

What, if any, stratification factors were used? Enter full details

What was the allocation ratio in each arm? e.g. 1:1

Method used to conceal allocation Enter full details

Were trial personnel blinded to the treatment received? Yes ☐ No ☐

Were trial participants blinded to the treatment received? Yes ☐ No ☐

If blinding of participants and/or trialists was not possible, please state why: Please provide full details

Figure 4.3 Excerpt from a trial-level data collection form for the STOPCAP M1 programme of IPD meta-analyses of therapies for metastatic prostate cancer.[94] *Source:* Based on Tierney JF, Vale CL, Parelukar WR, et al. Evidence Synthesis to Accelerate and Improve the Evaluation of Therapies for Metastatic Hormone-sensitive Prostate Cancer. *Eur Urol Focus* 2019;5(2):137–43.

or a quality threshold (e.g. based on an initial risk of bias examination based on published information; see Section 4.2.1), which trials must pass in order to be included. Further clarification and consideration of these issues may be required when more detailed engagement with trial investigators begins, and the likely shape and size of the available IPD emerges.

Given this set of eligible trials, how much IPD should be sought from them? As a general rule, the aim should be to maximise the quantity and quality of IPD available, in order to fulfil the project objectives and complete the planned analyses reliably. For conventional reviews, aggregate data would ordinarily be sought for *all* studies relevant to the question of interest. Similarly, and ideally, IPD should be sought from all the eligible trials, for all participants recruited to those trials, and for all relevant outcomes, even if they were not published or included in the original analyses. This will help circumvent the risk of publication bias, outcome reporting bias, attrition bias, and other data availability biases (Chapter 9).[46,58,95] For example, in trials of the effectiveness of recombinant human bone morphogenetic protein-2 for spinal fusion, the adverse event data were not reported sufficiently to allow a rigorous evaluation of safety,[96] whereas the collection of IPD allowed a complete, detailed, and in-depth analysis.[65] If it is not feasible or practical to seek IPD from all trials, the potential impact of these 'missing' trials should be taken into account (Chapter 9).

4.2.6 Deciding Which Variables Are Needed in the IPD

As for all systematic reviews, the pre-specified outcomes for the IPD meta-analysis project should be those judged to be most important and relevant to the objectives, even if ultimately there are insufficient data available to analyse all of them. While consideration of the participant-level variables required begins when the IPD meta-analysis questions are formulated, this should be re-visited before requesting IPD from trial investigators, so that they can be specified more precisely and ensure that the planned analyses can be completed satisfactorily. Trial publications can provide an initial guide as to which data might be available, but more variables may have been collected in a trial than is evident from a trial report. Often the trial protocol and the associated case report forms can provide a more reliable indication of which data have been recorded. Irrespective of whether these documents are available or not, it is useful to supply trial investigators with a provisional list of desired variables via a paper or online form, or as a detailed data dictionary (Section 4.2.7), so that trial teams can clarify precisely which data items they can provide. An example of the typical types of data requested from trial investigators is shown in Box 4.3.

In addition, it is important to anticipate what supplementary analyses might be needed in the IPD meta-analysis project to explore the main results. For example, for a question about the effects of chemotherapy on long-term cancer survival, it may be helpful to collect data which would allow the investigation of the effects of treatment on different (competing) causes of death, such as those due to cancer, treatment-related side effects or co-morbid conditions.

In many cases, it will only be necessary to collect outcomes and participant characteristics as defined in the individual trials. However, additional variables might be required to provide greater granularity (e.g. sub-scales in quality of life instruments), or to allow outcomes or other variables to be defined in a consistent way for each trial. For example, in an IPD meta-analysis of anti-platelet therapy for pre-eclampsia in pregnancy, data on systolic and diastolic blood pressure plus presence of proteinurea were collected. This was to allow the central research team to analyse pre-eclampsia according to both a pre-defined meta-analysis definition, as well as the individual trial definitions (of which there were many variations).[97] Furthermore, if the IPD are to be maintained in perpetuity, to address new questions that might arise, additional data may be requested to effectively 'future-proof' the database. For example, if there is a plan to use the IPD collected to produce

Box 4.3 Example of typical data obtained for trials to be included in an IPD meta-analysis project

At a minimum, the IPD requested for each trial would typically include variables that:

- 'Identify' participants, e.g.
  - De-identified participant ID (Section 4.4.1), centre ID
- Describe the participant population, facilitate data checking and allow analyses by participant characteristics, e.g.
  - Age, sex, demographic variables, disease or condition characteristics and key prognostic factors
- Describe the intervention, e.g.
  - Date of randomisation
  - Intervention allocation
  - If appropriate, the interventions participants received and the dates of administration
- Record all outcomes of interest and relevant to the objectives, e.g.
  - Survival, toxicity, pre-eclampsia, healing, hospital stay, last follow-up date
- Describe whether participants were excluded from the primary trial analysis and reasons, e.g.
  - Ineligible, protocol violation, missing outcome data, withdrawal, 'early' outcome

Source: Jayne Tierney and Lesley Stewart.

conditional treatment effects (Chapter 5), to identify predictors of treatment effect (Chapter 7), or to identify prognostic factors (Chapter 16), then it would be sensible to request more detailed baseline data than might be necessary if just the overall (unadjusted) effects of treatments were of interest. Having said that, it is important to avoid collecting extraneous data, as these will still need to be checked and managed, and if not used, this represents an unnecessary burden for the trial teams who have spent time preparing data. Of course, it may be easier for trial teams to provide a complete trial data file, and let the IPD meta-analysis research team extract what they need.

4.2.7 Developing a Data Dictionary for the IPD

In addition to preparing a list of variables that will be required for the analyses, it is important to consider carefully how best to define, collect and store these in an appropriate and unambiguous manner. The development of a detailed data dictionary for an IPD meta-analysis project effectively establishes the structure of the meta-analysis database, facilitates processing of IPD from each trial and ensures that the analyses can proceed as planned, with the greatest degree of flexibility. It also helps guide the trial teams in the preparation of IPD prior to transfer, and gives them the responsibility for modifying variables, lessening the likelihood of misinterpretation or coding errors. However, trial teams may not have the time to adhere to the data dictionary, and they should not be compelled to do so, particularly if their resources for preparing the IPD are limited. In such instances, it is advisable that the central research team accepts trial IPD in any (reasonable) workable form, and take responsibility for reformatting and re-coding it themselves, according to the data dictionary.

Table 4.1 provides an excerpt from a data dictionary used in an IPD meta-analysis examining the effects of chemoradiation for cervical cancer.[93] Age at randomisation was collected straightforwardly as a continuous variable, with a missing data code of 999. Tumour stage was collected as a categorical variable with a single code for each stage and sub-stage, and with a missing data code

Table 4.1 Excerpt from a data dictionary developed for an IPD meta-analysis of chemoradiation for cervical cancer.[93]

Variable	Variable name	Definition
Age at randomisation	Age	Numeric Age in years 999 = unknown
Tumour stage	TumStage	Numeric Tumour stage categories 1 = Stage Ia 2 = Stage Ib 3 = Stage IIa 4 = Stage IIb 5 = Stage IIIa 6 = Stage IIIb 7 = Stage IVa 8 = Stage IVb 9 = unknown
Performance status	PerfStat	Numeric Provide the data as defined in the trial and supply full details of the system used
Survival status	SurvStat	Numeric 0 = Alive 1 = Dead
Date of death or last follow-up	DOLF	Date in dd/mm/yy format unknown day = --/mm/yy unknown month = --/--/yy unknown date = --/--/--

Source: Claire Vale and Jayne Tierney.

of 9. This afforded the greatest flexibility for subsequent analysis, as the sub-stages could be used as supplied, or collapsed into broader-stage categories as needed. While trial eligibility criteria indicate which participants a trial intends to recruit, it is worth suggesting a wider range of possibilities in the data dictionary, because recruitment of some ineligible participants might be inevitable. This could arise, for example, if eligibility is predicated on a positive diagnostic test, and false positives are identified at subsequent review, or as a result of a later diagnostic procedure. In the aforementioned cervical cancer IPD meta-analysis, women with stage IVB stage were not eligible for any of the included trials. However, they were sometimes randomised erroneously, because initial clinical staging did not identify them as such, but subsequent surgical staging did, and so the data dictionary allowed for that possibility. If particular participant characteristics are collected on different scales, then it may be possible to convert to a common scale. In the cervical cancer IPD meta-analysis, the included trials recorded performance status on different scales, so in the data dictionary it was made clear that all were permitted, and these were later converted into a common meta-analysis scale.

The data dictionary should use accepted coding conventions wherever possible, not only to facilitate the provision of data by trial teams, but also to avoid errors. For example, for binary and time-to-event outcomes, 0 is most commonly used to indicate no event, and 1 to indicate an event has happened. For time-to-event outcomes such as survival in cancer, or time free of seizures in epilepsy, it is important to collect the three component variables that make up the outcome for each participant (Table 4.1). These would comprise: a variable that indicates whether an event has happened (e.g. a death or a seizure); another that provides the date the event happened (e.g. date of death or date of seizure) and finally one that describes the date that the participant was last assessed for the outcome of interest (e.g. the date last seen in clinic). If an event has not occurred, the latter allows the participant to be included in the analysis, and censored at that time-point. Together with the date of randomisation, these variables allow the time to event for each participant to be calculated, and provides the greatest flexibility for data checking (Section 4.5), risk of bias assessment (Section 4.6) and analysis (Part 2). Alternatively, the date of event and date of last follow-up (censoring time) can be collected as a composite. As a bare minimum, the collection of an indicator variable for the occurrence of an event (yes/no) and the time to event (or censoring) will suffice. In fact, the latter may be all that trial teams are able to provide, for example, if they originate from a country or institute bound by stringent data protection regulations, or if the data are downloaded from a repository that prohibits the supply of exact dates in order to help to preserve participant confidentiality.

Special care is needed to avoid ambiguity in the data dictionary, otherwise it will lead to ambiguity in the supplied IPD from each trial, and then the IPD meta-analysis database. For example, for an IPD meta-analysis of the effects of anti-platelet therapy for pre-eclampsia in pregnancy,[97] the data dictionary suggested that severe maternal morbidity be coded as a single variable. Unintentionally, this did not allow for the provision of more than one type of morbidity for an individual woman, which could occur, for example if she had eclampsia followed by a stroke (Table 4.2). In the same meta-analysis, a missing data code of 9 was used for gestation at randomisation, which meant that (although unlikely) any women randomised at nine weeks' gestation could potentially be regarded mistakenly as having missing gestation information (Table 4.2). Thus, an unambiguous missing data code such as 99 or, even better, a negative integer such as –9 would have been preferable. Furthermore, it is prudent to discriminate between different types of missing data, such as missing for the participant (e.g. –9 or 9), not applicable to the participant (e.g. –8 or 8) or not collected for the trial (e.g. –7 or 7). For example, in an IPD meta-analysis of progesterone for pre-term birth,[79] if a baby was stillborn, certain baby outcomes were coded as 8 to signify that they could not be collected, and as 9 to indicate a true missing value. Although this could be inferred from the birth data, coding the IPD in this way made it easier to calculate the proportions of missing data and to cross-check.

Table 4.2 Excerpt from a data dictionary developed for an IPD meta-analysis project the effects of anti-platelets for prevention of pre-eclampsia in pregnancy[97]

Variable	Definition	Issue
Severe maternal morbidity	1 = none 2 = stroke 3 = renal failure 4 = liver failure 5 = pulmonary oedema 6 = disseminated intravascular coagulation 7 = HELP syndrome 8 = eclampsia 9 = not recorded	Collection as a single variable did not allow for the provision of more than one morbidity for the same women
Gestation at randomisation	Gestation in completed weeks 9 = unknown	Woman could be randomised at 9 weeks gestation

Source: Lesley Stewart and Lisa Askie, based on the data dictionary used by Askie et al.[97]

4.3 Initiating and Maintaining Collaboration

Negotiating and maintaining collaborations with trial investigators and organisations from different countries, settings and disciplines can take considerable time and effort, and requires careful management,[43,44] but is critical to the success of collaborative IPD meta-analysis projects. In an era where the value of clinical data sharing is more widely appreciated, persuading trial investigators of the value of participating is becoming easier. However, it is worth remembering that not all trial investigators will be obliged by their funders to share their IPD, and it is perfectly reasonable that they may require persuading of the project's value and rigour before they agree to make their data available for meta-analysis. Also, whilst collection of IPD may be at the top of the IPD meta-analysis research team's agenda, it will not necessarily be a priority for the trial investigators, so perseverance, patience, tact and diplomacy must all be brought to bear.

Invitations to participate may need to be issued several times before receiving a reply. If no response is forthcoming from the first or corresponding author of the trial publication, it is worth seeking contact with other authors, or the data centre that hosts the trial (e.g. a trials unit or cooperative group) to trace an appropriate trial contact, particularly for older trials. In this context, careful logs of contact and the status of agreements should be maintained, especially if many studies are eligible for inclusion in the IPD meta-analysis project.

An initial correspondence can help prime trial investigators, letting them know at an early stage about the IPD project, and inviting their in principle support and agreement to collaborate. This may even take place during the planning phase, to provide an early opportunity to assess the feasibility of the approach (Section 3.4), to support a funding application (Section 3.9), or to inform a power calculation (Chapter 12). As the project moves forward, these early contacts can be repeated, particularly if some time has elapsed between initial contact, the award of funding and project start-up. Correspondence may be via a simple email or letter describing the nature of the collaboration they are being invited to join, with or without a project scope that outlines the project objectives and high-level methods (Section 3.3). This is a good time to seek key design features from trial investigators (Section 4.2.4), and thereby clarify understanding of each trial, and if need be, verify eligibility.

Subsequently, a more formal invitation to collaborate is usually accompanied by a draft protocol (Section 4.2.2), which may also include information on timelines, any funds available, the dissemination strategy and authorship policy for subsequent papers. Also, it can be useful to supply trial investigators with a provisional list of the variables required, or to provide them with the detailed data dictionary (Section 4.2.7), so that they might check which data items they will be able to share. If it transpires that certain key variables of interest (e.g. those that are hypothesised to modify treatment effect) have been collected in very few trials, then it may be necessary to document this and discuss how it impacts upon the IPD meta-analysis protocol and statistical analysis plan. The availability of data may even influence the decision to proceed with the project (e.g. if the potential power is considered very low; Chapter 12), or at least highlight whether the meta-analysis results will likely be better suited to informing the rationale and design of a new trial rather than influencing clinical practice.

At this stage, it may be worth giving trial investigators the opportunity to provide feedback on the draft protocol, and flag any important issues that may need further exploration and development in a subsequent version. This process also serves to emphasise to trial investigators that they are active members of the collaborative group, rather than being just passive providers of IPD, which may be important in securing their agreement to share data. That said, and as noted in Section 3.2.1, it is important that the central research team remain as independent and autonomous as possible, retaining the responsibility for deciding which methods and analytic approaches are appropriate to the project. Feedback on the protocol should also be sought from the project advisory group, including any patients or public representatives, which requires that a good lay summary of the project is available, and that additional explanatory material is provided, as required.

A data-sharing agreement outlining the nature of the collaboration, the responsibilities and obligations of each party, and intellectual property arrangements (Section 3.11) will usually be supplied with the finalised protocol. Normally this should be signed by both data provider and recipient before any trial IPD can be transferred. It is also useful to include a data transfer guide (Section 4.4.2), outlining the steps that should be taken to protect participant confidentiality and transfer data securely, as well as the detailed data dictionary, which describes the preferred format and coding for the IPD meta-analysis project (Section 4.2.7).

Usually, further communication back and forth between the IPD meta-analysis research team and trial personnel is required, to ensure appropriate understanding of the supplied IPD, and to resolve any queries arising from data harmonisation, checking (Section 4.5) or risk of bias assessment (Section 4.6). As the project will take place over a prolonged period, it is also good practice to give trial investigators regular updates on progress, for example, letting them know how many groups have agreed to collaborate, the status of data collection, and any deviations from the project timetable or protocol. This can be achieved via regular short newsletters, email updates or a project website (e.g. Figure 4.4). If trial investigators are unable to provide their IPD, or respond to queries in a timely manner, this can place extra time pressure on those undertaking data checking, harmonisation and analysis. Therefore, it is important to keep communicating key deadline dates for the project. Although it is wise to include some flexibility and contingency when setting these, any trials that fail to meet final deadlines may ultimately need to be excluded, so as not to jeopardise the successful delivery of the IPD meta-analysis results.

4.4 Obtaining IPD

Given that IPD meta-analyses are typically collaborative projects, trial investigators and their host institutes need to ensure that trial IPD are suitably de-identified, then transferred and stored securely, so as to preserve participant privacy, and that any unauthorised use is prohibited, as set out in the data-sharing agreement (Section 3.11).

4.4.1 Ensuring That IPD Are De-identified

It is important to request that data providers take steps to de-identify participants in their IPD, before transferring it to the meta-analysis research team, so as to minimise the risk of participants being re-identified and their confidentiality being breached.[98] De-identification generally involves the removal of all identifiers that could directly identify individuals, such as participant names and medical or hospital numbers. In an IPD meta-analysis project, this small degree of de-identification is the usual process followed by data providers, because the data recipients (i.e. the IPD project's central research team) will not have access to the full, original (identifying) data. However, the data protection legislation of the country from which the trial originates, or institutional requirements, may necessitate more stringent de-identification measures, for example, the removal or recoding of indirect or quasi-identifiers such as dates of birth, and the removal or redaction of free-text verbatim

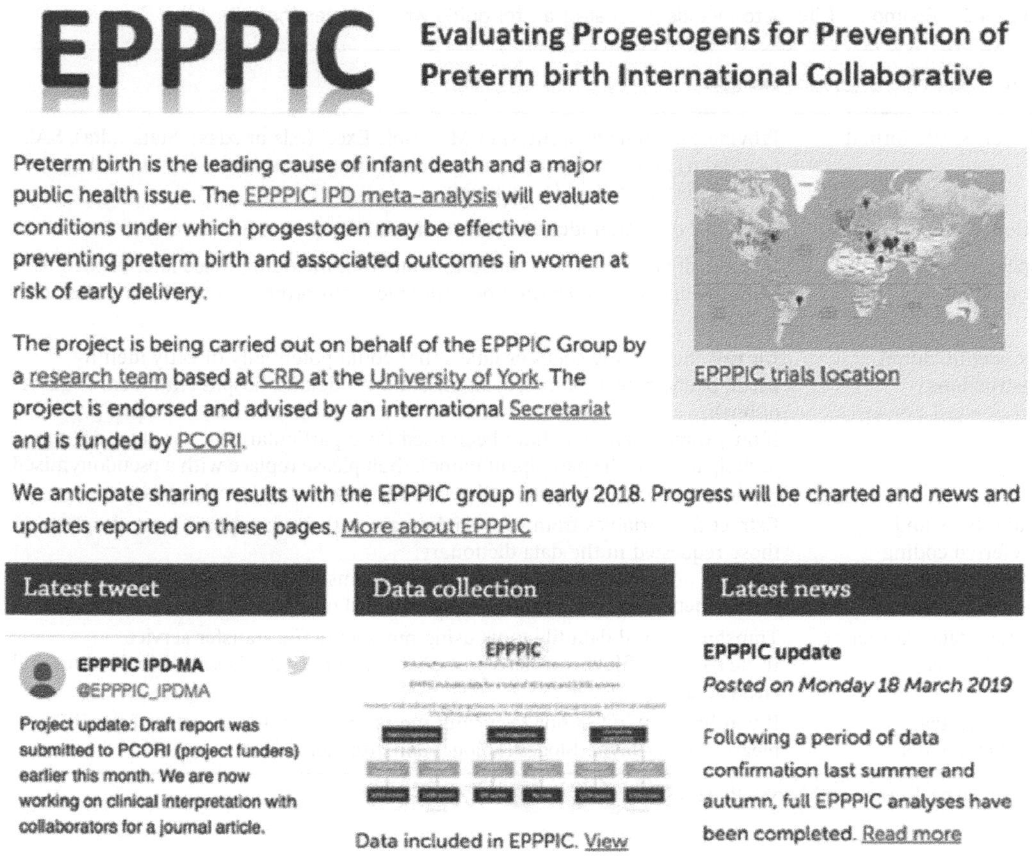
EPPPIC
Evaluating Progestogens for Prevention of Preterm birth International Collaborative
Preterm birth is the leading cause of infant death and a major public health issue. The EPPPIC IPD meta-analysis will evaluate conditions under which progestogen may be effective in preventing preterm birth and associated outcomes in women at risk of early delivery.
The project is being carried out on behalf of the EPPPIC Group by a research team based at CRD at the University of York. The project is endorsed and advised by an international Secretariat and is funded by PCORI.
EPPPIC trials location
We anticipate sharing results with the EPPPIC group in early 2018. Progress will be charted and news and updates reported on these pages. More about EPPPIC
Latest tweet
EPPPIC IPD-MA
@EPPPIC_IPDMA
Project update: Draft report was submitted to PCORI (project funders) earlier this month. We are now working on clinical interpretation with collaborators for a journal article.
Data collection
EPPPIC
Data included in EPPPIC. View
Latest news
EPPPIC update
Posted on Monday 18 March 2019
Following a period of data confirmation last summer and autumn, full EPPPIC analyses have been completed. Read more

Figure 4.4 Excerpts from the website https://www.york.ac.uk/crd/research/epppic/ for an IPD meta-analysis of the effects of progestogens for the prevention of preterm birth. *Source:* Evaluating Progestogens for Prevention of Preterm birth International Collaborative, © University of York.

terms. Direct identifiers may be replaced with new pseudonyms, and quasi-identifying dates may be removed or generalised to, for example, just the month and year so as to limit the risk of identification.[99] As the link between the shared IPD and original trial data is preserved, it remains feasible to consult with trial investigators on any issues that arise at the participant level, and update the IPD as needed.

Although with a lesser degree of de-identification or pseudonymisation there are risks that participants might be identified,[99] this is mitigated by the data provider and IPD project's central research team entering into a data-sharing agreement. This should specifically prohibit any attempt to identify individuals, and stipulate that the team receiving the data should have data privacy training, and will hold the data securely and use it appropriately (Section 3.11). Data recipients still need to sign data-sharing agreements to obtain IPD from more public sources, such as data-sharing platforms or repositories (Section 3.2.2),[100] but these data will usually have been subject to a greater degree of de-identification, because the risks to participant confidentiality are greater with such quasi-public data.[99] Full de-identification or anonymisation, involving the removal of all links between the de-identified IPD and the original datasets, limits the utility of the IPD for meta-analysis and therefore, is not recommended.

Table 4.3 Example of items to include in a data transfer guide when requesting IPD

Item	Example
Preferred file format	Provide electronic data file(s) in Microsoft Excel (.xls or .xlsx), Stata (.dta), SAS (.sas7bdat) or a delimited plain-text (.csv) format if possible. If you need to use another format, please let us know.
Filename instructions	Include a clear trial identifier in the name of any data files provided.
Specific trial population	Include all participants recruited to your trial, including those later classed as being ineligible, withdrawn, not evaluable, with protocol deviations, or lost to follow-up.
De-identification instructions	**Do not** include any codes or labels that could potentially directly identify participants, such as names, locations, address details, hospital numbers or dates of birth. If only direct identifiers have been used for a particular trial variable (e.g. the participant ID is the participant name), then please replace with a pseudonymised version for each participant and retain the key in case queries arise.
Data items and preferred coding	Extract the variables from your trial database that correspond most closely to those requested in the data dictionary. If this is not possible for some or all data items, please use your own codes, but define them clearly in your dataset documentation.
Secure data transfer instructions	Transfer the trial data file to us using our secure file transfer service. If the trial data file is transferred by email, ensure that it is secure and end-to-end encrypted.
Research team contact details	If you have any questions regarding the preparation and transfer of the IPD, please contact Jayne Bloggs (j.bloggs@institute.email).

Source: Jayne Tierney and Larysa Rydzewska.

4.4.2 Providing Data Transfer Guidance

It is useful to provide trial investigators, or their data contact, with a data transfer guide outlining how their IPD should be prepared and transferred securely (Table 4.3). In addition, the guide can be used to make data providers aware of how the central research team will subsequently manage, check and verify their data, and to encourage them to get in touch should any queries arise. It may also highlight whether there are any specific funds available to facilitate the preparation of trial data, and how to access these. If helpful, the guide can be accompanied by a template data file in the trial investigators preferred software package (such as Stata, R, SAS, or Excel), including all the variable names, but no actual data.

4.4.3 Transferring Trial IPD Securely

Based on the relevant data transfer guidance supplied by the central research team, secure data transfer can be achieved using a suitable file transfer site, for example, an institutional or suitable commercial file share service. Where a data file needs to be sent via email, ideally it should be end-to-end encrypted or otherwise password protected, with passwords sent separately (and ideally via a different communication medium, such as by post or by telephone). Although rare these days, if data need to be transferred using physical storage media, such as external disc drives or memory sticks, these should also be encrypted and sent using a delivery service that allows the package to be tracked and signed for upon delivery.

When data files are first received, it is important to ensure that they can be read and loaded into the preferred storage or analysis system before proceeding. For example, if a data file arrive electronically, it should be checked to ensure that any passwords provided work, and that it can be opened, is for the correct trial, and that the data have not been corrupted during transfer. It is important to thank relevant trial personnel for providing their data, and either confirm that they are as expected, or relay any issues that have arisen, as soon as possible.

4.4.4 Storing Trial IPD Securely

Once transferred, IPD need to be stored securely by the central research team, with access limited to those members responsible for data management, checking and analysis, or overall conduct. They should have appropriate expertise in the handling of participant data, as well as training in data protection, and also should be prohibited from copying data to any mobile devices, laptops, memory sticks or cloud servers that have not been set up for the secure storage of confidential data.

It is recommended that the central research team retain the original version of each trial data file exactly as supplied. This can be used for cross checking, and provides a back-up should any errors arise, for example, if the data file that the meta-analysis team are working on becomes corrupted. A copy of the file should be made prior to any changes, such as re-formatting, re-coding or re-defining variables (Section 4.5), being carried out. Firstly, the copy should be converted to the preferred software format (such as Stata, R or SAS) for the IPD meta-analysis project, which nowadays is a fairly straightforward process, because statistical packages can recognise or import data from multiple other sources, and if they do not, a specialist transfer package such as StatTransfer can be utilised. It is useful to add a numeric trial identifier and label to the trial data file, so that when IPD are being checked, harmonised, merged and analysed subsequently, each trial can be easily identified in the outputs, analyses and forest plots.

4.4.5 Making Best Use of IPD from Repositories

It may be possible or necessary to access IPD for one or more trials via a data-sharing repository or platform. For example, there is a reasonable likelihood that trial investigators conducting trials of newer therapies, or that have published results more recently, might have to comply with a funder-mandated data-sharing policy requiring that IPD are uploaded to a repository. As described in detail in Section 3.2.2, repositories may not include all trials of relevance to a particular meta-analysis, or the trials may be distributed across multiple platforms. Therefore, accessing trial IPD in this way can present challenges for the central collection, management, checking and analysis of data, and thereby potentially limit the ability to realise all the advantages generally associated with IPD meta-analysis projects.[45] The central research team may need to find ways to work around the issues.

The IPD from a repository may not contain all the variables required to conduct the planned analyses, or these may not be defined in a standard way across different repositories, making data harmonisation difficult. In such circumstances, it may be possible to get an investigator to upload a more appropriate dataset, if the IPD research team can persuade them of the value of doing so. For example, they might emphasise that this is important not only for the current IPD meta-analysis, but also for subsequent projects that may make use of their trial IPD, and therefore may ultimately prevent data providers receiving repeated requests for further data. However, this would take additional time and resource on the part of both the data provider and the central IPD meta-analysis research team.

In order to preserve participant confidentiality, often the IPD contained in a repository are subject to a greater degree of de-identification (Section 4.4.1) than might be required or expected of IPD obtained directly from investigators. This can limit the ability to thoroughly check data (Section 4.5) and assess risk of bias (Section 4.6), and moreover, the opportunity to query any anomalies is lost. Once again, it may be possible to query aspects of the trial, or its associated IPD, through additional contact with trial investigators (including the trial statistician), or to request that they run some validity or risk of bias checks on behalf of the research team. It should be noted though, that for some platforms, the associated data-sharing agreements require that all queries are mediated through them.

Provided appropriate data are available, are more or less in the same format across trials, and can be downloaded from the relevant repository to use locally, there should not be any restrictions to the analyses of IPD. However, if access to IPD (and therefore data management and analyses) are confined to within a platform, it will only be possible to download results (e.g. regression model parameter estimates and confidence intervals), and this will restrict the meta-analysis to a two-stage approach (Part 2).

4.5 Checking and Harmonising Incoming IPD

Checking IPD, and harmonisation across trials, are integral and necessary components of an IPD meta-analysis project. The checking process ensures that any missing data, or major errors in the supplied IPD, can be identified and brought diplomatically to the attention on the trial investigators. Often, the problems that arise turn out to be simple errors or reflect misunderstandings, which can be resolved readily, with major problems being rare. As well as preventing serious issues in the meta-analysis, checking the IPD also promotes a better understanding of each trial by the central research team, and their independent scrutiny of the IPD can enhance the IPD project's credibility.

Often trials will have collected and defined data items in a variety of ways, and it will be necessary to re-code or re-define certain variables to a common format, in preparation for meta-analysis. Depending on how data have been provided, and whether trial teams have followed the supplied data dictionary, this can be an involved process, as described next. Checking and harmonising data requires care and meticulous attention to detail, in order to avoid misunderstandings and the introduction of errors. Contact with those supplying data may be needed to resolve any uncertainties or sanction particular changes.

4.5.1 The Process and Principles

Data management is usually done in a number of steps, with queries back and forth to trial investigators or other data contacts, to resolve any issues and ensure accuracy (Figure 4.1), ultimately leading to trial data that are in the best possible shape for the IPD meta-analysis. Therefore, it is one of the most involved stages of an IPD project, and needs sufficient time and resources. Conducting the individual checking and harmonisation steps, and waiting for responses to queries across multiple trials, can take place over many months. As different members of the research team may handle different trials at different times, keeping track of the process and outputs can be challenging. Producing a detailed plan, and adopting a standardised approach to data checking and harmonisation, will help to ensure that the process is implemented consistently across trials, and between those managing the IPD. For example, using a checklist for all data checkers to follow, together with a common suite of statistical analysis code, can help to ensure and maintain consistency.

Regardless of the extent of checking and data transformation needed, it is always sensible to use formal database or statistical software code to carry out the different steps. The code and the associated outputs help to maintain a detailed log of the checks, and any conversions or modifications to the data, thereby providing a comprehensive and transparent audit trail for each trial. It is also important to record where checks have identified problems, how these were (or were not resolved), and equally to record where no problems were identified.

The information generated for each trial may be held on a number of forms, spreadsheets or as output from statistical software. A summary document is a useful means of bringing together the various elements of checking, querying and decision-making, and might include hyperlinks to the different outputs, together with correspondence from trial teams. Where resource allows, ideally two individuals would independently check each trial, blinded to the other's results, and compare and discuss the findings. At the very least, another research team member should review the checking results, and discuss problems arising. Any major or sensitive issues should be raised with senior research team members, prior to any dialogue with the trial investigators.

In the following sub-sections, we suggest a range of checks for IPD obtained from randomised trials evaluating treatment effects,[7,9,43,101] but most of these are applicable to other types of primary study.

4.5.2 Initial Checking of IPD for Each Trial

When IPD are received for a trial, and often before processing the data further, it is worth conducting some preliminary checks. For example, it is useful to confirm that all the participants randomised appear to have been included, and check that there are no obvious omissions or duplicates in the sequence of participant identifiers (if they have been provided). Similarly, it is helpful to check which outcomes, baseline covariates and other variables are included in the IPD, and whether any that are 'missing' were truly not collected in the trial (called *systematically missing variables*; Chapter 18) or were recorded, but not included in the IPD supplied. If the latter, then either more complete IPD should be requested again, or a full explanation for non-provision sought.

For time-to-event outcomes, it is worth checking that the extent of follow-up for each trial is sufficient for the condition and outcome of interest, and encouraging trial investigators to supply up-to-date follow-up information where possible.[7] Although short follow-up may not introduce bias, it might prevent a trial, and therefore an IPD meta-analysis, picking up benefits or harms of interventions that take a long time to accrue, such as late side effects of treatment or late recurrence of disease. For example, in an IPD meta-analysis evaluating the addition of chemotherapy local treatment for soft tissue sarcoma,[102] the median follow-up for survival was reported for seven of the included trials as being between 16 and 64 months,[46] which is rather short for this type of cancer. Trial investigators supplying IPD were asked to provide updated information, which extended the median follow-up for these trials to between 74 and 204 months,[46] and thus allowed a more reliable examination of the effects of chemotherapy in the long term (Figure 4.5).[102] Such updating may not be necessary if most or all events have already occurred, and may not be feasible if, for example, studies are very old, no longer obtaining follow-up information, or resources are limited.

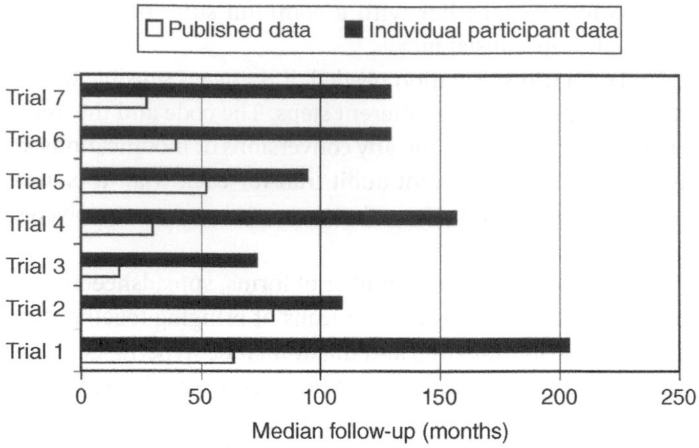

Figure 4.5 Median follow-up based on published aggregate data compared to updated obtained IPD for seven trials included in an IPD meta-analysis of adjuvant chemotherapy for soft tissue sarcoma.[46] *Source:* Stewart et al.[46], © 2006, John Wiley & Sons.

While ideally these checks should make use of database or statistical code, the value of scanning the data by eye should not be underestimated, as it can help members of the central research team get a feel for the trial as a whole, and even highlight unusual patterns or peculiarities.

4.5.3 Harmonising IPD across Trials

If data providers have followed the supplied data dictionary closely when preparing their IPD, much of the data harmonisation will have been done already, and minor adjustments may be all that are required. If trial investigators are unable or unwilling to prepare data according to suggested pre-specified formats, the central research team should accept data in whichever format is most convenient, and recode it as necessary.

Beyond simply aligning trial IPD to the data dictionary, there is also the opportunity to standardise definitions of outcomes or participant-level variables,[7,43] such as scoring or staging systems. For example, in an IPD meta-analysis examining the effects of chemotherapy for soft tissue sarcoma,[102] different definitions of histological grade were used in the included trials, but with input from trial investigators, it was possible to translate each of these into a high- or low-grade disease category, allowing exploration of treatment effectiveness according to grade.[43] It may also be necessary to construct new standardised variables for use in analyses. For example, in an IPD meta-analysis of the effects of antenatal diet and physical activity on maternal and foetal outcomes, the research team collected data on each woman's height, baseline weight and parity, as well as the gestational age at birth and foetal birthweight for each baby. This allowed researchers to generate a standardised meta-analysis definition of 'small for gestational age' (< 10th centile), using a bulk birthweight centile calculator.[103]

4.5.4 Checking the Validity, Range and Consistency of Variables

IPD should be checked for invalid, outlying or implausible values,[7,9,43] as these are the sorts of errors that can occasionally be missed during data input or checking of the original trials, or occasionally could arise as a result of variable recoding by the IPD meta-analysis project team. Such checks might highlight, for example, records of unusually old or young patients, or those with abnormally high or low levels of important biomarkers, which need to be queried with trial teams. Of course, such apparently implausible values may turn out to be accurate. For example, in a trial included in an IPD meta-analysis of neoadjuvant chemotherapy for cervical cancer,[104] some invalid codes were used for the brachytherapy (internal radiotherapy) variable (Figure 4.6), which were then queried and clarified as representing not applicable. When variables are related, checks should be carried out to ensure that they are coherent and consistent. For example, in a randomised trial, the recorded date of any event should follow the recorded date of randomisation and occur on or before the recorded date of last follow-up.

At this stage, it is also useful to perform a simple descriptive analysis of the IPD from each trial to provide, for example, the number of participants, distribution of baseline characteristics by treatment group and overall results for the main outcome(s). These can then be checked for concordance with relevant publications or, for unpublished trials, with any results that have been deposited in trial registers (e.g. ClinicalTrials.gov). However, it should be borne in mind that inconsistencies can arise if, for example, follow-up in a trial's IPD has been extended beyond that used to derive the reported results, or if the meta-analysis employs a different approach compared to the original trial analyses. When unexplained differences do arise, it is crucial to work with the original trial investigators to understand how and why they differ, and therefore, be in a position to report and explain any important discrepancies.

```
30/05/2002, 14:31:58 - Error record for N:\CERVIXNEO\DATA2\TRIAL22.DBF
Trial 22, patient reference 226: There is neither age, nor date of birth.
Trial 22, patient reference 231: Brachytherapy code -  7 - is not 0, 1, or 9.
Trial 22, patient reference 235: Brachytherapy code -  7 - is not 0, 1, or 9.
Trial 22, patient reference 245: Brachytherapy code -  7 - is not 0, 1, or 9.
Trial 22, patient reference 248: Brachytherapy code -  7 - is not 0, 1, or 9.
Trial 22, patient reference 254: Brachytherapy code -  7 - is not 0, 1, or 9.
Trial 22, patient reference 257: Brachytherapy code -  7 - is not 0, 1, or 9.
Trial 22, patient reference 276: Brachytherapy code -  7 - is not 0, 1, or 9.
Trial 22, patient reference 279: Brachytherapy code -  7 - is not 0, 1, or 9.
Trial 22, patient reference 282: Brachytherapy code -  7 - is not 0, 1, or 9.
Trial 22, patient reference 300: Brachytherapy code -  7 - is not 0, 1, or 9.
Trial 22, patient reference 304: Brachytherapy code -  7 - is not 0, 1, or 9.
Trial 22, patient reference 325: Brachytherapy code -  7 - is not 0, 1, or 9.
Trial 22, patient reference 332: Brachytherapy code -  7 - is not 0, 1, or 9.
Trial 22, patient reference 342: Brachytherapy code -  7 - is not 0, 1, or 9.
Trial 22, patient reference 363: Brachytherapy code -  7 - is not 0, 1, or 9.
Trial 22, patient reference 365: Brachytherapy code -  7 - is not 0, 1, or 9.
Trial 22, patient reference 366: Brachytherapy code -  7 - is not 0, 1, or 9.
Trial 22, patient reference 369: Brachytherapy code -  7 - is not 0, 1, or 9.
Trial 22, patient reference 386: Brachytherapy code -  7 - is not 0, 1, or 9.
Trial 22, patient reference 393: Brachytherapy code -  7 - is not 0, 1, or 9.
Trial 22, patient reference 402: Brachytherapy code -  7 - is not 0, 1, or 9.
Trial 22, patient reference 421: Brachytherapy code -  7 - is not 0, 1, or 9.
Trial 22, patient reference 430: There is neither age, nor date of birth.
Trial 22, patient reference 432: There is neither age, nor date of birth.
Trial 22, patient reference 436: There is neither age, nor date of birth.
Trial 22, patient reference 441: There is neither age, nor date of birth.
```

Figure 4.6 Summary of the data validity, range and consistency checks on IPD from a trial included in an IPD meta-analysis of neoadjuvant chemotherapy for cervical cancer[104] (N.B. The participant references are pseudonymised). *Source:* Based on Neoadjuvant Chemotherapy for Locally Advanced Cervical Cancer Meta-analysis C. Neoadjuvant chemotherapy for locally advanced cervical cancer: a systematic review and meta-analysis of individual patient data from 21 randomised trials. *European journal of cancer* 2003;39(17):2470–86.

4.6 Checking the IPD to Inform Risk of Bias Assessments

Similar to conventional aggregate data reviews, assessing the reliability (quality) of included trials is also an important feature of the checking phase of IPD meta-analysis projects. In such reviews, this is usually based on the *risk of bias*, a term that refers to the likelihood that included trials will generate biased results. In particular, the risk of bias assessment tool (RoB 2) can be used to evaluate potential bias in estimates of intervention effects from randomised trials.[91] It includes five domains to be considered for each eligible trial: the randomisation process; deviations from intended interventions; missing outcome data; measurement of the outcome; and selection of the reported result. Within each domain, assessments are guided by multiple signalling questions (with answers: yes, probably yes, probably no, no, or no information), allowing a risk of bias classification for that domain (low, high, or some concerns). Finally, an overall risk of bias judgement can be made (low, high, or some concerns) based on all domains (Section 4.7).

In aggregate data reviews, assessment of risk of bias is usually based on the information available in trial publications and other publicly accessible documents, such as trial registration entries or published protocols, sometimes supplemented by information requested from trial investigators. In an IPD meta-analysis project, it is common to obtain additional information from protocols, codebooks and forms, or direct from trial investigators, which can increase the clarity of risk of bias assessments compared to those based on trial reports alone.[48,105] As discussed in Sections 3.4 and 4.2.6, it may be helpful to undertake an initial risk of bias or quality assessment at the planning stages, before considering whether to obtain the IPD. However, the collection of IPD does allow a deeper and more reliable appraisal of data quality and risk of bias than is possible with aggregate data, because there is the opportunity to generate information directly from the IPD. There is also the potential to seek additional or updated trial IPD for inclusion in a meta-analysis, in order to reduce or remove the potential for bias in particular domains. For example, participants excluded from original trial analyses may be reinstated in the meta-analysis, or more appropriate statistical methods might be used. Therefore, an overall risk of bias assessment for each trial would be based on whether the design and conduct of the trial, and the quality of its final IPD (after correcting any data errors) are likely to lead to biased results when the IPD are analysed.

While assessing risk of bias in an IPD meta-analysis involves using many of the same domains and items listed in the RoB 2 tool,[91] some items are not relevant, because the IPD circumvents the issue. For example, the availability of IPD avoids reliance on a trial's original analysis methods and reported results. Table 4.4 lists the domains and signalling questions in the RoB 2 tool that are particularly relevant to an IPD meta-analysis project, and summarises how appraisal of the collected IPD, and other information harnessed through an IPD approach, can inform risk of bias judgements. These individual domains represent a useful starting point for assessing the risk of bias associated with each trial in an IPD meta-analysis project.

Ultimately, if the trial design, management or conduct are seriously flawed (e.g. failed randomisation, poor follow-up, or early stopping), this might lead to trials that are wholly or partially unreliable. Depending on the gravity of the issues, a trial may need to be excluded completely from the analyses or be the subject of sensitivity analysis; at the very least, the issues need to be brought to the attention of the reader in the IPD meta-analysis publication. The IPD project's central research team should have a plan in place for how they will deal with these sorts of occurrences. However, the objective of data checking is not to police trials or uncover fraud, and in our experience

Table 4.4 Domains in the Risk of Bias 2 tool[91] (RoB 2) of particular relevance to IPD meta-analysis projects

RoB 2 domains and signalling questions that are relevant to IPD meta-analysis projects	Additional information available from IPD
Domain 1: Randomisation process	
1.1 Was the allocation sequence random? 1.2 Was the allocation sequence concealed until participants were enrolled and assigned to interventions? 1.3 Did baseline differences between intervention groups suggest a problem with the randomisation process?	Assessing the pattern of randomisation using trial IPD may reveal instances where randomisation has failed, or may reassure that the randomisation process appears robust (Section 4.6.1). IPD can also be used to check balance across a full range of covariates (Section 4.6.1). Though formal testing is not recommended, visually, the distribution of each covariate by treatment group can help flag any systematic or unusual differences.
Domain 2: Deviations from the intended interventions (effect of assignment to intervention)	
2.1 Were participants aware of their assigned intervention during the trial? 2.2 Were carers and people delivering the interventions aware of participants' assigned intervention during the trial? 2.3 If Y/PY/NI to 2.1 or 2.2: Were there deviations from the intended intervention that arose because of the trial context? 2.4 If Y/PY to 2.3: Were these deviations likely to have affected the outcome? 2.5 If Y/PY/NI to 2.4: Were these deviations from intended intervention balanced between groups? 2.6 Was an appropriate analysis used to estimate the effect of assignment to intervention? 2.7 If N/PN/NI to 2.6: Was there potential for a substantial impact (on the result) of the failure to analyse participants in the group to which they were randomised?	Having IPD means that participants can be analysed by their allocated intervention, irrespective of how they were analysed in the original trial (Section 4.6.2). Then, provided that patients, those delivering treatments or outcome assessors are not aware of the treatments being given, and the outcomes are objective, this would mean there is no risk of bias in this domain. If the IPD do not enable analysis by the allocated intervention, there may be sufficient detail in the trial dataset to check whether participants who deviated from intended intervention did so for pre-specified or otherwise rational reasons.
Domain 3: Missing outcome data	
3.1 Were data for this outcome available for all, or nearly all, participants randomised? 3.2 If N/PN/NI to 3.1: Is there evidence that the result was not biased by missing outcome data? 3.3 If N/PN to 3.2: Could missingness in the outcome depend on its true value? 3.4 If Y/PY/NI to 3.3: Is it likely that missingness in the outcome depended on its true value?	Access to IPD provides opportunity to request data for participants completely excluded from the IPD dataset, and for any outcomes missing for particular individuals (Section 4.6.3). Also, the IPD obtained can be examined to check for any potential undisclosed exclusions (Section 4.6.3). Where all the relevant IPD are provided, any data that were not analysed in the trial can be reinstated in the meta-analysis, as appropriate. Also, methods for dealing with missing outcome data (e.g. mixed models) can be implemented, even if not undertaken by trial investigators in the original analysis.
Domain 4: Measurement of the outcome	
4.1 Was the method of measuring the outcome inappropriate? 4.2 Could measurement or ascertainment of the outcome have differed between intervention groups?	Access to IPD offers some opportunities to redress situations where inappropriate measurement may have been used. For example, component participant-level data can be used to construct a new composite outcome (Section 4.6.4) and this may also reduce heterogeneity across trials. Even if a range of

(*Continued*)

Table 4.4 (Continued)

RoB 2 domains and signalling questions that are relevant to IPD meta-analysis projects	Additional information available from IPD
4.3 If N/PN/NI to 4.1 and 4.2: Were outcome assessors aware of the intervention received by study participants? 4.4 If Y/PY/NI to 4.3: Could assessment of the outcome have been influenced by knowledge of intervention received? 4.5 If Y/PY/NI to 4.4: Is it likely that assessment of the outcome was influenced by knowledge of intervention received?	instruments have been used in trials, a more appropriate one may be obtained via the IPD.
Domain 5: Selection of the reported result	
5.1 Were the data that produced this result analysed in accordance with a pre-specified analysis plan that was finalized before unblinded outcome data were available for analysis?	As new analyses are carried out according to the IPD meta-analysis project protocol and SAP, this domain is not applicable.

Y: yes, PY: probably yes, N: no, PY: probably no, NI: no information. Note that in RoB 2, Domain 2 has an additional/alternative series of signalling questions for risk of bias arising from deviations from interventions in terms of adhering to interventions. The additional information that may be available from the IPD is similar to those given for the effect of assignment to the intervention in the table. Domain 5 has a sub-list of questions that are not listed, because they are not relevant to IPD meta-analysis projects.
Source: Based on Sterne JAC, Savovic J, Page MJ, et al. RoB 2: a revised tool for assessing risk of bias in randomised trials. *BMJ* 2019;366:l4898

wholesale fabrication of trial data is uncommon. Also, note that this is probably less likely to occur in large, complex or multicentre trials, where collusion between multiple parties would be required. Nevertheless, sometimes trials are encountered where it is suspected that the data have been purposefully manipulated or falsified, so such trials would need to be excluded from the analyses, and the reasons for doing so described in the meta-analysis report.

Details of ways to evaluate the IPD in relation to the relevant RoB 2 domains are provided in the following sections. Findings of risk of bias and data checking can usefully be presented using a modified version of the 'traffic light' table used for standard risk of bias assessments (Section 4.7).

4.6.1 The Randomisation Process

For randomised trials, it is important to check that the methods of sequence generation and allocation concealment appear robust. This will help guard against the inclusion of non-randomised trials, or non-randomised participants, in the IPD meta-analysis project. While a description of the methods can be gleaned from trial documentation and/or trial personnel, interrogating the IPD directly can highlight any unusual allocation patterns that may need further investigation.[7,9,43]

A simple method of checking the pattern of allocation is to look at the cumulative number of participants randomised into each treatment group over time. For example, Figure 4.7 shows the pattern for a trial included in an IPD meta-analysis evaluating the effects of chemoradiation for cervical cancer.[93] There are a similar number of participants allocated to each group throughout, and the curves cross frequently, which is what we would expect in a trial with robust randomisation procedures. It should be noted that for smaller trials, greater separation of curves and less crossing over might be expected, even if they are properly randomised, particularly if a simple method of

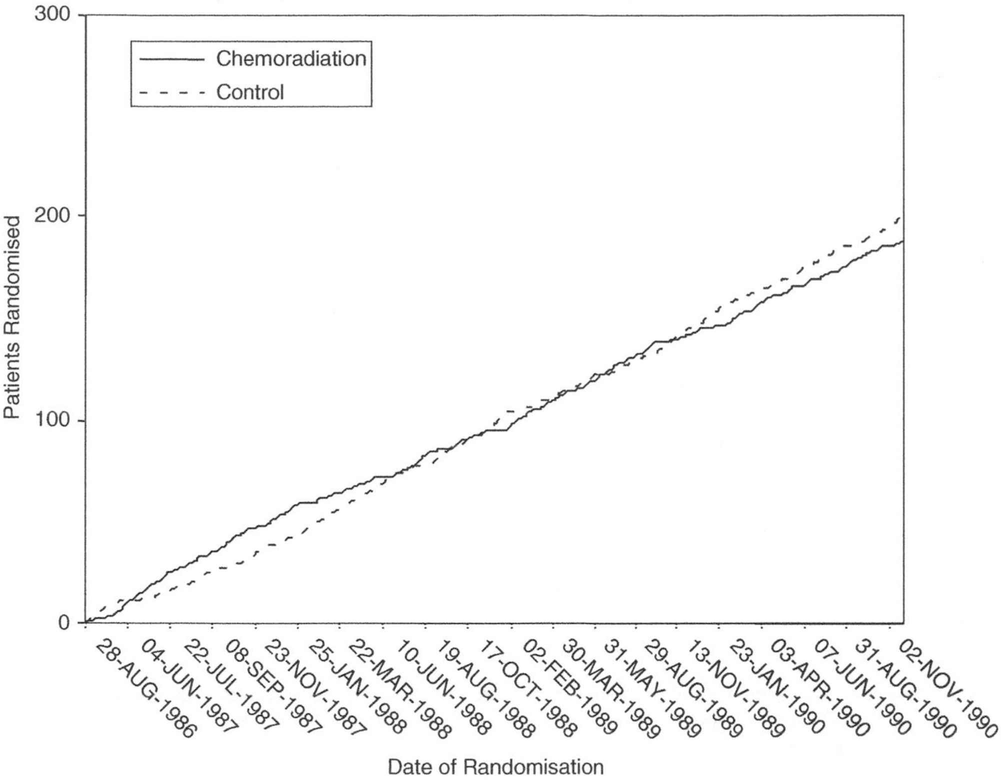

Figure 4.7 The cumulative number of participants randomised to the intervention and control groups in a trial included in an IPD meta-analysis of chemoradiation for cervical cancer.[93] *Source:* Based on Chemoradiotherapy for Cervical Cancer Meta-Analysis Collaboration. Reducing uncertainties about the effects of chemoradiotherapy for cervical cancer: a systematic review and meta-analysis of individual patient data from 18 randomized trials. *Journal of clinical oncology: official journal of the American Society of Clinical Oncology* 2008;26(35):5802–12.

randomisation was used. Also, where the allocation ratio is not 1:1, the curves would not be expected to cross, but rather would be expected to track one another.

A similar pattern is seen in the early stages of a trial included in an IPD meta-analysis of chemotherapy versus radiotherapy for multiple myeloma, but for a short time period all the participants were allocated to the chemotherapy group (Figure 4.8).[7] The trial investigator explained that this was when the radiotherapy machine had broken down, and all participants were given chemotherapy. As this particular cohort of participants were not randomly allocated to treatment, they were excluded from the IPD, thereby still allowing the trial to be included in the IPD meta-analysis.

Figure 4.9 shows another example of how treatment allocation can be plotted, and was used to examine the pattern of assignment in a trial from another IPD meta-analysis project. In this case, all participants except one were allocated to one intervention (arm 1) in the first months of the trial, and participants were allocated to the other intervention (arm 0) mostly in the final months. The trial investigator was unable to explain the pattern, agreed that it was not consistent with randomisation, and that the trial should be excluded from the meta-analysis. As this was a single-centre trial, where treatments were supplied in independently pre-prepared trial packs (with no indication of the treatment they contained), it was speculated that these had not been mixed sufficiently.

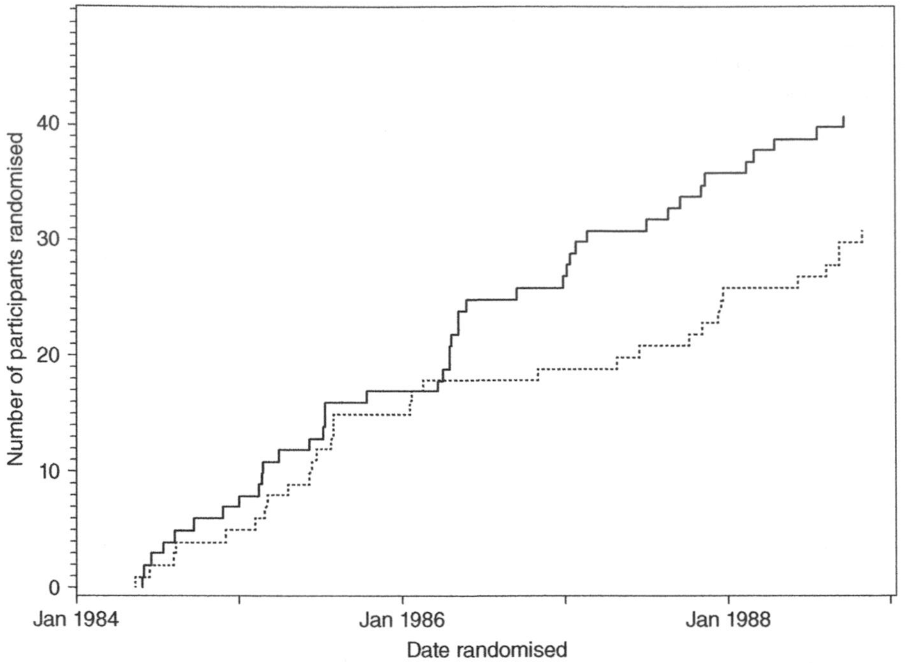

Figure 4.8 The cumulative number of participants allocated to chemotherapy or radiotherapy in a trial included in an IPD meta-analysis of treatments for multiple myeloma. *Source:* Stewart et al.,[7]. © 1995, John Wiley & Sons.

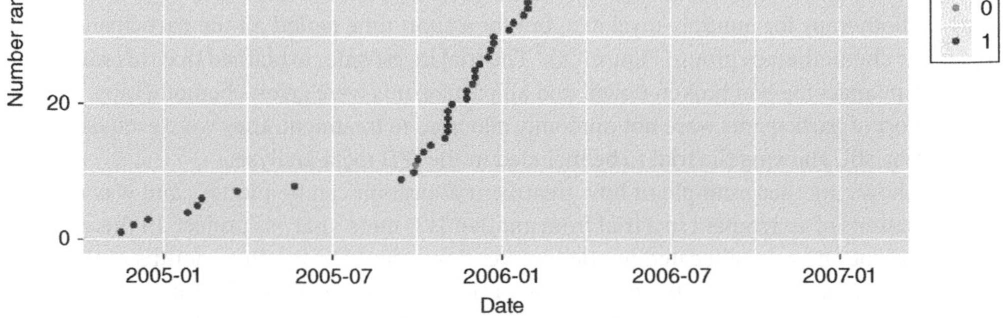

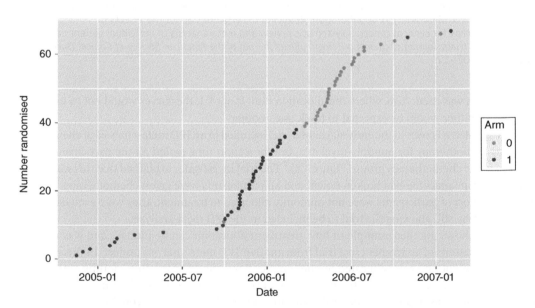

Figure 4.9 Date (shown by year-month) participants were allocated to treatment and control in a trial excluded from an IPD meta-analysis, because participants in one group ('arm 1') were generally recruited earlier than those in the other group ('arm 0'). *Source:* Lesley Stewart.

As statistical software and database packages allow dates to be converted to days of the week, another simple check is to look at the number of participants allocated to the research and control groups on each day of the week.[7,106] This method would highlight, for example, if participants were being allocated to treatment on particular clinic days (pseudo-random allocation) or if participants were being allocated on the weekends, which would be unusual for trials in chronic conditions in many countries. For example, in a trial included in an IPD meta-analysis examining pre-operative chemotherapy for lung cancer,[88] there were no weekend randomisations, and the numbers randomised to each treatment group were well balanced on the weekdays (Figure 4.10(a)). In contrast, for a trial included in an IPD meta-analysis examining post-operative radiotherapy for lung cancer,[107] there appeared to be an unusually high number of weekend randomisations, and large imbalances in the number of participants allocated to each group on each day (Figure 4.10(b)). When this was brought to the attention of the trial investigator, they discovered problems with the management of the trial data, and went back to individual participant records, to ensure that the appropriate information was supplied, and the issues were resolved.

As mentioned in Section 4.4.1, if the dates of randomisation have been redacted from trial IPD for de-identification purposes, it will not be feasible for the central research team to employ these checking procedures, but the trial statistician may be able to run these on their behalf. Moreover, it is still possible to visually check whether baseline characteristics appear reasonably balanced by group, as we would expect with a robust randomisation process. However, balance will never be perfect, and imbalances may be more pronounced in small trials or those with simple (i.e. non-stratified) randomisation methods; indeed we might be concerned if everything appeared too perfectly balanced. Note that we do not advocate statistical tests of baseline balance.[108]

4.6.2 Deviations from the Intended Interventions

While robust randomisation procedures should ensure the unbiased assignment to, and comparison of, participants between treatment groups, this can only be guaranteed if all participants are analysed according to the treatments initially assigned: an intention-to-treat approach.[109–111] Even if a trial has not been analysed appropriately, as long as the IPD have been provided with the original treatment allocation recorded, then participants can be grouped according to this treatment allocation, rather than the treatment they received, enabling an intention-to-treat analysis of effectiveness.[109–111] However, there may be value in conducting certain analyses based on a subset of participants randomised, such as an analysis of toxicity in just those who received most of their allocated treatment, or sensitivity analyses according to treatment received, to explain differences between published trial results and those used in the meta-analysis.

There may be sufficient detail in the trial dataset to check whether participants who deviated from intended interventions did so for pre-specified or otherwise rational reasons. For example, if the data indicate that a participant had experienced an adverse event, this might explain why treatment was stopped early, and would also need to be considered in any analysis of adverse outcomes. It may also be possible to assess whether deviations from planned treatment are similar, and for comparable reasons across treatment groups (more so than with aggregate data).

If a treatment is a major procedure, such as surgery, or particularly toxic, then those delivering treatments and participants will usually be aware of the assigned treatment. Provided that outcomes are objectively measured or 'hard', such as mortality, this is unlikely to introduce bias. However, a carer might inadvertently or otherwise deliver a treatment or measure a more subjective outcome, such as an adverse effect, differently if they are aware of which treatment a participant received. Similarly, if a participant is aware of their assigned treatment, it might influence a patient-reported

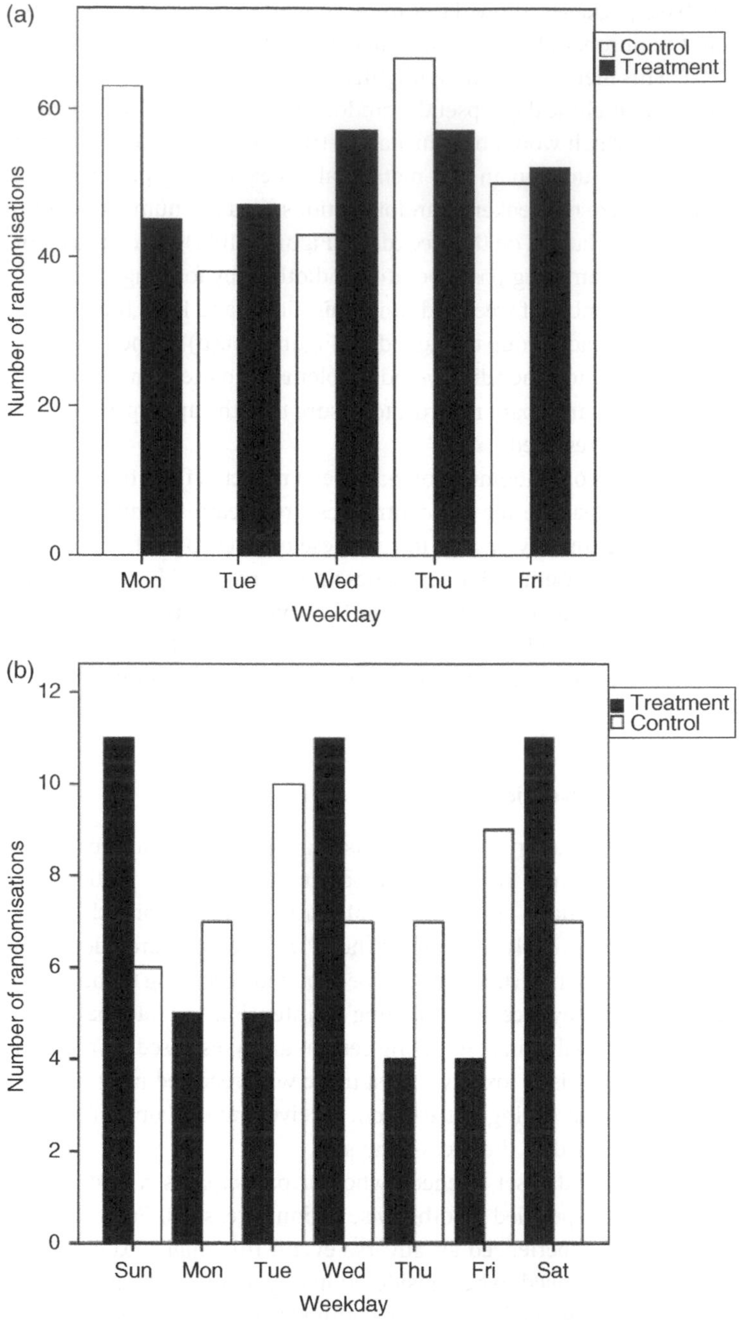

Figure 4.10 Days of the week participants were allocated to treatment and control groups in a trial included in (a) an IPD meta-analysis of pre-operative chemotherapy for non-small cell lung cancer,[88] and (b) an IPD meta-analysis of post-operative radiotherapy for non-small cell lung cancer.[107] *Source:* (a) Based on NSCLC Meta-Analysis Collaborative Group. Preoperative chemotherapy for non-small cell lung cancer: a systematic review and meta-analysis of individual participant data. *Lancet* 2014;383:1561–71. (b) Based on PORT Meta-analysis Trialists Group. Postoperative radiotherapy in non-small-cell lung cancer: systematic review and meta-analysis of individual patient data from nine randomised controlled trials. *The Lancet* 1998;352(9124):257–63.

outcome, such as pain or quality of life. Therefore, in this scenario, there is a potential for bias in this domain, which cannot be alleviated by the collection of IPD. However, the contact with trial teams, that is intrinsic to collaborative IPD meta-analyses, can provide useful clarification of the methods used to blind participants, carers or outcome assessors, to help determine whether these are appropriate, and therefore allow the risk of bias to be judged with more accuracy.

4.6.3 Missing Outcome Data

If participants drop out or are actively excluded from the analysis of a trial in substantial numbers and/or disproportionately by group, this could lead to quite considerable imbalances between intervention and control groups. More importantly, it could lead to incomplete outcome data and potentially attrition bias. For example, an examination of 14 cancer IPD meta-analyses, incorporating 133 trials, found that between 0% and 38% of randomised participants were excluded from the original trial survival analyses, with the largest proportion often being excluded from the treatment groups (Figure 4.11). In one of these projects examining the effects of chemotherapy for soft tissue sarcoma,[112] the evidence for a benefit of chemotherapy on survival was stronger when it was based just on participants included in the original trial analyses (hazard ratio = 0.85; 95% CI: 0.72 to 1.00, $p = 0.06$), compared to when all possible participants were included (hazard ratio = 0.90, 95% CI: 0.77 to 1.04, $p = 0.16$).

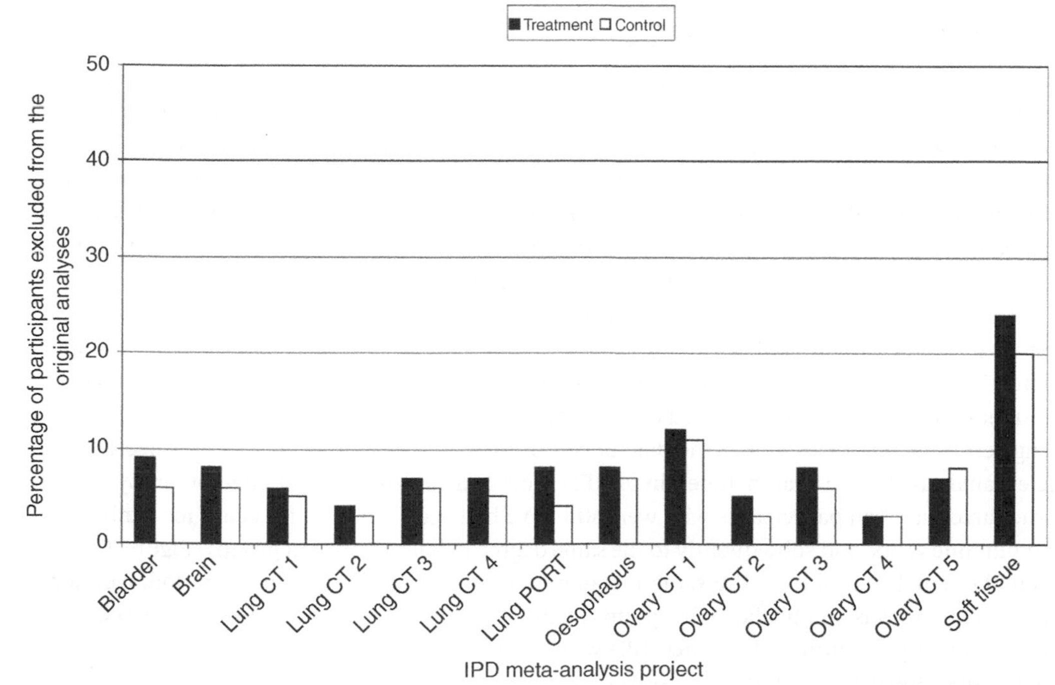

Figure 4.11 Percentage of participants excluded from the original analyses of trials included in 14 IPD meta-analysis projects in the cancer field.[112] *Source:* Jayne Tierney, reproduced with permission from Tierney and Stewart.[112]

Therefore, it is important to check that data on all, or as many as possible, participants recruited to a trial are included in an IPD meta-analysis (assuming that all the individuals meet the IPD meta-analysis inclusion criteria for population and setting). If good records are maintained for a trial, it is possible to recover data on participants who were excluded from the original trial analyses, as part of the IPD collection process, and incorporate them into the meta-analysis. For example, in the same 14 cancer meta-analyses described previously, when IPD were collected, approximately 1,800 participants who had been excluded from the original trial analyses were re-instated, and without them most meta-analysis results would have been biased towards the research intervention, albeit to a small degree in most cases.[112]

A major advantage of IPD meta-analysis is the ability to include all outcomes of relevance to the meta-analysis, irrespective of whether they have been published or not, thereby overcoming the potential biases associated with differential reporting of outcomes,[113] and providing a more balanced view of benefits and harms. For example, in a systematic review of laparoscopic versus open surgery for the repair of inguinal hernia, based on the available published aggregate data from three trials, the risk of persistent pain was found to be significantly greater with laparoscopic repair (odds ratio = 2·03, 95% CI: 1·03 to 4·01).[114] However, when IPD were collected, data were available for a further 17 trials that had not published results for this outcome, and the combined meta-analysis results showed that the risk of persistent pain was actually *lower* with laparoscopic repair (odds ratio = 0·54, 95% CI: 0·46 to 0·64). Recognising that some outcomes measured in trials may not be reported, it is always worth checking trial protocols, registry entries and with trial investigators to firmly establish which outcomes can be made available when IPD are provided.[115]

4.6.4 Measurement of the Outcome

Direct access to IPD does not usually allow the assessment of whether the measurement or ascertainment of outcomes differed between intervention groups. However, contact with trial investigators can provide useful clarification of the methods used, to help determine whether these are appropriate, and therefore allow the risk of bias associated with, for example, differential outcome assessments to be judged with more certainty. If the IPD are sufficiently detailed, outcomes may be defined more appropriately or consistently across trials. For example, a new standardised composite outcome might be constructed from a series of component variables.

For time-to-event outcomes, such as survival or time to relief of symptoms, bias can occur if certain participants are followed-up for a longer duration than others, such that event rates appear higher. Therefore, for these outcomes, it is also desirable to check that follow-up is balanced by treatment group. This can be achieved by selecting those trial participants who are event-free, then using censoring as the event and the date of censoring as the time-to-event in a 'reverse Kaplan-Meier' analysis. In one trial included in an IPD meta-analysis of adjuvant chemotherapy for soft tissue sarcoma,[102] all participants who were still alive had been followed for death for a minimum of about nine years, and subsequently to the same degree in both treatment groups (Figure 4.12(a)). In another smaller trial from the same meta-analysis, although participants were followed for a long time, there was an imbalance by group (Figure 4.12(b)), which became less of an issue when the trial investigator provided updated IPD with extended follow-up (Figure 4.12(c)).

Trials that stop early can produce results that are overly in favour of treatment or control,[117] and therefore introduce bias into a subsequent meta-analysis. For those based on time-to-event outcomes, obtaining IPD with updated follow-up can go some way to addressing this issue. For example, in an IPD meta-analysis examining adjuvant chemotherapy for locally advanced bladder

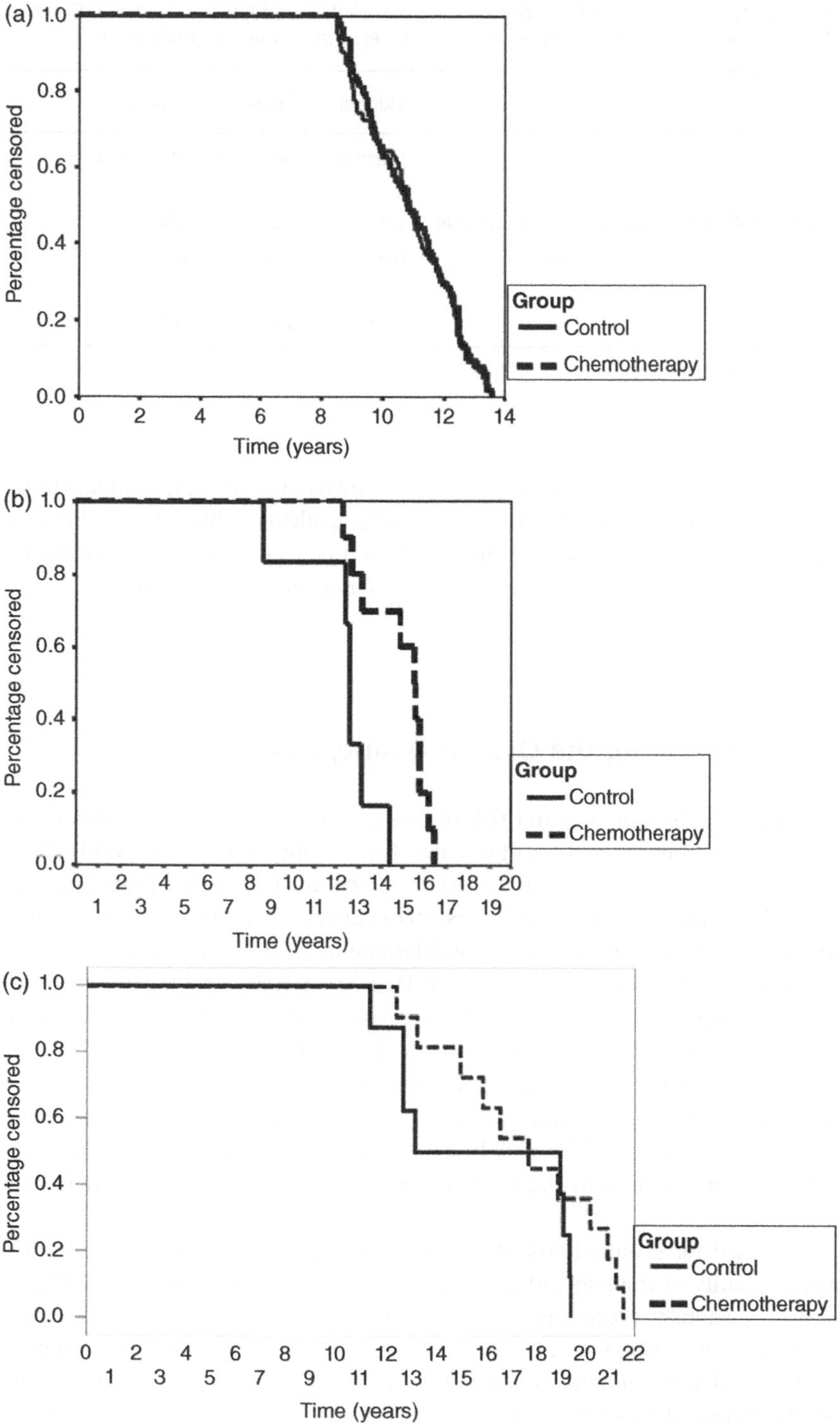

Figure 4.12 'Reverse' Kaplan-Meier analysis of participants who are event-free for (a) a trial with balanced follow-up, and (b) a trial with imbalanced follow-up that was (c) subsequently updated with longer follow-up when IPD were collected. Each was included in an IPD meta-analysis of adjuvant chemotherapy for soft tissue sarcoma.[102] *Source*: Sarcoma Meta-Analysis Collaboration. Adjuvant chemotherapy for localised resectable soft-tissue sarcoma of adults: meta-analysis of individual data. *Lancet* 1997;350(9092):1647–54.

Table 4.5 Alleviating potential bias in trials that stopped early for perceived benefit (included in an IPD meta-analysis of adjuvant chemotherapy for locally advanced bladder cancer) through updated follow-up

Trial	Skinner	Studer	Stockle
Outcome analysed	Survival	Survival	Disease-free survival
% participants with updated follow-up since published analysis	100	22	100
Hazard ratio estimated from published statistics or Kaplan-Meier curves	0.65	0.86	0.39
Hazard ratio derived from IPD	0.75	1.02	0.45

Source: Jayne Tierney, adapted with permission.[118]

cancer, three of the included trials were stopped early, because they had interim results in favour of adjuvant treatment. However, the IPD meta-analysis project helped alleviate this potential bias, as it included IPD with updated follow-up for the three trials, which produced results that were less in favour of adjuvant treatment (Table 4.5).[118] IPD also allows non-proportional hazards (non-constant hazard ratios) to be examined (see Chapter 5).

4.7 Assessing and Presenting the Overall Quality of a Trial

The results of validity checking (Section 4.5) and risk of bias assessment (Section 4.6) should be considered together in order to build up an overall picture of the quality of each trial's IPD. This should include reflections on the quality of the trial design and conduct (from the ROB 2 assessment), checks of IPD obtained, and any unresolved errors or concerns therein. If it is concluded that the IPD from a particular trial is likely to introduce considerable bias into an IPD meta-analysis, then it is may be sensible to exclude it. For example, in an IPD meta-analysis of post-operative therapy for non-small-cell lung cancer,[107] a trial was excluded because it 'failed' the data checks,[101] and it is certainly worth highlighting any such exclusions in the relevant meta-analysis publication. However, such situations need to be handled sensitively with trial investigators, who will have invested time and effort in supplying the data, and may have been unaware that issues would emerge. Alternatively, the impact of risk of bias may be explored through sensitivity analysis, such as examining how meta-analysis conclusions change according to whether or not trials have risk of bias concerns (Chapter 9).

The 'traffic light' table used for standard risk of bias assessment can be usefully adapted for summarising the overall quality of trials included in an IPD meta-analysis. This would include all the domains described previously, except the "selection of the reported results" domain, which is not applicable to IPD projects (Section 4.6), because the trial IPD are re-analysed according to the meta-analysis protocol and SAP. Adopting this structure means that the information is readily comparable with a standard risk of bias table, but can easily be extended to incorporate columns for additional project-specific IPD checks that are deemed particularly important. For example, it is useful to include an additional column to indicate whether there were any residual concerns

Table 4.6 Excerpt of a RoB2 table for an IPD meta-analysis of adjuvant chemotherapy for locally advanced bladder cancer based on a single trial and the main outcome of overall survival (Tierney et al., in preparation).

Risk of Bias Domain	1) Randomisation process	2) Deviations from the intended interventions	3) Missing outcome data	4) Measurement of the outcome	5) Overall risk of bias judgement
Trial EORTC 30994					
	LOW RISK ***Was allocation sequence random?*** YES: Minimisation, stratified by institution, pathological T stage and lymph node status. Also, IPD checks show that the pattern of allocation is steady by treatment group and over time; there were no obvious imbalances by group on any day of the week; and there were few weekend randomisations. ***Was allocation sequence concealed?*** YES: Randomisation was done centrally at the EORTC headquarters. ***Did baseline differences suggest a problem?*** NO: IPD checks show no obvious imbalance by treatment group in baseline characteristics.	LOW RISK ***Were participants aware of their assigned intervention during the trial?*** YES: Blinding not possible in a chemotherapy versus none trial, but awareness cannot affect survival outcome. ***Were carers and people delivering the interventions aware of participants' assigned intervention during the trial?*** YES: Blinding not possible in a chemotherapy versus none trial, but awareness is unlikely to affect how these treatments were given. ***Were there deviations from the intended intervention that arose because of the trial context?*** NO: There were no deviations from because of the context. ***Was an appropriate analysis used to estimate the effect of assignment to intervention?***YES: An intention-to-treat analysis of all randomised patients was derived from the IPD.	LOW RISK ***Were data available for all, or nearly all, participants randomised?*** YES: Data were provided for all patients randomised.	LOW RISK ***Was method of measuring the outcome inappropriate?*** NO: Overall survival was derived from the IPD according to the meta-analysis protocol and SAP. ***Could measurement of the outcome have differed between intervention groups?*** NO: Checks of the IPD revealed that follow-up of participants was balanced by treatment group. ***Outcome assessor aware of intervention received?*** YES: This cannot affect the overall survival outcome.	LOW RISK

Source: Sarah Burdett and Jayne Tierney.

about data quality once the data checking and correction procedures had been completed, and which might impact on the trustworthiness of a trial. Often these risk of bias 'traffic light' tables will be almost completely green (low risk of bias), as any trials that fail data checking or have serious bias issues would likely be excluded from the IPD meta-analysis project completely. Note that assessments should be based on the fullest information possible, thereby considering the trial design and conduct based on all trial documentation and contact with investigators, plus the results of checks of the IPD. A more detailed risk of bias table might be included in an appendix to provide fuller information on this data checking process (Table 4.6), and show how individual judgements have been arrived at. It also provides an opportunity to flag less serious or unclear bias issues.

4.8 Verification of Finalised Trial IPD

Once a trial's IPD has been processed, checked and all issues resolved as far as possible, it is useful to give trial investigators a final opportunity to verify their data prior to it being used in any meta-analysis. This is most easily achieved by sending a descriptive summary of the finalised data for each trial, any amendments made to the original data provided, and results of the primary analyses (Figure 4.13 gives an example), but offering the option to supply a copy of the full checked IPD, if required. Such a document may be useful if investigators raise queries about differences between trial data presented in the original trial publication and in the IPD meta-analysis.

4.9 Merging IPD Ready for Meta-Analysis

After verification, the finalised dataset for each trial is ready to be used within subsequent IPD meta-analyses. At this stage, it is helpful to merge the final IPD from all trials into a single dataset. Although statistical methods for IPD meta-analysis can still be applied if trial datasets are located locally in different files, a single dataset that houses all the IPD is more convenient and potentially makes analyses faster. For example, Box 1.1 (Chapter 1) shows an example dataset containing IPD from 10 trials after data checking, harmonisation, verification and merging. Most statistical packages, such as Stata, SAS and R, have built-in commands for merging datasets from different files, and these generally require the datasets to share common variable names, which will have been achieved at the data harmonisation stage (Section 4.5.3). Not all variables in every trial dataset need to be merged, and the statistician can restrict the variables to just those to be used in particular statistical analyses. It is important to check that no errors are introduced when merging the datasets. Therefore, it is sensible to calculate summary statistics (e.g. number of participants in each group, mean age, proportion of women, overall treatment effect) for each trial before (in the pre-merge dataset) and after (in the merged dataset), to ensure they agree exactly. A single dataset comprising IPD from all trials will not be achievable if the IPD for some can only be accessed remotely, but the central research team can still proceed with a two-stage meta-analysis as described in Chapter 5.

Summary of data held for trial [Trial name or number]

(1) Contact and publication details
Main trial contact: [*Name*]
Author representing trial: [*Name*]

Main trial publication (this is the paper that will be cited in the final IPD report):
[*Citation*]

(2) Documentation held for trial

Available	Yes	No
Protocol		
Ethics approval documentation		
Data sharing agreement		
....		

(3) Trial characteristics
to be used in analysis of potential trial-level effect modifiers

Intended dose of active drug:
Geographical location:

(4) Baseline participant characteristics calculated from 'finalised' IPD

Example characteristics	Baseline characteristics as determined from the IPD		Baseline characteristics as reported in main publication	
	Intervention	Control	Intervention	Control
Number randomised				
Age (Mean)				
Smoking (*n*)				
Chronic Hypertension (*n*)				
.....				

Baseline characteristics not collected/available in the individual-level dataset:

- Chronic diabetes
- Ethnicity
- ....

(5) Individual trial outcomes as calculated from the finalised IPD
The table below show the data as they are coded/re-coded in the IPD meta-analysis format and reflect any changes made to data agreed in response to data checking.

Outcomes	Treatment Events/N	Control Events/N	Estimate*	95% CI
Delivery < 34 weeks			RR	
Pregnancy duration (time to birth)	-	-	HR	
Neonatal death			RR	
....				

** Note any important differences between the meta-analusis project calclations and the trial publication and whether these have been confirmed with the trial investigator. For example, in trials of twin pregnancies whether preterm birth is treated as a maternal outcome (1 event) or as a baby outcome (2 events).

(6) Variables (covariates and outcomes) with over 20% missing data.
This may influence if trials are used in certain analyses.

	Percentage of missing data	
Variable	Treatment X (n)	Control (n)
Maternal BMI		
Birthweight		

(7) Risk of bias assessment
Five domains including selection bias, performance bias, detection bias, attrition bias and availability biad were rated as low, unclear or high risk of bias.

Selection bias	Performance bias	Detection bias	Attrition bias	Availability bias
Low	Low	Low	Low	Low

Footnotes can be used to explain risk of bias domains or to provide a citation to an explanatory publication

Figure 4.13 Example of items to include in summary of finalised trial IPD for verification by a trial investigator. *Source:* Ruth Walker and Lesley Stewart.

4.10 Concluding Remarks

There is no doubt that development of the project protocol, managing a large-scale collaboration and carefully collecting, processing and checking data is a lengthy and resource-intensive phase of an IPD meta-analysis project. However, these aspects are key to ensuring that the approach is scientifically rigorous and truly collaborative, and that the privacy of the participants in the included trials is maintained. Importantly, it also ensures that the collated IPD is as accurate, up to date, reliable and comprehensive as it can be, and that it is well understood by the central research team. In all, this provides a necessary solid foundation for the statistical analysis part of the IPD project that follows.

Part I References

1 Higgins JPT, Thomas J, Chandler J, et al., *editors. Cochrane Handbook for Systematic Reviews of Interventions (2nd edition).* Chichester, UK: Wiley 2019.

2 Leeflang MM, Deeks JJ, Takwoingi Y, et al. Cochrane diagnostic test accuracy reviews. *Syst Rev* 2013;2:82.

3 Riley RD, Moons KGM, Snell KIE, et al. A guide to systematic review and meta-analysis of prognostic factor studies. *BMJ* 2019;364:k4597.

4 Debray TP, Damen JA, Snell KI, et al. A guide to systematic review and meta-analysis of prediction model performance. *BMJ* 2017;356:i6460.

5 Glass GV. Primary, secondary, and meta-analysis of research. *Educ Res* 1976;5(10):3–8.

6 Riley RD, Lambert PC, Abo-Zaid G. Meta-analysis of individual participant data: rationale, conduct, and reporting. *BMJ* 2010;340:c221.

7 Stewart LA, Clarke MJ. Practical methodology of meta-analyses (overviews) using updated individual patient data. *Cochrane Working Group. Stat Med* 1995;14(19):2057–2079.

8 Stewart LA, Parmar MK. Meta-analysis of the literature or of individual patient data: is there a difference? *Lancet* 1993;341.

9 Tierney JF, Vale C, Riley R, et al. Individual participant data (IPD) meta-analyses of randomised controlled trials: guidance on their use. *PLoS Med* 2015;12(7):e1001855.

10 Loder E. Data sharing: making good on promises. *BMJ* 2018;360:k710.

11 Advanced Ovarian Cancer Trialists Group. Chemotherapy in advanced ovarian cancer: an overview of randomised clinical trials. *BMJ* 1991;303(6807):884–893.

12 Non-small Cell Lung Cancer Collaborative Group. Chemotherapy in non-small cell lung cancer: a meta-analysis using updated data on individual patients from 52 randomised clinical trials. *BMJ* 1995;311(7010):899–909.

13 Clarke M, Stewart L, Pignon JP, et al. Individual patient data meta-analysis in cancer. *Br J Cancer* 1998;77(11):2036–2044.

14 Oxman AD, Clarke MJ, Stewart LA. From science to practice. Meta-analyses using individual patient data are needed. *JAMA* 1995;274(10):845–846.

15 Early Breast Cancer Trialists' Collaborative Group. Tamoxifen for early breast cancer: an overview of the randomised trials. *Lancet* 1998 351:1451–1467.

16 O'Rourke K. An historical perspective on meta-analysis: dealing quantitatively with varying study results. *J R Soc Med* 2007;100(12):579–582.

17 Green AK, Reeder-Hayes KE, Corty RW, et al. The project data sphere initiative: accelerating cancer research by sharing data. *The Oncologist* 2015;20(5):464–e20.

18 Glasziou P, Altman DG, Bossuyt P, et al. Reducing waste from incomplete or unusable reports of biomedical research. *Lancet* 2014;383(9913):267–276.

Individual Participant Data Meta-Analysis: A Handbook for Healthcare Research, First Edition.
Edited by Richard D. Riley, Jayne F. Tierney, and Lesley A. Stewart.

19 Ross JS, Krumholz HM. Ushering in a new era of open science through data sharing: the wall must come down. *JAMA* 2013;309(13):1355–1356.

20 Krumholz HM, Ross JS, Gross CP, et al. A historic moment for open science: the Yale University Open Data Access project and medtronic. *Ann Intern Med* 2013;158(12):910–911.

21 Krumholz HM. Open science and data sharing in clinical research: basing informed decisions on the totality of the evidence. *Circ Cardiovasc Qual Outcomes* 2012;5(2):141–142.

22 Krumholz HM. Why data sharing should be the expected norm. *BMJ* 2015;350:h599.

23 Loder E, Groves T. The BMJ requires data sharing on request for all trials. *BMJ* 2015;350:h2373.

24 Taichman DB, Backus J, Baethge C, et al. Sharing clinical trial data: a proposal from the International Committee of Medical Journal Editors. *Chin Med J (Engl)* 2016;129(2):127–128.

25 Hingorani AD, Windt DA, Riley RD, et al. Prognosis research strategy (PROGRESS) 4: stratified medicine research. *BMJ* 2013;346:e5793.

26 Morere JF. Oncology in 2012: from personalized medicine to precision medicine. *Target Oncol* 2012;7(4):211–212.

27 Krumholz HM, Waldstreicher J. The Yale Open Data Access (YODA) Project – a mechanism for data sharing. *N Engl J Med* 2016;375(5):403–405.

28 Kalter J, Sweegers MG, Verdonck-de Leeuw IM, et al. Development and use of a flexible data harmonization platform to facilitate the harmonization of individual patient data for meta-analyses. *BMC Research Notes* 2019;12(1):164.

29 Ross JS, Waldstreicher J, Bamford S, et al. Overview and experience of the YODA Project with clinical trial data sharing after 5 years. *Sci Data* 2018;5:180268.

30 Hee SW, Dritsaki M, Willis A, et al. Development of a repository of individual participant data from randomized controlled trials of therapists delivered interventions for low back pain. *Eur J Pain* 2017;21(5):815–826.

31 van Middelkoop M, Arden NK, Atchia I, et al. The OA Trial Bank: meta-analysis of individual patient data from knee and hip osteoarthritis trials show that patients with severe pain exhibit greater benefit from intra-articular glucocorticoids. *Osteoarthr Cartil* 2016;24(7):1143–1152.

32 Riley RD, van der Windt D, Croft P, et al., *editors. Prognosis Research in Healthcare: Concepts, Methods and Impact.* Oxford, UK: Oxford University Press 2019.

33 Riley RD, Debray TPA, Fisher D, et al. Individual participant data meta-analysis to examine interactions between treatment effect and participant-level covariates: statistical recommendations for conduct and planning. *Stat Med* 2020;39(15):2115–2137.

34 Egger M, Davey Smith G, Altman DG. *Systematic Reviews in Health Care: Meta-analysis in Context.* London: BMJ Publishing Group 2001.

35 Whitehead A. *Meta-analysis of Controlled Clinical Trials.* West Sussex, UK: Wiley 2002.

36 Cooper H, Hedges LV, Valentine JC, *editors. The Handbook of Research Synthesis and Meta-Analysis (3rd edition).* New York: Russell Sage Foundation 2019.

37 Schmid CH, Stijnen T, *White IR, editors.* Handbook of Meta-Analysis. New York: Chapman and Hall/CRC 2020.

38 Brown H, Prescott R. *Applied Mixed Models in Medicine (3rd edition).* Chichester, UK: Wiley 2015.

39 Altman DG. *Practical Statistics for Medical Research.* London, UK: Chapman and Hall 1991.

40 Montgomery DC, Peck EA, Vining GG. *Introduction to Linear Regression Analysis (3rd edition).* New York: Wiley 2001.

41 Harrell FE, Jr. *Regression Modeling Strategies: With Applications to Linear Models, Logistic and Ordinal Regression, and Survival Analysis (2nd edition).* New York: Springer 2015.

42 O'Connor D, Green S, Higgins JPT. Defining the review question and developing criteria for including studies. In: Higgins JPT, Green S, eds. *Cochrane Handbook for Systematic Reviews of Interventions*. Chichester, UK: Wiley 2008:81–94.

43 Stewart LA, Tierney JF. To IPD or not to IPD? Advantages and disadvantages of systematic reviews using individual patient data. *Eval Health Prof* 2002;25(1):76–97.

44 Tierney JF, Stewart LA, Clarke M. Individual participant data. In: Higgins JPT, Chandler TJ, Cumpston M, et al., eds. *Cochrane Handbook for Systematic Reviews of Interventions*. London, UK: Cochrane 2019.

45 Rydzewska LHM, Stewart LA, Tierney JF. Clinical data repositories through a systematic reviewer lens. 2021 (submitted).

46 Stewart L, Tierney J, Burdett S. Do systematic reviews based on individual patient data offer a means of circumventing biases associated with trial publications? In: Rothstein H, Sutton A, Borenstein M, eds. *Publication Bias in Meta-Analysis: Prevention, Assessment and Adjustments*. Chichester: Wiley 2005:261–286.

47 Tierney JF, Fisher DJ, Burdett S, et al. Comparison of aggregate and individual participant data approaches to meta-analysis of randomised trials: an observational study. *PLoS Med* 2020;17(1): e1003019.

48 Vale CL, Tierney JF, Burdett S. Can trial quality be reliably assessed from published reports of cancer trials: evaluation of risk of bias assessments in systematic reviews. *BMJ* 2013;346:f1798.

49 Ensor J, Burke DL, Snell KIE, et al. Simulation-based power calculations for planning a two-stage individual participant data meta-analysis. *BMC Med Res Methodol* 2018;18(1):41.

50 Simmonds MC. Statistical methodology for individual patient data meta-analysis. PhD Thesis, University of Cambridge 2006.

51 Burke DL, Ensor J, Riley RD. Meta-analysis using individual participant data: one-stage and two-stage approaches, and why they may differ. *Stat Med* 2017;36(5):855–875.

52 Fisher DJ, Carpenter JR, Morris TP, et al. Meta-analytical methods to identify who benefits most from treatments: daft, deluded, or deft approach? *BMJ* 2017;356:j573.

53 Higgins JP, Whitehead A, Turner RM, et al. Meta-analysis of continuous outcome data from individual patients. *Stat Med* 2001;20(15):2219–2241.

54 Whitehead A, Omar RZ, Higgins JP, et al. Meta-analysis of ordinal outcomes using individual patient data. *Stat Med* 2001;20(15):2243–2260.

55 Tudur-Smith C, Williamson PR, Marson AG. Investigating heterogeneity in an individual patient data meta-analysis of time to event outcomes. *Stat Med* 2005;24(9):1307–1319.

56 Debray TP, Moons KG, van Valkenhoef G, et al. Get real in individual participant data (IPD) meta-analysis: a review of the methodology. *Res Synth Methods* 2015;6(4):293–309.

57 Morris TP, Fisher DJ, Kenward MG, et al. Meta-analysis of Gaussian individual patient data: two-stage or not two-stage? *Stat Med* 2018;37(9):1419–1438.

58 Ahmed I, Sutton AJ, Riley RD. Assessment of publication bias, selection bias and unavailable data in meta-analyses using individual participant data: a database survey. *BMJ* 2012;344:d7762.

59 Riley RD, Lambert PC, Staessen JA, et al. Meta-analysis of continuous outcomes combining individual patient data and aggregate data. *Stat Med* 2008;27(11):1870–1893.

60 Stewart LA, Clarke M, Rovers M, et al. Preferred reporting items for systematic review and meta-analyses of individual participant data: the PRISMA-IPD Statement. *JAMA* 2015;313(16):1657–1665.

61 Fisher DJ. Two-stage individual participant data meta-analysis and generalized forest plots. *Stata J* 2015;15(2):369–396.

62 Clarke M, Godwin J. Systematic reviews using individual patient data: a map for the minefields? *Ann Oncol* 1998;9(8):827–833.

63 Tudur Smith C, Marcucci M, Nolan SJ, et al. Individual participant data meta-analyses compared with meta-analyses based on aggregate data. *Cochrane Database Syst Rev* 2016;9:MR000007.

64 Tudur Smith C, Clarke M, Marson T, et al. A framework for deciding if individual participant data are likely to be worthwhile. *Cochrane Database Syst Rev* 2015;10(Supplement (Abstracts from the 23rd Cochrane Colloquium)):RO 6.1, 26.

65 Simmonds MC, Brown JV, Heirs MK, et al. Safety and effectiveness of recombinant human bone morphogenetic protein-2 for spinal fusion: a meta-analysis of individual-participant data. *Ann Intern Med* 2013;158(12):877–889.

66 Tierney JF, Fisher DJ, Vale CL, et al. A framework for prospective, adaptive meta-analysis (FAME) of aggregate data from randomised trials. *PLoS Med* in press.

67 Thomas J, Askie LM, Berlin JA, et al. Chapter 22: Prospective approaches to accumulating evidence. In: Higgins JPT, Thomas J, Chandler J, et al., eds. *Cochrane Handbook for Systematic Reviews of Interventions*. Cochrane Version 61 (updated September 2020). Available from www.training.cochrane.org/handbook2020. Cochrane 2020.

68 Siemieniuk RA, Bartoszko JJ, Ge L, et al. Drug treatments for covid-19: living systematic review and network meta-analysis. *BMJ* 2020;370:m2980.

69 Pogue JM, Yusuf S. Cumulating evidence from randomized trials: utilizing sequential monitoring boundaries for cumulative meta-analysis. *Control Clin Trials* 1997;18(6):580–593; discussion 661–666.

70 Simmonds MC, Higgins JP. Covariate heterogeneity in meta-analysis: criteria for deciding between meta-regression and individual patient data. *Stat Med* 2007;26(15):2982–2999.

71 Burke DL, Billingham LJ, Girling AJ, et al. Meta-analysis of randomized phase II trials to inform subsequent phase III decisions. *Trials* 2014;15:346.

72 Sutton AJ, Cooper NJ, Jones DR, et al. Evidence-based sample size calculations based upon updated meta-analysis. *Stat Med* 2007;26(12):2479–2500.

73 IOM (Institute of Medicine). 2011. *Finding What Works in Health Care: Standards for Systematic Reviews*. Washington, DC: The National Academies Press.

74 Nevitt SJ, Marson AG, Davie B, et al. Exploring changes over time and characteristics associated with data retrieval across individual participant data meta-analyses: systematic review. *BMJ* 2017;357:j1390.

75 Veroniki AA, Ashoor HM, Le SPC, et al. Retrieval of individual patient data depended on study characteristics: a randomized controlled trial. *J Clin Epidemiol* 2019;113:176–188.

76 Renfro LA, Shi Q, Sargent DJ. Mining the ACCENT database: a review and update. *Chinese Clin Oncol* 2013;2(2):18.

77 Wilson RC, Butters OW, Avraam D, et al. DataSHIELD – New directions and dimensions. *Data Sci J* 2017;16:21.

78 Rodgers M, Marshall D, Simmonds M, et al. Intensive behavioural interventions based on applied behaviour analysis for young autistic children: a systematic review and cost-effectiveness analysis. *Health Technol Assess* 2020;24(35):1.

79 The EPPPIC Group. Evaluating progestogens for prevention of preterm birth international collaborative (EPPPIC) individual participant data (IPD): meta-analysis of individual participant data from randomised controlled trials. Lancet (in press).

80 Mental Health Research Network and INVOLVE. Budgeting for involvement: Practical advice on budgeting for actively involving the public in research studies. London, UK: Mental Health Research Network, and Eastleigh, UK: INVOLVE 2013

81 Obtaining funding for IPD meta-analyses: Top tips for a successful application. 19th Cochrane Colloquium. Madrid, Spain: Wiley-Blackwell 2011.

82 NCRI, National Cancer Intelligence Network, onCore UK. Summary of responses to consultation on 'Access to Samples and Data for Cancer Research' (available at http://www.ncri.org.uk/wp-content/uploads/2013/09/Initiatives-Biobanking-2-responses.pdf). 2009.

83 Kalkman S, van Delden J, Banerjee A, et al. Patients' and public views and attitudes towards the sharing of health data for research: a narrative review of the empirical evidence. *J Med Eth* 2019.

84 Phillips RS, Sung L, Ammann RA, et al. Predicting microbiologically defined infection in febrile neutropenic episodes in children: global individual participant data multivariable meta-analysis. *Br J Cancer* 2016;114(6):623–630.

85 Phillips B, Ranasinghe N, Stewart LA. Ethical and regulatory considerations in the use of individual participant data for studies of disease prediction. *Arch Dis Childh* 2013;98(7):567–568.

86 Seidler AL, Hunter KE, Cheyne S, et al. A guide to prospective meta-analysis. *BMJ* 2019;367:l5342.

87 Askie LM, Darlow BA, Finer N, et al. Association between oxygen saturation targeting and death or disability in extremely preterm infants in the Neonatal Oxygenation Prospective Meta-analysis Collaboration. *JAMA* 2018;319(21):2190–2201.

88 NSCLC Meta-analysis Collaborative Group. Preoperative chemotherapy for non-small cell lung cancer: a systematic review and meta-analysis of individual participant data. *Lancet* 2014;383:1561–1571.

89 Cholesterol Treatment Trialists Collaboration, Baigent C, Blackwell L, et al. Efficacy and safety of more intensive lowering of LDL cholesterol: a meta-analysis of data from 170,000 participants in 26 randomised trials. *Lancet* 2010;376(9753):1670–1681.

90 NSCLC Meta-analyses Collaborative Group. Adjuvant chemotherapy, with or without postoperative radiotherapy, in operable non-small-cell lung cancer: two meta-analyses of individual patient data. *Lancet* 2010;375(9722):1267–1277.

91 Sterne JAC, Savovic J, Page MJ, et al. RoB 2: a revised tool for assessing risk of bias in randomised trials. *BMJ* 2019;366:l4898.

92 Lefebvre C, Glanville J, Briscoe S, et al. Chapter 4: Searching for and selecting studies. In: Higgins JPT, Thomas J, Chandler J, et al., eds. *Cochrane Handbook for Systematic Reviews of Interventions version 60* (updated July 2019). Available from www.training.cochrane.org/handbook. Cochrane 2019.

93 Chemoradiotherapy for Cervical Cancer Meta-Analysis Collaboration. Reducing uncertainties about the effects of chemoradiotherapy for cervical cancer: a systematic review and meta-analysis of individual patient data from 18 randomized trials. *J Clin Oncol* 2008;26(35):5802–5812.

94 Tierney JF, Vale CL, Parelukar WR, et al. Evidence synthesis to accelerate and improve the evaluation of therapies for metastatic hormone-sensitive prostate cancer. *Eur Urol Focus* 2019;5(2):137–143.

95 Vale CL, Tierney JF, Stewart LA. Effects of adjusting for censoring on meta-analyses of time-to-event outcomes. *Int J Epidemiol* 2002;31(1):107–111.

96 Rodgers MA, Brown JV, Heirs MK, et al. Reporting of industry funded study outcome data: comparison of confidential and published data on the safety and effectiveness of rhBMP-2 for spinal fusion. *BMJ* 2013;346:f3981.

97 Askie LM, Duley L, Henderson-Smart DJ, et al. Antiplatelet agents for prevention of pre-eclampsia: a meta-analysis of individual patient data. *Lancet* 2007;369(9575):1791–1798.

98 Ohmann C, Banzi R, Canham S, et al. Sharing and reuse of individual participant data from clinical trials: principles and recommendations. *BMJ Open* 2017;7(12):e018647.

99 El Emam K, Rodgers S, Malin B. Anonymising and sharing individual patient data. *BMJ* 2015;350:h1139.

100 Banzi R, Canham S, Kuchinke W, et al. Evaluation of repositories for sharing individual-participant data from clinical studies. *Trials* 2019;20(1):169.

101 Burdett S, Stewart LA. A comparison of the results of checked versus unchecked individual patient data meta-analyses. *Int J Technol Assess Health Care* 2002;18(3):619–624.

102 Sarcoma Meta-analysis Collaboration. Adjuvant chemotherapy for localised resectable soft-tissue sarcoma of adults: meta-analysis of individual data. *Lancet* 1997;350(9092):1647–1654.

103 Rogozinska E, Marlin N, Jackson L, et al. Effects of antenatal diet and physical activity on maternal and fetal outcomes: individual patient data meta-analysis and health economic evaluation. *Health Technol Assess* 2017;21(41):1–158.

104 Neoadjuvant Chemotherapy for Locally Advanced Cervical Cancer Meta-analysis C. Neoadjuvant chemotherapy for locally advanced cervical cancer: a systematic review and meta-analysis of individual patient data from 21 randomised trials. *Eur J Cancer* 2003;39(17):2470–2486.

105 Mhaskar R, Djulbegovic B, Magazin A, et al. Published methodological quality of randomized controlled trials does not reflect the actual quality assessed in protocols. *J Clin Epidemiol* 2012;65 (6):602–609.

106 Stewart LA, Tierney J, Clarke M. Chapter 18: Reviews of individual patient data. In: Higgins JPT, Green S (editors), Cochrane Handbook for Systematic Reviews of Interventions Version 5.1.0 (updated March 2011). The Cochrane Collaboration, 2011; Available from: www.handbook.cochrane.org.

107 PORT Meta-analysis Trialists Group. Postoperative radiotherapy in non-small-cell lung cancer: systematic review and meta-analysis of individual patient data from nine randomised controlled trials. *Lancet* 1998;352(9124):257–263.

108 Senn S. Testing for basline balance in clinical trials. *Stat Med* 1994;13:1715–1726.

109 Altman DG. Randomisation. *BMJ* 1991;302:1481–1482.

110 Lachin JM. Statistical considerations in the intent-to-treat principle. *Control ClinTrials* 2000;21:167–189.

111 Schulz K, F., Grimes DA. Sample size slippages in randomised trials: exclusions and the lost and wayward. *Lancet* 2002;359:781–785.

112 Tierney JF, Stewart LA. Investigating patient exclusion bias in meta-analysis. *Int J Epidemiol* 2005;34(1):79–87.

113 Kirkham JJ, Dwan KM, Altman DG, et al. The impact of outcome reporting bias in randomised controlled trials on a cohort of systematic reviews. *BMJ* 2010;340:c365.

114 McCormack K, Grant A, Scott N. Value of updating a systematic review in surgery using individual patient data. *Br J Surg* 2004;91(4):495–499.

115 Dwan K, Altman DG, Cresswell L, et al. Comparison of protocols and registry entries to published reports for randomised controlled trials. *Cochrane Database Syst Rev* 2011(1):MR000031.

116 Advanced Bladder Cancer Meta-analysis C. Neoadjuvant chemotherapy in invasive bladder cancer: a systematic review and meta-analysis. *Lancet* 2003;361(9373):1927–1934.

117 Green SJ, Fleming TR, Emerson S. Effects on overviews of early stopping rules for clinical trials. *Stat Med* 1987;6(3):361–369.

118 Advanced Bladder Cancer Meta-analysis Collaboration. Adjuvant chemotherapy in invasive bladder cancer: a systematic review and meta-analysis of individual patient data. Advanced Bladder Cancer (ABC) Meta-analysis Collaboration. *Eur Urol* 2005;48(2):189–199.

Part II

Fundamental Statistical Methods and Principles

5

The Two-stage Approach to IPD Meta-Analysis

Richard D. Riley, Thomas P.A. Debray, Tim P. Morris, and Dan Jackson

Summary Points

- In an IPD meta-analysis of multiple randomised trials, statistical methods are needed to synthesise the IPD and produce summary meta-analysis results.
- A two-stage approach can be used for meta-analysis. The first stage typically involves a standard regression analysis in each trial separately to produce aggregate data, whilst the second stage uses well-known (e.g. inverse-variance weighted) meta-analysis methods to combine this aggregate data and produce summary results and forest plots.
- For synthesis of randomised trials evaluating a treatment effect, the first stage produces estimates of treatment effect for each trial. Adjustment for key prognostic factors is recommended within each trial, and each trial's analysis should be appropriate for its design (e.g. accounting for any cluster randomisation, repeated measurements, etc).
- In the second stage, the treatment effect estimates obtained from the first stage are combined assuming either a common-effect or a random-effects model. A common treatment effect model assumes that the true treatment effect is the same in every trial. A random treatment effects model allows for between-trial heterogeneity in the true treatment effect, and is more plausible because included trials often differ in their characteristics.
- A frequentist or Bayesian estimation framework can be used. Bayesian estimation is appealing, to produce direct probabilistic statements that account for all parameter uncertainty, and to include prior distributions for the between-trial variance. In a frequentist framework, restricted maximum likelihood (REML) estimation is recommended for fitting the random-effects model in the second stage, with confidence intervals derived using the approach of Hartung-Knapp-Sidik-Jonkman.
- Heterogeneity can be summarised by the estimate of between-trial variance of true treatment effects, and a 95% prediction interval for the potential true treatment effect in a new trial.
- A meta-regression extends the random-effects model by including trial-level covariates (that define subgroups of trials) that may explain between-trial heterogeneity. However, meta-regression usually has low power and should be interpreted cautiously.
- For trials that do not provide their IPD, aggregate data (such as treatment effect estimates and their variances) might be obtainable from publications or from trial investigators. If appropriate, such aggregate data can be included in the second stage of the two-stage meta-analysis, alongside the aggregate data derived directly from IPD trials.

Individual Participant Data Meta-Analysis: A Handbook for Healthcare Research, First Edition.
Edited by Richard D. Riley, Jayne F. Tierney, and Lesley A. Stewart.

5.1 Introduction

There are two statistical approaches for conducting an IPD meta-analysis: a two-stage or a one-stage approach.[1,2] For example, consider an IPD meta-analysis of randomised trials to summarise a treatment effect. In the two-stage approach, the first stage analyses the IPD separately for each trial to obtain relevant aggregate data (i.e. treatment effect estimates and their variances), and then the second stage combines this aggregate data to produce summary results (i.e. a summary treatment effect estimate and its confidence interval). The alternative one-stage approach produces summary results by analysing the IPD from all trials together in a single step using an appropriate statistical model.[3]

The two-stage approach is often preferred to a one-stage analysis,[4,5] for a number of reasons. In particular, the second stage uses well-known meta-analysis methods that are relatively straightforward and well documented, for example in the *Cochrane Handbook for Systematic Reviews of Interventions*.[6] This makes the two-stage approach accessible to a broad set of researchers (including non-statisticians), and in most situations it performs at least as well as a one-stage approach (Chapter 8),[7] whilst often being computationally faster and naturally separating within-trial information from across-trial information, which is important (Chapter 7). The second stage also provides a convenient framework for incorporating aggregate data from any trials not providing their IPD.[8] Further, even when IPD are available from all trials, a two-stage approach will be necessary if some trials only permit remote access to their IPD (e.g. via a remote server located at the trial's host institution), such that their IPD cannot be merged directly with IPD from other trials.

In this chapter we describe the two-stage approach to IPD meta-analysis, covering the specification, estimation and application of various statistical models that can be used in the first and second stages. We focus on estimating a summary treatment effect using IPD from multiple randomised trials, but the key principles also apply to other research questions that aim to summarise a single effect or measure of interest, such as a treatment-covariate interaction (Chapter 7), the prognostic effect of a biomarker (Chapter 16) or the discrimination performance of a prognostic model (Chapter 17).

5.2 First Stage of a Two-stage IPD Meta-Analysis

Let us assume that IPD are available from a total of S parallel-group randomised trials that each compares a particular treatment to a control group. Let i denote trial ($i = 1$ to S), j denote participant, and y_{ij} denote the outcome value of interest, recorded for each participant in each trial. Outcome data may be continuous (e.g. blood pressure), binary (e.g. pre-eclampsia during pregnancy, yes or no), multinomial (e.g. type of delivery at birth), ordinal (e.g. severity of disease), count (e.g. number of infections during hospital stay), rate (e.g. number of hospital admissions within a particular follow-up period), or time-to-event (e.g. time to death following treatment for cancer). For all trials let x_{ij} denote the treatment group allocation for participant j in trial i (typically 1 for treatment and 0 for control), and let z_{1ij}, z_{2ij}, z_{3ij}... denote values of other participant-level covariates of interest (e.g. prognostic factors such baseline age, blood pressure, and stage of disease). An example of the format of such IPD from a randomised trial is shown in Table 5.1, as finalised after the cleaning and harmonisation process described in Chapter 4.

In the two-stage approach to IPD meta-analysis, the first stage requires a separate analysis in each trial to derive a treatment effect estimate and its variance. So, for example, if there are 10 trials providing their IPD, the first stage will produce 10 treatment effect estimates and 10 corresponding variances. Typically, the treatment effect estimate of interest will be a difference in means (for

Table 5.1 Example of hypothetical IPD for one trial similar to those received from the International Weight Management in Pregnancy (i-WIP) Collaborative Group, who obtained IPD from $S = 36$ trials (12,447 women),[24] to investigate whether diet and lifestyle interventions improve outcomes during pregnancy.

		Prognostic (adjustment) factors			**Continuous outcome**	**Binary outcome**
Participant ID	**Treatment group (x_{ij}), 1 = treatment 0 = control**	**Weight at baseline (z_{1ij}), *kg***	**Age at baseline (z_{2ij}), *years***	**BMI at baseline (z_{3ij})**	**Weight at end of follow-up (y_{ij}), *kg***	**Composite maternal outcome, (y_{ij}) 1 yes, 0 no**
1	0	52.18	31	29.95	62.30	0
2	1	54.34	30	20.89	66.50	0
3	0	56.22	33	20.35	73.11	1
⋮	⋮	⋮	⋮	⋮	⋮	⋮
227	0	56.11	29	22.31	70.51	1
228	1	56.09	33	27.06	64.28	1
229	1	57.19	30	20.05	65.26	0

Source: Richard Riley.

continuous outcomes), an odds ratio or risk ratio (for binary, ordinal or multinomial outcomes), an incidence or incidence rate ratio (for count and rate outcomes, respectively), or a hazard ratio (for time-to-event outcomes). The same effect measure should be estimated in each of the trials so they can be combined sensibly in the second stage (Section 5.3); for example, it would be inappropriate to combine odds ratios in some trials with hazard ratios in other trials. Hence, the first stage needs to apply the same (or similar) analysis method within in each trial, so that the same effect measure is estimated.

In general, the most suitable approach for deriving treatment effect estimates and variances is by fitting a regression model to the IPD in each trial. The regression model must be suitable for the outcome of interest, such as a linear, logistic or Cox regression for continuous, binary and time-to-event outcomes, respectively. Regression also enables adjustment for prognostic factors, and enables additional complexities in each trial's design to be accounted for, such as multiple centres, cluster randomisation, or repeated measures per individual. The key principles of regression modelling are now described.

5.2.1 General Format of Regression Models to Use in the First Stage

Table 5.2 provides the basic format of regression models to be used in the first stage of a two-stage IPD meta-analysis; equations are shown for different outcome types and for simplicity they include just a single covariate for treatment (though adjustment for prognostic factors is recommended in practice; see Section 5.2.4). With the exception of time-to-event outcomes, the models shown are general or generalised linear regression models. They involve specifying the conditional distribution of the outcome data (e.g. $y_{ij} \sim N(\mu_{ij}, \sigma_i^2)$ or $y_{ij} \sim \text{Bernoulli}(p_{ij})$) and a link function, g, which maps the expected (E) value of y_{ij} (i.e. $E(y_{ij})$) to a particular scale, which is then modelled ('regressed') against one or more covariates. Extending the models shown in Table 5.2 to allow for multiple covariates (i.e. treatment and prognostic factors), the regression component to fit in each trial separately can be written as:

$$g\left(E\left(y_{ij}\right)\right) = \alpha_i + \theta_i x_{ij} + \beta_{1i} z_{1ij} + \beta_{2i} z_{2ij} + \cdots \tag{5.1}$$

This format can equivalently be expressed in matrix notation, containing a vector of participant outcome values, a vector of unknown parameter values, and a design matrix linking the participant covariate values to the corresponding parameters.[9–11] For multinomial or ordinal outcomes, y_{ij} becomes y_{ijC} because C is additionally needed to denote category (Table 5.2). Note that the subscript i is really redundant in model (5.1), as the model is fitted in each trial separately; however, we retain subscript i to emphasise that each estimated parameter relates to a particular trial (this is important for setting up the second stage, Section 5.3).

The link function, g, takes different forms depending on the type of outcome data. For a linear regression model of continuous outcomes this is simply $g(E(y_{ij})) = E(y_{ij})$, such that no transformation (i.e. a natural link) is applied. For a logistic regression model of a binary outcome this is $\ln\left(\frac{E(y_{ij})}{1-E(y_{ij})}\right)$ or equivalently $\ln\left(\frac{p_{ij}}{1-p_{ij}}\right)$, which is a logit link function expressing the log-odds of the outcome occurring (where p_{ij} denotes the probability that the outcome occurs, also known as the outcome *event* probability). For a Poisson regression model of a count outcome, the transformation is $\ln(E(y_{ij}))$, known as the log link function.*

The parameter α_i represents the expected value of the outcome (on the transformed scale) in trial i for a participant whose covariate values are all zero; for binary outcomes, this represents a transformation of the baseline event risk. The main parameter of interest is θ_i, which denotes the treatment effect in trial i; this is the mean difference in the $g(E(y_{ij}))$ value for treatment and control groups. The parameters $\beta_{1i}, \beta_{2i}, \beta_{3i}, \ldots$ represent the effect of a one-unit increase in the corresponding covariate $z_{1ij}, z_{2ij}, z_{3ij} \ldots$ on the value of $g(E(y_{ij}))$ in trial i.

For time-to-event outcomes, the basic framework shown in model (5.8) is known as a Cox proportional hazards regression,[12] and it models how covariates impact the hazard (rate) of the outcome event over time. This requires outcome data about whether the event occurred or not, alongside the time of the event or end of follow-up.

5.2.2 Estimation of Regression Models Applied in the First Stage

Regression models used in the first stage are typically fitted (i.e. the unknown parameters of the model equation are estimated) using maximum likelihood (ML) estimation, which aims to yield parameter estimates that maximise the probability of observing the available data, conditional on the distributional assumptions made. For continuous outcomes, this will obtain the same estimates as ordinary least squares estimation. To indicate that a regression model has been estimated, parameters are expressed with a 'hat', for example:

$$g\left(E\left(y_{ij}\right)\right) = \hat{\alpha}_i + \hat{\theta}_i x_{ij} + \hat{\beta}_{1i} z_{1ij} + \hat{\beta}_{2i} z_{2ij} + \cdots$$

---

* In this book, we use ln and log interchangeably, with both referring to the natural log transformation (i.e. $\ln(x) = \log(x) = \log_e(x)$ in this book).

Table 5.2 Basic format of the regression model to be fitted separately within each trial in the first stage of the two-stage IPD meta-analysis approach, where the aim is to estimate a treatment effect (θ_i) from parallel-group randomised trials with continuous, binary, ordinal, count, or time-to-event data, where i denotes trial, j denotes participant, and y_{ij} denotes the outcome value.

Outcome type (y_{ij})	**Model type**	**Basic* regression model (for participant j in trial i) to be fitted in each trial separately, including a single covariate (x_{ij} = 1 for treatment group or x_{ij}=0 for control group)**	**Model number**
Continuous	Linear regression	$y_{ij} \sim N\left(\mu_{ij}, \sigma_i^2\right)$ $\mu_{ij} = \alpha_i + \theta_i x_{ij}$ NB σ_i^2 specifies that the residual variance is common to the control and treatment groups in trial i; alternatively it could be stratified by trial and treatment group by specifying σ_{ij}^2	(5.2)
Binary	Logistic regression	$y_{ij} \sim \text{Bernoulli}(p_{ij})$ $\text{logit}(p_{ij}) = \alpha_i + \theta_i x_{ij}$	(5.3)
Ordinal (with $C = 1$ to k ordered categories, from worst (1) to best (k))	Logistic regression (proportional odds model)	$y_{ijC} \sim \text{multinomial}\left(p_{ijC}\right)$ where $p_{ijk} = 1 - \sum_{C=1}^{k-1} p_{ijC}$ $\text{logit}(Q_{ijC}) = \alpha_{iC} + \theta_i x_{ij}$ for $C = 1$ to $(k - 1)$ where $Q_{ijC} = p_{ij1} + \ldots + p_{ijC}$ and $Q_{ijk} = 1$ and $\alpha_{i1} \leq \alpha_{i2} \leq \ldots \leq \alpha_{i(k-1)}$ NB assumes proportional odds, such that the treatment effect is common (the same) for each category 1 to $(k - 1)$	(5.4)
Multinomial (with $C = 1$ to k categories, and category k chosen as the reference)	Logistic regression	$y_{ijC} \sim \text{multinomial}\left(p_{ijC}\right)$ where $p_{ijk} = 1 - \sum_{C=1}^{k-1} p_{ijC}$ $\ln\left(\frac{p_{ijC}}{p_{ijk}}\right) = \alpha_{iC} + \theta_{iC} x_{ij}$ for $C = 1$ to $(k-1)$	(5.5)
Count	Poisson regression	$y_{ij} \sim \text{Poisson}(\mu_{ij})$ $\ln(\mu_{ij}) = \alpha_i + \theta_i x_{ij}$	(5.6)
Incidence rate	Poisson regression	$y_{ij} \sim \text{Poisson}(\mu_{ij})$ $\ln(\mu_{ij}) = \alpha_i + \theta_i x_{ij} + \ln(t_{ij})$ where $\ln(t_{ij})$ is an offset term for the log of the observed time (t_{ij}) at risk (i.e. the log of the follow-up time)	(5.7)
Time-to-event	Cox regression (proportional hazards model)	y_{ij} distribution unspecified $h_{ij}(t) = h_{0i}(t)\exp(\theta_i x_{ij})$ NB assumes proportional hazards, such that the treatment effect is common (the same) at all time points	(5.8)

* Adjustment for pre-defined prognostic factors is also recommended in practice (Section 5.2.4).
Source: Richard Riley.

As the chosen regression model is estimated in each trial separately, a separate estimate of each parameter (i.e. $\hat{\alpha}_i, \hat{\theta}_i, \hat{\beta}_{1i}, \hat{\beta}_{2i}, \ldots$) is obtained for each trial. This process is also known as *stratifying* the estimation by trial, and implies that no information is shared across trials; for example, the treatment effect estimate in trial 1 is estimated solely from the IPD in trial 1, and so is independent of the IPD from other trials. For continuous outcomes, restricted maximum likelihood (REML) estimation should be the default,[13] as this removes downward bias (i.e. estimated values that are less than they ought to be) in ML estimates of residual variances, which is a particular concern when the number of participants is small.

To facilitate the second stage of the IPD meta-analysis (Section 5.3), each trial's treatment effect estimate is required together with an estimate of its variance, in order to quantify the uncertainty of the estimate; we refer to these variances as $\text{var}(\hat{\theta}_i) = s_i^2$. Smaller variances indicate more precise estimates (less uncertainty) and, in the second stage of the two-stage IPD meta-analysis, we weight by these variances when combining treatment effect estimates in the meta-analysis (Section 5.3). Variances of the regression model's main parameter estimates (such as $\hat{\alpha}_i, \hat{\theta}_i, \hat{\beta}_{1i}, \hat{\beta}_{2i}, \ldots$ in model (5.1)) are typically obtained by the inverse of Fisher's information matrix. These are routinely calculated by statistical software, although usually the *standard error* of each parameter estimate is shown, which is the square root of the variance. Note that the variance of a parameter estimate is itself an estimate; therefore, when expressing the variance of a treatment effect estimate, we could also add a 'hat' to s_i^2 and rather write $\hat{s}_i^2$. However, we refrain from such notation in this book, as the variances are typically assumed known in the second stage of the two-stage IPD meta-analysis (Section 5.3). Ignoring the uncertainty in variance estimates is a potential criticism of the two-stage approach.[14,15]

An example of a dataset obtained by applying the first stage of a two-stage IPD meta-analysis is shown in Table 5.3, which corresponds to the setting described in Box 5.1.

5.2.3 Regression for Different Outcome Types

5.2.3.1 Continuous Outcomes

If the outcome, y_{ij}, is continuous (e.g. blood pressure) then a linear regression model can be fitted in each trial separately to estimate the treatment effect (θ_i), which denotes the difference in the mean outcome value for the treatment and control groups. The model residuals (e_{ij}) denote the difference between an individual's observed outcome value and that predicted by the fitted model equation (e.g. the estimated $\alpha_i + \theta_i x_{ij}$ component in model (5.2)). These residuals are assumed normally distributed with a mean of zero and a variance of σ_i^2, and so an equivalent way of writing model (5.2) is:

$$y_{ij} = \alpha_i + \theta_i x_{ij} + e_{ij}$$
$$e_{ij} \sim N(0, \sigma_i^2)$$

The σ_i^2 parameter is the residual variance; as for other parameters, it is estimated separately for each trial and so is stratified by trial. However, σ_i^2 is assumed to be common (i.e. the same) for control and treatment groups in the same trial. Alternatively, the residual variance could be stratified by treatment group by replacing σ_i^2 with σ_{ij}^2. Differences in residual variances for distinct groups is also known as heteroscedasticity, and this may be more plausible than common variances.[17,18] Availability of IPD allows heteroscedasticity to be modelled more easily than when only published aggregate data are available; at the very least, the impact of assuming σ_i^2 rather than σ_{ij}^2 can be examined. Further discussion of residual variance specification is given in Section 6.2.5.

If the outcome of interest represents a change from baseline (e.g. a change in blood pressure since start of the trial), we recommend the final outcome value to be modelled as y_{ij} and adjusted for the baseline value (y_{0ij}) as a covariate. This approach is known as analysis of covariance (ANCOVA), and is detailed as model (5.9) in Box 5.1, alongside a case study. Alternative approaches have been

Table 5.3 Example of aggregate data calculated for each trial in the first stage of a two-stage IPD meta-analysis; results correspond to the pregnancy example of Rogozinska et al. described in Box 5.1,[16] where the treatment effect corresponds to the mean difference in final weight (kg) for treatment (diet and lifestyle interventions) versus control (usual care) after adjusting for baseline weight.

Trial	Sample size	Intervention type	Treatment effect estimate: mean difference in final weight ($\hat{\theta}_i$)	Standard error of treatment effect estimate (s_i)	Variance of treatment effect estimate (s_i^2)	95% confidence interval for the treatment effect
Khoury 2005	198	Diet	−0.620	0.502	0.252	−1.604, 0.364
Vitolo 2011	292	Diet	−0.508	0.444	0.197	−1.379, 0.362
Walsh 2012	622	Diet	−0.765	0.358	0.128	−1.467, −0.063
Wolff 2008	56	Diet	−2.199	1.136	1.291	−4.425, 0.028
Baciuk 2008	69	Exercise	−1.665	1.319	1.741	−4.251, 0.921
Barakat 2008	140	Exercise	−0.473	0.593	0.351	−1.635, 0.689
Barakat 2012a	279	Exercise	−1.579	0.488	0.238	−2.535, −0.623
Haakstad 2011	82	Exercise	−0.725	0.842	0.709	−2.375, 0.926
Khaledan 2010	39	Exercise	−0.675	0.680	0.463	−2.008, 0.658
Nascimento 2011	80	Exercise	−0.466	0.942	0.887	−2.313, 1.380
Ong 2009	12	Exercise	−0.568	1.300	1.689	−3.115, 1.980
Oostdam 2012	80	Exercise	0.135	0.951	0.903	−1.728, 1.998
Perales 2014	164	Exercise	−1.197	0.675	0.456	−2.521, 0.127
Prevedel 2003	39	Exercise	0.077	0.853	0.728	−1.596, 1.749
Ruiz 2013	927	Exercise	−1.074	0.264	0.070	−1.592, −0.556
Stafne 2012	725	Exercise	−0.258	0.187	0.035	−0.625, 0.108
Yeo 2000	14	Exercise	−1.393	2.068	4.277	−5.446, 2.660
Yeo unpublished	16	Exercise	−0.082	1.368	1.871	−2.763, 2.599
Renault 2013	376	Exercise and Mixed	−1.041	0.508	0.258	−2.038, −0.045
Althuizen 2012	191	Mixed	0.450	0.994	0.988	−1.498, 2.399
Bogaerts 2012	197	Mixed	−3.221	1.046	1.094	−5.271, −1.170
Dodd 2014	1586	Mixed	−0.103	0.277	0.076	−0.645, 0.439
Guelinckx 2010	168	Mixed	0.184	1.086	1.179	−1.944, 2.312
Harrison 2013	213	Mixed	−0.569	0.419	0.175	−1.389, 0.252
Hui 2011	183	Mixed	−1.158	0.891	0.795	−2.905, 0.589
Jeffries 2009	232	Mixed	−0.788	0.529	0.279	−1.825, 0.248
Luoto 2011	382	Mixed	−0.703	0.551	0.303	−1.782, 0.376
Petrella 2013	61	Mixed	−3.749	1.502	2.256	−6.693, −0.805

(Continued)

Table 5.3 (Continued)

Trial	Sample size	Intervention type	Treatment effect estimate: mean difference in final weight ($\hat{\theta}_i$)	Standard error of treatment effect estimate (s_i)	Variance of treatment effect estimate (s_i^2)	95% confidence interval for the treatment effect
Phelan 2011	389	Mixed	−0.515	0.466	0.218	−1.429, 0.399
Poston unpublished	415	Mixed	−0.173	0.528	0.279	−1.209, 0.863
Rauh 2013	226	Mixed	−1.675	0.607	0.369	−2.866, −0.484
Sagedal unpublished	575	Mixed	−0.768	0.416	0.173	−1.584, 0.047
Vinter 2011	292	Mixed	−1.133	0.617	0.381	−2.342, 0.077

Source: Richard Riley.

discussed and debated, including modelling y_{ij} as the change score (outcome value at baseline minus outcome value at follow-up), or modelling y_{ij} as the final outcome value without adjustment for baseline value.[19–21] Although in principle all methods produce unbiased treatment effect estimates in randomised trials,[22,23] ANCOVA is preferred because, by adjusting for baseline outcome values, it is generally more efficient (i.e. it produces the smallest standard error of treatment effect estimates).[19,24,25] In contrast, modelling just the final outcome value is the worst approach, as by ignoring and not adjusting for baseline it loses efficiency and does not account for any correlation between baseline and follow-up values. Modelling the change score also ignores the correlation between baseline and follow-up, and loses information about baseline imbalances. A major advantage of having IPD is being able to implement the ANCOVA approach, as it is often neglected in published trials. White and Thompson discussed various options for including participants with missing baseline values (rather than performing a complete case analysis) in ANCOVA,[26] including mean imputation and the missing indicator method.

Sometimes continuous outcomes may not be recorded on the same scale in each trial; for example, multiple scales exist for subjective measures like pain, depression, and quality of life. This creates a problem for meta-analysis, as then the first stage will produce treatment effect estimates that relate to different scales in each trial. If the relationship between scales is known, it may be possible to transform participant outcome values from one scale to another within the IPD. Whitehead also highlighted the opportunity to model a standardised treatment difference in each trial,[27] by transforming the outcome responses to a standard normal distribution (i.e. a $N(0,1)$ distribution), by taking $(y_{ij} - \text{mean}(y_{ij}))/s_i$, where s_i is the standard deviation of outcome values observed in the trial. This standardisation ensures that the treatment effects in each trial are now on the same scale, but comes at the considerable expense of making the summary treatment effect (from subsequent meta-analysis) hard to interpret. The value of s_i is also an estimate, and White and Thomas

Box 5.1 Applied example of the first stage of a two-stage IPD meta-analysis of randomised trials with a continuous outcome. Case study based on the IPD meta-analysis project of Rogozinska et al.[16]

The International Weight Management in Pregnancy (i-WIP) Collaborative Group obtained IPD from 36 trials (12,447 women),[16] to investigate whether antenatal diet and lifestyle interventions improve outcomes during pregnancy. After lengthy data cleaning, harmonisation and quality checking, a two-stage IPD meta-analysis was applied. A main outcome was whether interventions reduced excessive weight gain, for which 33 trials and a total of 9,320 women were available. The IPD for one of the trials is illustrated in Table 5.1.

Weight was recorded as a continuous outcome (in kg), available at baseline (i.e. confirmation of pregnancy) and follow-up (i.e. last available weight recorded before delivery). In the first stage of the two-stage IPD meta-analysis approach the IPD for each trial was analysed separately, using an analysis of covariance (ANCOVA) model to estimate the treatment effect (i.e. difference in final weight in kg for those in the intervention group compared to the control group) after adjusting for baseline weight. In trials with a parallel-group design, the applied ANCOVA model can be written as:

$$\begin{aligned} y_{ij} &= \alpha_i + \theta_i x_{ij} + \beta_{1i} y_{0ij} + e_{ij} \\ e_{ij} &\sim N\left(0, \sigma_i^2\right) \end{aligned} \tag{5.9}$$

Here, y_{ij} is the weight value at end of follow-up (i.e. before delivery) for the jth participant in trial i; x_{ij} is 1 for treatment and 0 for control; y_{0ij} is the participant's baseline weight; and σ_i^2 is the residual variance in trial i. The ANCOVA model was adapted for two trials with a cluster trial design (i.e. randomisation at the cluster rather than participant-level), with random intercepts to account for the clustering. Restricted maximum likelihood (REML) estimation was used to fit the model in each trial, and the estimate of the treatment effect, θ_i, was recorded alongside its variance. The trial results are summarised in the dataset shown in Table 5.3, ready to be used for meta-analysis in the second stage (Box 5.5). Allowing for a separate residual variance (σ_{ij}^2) for each of treatment and controls groups did not materially alter the findings.

Sources: Richard Riley; Rogozinska E, Marlin N, Jackson L, et al. Effects of antenatal diet and physical activity on maternal and fetal outcomes: individual patient data meta-analysis and health economic evaluation. *Health Technol Assess* 2017;21(41):1–158.

described how standard errors of standardised mean differences should account for this.[28] Other options for standardisation are discussed by Murad et al. and Borenstein et al.,[29,30] including extensions to ANCOVA situations.

If some trials provide outcome values for each of multiple scales, then the treatment effect estimates for each available scale could be calculated, and then (in the second stage) a multivariate meta-analysis used to produce a summary result for each scale, whilst accounting for their correlation. This framework does not require all trials to provide all measurement scales and still produces a separate meta-analysis result for each scale. Chapter 13 discusses multivariate meta-analysis in detail.

5.2.3.2 Binary Outcomes

When modelling a binary outcome ($y_{ij} = 0$ or 1), such as onset of pre-eclampsia during pregnancy, the conditional outcome distribution is a Bernoulli distribution and usually a logit link function is applied to form a logistic regression (model (5.3)). The outcome 'event' (e.g. death) is typically coded as $y_{ij} = 1$ and the absence of an event as $y_{ij} = 0$, so that the logit function models the log-odds of the event (denoted by logit(p_{ij}), where p_{ij} is the probability of having the event) conditional on included covariates, such as the treatment covariate (x_{ij}: 1 for treated, 0 for control) and prognostic factors. Then the treatment effect is $\exp(\theta_i)$, which represents an odds ratio, and reveals how much the odds of the outcome event are reduced (or increased) for the treatment compared to the control group in the ith trial. A case study is given in Box 5.2. An alternative to logistic regression is to use a log-link function, so that $\exp(\theta_i)$ represents the risk ratio, which is usually more clinically meaningful and might offer some theoretical advantages,[31] although can suffer from more model fitting problems that lead to non-convergence or erroneous final parameter estimates.

Box 5.2 Applied example of the first stage of a two-stage IPD meta-analysis of randomised trials with a binary outcome. Case study based on the IPD meta-analysis project of Rogozinska et al.[16]

Let us return to the example in Box 5.1. A binary outcome of interest was a composite maternal adverse outcome (any of gestational diabetes, pre-eclampsia, pregnancy-induced hypertension, preterm birth or Caesarean section), for which IPD from 24 trials containing 8852 women with 3733 adverse maternal events. The IPD from each trial was of the format shown in Table 5.1.

In the first stage the IPD for each trial was analysed separately, using a logistic regression model to estimate the treatment effect (i.e. log odds ratio) and its variance. In trials with a parallel-group design, the model that was fitted can be written as:

$$y_{ij} \sim \text{Bernoulli}\left(p_{ij}\right)$$
$$\text{logit}\left(p_{ij}\right) = \alpha_i + \theta_i x_{ij}$$

Here, y_{ij} is 1 for participants that had the composite outcome event and 0 otherwise; p_{ij} is the outcome event probability for the jth participant in trial i; x_{ij} denotes the treatment group (i.e. 1/0 for treatment/control); α_i denotes the log-odds of the outcome event in the control group in trial i; and θ_i denotes the treatment effect in trial i. The model was fitted in each trial using maximum likelihood (ML) estimation. If a trial had zero events in either the treatment or control groups, the approach of Sweeting et al. was applied (as a continuity correction) to allow model estimation (Section 5.2.3.2). The model was adapted for trials with a cluster trial design (i.e. randomisation at the cluster rather than participant-level), with random intercepts to account for the clustering (Section 5.2.5). The trial results were summarised in a dataset (similar to that shown in Table 5.3, except the treatment effect estimates were log odds ratios) ready to be used for meta-analysis in the second stage (Box 5.6). First-stage analyses were also repeated with adjustment for age, to provide treatment effects conditional of this pre-defined prognostic factor.

Sources: Richard Riley; Rogozinska E, Marlin N, Jackson L, et al. Effects of antenatal diet and physical activity on maternal and fetal outcomes: individual patient data meta-analysis and health economic evaluation. *Health Technol Assess* 2017;21(41):1–158.

When IPD are not available, two-by-two tables are often reported in each trial indicating the number of participants with and without the outcome event in each of the two treatment groups. If only the treatment covariate (x_{ij}) is to be included in the regression model within the first stage, then the necessary IPD can be fully reconstructed from these two-by-two tables (Section 6.4.1 demonstrates this) and model (5.3) can be fitted. However, IPD meta-analysis projects are usually interested in modelling other participant-level variables in addition to treatment and outcome; in particular, to adjust treatment effects for prognostic factors (Section 5.2.4), to account for clustering (e.g. if there are multiple centres, Section 5.2.5) or to examine treatment-covariate interactions (Chapter 7). It is harder to reconstruct IPD including such participant-level covariates, though options do exist (Section 5.6).

A problem occurs in trials that have no outcome events (or no non-events) in either the treatment group or the control group, as then the treatment effect estimate (e.g. log odds ratio or log risk ratio) and its variance cannot be calculated because the regression model cannot be fitted.[32–34] Then, the meta-analyst is faced with either throwing such trials away (which might be viewed as research waste) or adding extra information to their data to allow estimates to be derived. Traditionally, the latter is addressed in a particular trial by using a continuity correction, where a small number is added to each cell of the trial's two-by-two table (i.e. that which tabulates the number of events and non-events for the treatment and control groups). Traditionally 0.5 is the value added,[35] but Sweeting et al. suggest that a 'treatment arm' continuity correction is more appropriate,[33] which adds 1/(sample size of the opposite treatment group) to the number of event and non-events. In the IPD context, a similar approach is to add two extra participants to each group in a trial if it has zero events in either of the groups; one of the added participants has the event and the other does not have the event in each group. Then, a weighted regression analysis can be performed to analyse the extended IPD, with all participants weighted equally except the four added participants, who are given a weight according to Sweeting correction (i.e. 1/(sample size of the opposite treatment group)). However, this approach becomes problematic when adjusting for prognostic factors or extending to non-binary variables. For this reason, a more general approach is to adopt Firth regression,[36] which is a penalisation method that reduces small sample bias for non-linear models such as logistic regression, and resolves problems related to separation. Alternatively, researchers may revert to a one-stage IPD meta-analysis approach (Chapter 6),[14,34] and placing random effects on parameters (rather than stratifying parameters by trial) so that estimation of trial-specific terms are avoided.

Occasionally the IPD for a trial may have no outcome events in either of the treatment or control groups (so-called 'double-zero' trials). Although approaches have been suggested to include such trials,[37] we generally recommend that they be removed from the IPD meta-analysis entirely when relative effects are of interest (i.e. odds or risk ratios). Although double-zero trials provide information about the absolute (baseline) risk in the population, they provide negligible information about the treatment effect measured by an odds or risk ratio, unless the analyst is willing to allow between-trial borrowing of information about baseline risk (e.g. using a random effect on the intercept in a one-stage model (Section 6.2.4)), or to specify a between-trial relationship between the baseline risk and the treatment effect (such as a bivariate normal distribution; Section 6.2.4.3). Double-zero trials are more useful where estimates of (or differences in) absolute risk are also interest.

5.2.3.3 Ordinal and Multinomial Outcomes

The logistic regression framework for a binary outcome can be extended to model ordinal outcome data via a proportional odds model (model (5.4)),[27,38,39] which accounts for the multinomial and ordered nature of the data. Ordinal data relates to categories (e.g. of pain levels) that are ordered, say from worst (unbearable pain) to best (no pain), with a total of $C = 1$ to k categories in each trial. Here, the outcome value, y_{ijC}, for participant j in trial i takes the value of their outcome category (C). So, for example, $y_{ijC} = 1$ if their outcome category is 1, $y_{ijC} = k$ if their outcome is category k, and so on. The underlying distribution of y_{ijC} is multinomial, with p_{ijC} denoting the probability of falling in category C. For categories $C = 1$ to $(k - 1)$, model (5.4) models the cumulative probability (Q_{ijC}) of the outcome falling in categories 1 to C, and the proportional odds framework means that the treatment effect (θ_i) is assumed to be common (i.e. the same) regardless of the category, with $\exp(\theta_i)$ expressing the odds ratio (i.e. how the odds of being in a worse outcome category are changed by being in the treatment rather than the control group for participants in trial i). Detailed examples are given by Whitehead.[27]

Note that the proportional odds modelling approach of model (5.4) is consistent with assuming the existence of a latent (i.e. unobserved) continuous outcome variable (e.g. continuous pain score), which has been categorised into the groups (e.g. unbearable pain, ... , no pain).[27] It is preferable to analyse continuous outcomes on their continuous scale, and so outcomes should be requested on their continuous scale. However, some trials may only record continuous outcomes as ordered categories (e.g. of severity), thereby enforcing an ordinal outcome analysis. Different trials may have used different cut-points to define the categories,[27,38] but the proportional odds approach can still be used in this situation because (i) each trial is analysed separately in the first stage of a two-stage IPD meta-analysis, and (ii) under the proportional odds assumption, the odds ratios from each trial will have a similar interpretation and so can be combined in a meta-analysis in the second stage (Section 5.3).

Some multinomial outcomes are not ordered, such that it is not appropriate to order them from worst to best (or most to least severe). For example, in dementia patients followed for six months, a multinomial outcome may be living (i) in own home, (ii) with family, (iii) in a care home, or (iv) in hospital; these four categories are difficult to place in order of severity. Then, proportional odds model (5.4) is inappropriate, and the framework of model (5.5) is preferable. Here, for categories $C = 1$ to $(k - 1)$, the probability (p_{ijC}) of being in category C is modelled relative to the probability of being in reference category (k). Now the treatment effect (θ_{iC}) is category-specific, with $\exp(\theta_{iC})$ expressing the odds ratio (i.e. how the probability of being in category C relative to the probability of being in category k are changed by being in the treatment rather than the control group for participants in trial i). This approach can also be used for ordered outcomes, if the proportional odds assumption is considered too restrictive.

As for binary outcomes, sometimes IPD can be partly reconstructed from aggregate data for ordinal and multinomial outcomes, given the number of participants in each outcome category for each treatment group.

5.2.3.4 Count and Incidence Rate Outcomes

For outcome data that are counts (e.g. number of asthma events within six months), y_{ij} is the number of outcome occurrences (events) for participant j in trial i, and the outcome distribution (conditional on included covariates in the regression model) is a Poisson distribution. The main model for count outcome data is a Poisson regression with a log-link (model (5.6)), such that the treatment effect ($\exp(\theta_i)$) represents the ratio of expected counts in the treatment and control group. If follow-up length differs per individual, then the model can be extended to include an offset term for the log length of follow-up (model (5.7)), such that $\exp(\theta_i)$ is now the incidence rate ratio. Several extensions have been described that, for instance, allow for data with many zeros by introducing a discrete point mass (hierarchical zero-inflated Poisson regression).[40–42] Poisson regression can also be used to (approximately) model binary outcomes in order to estimate risk ratios.[43]

If each trial provides total number of events and total follow-up time, then model (5.7) can be fitted even without the IPD.[14] So, as for binary and ordinal outcomes, a key statistical advantage of obtaining IPD is having information to include (adjust for) other participant-level covariates in the regression model. Additionally, model (5.7) assumes the rate in each treatment group is a constant throughout the whole follow-up period, but availability of IPD (including time of events for each individual) allows this assumption to be relaxed. In fact, by splitting the time-scale into intervals defined by distinct event times, the Poisson regression approach can be used to fit a Cox regression (model (5.8)),[44] which does not require assumptions about the shape of the hazard function, as now described for time-to-event outcomes.

5.2.3.5 Time-to-Event Outcomes

Participants in randomised trials are not always followed for the same length of time, and many will not experience the outcome event of interest during their trial follow-up. For example, a participant may choose to withdraw from the trial before having the outcome event of interest, may be lost to follow-up (e.g. if they move to a different county), or reach the trial end without an outcome event. Such participants are usually assumed to be right censored, indicating that any outcome event could only occur after their censoring time (i.e. their last follow-up time). It is often assumed that censoring is non-informative, such that the reason for censoring is independent to the outcome event occurrence. When (right) censoring occurs, it is inappropriate to simply exclude participants who are censored, as they contain valuable information in that there was no outcome event up to their final follow-up time. Time-to-event (survival) models are used to include such participants in the statistical analysis up to their censoring time. Therefore, the outcome value, y_{ij}, is the time to event (e.g. death) or censoring for the jth participant in trial i, and a further variable is needed to denote whether the participant did or did not have the event by that time.

To analyse such outcome data in the first stage of a two-stage IPD meta-analysis, appropriate statistical methods for analysing time-to-event data are needed. These most commonly utilise hazard functions ($h_{ij}(t)$), which quantify the instantaneous risk of experiencing the outcome event at time t conditional on the outcome event having not already occurred prior to time t. This is shown in model (5.8), where $h_{ij}(t)$ is the hazard rate over time t for the jth participant in trial i, $h_{0i}(t)$ is the baseline hazard (i.e. the hazard rate for those in the reference category, here control group) in trial i, and θ_i denotes the log hazard ratio (i.e. the treatment effect) in trial i.

To fit this model, the hazard function (or related measures like the survival or cumulative hazard function) could be modelled parametrically, based on assuming the time-to-event data arise from a particular distribution (e.g. Weibull). However, parametric distributions are often not flexible enough to model complex shapes of the baseline hazard ($h_{0i}(t)$) in a trial. To address this, Cox proposed the proportional hazards regression model.[12] The advantage of Cox regression is that, through ML estimation of the partial likelihood, the approach avoids estimating $h_0(t)$ entirely and places no constraints on its actual shape, whilst still providing other parameter estimates of interest, such as the treatment effect. Usually the hazard functions for treatment and control groups are assumed proportional, such that estimated hazard ratios are assumed constant over time. This can be examined, for example by extending model (5.8) by including a (non-linear) interaction between log time and the treatment effect (log hazard ratio). As for binary outcomes, when there are few events in some trials adaptions of Firth's correction are important to reduce small sample bias in the estimated treatment effect.[45]

5.2.4 Adjustment for Prognostic Factors

The availability of IPD provides the potential to adjust for prognostic factors, which is unlikely to be possible in a conventional meta-analysis of published aggregate data. In the first stage of the two-stage approach, an adjusted treatment effect for a particular trial can be obtained by fitting a regression model including the treatment variable alongside prognostic factors, as in model (5.1). Such a treatment effect is also known as a *conditional* treatment effect. An alternative approach is standardisation, which obtains a *marginal* treatment effect accounting for prognostic factors. This is obtained by fitting a regression model such as model (5.1) and then standardising the results by summing or integrating over the observed distribution of prognostic factors in the trial. This can be achieved by making predictions assuming all participants were assigned to treatment and then assuming all participants were assigned to control, and forming an appropriate contrast of the predictions to obtain the adjusted treatment effect. This method is sometimes termed 'marginalisation' or 'G-computation'.

In this book we focus on obtaining conditional treatment effects (both at the trial level and the meta-analysis level), and the term 'adjusted treatment effect' refers to a conditional treatment effect. As trials randomise participants into treatment and control groups, the adjustment for prognostic (confounding) factors might be deemed unnecessary. This may be short-sighted, however.[47–53] Firstly, adjusting for pre-specified prognostic factors by fitting model (5.1) allows inferences about treatment effect to be made conditional on values of participant-level covariates. This aligns with the drive toward personalised medicine where treatment decisions are ideally tailored to each individual patient given their particular characteristics and outcome risks (Sections 7.8.4 and 7.11). Hence, to guide clinical practice at the patient level, a conditional treatment effect is a more relevant estimand (target parameter) than an unadjusted treatment effect, whilst marginal treatment effects are more relevant to population-level decision making.

Secondly, conditional and unadjusted treatment effects can be very different from each other, and so the decision (of whether to adjust for prognostic factors or not) is not necessarily an arbitrary one. In some statistical models, such as linear regression and binomial regression with a log-link, the treatment effect is the same regardless of whether prognostic factors are included or not. However, for models that examine non-collapsible measures (most notably logistic regression and Cox regression, which model odds ratios and hazard ratios, respectively), if the treatment is beneficial the unadjusted or marginal treatment effect will be closer to 1 than the conditional treatment effect.[3,54–56] In such models, if a conditional treatment effect is of interest, omission of prognostic factors from a trial analysis may have an important impact on the trial's treatment effect estimate. The difference between conditional and marginal or unadjusted estimates may sometimes be small,[54] but can be large when the conditional estimate adjusts for strong prognostic factors. For example, in a randomised trial of azathioprine versus placebo in participants with primary biliary cirrhosis,[57] a Cox regression produced an unadjusted treatment effect estimate that is inconclusive about whether azathioprine is beneficial (HR = 0.83, 95% CI: 0.57 to 1.22, p = 0.348); however, after adjusting for the strong prognostic factor of baseline serum bilirubin concentration (suitably modelled on its continuous scale), the adjusted treatment effect estimate was substantially larger and suggests strong evidence that azathioprine is beneficial after accounting for bilirubin (HR = 0.61, 95% CI: 0.41 to 0.91, *p*-value = 0.015). Hence, a subsequent meta-analysis of unadjusted treatment effect estimates may produce very different results to a meta-analysis of adjusted estimates; similarly, the amount of between-trial heterogeneity in treatment effect will often be different depending on whether unadjusted or adjusted treatment effect estimates are combined.[58,59] In clinical practice, measuring prognostic factors like bilirubin is usually a key part of patient care and decision making, and so the conditional treatment effect provides a better reflection of actual practice.

Thirdly, adjustment for prognostic factors may gain power to detect a genuine treatment effect (as prognostic factors may explain variation in outcomes across participants).[50–53] This was discussed in Section 5.2.3.1, where ANCOVA was recommended for analysing trials with a continuous outcome whilst adjusting for baseline value of the outcome.[23] Fourth, when the main focus is on extending beyond the overall treatment effect, such as estimating treatment-covariate interactions (Chapter 7) or dose-response associations across participants within trials, adjustment for prognostic factors is important to reduce the potential for confounding.[60,61]

Given these reasons, we generally recommend that IPD meta-analyses adjust for key prognostic factors, and – assuming the focus is on informing clinical practice at the patient level – to summarise conditional treatment effects (i.e. θ_i from model (5.1)). Ideally, the set of prognostic factors should be pre-specified in the analysis plan, and it is sensible to restrict to a small number of strong prognostic factors that are likely to be routinely recorded (e.g. age, stage of disease, baseline value of the corresponding continuous outcome, etc) by trials in the IPD meta-analysis. It may help to focus on those prognostic factors identified from systematic reviews,[62] and those used within the design of some trials (e.g. as stratification factors). Applied examples are given for a continuous outcome in Box 5.1, where adjustment is made for baseline SBP, and for a time-to-event outcome in Box 5.3, where adjustment is made for prognostic factors of age, BMI, SBP, and smoking.

When including prognostic factors that are recorded on a continuous scale, they should be analysed on their continuous scale, as dichotomisation or categorisation is arbitrary and loses power.[57,63,64] Thus, adjustment for continuous prognostic factors should at least assume a linear trend. For example, in the aforementioned trial examining azathioprine versus placebo, the treatment effect was larger (HR = 0.61, 95% CI: 0.41 to 0.91, $p = 0.015$) when bilirubin was included as a linear effect, rather than when dichotomised at the median (HR = 0.76, 95% CI: 0.51 to 1.12, $p = 0.17$).[57] It is also possible to allow for non-linear prognostic effects in each trial. For example, if age is considered an important prognostic factor, then, rather than assuming a linear effect of age, one could fit trial-specific non-linear associations by including a restricted cubic spline term for age, with a pre-specified number of knots.[65–67] Alternative options are generalised additive models or fractional polynomials.[68–70] In the aforementioned azathioprine trial, allowing for a non-linear rather than a linear effect of bilirubin gave almost identical results, which is reassuring.[57] Allowing for non-linear (rather than linear) trends in prognostic factors may be more important when the focus is on the prognostic effect itself (Chapter 16) or on treatment-covariate interactions (Chapter 7).

5.2.5 Dealing with Other Trial Designs and Missing Data

So far we have focused on regression models for analysing randomised trials with a parallel-group design, where participants are randomly allocated to one of two groups. However, some trials in the IPD meta-analysis may have a different or more complex design that requires the regression models of Table 5.2 to be modified or extended accordingly (in addition to including prognostic factors). In particular, some trials may have a cluster randomised design, where the randomisation is at the

Box 5.3 Applied example of the first stage of a two-stage IPD meta-analysis of randomised trials with a time-to-event outcome. Case study based on an extension of IPD meta-analysis project of Wang et al.[46] as described by Crowther et al.[44]

Wang et al. performed an IPD meta-analysis of trials in participants with hypertension to investigate to what extent lowering systolic blood pressure (SBP) contributed to cardiovascular prevention.[46] They selected randomised trials that tested active antihypertensive drugs against placebo or no treatment. Ten trials (with a parallel-group design) were ultimately included, which provided IPD for a total of 28,581 participants. Crowther et al. used this IPD to summarise the effect of anti-hypertensive drugs in regard to all-cause mortality.[44] The IPD for each trial had the following format, taking trial 1 as an example (hypothetical data shown for illustration):

		Prognostic factors			Time-to-event outcome	
Participant ID	**Treatment group, x_{ij} (1 treatment, 0 control)**	**Age at baseline, *years***	**BMI at baseline**	**SBP at baseline, *mmHg***	**Dead (1 yes, 0 no)**	**Follow-up time, years**
1	1	49	26.02	176	0	5.48
2	1	47	23.60	148	0	5.24
3	0	48	26.03	144	1	0.97
⋮	⋮	⋮	⋮	⋮	⋮	⋮
337	0	35	25.94	144	0	2.92
338	0	40	24.34	164	0	4.99
339	1	45	27.35	141	0	3.69

In the first stage of the two-stage IPD meta-analysis approach the IPD for each trial was analysed separately, using a Cox regression model to estimate the unadjusted treatment effect (i.e. log hazard ratio) and its variance, as follows:

$$h_{ij}(t) = h_{0i}(t)\exp(\theta_i x_{ij})$$

Here, $h_{ij}(t)$ is the hazard rate over time, t, for the jth participant in trial i, $h_{0i}(t)$ is the baseline hazard (for those in the control group) in trial i, and θ_i denotes the log hazard ratio (i.e. the treatment effect) in trial i. The model was fitted using maximum likelihood (ML) estimation of the IPD in each trial separately, and the trial results were summarised in a dataset (similar to that shown in Table 5.3 except the treatment effect estimates were log hazard ratios) ready to be used for meta-analysis in the second stage. The trial-specific estimates are shown in Box 5.4. The first stage was also repeated to obtain conditional treatment effects, after adjusting for the following pre-specified prognostic factors measured at baseline: age, body mass index, SBP, and smoking status.

Sources: Richard Riley; Wang JG, Staessen JA, Franklin SS, et al. Systolic and diastolic blood pressure lowering as determinants of cardiovascular outcome. Hypertension 2005;45(5):907–13 ; Crowther MJ, Riley RD, Staessen JA, et al. Individual patient data meta-analysis of survival data using Poisson regression models. *BMC Med Res Methodol* 2012;12:34.

cluster (e.g. hospital, practice) rather than participant level.[71–73] This was the situation in the applied examples of Box 5.1 and Box 5.2, and the analysis of such trials must account for the nesting of participants within clusters.

To analyse a cluster randomised trial with a binary outcome, model (5.3) can be modified as follows:

$$\text{logit}\left(p_{ikj}\right) = \alpha_{ik} + \theta_i x_{ikj}$$

As before, i denotes trial, j denotes participant, and y_{ij} denotes the binary outcome value. Additionally, k denotes the cluster within trial i, and the log-odds of the outcome event in each control group cluster is allowed to be different (α_{ik}). Often the α_{ik} are assumed drawn from a normal distribution with mean α_i (the average control group log-odds across clusters in trial i) and between-cluster variance τ_k^2. After model estimation, the treatment effect estimate ($\hat{\theta}_i$) summarises the average difference in the log-odds of the outcome event (i.e. the log odds ratio) for those in a treatment cluster ($x_{ikj} = 1$) compared to those in a control cluster ($x_{ikj} = 0$). This treatment effect estimate can be taken forward for meta-analysis in the second stage, alongside those obtained for other trials (Section 5.3).

The analysis and modelling strategy for each trial may also need adapting to handle other complexities. For example, some trials involve multiple centres, such that their analysis might require clustering of participants within centres to be accounted for,[74,75] and a decision made on whether treatment effects in each centre are assumed common or random.[76,77] Some trials may include three or more treatment groups, so that two or more treatment effect parameters are then required in the analysis model. Chapter 14 describes multiple treatment comparisons in the context of a network IPD meta-analysis.

Some trials may have missing outcome values for some participants, with little or no missing data in covariates included in the analysis. Then, if missing outcomes are considered 'missing at random' (that is, that the probability of being missing depends only on the observed data for included covariates such as treatment and prognostic factors), Sullivan et al. recommend generally using complete-case analysis for a single outcome or a likelihood-based approach for multiple outcomes (e.g. linear mixed model for multiple continuous outcomes).[78] They note that for randomised trials aiming to estimate a treatment effect, "multiple imputation can be inferior to complete-case analysis and likelihood-based approaches, adding in unnecessary simulation error" and that complete-case analysis "is optimal when missing data are restricted to a univariate outcome and variables associated with missingness are included as covariates in the analysis model".[78] This agrees with Groenwold et al., who state that for randomised trials "complete-case analysis with covariate adjustment and multiple imputation yield similar estimates in the event of missing outcome data, as long as the same predictors of missingness are included. Hence, complete case analysis with covariate adjustment can and should be used as the analysis of choice more often".[79] The missing at random assumption is more plausible when prognostic factors are included as adjustment covariates in the analysis model (or the imputation model[80]), which gives further weight to our recommendation to include a pre-defined set of prognostic factors (Section 5.2.4).

Note that missing outcomes in the analysis of time-to-event data are handled naturally through censoring. If missing outcomes or censoring is informative (i.e. cannot be considered missing at random even after accounting for covariates), alternative approaches to complete-case analysis are required. Multiple imputation might be the most flexible approach to allow for potential missing not at random mechanisms.[81] Where multiple imputation is used, it is important to impute separately for each randomised group as this offers greater robustness.[78] Multiple imputation is described in detail in Chapter 18. Trials without the outcome of interest for any participants (i.e. the outcome is systematically missing) could still be included using a multivariate meta-analysis approach which borrows strength from other correlated outcomes that are available (Chapter 13).[82]

Where conditional treatment effects are of interest for meta-analysis and the pre-defined prognostic (adjustment) factors are systematically missing in some trials, then it is sensible to use the subset of factors that are consistently recorded. In particular, for treatment effects defined by odds ratios or hazard ratios, adjusting for different sets of prognostic factors is problematic due to non-collapsibility (Section 5.2.4); it will make the subsequent summary meta-analysis result hard to interpret and impact upon (often increase) the between-trial heterogeneity in treatment effect. Even for collapsible measures (such as mean differences and risk ratios), the weighting of a particular trial in the meta-analysis may be influenced by whether a full or reduced set of prognostic factors is used, and so it is better to be consistent across trials. Rather than just using those prognostic factors routinely recorded, an alternative approach is to apply a multivariate meta-analysis of partially and fully adjusted estimates, or multilevel multiple imputation; these methods are described in Chapter 18.[83–86]

Partially missing prognostic factor values in a trial can be handled (in each trial separately) by using mean imputation or the missing indicator method, which – although rightly criticised for use in other medical research applications – is actually appropriate for randomised trials aiming to estimate a treatment effect.[78,87] Again, multiple imputation is a possible alternative (Chapter 18), for example to utilise additional prognostic factors and outcomes available in the IPD, or even to consider missing not at random assumptions.[78]

5.3 Second Stage of a Two-stage IPD Meta-Analysis

At the end of the first stage of a two-stage IPD meta-analysis, the treatment effect estimates ($\hat{\theta}_i$) and their variances (i.e. $\text{var}(\hat{\theta}_i) = s_i^2$) have been derived for all trials, ready to be combined using a meta-analysis in the second stage, as now described. Other parameters estimated in each trial (e.g. intercepts, prognostic effects, etc) are not used in the second stage unless a multivariate approach is used, which is considered in Chapter 13.

5.3.1 Meta-Analysis Assuming a Common Treatment Effect

Recall that the $\hat{\theta}_i$ represent mean differences for continuous outcomes; log odds ratios or log risk ratios for binary (or ordinal) outcomes; log incidence (rate) ratios for count outcomes; and log hazard ratios for time-to-event outcomes. We assume that the $\hat{\theta}_i$ have the same interpretation in each trial: for example, they all represent unadjusted treatment effects or, preferably, conditional treatment effects with adjustment for the same set of pre-defined prognostic factors (Section 5.2.4). This is important to aid interpretation of the summary meta-analysis result.

The simplest approach to meta-analysis is to assume that the $\hat{\theta}_i$ are all estimates of a common treatment effect, represented as θ. In other words, the true treatment effect is assumed to be the same for each trial, such that the observed trial estimates only differ due to chance. This implies that, if all trials had an infinite sample size, there would be no differences due to chance and the differences in trial estimates would completely disappear.

A meta-analysis model with a common treatment effect can be written as:[88]

$$\hat{\theta}_i \sim N(\theta, s_i^2) \tag{5.10}$$

This assumes treatment effect estimates ($\hat{\theta}_i$) from the first stage are normally distributed (which is plausible if trials are not small), and that their variances (s_i^2) are known (such that the uncertainty of the variance estimates is ignored). In the meta-analysis literature this approach has been loosely termed a *fixed-effect meta-analysis*. However, the word 'fixed' is ambiguous; statistically speaking, a parameter can be called fixed even when stratified by trial (i.e. estimated separately in each trial) and so the word 'fixed' does not necessarily imply a parameter is common to all trials.[89] Therefore, in this book we refer to model (5.10) as a *common-effect meta-analysis*, which makes it explicit that we are assuming the effect of interest is common (the same) for all trials. A broader discussion on the specification and assumptions of fixed-effect(s) meta-analysis models is given by Rice et al.[89]

ML estimation can be used to fit model (5.10). This leads to the following analytic solutions for the summary treatment effect estimate ($\hat{\theta}$) and its variance ($\text{var}(\hat{\theta})$),

$$\hat{\theta} = \frac{\sum_{i=1}^{S} \hat{\theta}_i w_i}{\sum_{i=1}^{S} w_i} \tag{5.11}$$

$$\text{var}\left(\hat{\theta}\right) = \frac{1}{\sum_{i=1}^{S} w_i} \tag{5.12}$$

where S is the total number of trials in the IPD meta-analysis. Model (5.11) reveals that the summary result, $\hat{\theta}$, is simply a weighted average, where the weight of each trial, w_i, is defined by:

$$w_i = \frac{1}{s_i^2} \tag{5.13}$$

The meta-analysis will give more weight to the $\hat{\theta}_i$ from those trials with smallest s_i^2 values (i.e. those trials with more precise treatment effect estimates), which are generally those with the largest numbers of participants or outcome events. An applied example is given in Box 5.4, where model (5.10) is used to summarise the effect of anti-hypertensive treatment on mortality rate, building on the first stage introduced in Box 5.3.

5.3.2 Meta-Analysis Assuming Random Treatment Effects

Usually the assumption of a common treatment effect will be inappropriate, as the true effect of a treatment is likely to vary across trials. This is known as *between-trial heterogeneity* in treatment effect, and it occurs when the distribution of any treatment effect modifiers (i.e. methodological, clinical or participant-level characteristics that influence the magnitude of a treatment's effect) varies across trials included in the IPD meta-analysis. Examples of potential effect modifiers include follow-up length, the dose of the treatment, the type of intervention in the control group (e.g. usual care), trial quality (risk of bias), and participant-level covariates that interact with treatment response.

To allow for between-trial heterogeneity in treatment effect, the θ_i can be made *random*,[89,90] such that the true treatment effects are allowed to be different but assumed to be drawn from a particular distribution, such as a normal distribution.[15] Then, the goal for meta-analysis is to summarise this distribution, for example according to its mean and variance. Extending model (5.10), we can write a meta-analysis model with random treatment effects as follows:[88]

$$\begin{aligned} \hat{\theta}_i &\sim N\left(\theta_i, s_i^2\right) \\ \theta_i &\sim N\left(\theta, \tau^2\right) \end{aligned} \tag{5.14}$$

Box 5.4 Applied example of the second stage of a two-stage IPD meta-analysis for a time-to-event outcome, assuming a common treatment effect. Case study based on an extension of the IPD meta-analysis project of Wang et al.,[46] as described by Crowther et al.[44]

Let us return to the example of Box 5.3, where the first stage had derived unadjusted log hazard ratio estimates and their variances for each of 10 randomised trials examining the effect of anti-hypertensive treatment in regard to all-cause mortality.[44] Using this data, in the second stage we assumed a common treatment effect and so fitted meta-analysis model (5.10) using ML estimation. The summary treatment effect estimate is a hazard ratio of 0.88 (95% CI: 0.79 to 0.98), providing strong evidence that anti-hypertensive treatment reduces the rate of all-cause mortality compared to the control group. There is no observed between-trial heterogeneity in the treatment effect ($\hat{\tau}^2 = 0$, $I^2 = 0\%$), and so results are the same when rather fitting a random treatment effects meta-analysis model. The results are shown on the forest plot below. When repeating the approach after adjustment for pre-defined prognostic factors of age, BMI, SBP, and smoking, the summary results are very similar (hazard ratio of 0.87; 95% CI: 0.78 to 0.97).

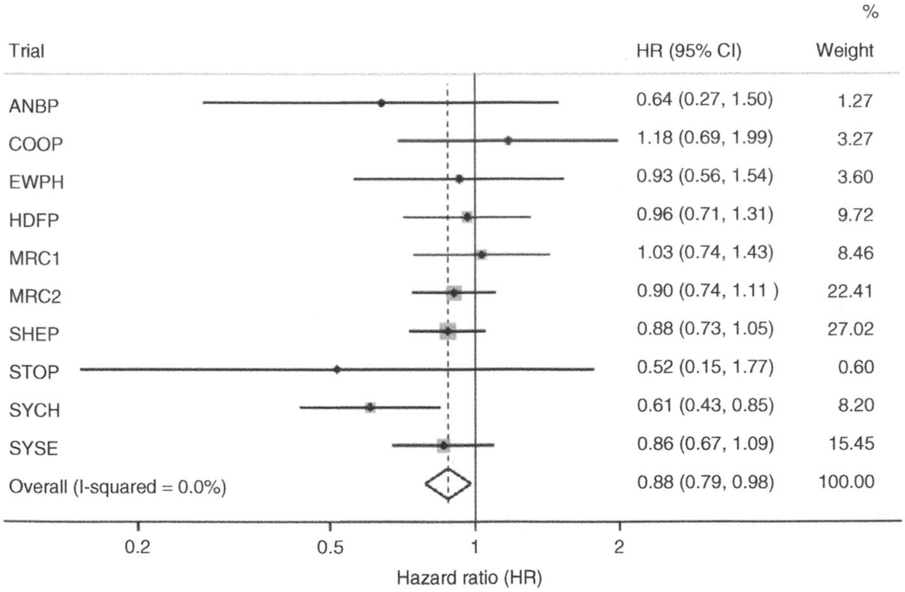

Crowther et al. extended this analysis to show that the hazard ratio may not be constant over time, with anti-hypertensive treatment potentially more effective in the first year after treatment begins. When restricting the length of follow-up to the first year and re-performing the two-stage IPD meta-analysis, the summary hazard ratio is 0.66 (95% CI: 0.52 to 0.85). When considering follow-up information from year one onwards, the summary hazard ratio is 0.93 (95% CI: 0.83 to 1.04).

Sources: Richard Riley; Wang JG, Staessen JA, Franklin SS, et al. Systolic and diastolic blood pressure lowering as determinants of cardiovascular outcome. Hypertension 2005;45(5):907–13 ; Crowther MJ, Riley RD, Staessen JA, et al. Individual patient data meta-analysis of survival data using Poisson regression models. *BMC Med Res Methodol* 2012;12:34.

As for model (5.10), the s_i^2 estimates are assumed to be known. Of key interest is θ, which denotes the mean (average) treatment effect, and τ^2, which denotes the between-trial variance of the true treatment effects. When $\hat{\tau}^2$ equals zero (i.e. there is no observed between-trial heterogeneity in treatment effect), model (5.14) reduces to the common-effect meta-analysis of model (5.10).

Model (5.14) is often loosely termed a *random-effects meta-analysis*; however, it is more explicit to refer to it as a random treatment effects meta-analysis (indeed, in subsequent chapters we introduce IPD meta-analysis models that place random effects on multiple parameters, not just the treatment effect). Usually the main interest is estimating the average treatment effect θ, which we also refer to as the summary treatment effect in this book. Conditional on having an estimate of τ^2, the ML estimation solution for $\hat{\theta}$ is again a weighted average of the treatment effect estimates,

$$\hat{\theta} = \frac{\sum_{i=1}^{S} \hat{\theta}_i w_i^*}{\sum_{i=1}^{S} w_i^*} \tag{5.15}$$

$$\text{var}(\hat{\theta}) = \frac{1}{\sum_{i=1}^{S} w_i^*} \tag{5.16}$$

where S is the total number of trials in the IPD meta-analysis and the weights are:

$$w_i^* = \frac{1}{s_i^2 + \hat{\tau}^2} \tag{5.17}$$

The analytic solution for the summary treatment effect (equation (5.15)) is similar to that when assuming a common treatment effect (equation (5.10)), except each trial's weight (w_i^*) now depends on the sum of two estimated variances: the variance of the trial's treatment effect estimate (s_i^2) and the between-trial variance of treatment effect (τ^2). Hence, τ^2 must also be estimated in order to derive the summary treatment effect estimate ($\hat{\theta}$) when assuming random treatment effects (Section 5.3.6).

Model (5.16) reveals that if the estimate of τ^2 is greater than zero, then the estimated variance of the summary treatment effect will be larger when assuming the true treatment effects are random rather than common. This is intuitive, as heterogeneity in treatment effects reflects unexplained variability in the trial effect estimates beyond chance (i.e. beyond the variances defined by s_i^2), and thus the random treatment effects model accounts for more variability, which leads to wider confidence intervals. In this situation, the w_i^* weights (equation (5.17)) for each trial will be more similar to each other than the w_i weights (equation (5.13)), such that larger and smaller trials will be more equally weighted when assuming random rather than common treatment effects. Some readers may view this as controversial, but it is a consequence of allowing for the heterogeneity in treatment effects, and estimating the average of a distribution of true treatment effects, rather than a single common treatment effect. A more equal weighting is of most concern when smaller trials are at a higher risk of bias, as then the distribution of true treatment effects is potentially distorted by the smaller trials. Sensitivity analyses excluding trials at high risk of bias are important in this situation (Chapter 9).

Box 5.5 gives an applied example where random treatment effects are assumed and so meta-analysis model (5.14) is used to summarise the effect of interventions to reduce excessive weight gain during pregnancy, building on the first-stage analyses described in Box 5.1.

5.3.3 Forest Plots and Percentage Trial Weights

The results from a two-stage IPD meta-analysis can be presented graphically on a forest plot. Examples are shown in Box 5.4 and Box 5.5. A forest plot provides the trial-specific estimates (as boxes) and their confidence intervals (via a horizontal line around the boxes) from the first stage, and the summary meta-analysis result (the centre of a diamond at the base of the plot) and its confidence interval (the width of the diamond). Additional information can also be displayed, such as trial names, number of participants and events, heterogeneity statistics, and percentage weight of each trial. The percentage weights reveal the relative contribution of each trial toward the summary meta-analysis result. This is important for transparency, and especially pertinent when some trials are potential outliers or at high risk of bias. Trial weights are also reflected by the proportional size of each trial's box (i.e. larger boxes can be used to denote trials with more weight). They are easily calculated. In the random treatment effects meta-analysis of model (5.14) the percentage weight of trial i is $100 \times \frac{w_i^*}{\sum_{i=1}^{S} w_i^*}$. For the common treatment effect meta-analysis of model (5.10), the percentage weight of trial i is $100 \times \frac{w_i}{\sum_{i=1}^{S} w_i}$.

5.3.4 Heterogeneity Measures and Statistics

It is also important to report (e.g. within a forest plot or accompanying tables and text) measures that quantify the between-trial heterogeneity of treatment effects. Fundamentally, after fitting model (5.14), the estimate of τ^2 should be reported, as this is a direct measure of the variance of treatment effect across trials. It may be preferable to report $\hat{\tau}$, the estimated between-trial standard deviation of treatment effects, as this is on the same scale as the meta-analysis (i.e. mean difference

Box 5.5 Applied example of the second stage of a two-stage IPD meta-analysis of randomised trials with a continuous outcome, assuming a random treatment effect. Case study based on the IPD meta-analysis project of Rogozinska et al.[16]

Let us return to the example introduced in Box 5.1. Treatment effect estimates derived in the first stage are shown in Table 5.3, as obtained by an analysis of covariance model (i.e. adjusting for baseline weight). In the second stage, we combined these estimates using meta-analysis model (5.14), which assumes the treatment effects are random. The model was fitted using REML estimation (Section 5.3.6), and a 95% confidence interval for the summary effect was derived using the Hartung-Knapp-Sidik-Jonkman (HKSJ) approach (Section 5.3.7).

The results are shown on the following forest plot. The summary treatment effect indicates that, on average across trials, the mean difference in weight gain (after adjusting for baseline weight) is −0.70kg (95% CI: −0.92 to −0.48). This provides strong evidence that the class of interventions reduce weight gain by, on average, 0.70 kg more than control by the last recorded weight before birth. There was heterogeneity in the treatment effects across trials ($\hat{\tau}^2$ =0.059), with an approximate 95% prediction interval of −1.24 to −0.16 for the treatment effect in a new trial. This suggests that the class of interventions are likely to be beneficial in most settings, although the magnitude of effect may vary considerably due to unexplained causes of heterogeneity. The summary results are similar for each sub-type of intervention (diet: −0.72 (95% CI: −1.48 to 0.04); exercise: −0.71 (95% CI: −1.12 to −0.30); mixed approach: −0.68 (95% CI: −1.11 to −0.26)).

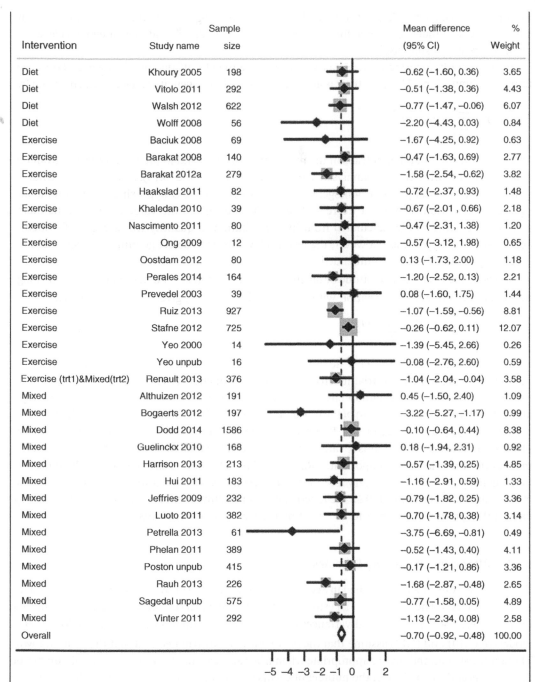

Intervention	Study name	Sample size	Mean difference (95% CI)	% Weight
Diet	Khoury 2005	198	−0.62 (−1.60, 0.36)	3.65
Diet	Vitolo 2011	292	−0.51 (−1.38, 0.36)	4.43
Diet	Walsh 2012	622	−0.77 (−1.47, −0.06)	6.07
Diet	Wolff 2008	56	−2.20 (−4.43, 0.03)	0.84
Exercise	Baciuk 2008	69	−1.67 (−4.25, 0.92)	0.63
Exercise	Barakat 2008	140	−0.47 (−1.63, 0.69)	2.77
Exercise	Barakat 2012a	279	−1.58 (−2.54, −0.62)	3.82
Exercise	Haakslad 2011	82	−0.72 (−2.37, 0.93)	1.48
Exercise	Khaledan 2010	39	−0.67 (−2.01 , 0.66)	2.18
Exercise	Nascimento 2011	80	−0.47 (−2.31, 1.38)	1.20
Exercise	Ong 2009	12	−0.57 (−3.12, 1.98)	0.65
Exercise	Oostdam 2012	80	0.13 (−1.73, 2.00)	1.18
Exercise	Perales 2014	164	−1.20 (−2.52, 0.13)	2.21
Exercise	Prevedel 2003	39	0.08 (−1.60, 1.75)	1.44
Exercise	Ruiz 2013	927	−1.07 (−1.59, −0.56)	8.81
Exercise	Stafne 2012	725	−0.26 (−0.62, 0.11)	12.07
Exercise	Yeo 2000	14	−1.39 (−5.45, 2.66)	0.26
Exercise	Yeo unpub	16	−0.08 (−2.76, 2.60)	0.59
Exercise (trt1)&Mixed(trt2)	Renault 2013	376	−1.04 (−2.04, −0.04)	3.58
Mixed	Althuizen 2012	191	0.45 (−1.50, 2.40)	1.09
Mixed	Bogaerts 2012	197	−3.22 (−5.27, −1.17)	0.99
Mixed	Dodd 2014	1586	−0.10 (−0.64, 0.44)	8.38
Mixed	Guelinckx 2010	168	0.18 (−1.94, 2.31)	0.92
Mixed	Harrison 2013	213	−0.57 (−1.39, 0.25)	4.85
Mixed	Hui 2011	183	−1.16 (−2.91, 0.59)	1.33
Mixed	Jeffries 2009	232	−0.79 (−1.82, 0.25)	3.36
Mixed	Luoto 2011	382	−0.70 (−1.78, 0.38)	3.14
Mixed	Petrella 2013	61	−3.75 (−6.69, −0.81)	0.49
Mixed	Phelan 2011	389	−0.52 (−1.43, 0.40)	4.11
Mixed	Poston unpub	415	−0.17 (−1.21, 0.86)	3.36
Mixed	Rauh 2013	226	−1.68 (−2.87, −0.48)	2.65
Mixed	Sagedal unpub	575	−0.77 (−1.58, 0.05)	4.89
Mixed	Vinter 2011	292	−1.13 (−2.34, 0.08)	2.58
Overall			−0.70 (−0.92, −0.48)	100.00

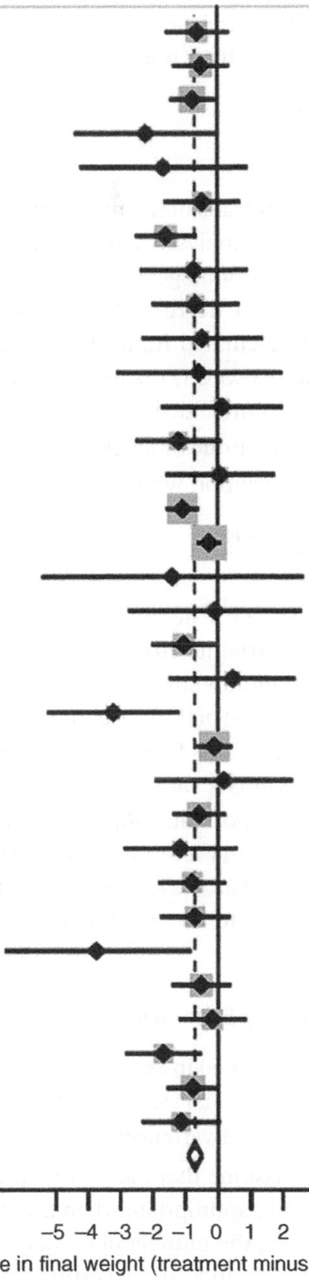

Sources: Richard Riley; Rogozinska E, Marlin N, Jackson L, et al. Effects of antenatal diet and physical activity on maternal and fetal outcomes: individual patient data meta-analysis and health economic evaluation. *Health Technol Assess* 2017;21(41):1–158.

for continuous outcomes, log odds ratio for binary outcomes, log hazard ratio for time-to-event outcomes, etc). A confidence interval for $\hat{\tau}$ might also be calculated,[91–94] and may often be wide, as $\hat{\tau}$ is often imprecisely estimated.[95]

Two commonly reported heterogeneity measures are the Q-statistic and I^2; however, both have important limitations. The Q-statistic is also known as the heterogeneity test statistic, and given by,

$$Q = \sum_{i=1}^{S} w_i \left(\hat{\theta}_i - \hat{\theta}\right)^2$$

where S is the total number of trials in the meta-analysis, and $\hat{\theta}$ and w_i are those obtained from the common treatment effect meta-analysis model (equations (5.11) and (5.13), respectively).[96] Under a null hypothesis assumption of homogeneity of treatment effects, Q approximately follows a chi-squared distribution with $S - 1$ degrees of freedom. Thus, given the value of Q from the meta-analysis, a p-value can be calculated from this distribution to quantify the strength of evidence against the null hypothesis. However, the test has low power to detect genuine between-trial heterogeneity, and so is not recommended.

Alongside the absolute magnitude of heterogeneity ($\hat{\tau}^2$), it can also be helpful to report the magnitude of $\hat{\tau}^2$ relative to the variation within each trial (i.e. the s_i^2) given by the I^2 statistic,

$$I^2 = 100\% \times \frac{(Q - (S - 1))}{Q}$$

with I^2 set to zero if $Q < (S - 1)$. I^2 describes the percentage of variability in treatment effect estimates that is due to between-trial heterogeneity rather than chance. The value of I^2 should not be used to decide between a common-effect or random-effects meta-analysis. Another common mistake is to interpret I^2 as a measure of the (absolute) amount of heterogeneity (i.e. to consider I^2 as an estimate of τ^2). This is dangerous, as I^2 depends on the size of the within-trial variances; for example, if all trials are small and thus s_i^2 values are large, I^2 can be small (i.e. close to 0%) even when the magnitude of τ^2 is large and important.[97] Rather, I^2 should be viewed as a measure of the impact of heterogeneity (τ^2) on the summary treatment effect estimate, with the impact small if I^2 is close to 0% and large if I^2 is close to 100%. The heterogeneity of treatment effects can also be quantified by using a 95% prediction interval for the treatment effect in a new trial (Section 5.3.10).

5.3.5 Alternative Weighting Schemes

The meta-analysis models described in Sections 5.3.1 and 5.3.2 are known as inverse variance meta-analysis methods. They combine trial estimates of treatment effect (i.e. $\hat{\theta}_i$), with weights accounting for the inverse of their estimated variances (i.e. s_i^2). Both the common-effect and random-effects models of (5.10) and (5.14) assume that the $\hat{\theta}_i$ are normally distributed and that the s_i^2 are known. Though these assumptions are appropriate when trials are reasonably large (in terms of number of participants and, if applicable, the number of events), they are more tenuous when trials are small or outcome events are rare;[6,32,33] indeed, trial estimates of treatment effects and their variances may even be biased in such situations.[98]

To address this, other two-stage approaches have been proposed that use a different weighting scheme, such as the Mantel-Haenszel and Peto methods.[99,100] For example, the Peto method combines log odds ratio estimates (derived using an approximate method) using model (5.11),[99] but with w_i equal to the hypergeometric variance of the event count in the treatment group. For time-to-event outcomes, an extension to the Peto method is to calculate log hazard ratio estimates and variances based on the log-rank statistics in each trial, and then apply model (5.11). Simulation results suggest that, compared to the inverse variance method, the Peto method works well when treatment effects are small, event risks are <1%, and when treatment and control group sizes within trials are balanced (i.e. similar numbers allocated to each).[6,32] A key advantage is that it does not require continuity corrections in trials with a zero event in either treatment or control groups. However, this issue can also be addressed by applying a one-stage IPD meta-analysis model (Chapter 6), which is our preference as it can be more easily extended to more complex models, such as including prognostic factors and treatment-covariate interactions (Chapter 7).

5.3.6 Frequentist Estimation of the Between-Trial Variance of Treatment Effect

When assuming random treatment effects, the summary treatment effect estimate of $\hat{\theta}$ (equation (5.15)) depends on $\hat{\tau}^2$, the estimated between-trial variance of the treatment effect. There are various methods available for estimating τ^2, and importantly the choice can impact the meta-analysis results.[101] Traditionally the most popular method of estimating τ^2 is the non-iterative, non-parametric methods of moments estimator of DerSimonian and Laird,[96] due to its speed and availability in non-sophisticated statistical packages, such as RevMan.[102] It also avoids the assumption of normally distributed effects as written in model (5.14), as it simply uses the Q-statistic and the weights (w_i) from the common treatment effect model (5.13). Other non-iterative estimators have been proposed, which have been shown to improve upon DerSimonian and Laird in some - situations.[103,104] Iterative methods are also available,[101,103] including ML and REML estimation, which simultaneously estimate τ^2 and θ until convergence. REML improves upon ML estimation,[13,105,106] as it penalises for the number of parameters being estimated simultaneously, and provides larger (approximately unbiased) between-trial variance estimates, whereas ML tends to produce downwardly biased between-trial variances, especially when the number of trials in the meta-analysis is small.

In a review, Veroniki et al. found 16 different estimation methods for the between-trial variance of treatment effect.[107] Langan et al. conducted a large simulation study to compare many of these methods,[95] and concluded that "the DerSimonian-Laird estimator is negatively biased in scenarios with small trials and in scenarios with a rare binary outcome", and recommend that researchers use REML, as it outperforms other methods and is routinely available in most software packages. Although it assumes normality of the between-trial variance of treatment effects, REML is quite robust to deviations from this assumption.[103] It is also consistent with recommendations to use REML for estimation of one-stage IPD meta-analyses (Chapter 6).[108]

Therefore, generally we recommend REML for fitting meta-analysis models assuming random treatment effects, and this is used when applying model (5.14) in Box 5.4 and Box 5.5. However, it is not perfect; as for other estimation methods, it has poor properties when trial sizes are small or the event of interest is rare. In situations where REML does not converge, the Paule Mandel approach is a viable alternative.[95,109] We agree with Langan et al. that, especially in meta-analyses of few trials, any heterogeneity variance estimate "should not be used as a reliable gauge for the extent of heterogeneity in a meta-analysis".[95]

5.3.7 Deriving Confidence Intervals for the Summary Treatment Effect

After estimation of a two-stage IPD meta-analysis model, confidence intervals can be derived for the summary treatment effect (θ) based on large-sample inference that assumes parameter estimates are approximately normally distributed. For example, following estimation of either models (5.10) or (5.14), a standard ('Wald-based') confidence interval for the summary treatment effect can be calculated using

$$\hat{\theta} \pm z_{1-\frac{\alpha}{2}}\sqrt{\text{var}(\hat{\theta})},$$

where $\hat{\theta}$ is the estimated summary (average) treatment effect, $\text{var}(\hat{\theta})$ is its variance, and $z_{1-\frac{\alpha}{2}}$ is the critical value of the standard normal distribution, which equals 1.96 when α is 0.05 (i.e. a 95% confidence interval is desired). However, this approach does not account for the uncertainty in variance estimates, and so is likely to give confidence intervals that are too narrow.[110] To address this, Hartung and Knapp[111,112] (and also independently Sidik and Jonkman[113]) suggest using a modified confidence interval of:

$$\hat{\theta} \pm t_{S-1,1-\frac{\alpha}{2}}\sqrt{\text{var}_{\text{HKSJ}}(\hat{\theta})}$$

Here, S is the total number of trials in the IPD meta-analysis, $t_{S-1,1-\frac{\alpha}{2}}$ is the critical value of a t-distribution with $S-1$ degrees of freedom, and $\text{var}_{\text{HKSJ}}(\hat{\theta}) = q\,\text{var}(\hat{\theta})$ is the Hartung-Knapp-Sidik-Jonkman (HKSJ) modified estimate of the variance of the summary result, where

$$q = \frac{1}{S-1}\sum_{i=1}^{S} w_i^*\left(\hat{\theta}_i - \hat{\theta}\right)^2$$

and $w_i^* = 1/\left(\text{var}(\hat{\theta}_i) + \hat{\tau}^2\right)$ and $\hat{\tau}^2$ is the estimate of between-trial variance of treatment from the chosen estimation method (e.g. REML). When $\hat{\tau}^2 > 0$, the HKSJ confidence interval will usually be wider than the standard confidence interval because it is based on the t-distribution, which has larger critical values ($t_{S-1,1-\frac{\alpha}{2}}$) than the standard normal distribution ($z_{1-\frac{\alpha}{2}}$). However, if q is less than 1 (as is necessarily the case when the DerSimonian and Laird estimator is used and $\hat{\tau}^2$ is truncated to zero[114]), then the HKSJ interval may be shorter than the standard confidence interval. This contradicts the premise of the approach, which is to widen confidence intervals to account for additional uncertainty. There are a variety of potential options to address this,[115] including the suggestion of Rover et al. to set $q = 1$ if the above model gives $q < 1$,[116] or only using the HKSJ correction when τ^2 is estimated greater than zero.[115] Another cautious option, but less conservative than the first of these suggestions, is to derive confidence intervals based on both the standard method and the HKSJ method, and then select the confidence interval which is widest (or even present both). This was suggested by Van Aert and Jackson,[117] on the grounds that it is equivalent to using a less severe constraint than ensuring $q \geq 1$, and we also advocate this.

Many other approaches to confidence interval derivation have been proposed.[118–120] Partlett and Riley compared many of the available options in a simulation study, and conclude that the HKSJ method performs well in terms of coverage of 95% confidence intervals across a wide range of scenarios and outperforms other methods (including the aforementioned Rover modified method), especially when heterogeneity was large and/or trial sizes were similar. In particular, the standard confidence interval approach has coverage considerably less than 90% when the number of trials is five or fewer. Other simulations give similar conclusions,[95,121] and show that the HKSJ method performs well regardless of the method used to estimate the between-trial variance of treatment effect.[95] However, the coverage of the HKSJ method is slightly too low when the heterogeneity is small relative to the average within-trial variance ($I^2 < 30\%$) and the trial sizes are quite varied.[122]

In summary, we generally recommend taking the HKSJ approach for deriving confidence intervals for the summary treatment effect following estimation of the random-effects meta-analysis model (5.14); however, if the standard method for deriving confidence intervals gives a wider interval than the HKSJ approach, then the standard confidence interval should (also) be presented.[117]

5.3.8 Bayesian Estimation Approaches

5.3.8.1 An Introduction to Bayes' Theorem and Bayesian Inference

Meta-Analysis models, including those of models (5.10) and (5.14), can be fitted using a Bayesian framework. Bayesian statistics is based on a publication by Thomas Bayes,[123] which introduced what is now known as Bayes' theorem. Given some data and an unknown parameter θ (e.g. a treatment effect), Bayes' theorem can be expressed mathematically as

$$p(\theta|\text{data}) = \frac{p(\text{data}|\theta)\; p(\theta)}{p(\text{data})}$$

where $p(\theta|\text{ data})$ is the *posterior probability distribution* of θ given the data, and $p(\theta)$ is the *prior probability* distribution of θ. Furthermore, $p(\text{data}|\;\theta)$ is the probability (or *likelihood*) of the data given parameter θ, which is the basis of frequentist statistical inference (such as ML estimation). Finally, $p(\text{data})$ is the overall probability of the observed data occurring. As $p(\text{data})$ is a constant, Bayes' theorem can also be expressed just in terms of those components including θ:

$$p(\theta|\text{data}) \propto p(\text{data}|\theta)\; p(\theta)$$

Bayes' theorem is an uncontroversial mathematical result about conditional probabilities. However, it is the use of this result to make probabilistic inferences about θ that creates tensions with the frequentist estimation approach described so far in this chapter. Given the data, the frequentist approach makes inferences about the value of θ from the likelihood, $p(\theta \mid \text{data})$, using an argument: how plausible are the data given different values of θ? For example, with ML or REML estimation, the value of θ that is most plausible for the observed data becomes the estimated value ($\hat{\theta}$).

However, the Bayesian approach is to make inferences about θ from the posterior distribution, $p(\theta|\text{data})$, which takes into account both the data and the prior beliefs about θ. This allows θ to be summarised according to its posterior distribution; for example, the mean and variance could be reported. Moreover, direct probability statements about θ can be made, such as the probability that θ is in the direction of a beneficial treatment effect (e.g. probability $\theta < 0$ when θ is a log odds ratio and the outcome is adverse), or the probability that θ is greater than some clinically relevant amount (e.g. $\exp(\theta) < 0.8$, such that the odds of an adverse outcome event are reduced by at least 20%). These can be calculated by the proportion of the posterior distribution for θ that falls below (or above) the value of interest. We can also derive a 95% probability (or so-called *credibility* or *credible*) interval for θ, giving a range within which there is a 95% probability the true value of θ lies. For all these reasons, the Bayesian approach is highly appealing, and has become the standard analysis method for clinical decision making (e.g. within reports conducted by the National Institute for Clinical Excellence (NICE)).

5.3.8.2 Using a Bayesian Meta-Analysis Model in the Second Stage

In the second stage of the two-stage IPD meta-analysis, a Bayesian approach to meta-analysis can be used. This has a likelihood defined by model (5.10) or model (5.14), when assuming common or random treatment effects, respectively. In addition, prior distributions are required for the unknown model parameters, such as τ^2 and θ in model (5.14). Where no (reliable) prior information exists, non-informative prior distributions should be chosen so that the posterior distribution is mainly driven by the likelihood (i.e. the meta-analysis data).[124,125] For example, using a prior distribution such as $\theta \sim N(0, 1000000)$ indicates vague prior information about the summary treatment effect. A realistically vague prior distribution may be preferred, such that the distribution reflects only plausible values of the treatment. For example, odds ratios, risk ratios or hazard ratios below 0.1 are rare for treatment effects, and so assuming θ (i.e. log odds ratio, log risk ratio or log hazard ratios) has a prior distribution of $N(0,100)$ already allows for extreme treatment effects, such that a variance of 100 is more sensible than 1000000.

Although non-informative prior distributions for the treatment effect parameter(s) can usually be selected, the choice of prior distributions for dispersion parameters (such as the between-trial variance) is more problematic and they tend to be quite informative, especially when the number of trials is limited. Consider, for instance, a prior $\tau \sim \text{uniform}(0,100)$ for a binary outcome; this puts a lot of density mass to extreme values, and so a more realistic vague prior distribution (e.g. $\tau \sim \text{uniform}(0,5)$) might be considered.[126] However, in meta-analyses with small numbers of trials (such as 10 or less), even realistically vague prior distributions for τ may be informative.[127]

To address this, Turner et al. and Rhodes et al. derived informative prior distributions for τ^2 for a range of different clinical settings with binary or continuous outcome types, respectively, based on empirical evidence of the estimated value of τ^2 in Cochrane reviews of intervention effects.[128–130] For example, for the clinical setting of Box 5.2, where non-pharmacological interventions are compared to control in regards to the odds of adverse maternal outcome events in pregnancy, Turner et al. suggest using $\tau^2 \sim \text{log-normal}(-2.89, 1.91^2)$. Thus the corresponding Bayesian framework for model (5.14) can be written as:

$$
\begin{aligned}
&\text{Likelihood:} && \hat{\theta}_i \sim N(\theta_i, s_i^2) \\
& && \theta_i \sim N(\theta, \tau^2) \\
&\text{Prior distributions:} && \tau^2 \sim \text{log-normal}(-2.89, 1.91^2) \\
& && \theta \sim N(0, 1000000)
\end{aligned}
\qquad (5.18)
$$

Such Bayesian meta-analysis models can be fitted within specialist software such as WinBUGS, JAGS, OpenBUGS, or Stan, and also more general statistical software such as R, Stata, SAS and MLwiN, and packages therein (e.g. *bayesmeta* in R). The estimation typically utilises a Markov Chain Monte Carlo (MCMC) procedure (such as Gibbs sampling) that, after a burn-in procedure (e.g. 100,000) and convergence checks, draws samples (e.g. 100,000) directly from the joint posterior distribution of parameters to make subsequent inferences. Where empirical evidence for the choice of prior distributions for τ^2 is lacking, it is important to assess the sensitivity of meta-analysis results to the choice of prior distribution for τ^2 using a range of different prior distributions.[131] The use of an inverse gamma prior distribution is best avoided, as it is can be extremely influential.[132]

The posterior distribution for each parameter in the meta-analysis (e.g. θ) naturally accounts for the uncertainty of other parameters (e.g. τ^2); thus there is no need for post-estimation corrections when deriving credible intervals for θ, unlike when deriving confidence intervals following frequentist estimation (Section 5.3.7). However, it should be noted that model (5.18) still assumes that s_i^2 are known, and so not all uncertainty is being accounted for. This might be addressed by also putting a distribution on the s_i^2, perhaps on the log scale.[133]

5.3.8.3 Applied Example

Using WinBUGS, we applied the Bayesian random treatment effects meta-analysis model (5.18) within the second stage of the two-stage IPD meta-analysis introduced in Box 5.2, examining interventions to reduce gestational weight gain. Following a suitable burn-in of 100,000 samples, posterior inferences were based on a further 100000 samples. The posterior distributions for τ^2 and θ are shown in Figure 5.1. The mean (median) of the posterior distribution for τ^2 is 0.025 (0.017), with a 95% credible interval for τ^2 of 0 to 0.096. The mean of the posterior distribution for the summary odds ratio ($\exp(\theta)$) is 0.91, with a 95% credible interval of 0.79 to 1.02. When using a frequentist approach with REML estimation (and HKSJ confidence interval derivation), the estimate of τ^2 is 0.014, and the summary odds ratio is 0.91 (95% CI: 0.80 to 1.04). These results are very similar to those from the Bayesian approach, which is perhaps not surprising given there are 23 trials, and so the posterior distribution is dominated by the likelihood (i.e. the IPD meta-analysis data), and the influence of the prior distributions is small.

However, unlike the frequentist approach, the Bayesian analysis allows us to make direct probability statements about the parameters of interest, which may better inform clinical decision making. For example, there is a large probability of 0.949 that the class of interventions (diet, exercise, mixed) are, on average, effective at reducing the odds of adverse maternal outcome events compared to control (i.e. $\text{prob}(\exp(\theta) < 1) = 0.949$). However, there is a probability of only 0.44 that the summary odds ratio is less than 0.90. Hence, if a reduction in odds of adverse maternal outcome events by at least 10% compared to control is deemed important (e.g. in terms of clinical benefit or for adequate cost effectiveness), there is just a 44% chance the interventions achieve this.

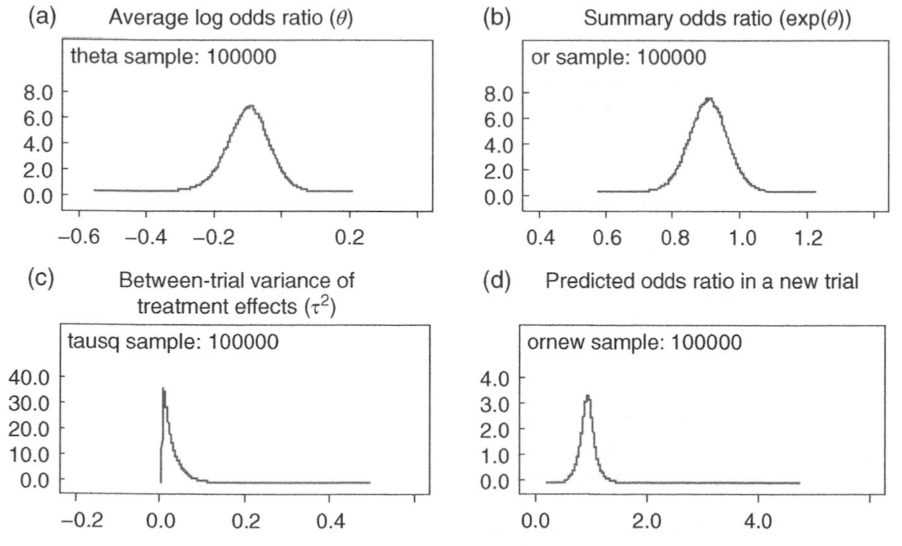

Figure 5.1 Posterior distributions after applying a Bayesian random treatment effects meta-analysis model (model (5.18)) in the second stage of the two-stage IPD meta-analysis introduced in Box 5.2, to examine the effect of interventions to reduce the odds of adverse maternal outcomes during pregnancy. Case study is based on data extracted from the IPD meta-analysis report of Rogozinska et al.[16] *Sources:* Richard Riley; Rogozinska E, Marlin N, Jackson L, et al. Effects of antenatal diet and physical activity on maternal and fetal outcomes: individual patient data meta-analysis and health economic evaluation. *Health Technol Assess* 2017;21 (41):1–158.

5.3.9 Interpretation of Summary Effects from Meta-Analysis

The interpretation of the summary treatment effect should change according to whether common or random treatment effects are assumed.[90,134] We illustrate this using two hypothetical IPD meta-analyses (Example 1 and Example 2 in Figure 5.2), modified from Riley et al.[134] In each meta-analysis, treatment effect estimates (standardised mean differences) are computed in the first stage from 10 trials, and then synthesised using a meta-analysis model in the second stage. Negative treatment effect estimates indicate a greater blood pressure reduction for participants in the treatment group than the control group. Example 1 evaluates treatment A and Example 2 evaluates treatment B; the sets of trials are different, but their settings and populations can be assumed similar. The two meta-analyses give identical summary treatment effect estimates of −0.33 with a standard 95% confidence interval of −0.48 to −0.18. Therefore, a naïve interpretation is that the clinical conclusions about the two treatments should be the same; however, this is incorrect.

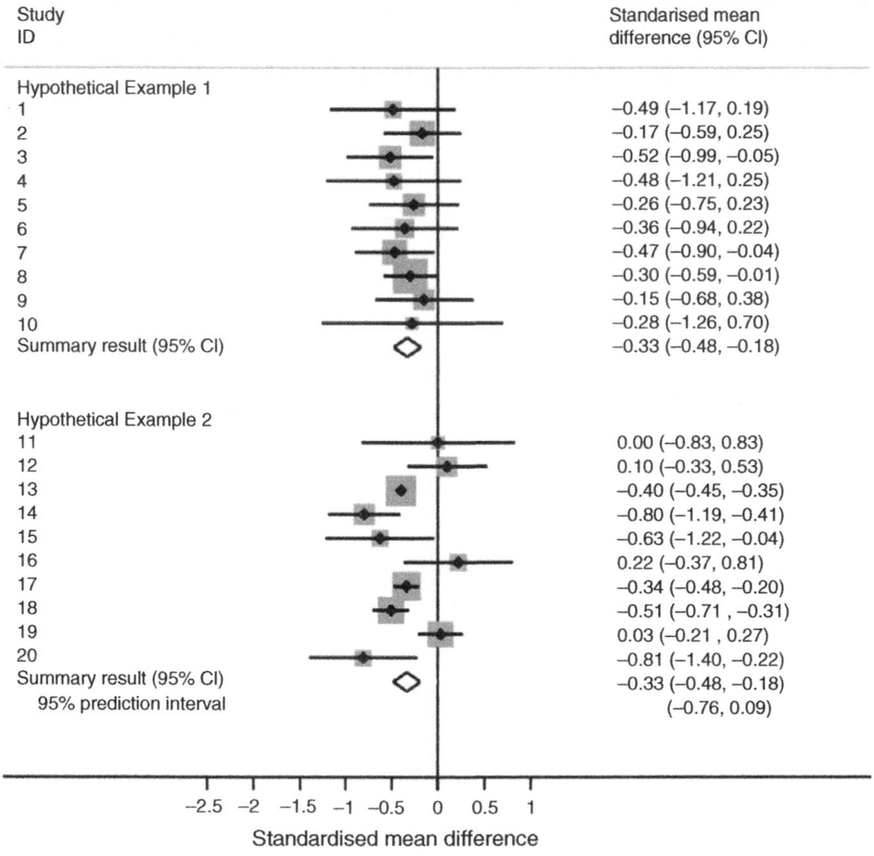

Figure 5.2 Forest plots of two hypothetical meta-analyses that give the same summary estimate (centre of the diamond) and its 95% confidence interval (width of the diamond). Example 1 has no observed between-trial heterogeneity in treatment effect, whereas Example 2 has large heterogeneity. A common treatment effect meta-analysis model is used for Example 1 model (5.10), and a random treatment effects meta-analysis model for Example 2 model (5.14). *Sources:* Richard Riley; figure is adapted from that shown in Figure 1 of Riley et al.[134]

In Example 1 the researchers decided to assume a common treatment effect. There is no observed between-trial heterogeneity in the true treatment effect ($\hat{\tau}^2 = 0$), which is reflected by a narrow scatter of treatment effect estimates across trials, with large overlap in their confidence intervals. Thus, the summary result of −0.33 provides the best estimate of the assumed common treatment effect, and the 95% confidence interval of −0.48 to −0.18 depicts the uncertainty around this estimate. As the confidence interval is all well below zero, there is strong evidence that the treatment is more effective than control.

In Example 2 the researchers decided to assume random treatment effects. There is observed heterogeneity in the treatment effect ($\hat{\tau}^2 > 0$), which is reflected by a wide scatter of treatment effect estimates across trials, with little overlap in their confidence intervals (in contrast to Example 1). Here, the summary result of −0.33 provides an estimate of the *average* treatment effect. The 95% confidence interval of −0.48 to −0.18 depicts the uncertainty around this average treatment effect estimate. As the confidence interval is all well below zero, there is strong evidence that on *average* the treatment effect is beneficial.

Hence, despite having identical summary results, Examples 1 and 2 lead to different interpretations. Based on the observed evidence, the effect of treatment A is likely to be the same in the populations and settings covered by the trials in the meta-analysis of Example 1. In contrast, the observed evidence suggests that the effect of treatment B may vary considerably across the populations and settings covered by the trials in the meta-analysis of Example 2. This clarification is not immediately evident from the summary results themselves and highlights the need for researchers to quantify the impact of heterogeneity, for example using prediction intervals, as now described.[90]

5.3.10 Prediction Interval for the Treatment Effect in a New Trial

> *"Predictive distributions are potentially the most relevant and complete statistical inferences to be drawn from random-effects meta-analyses."*[90]

After fitting a random treatment effects meta-analysis model (such as models (5.14) and (5.18)) and summarising the average effect (θ) and its confidence (credible) interval, Higgins et al. suggest to also provide a prediction interval for the effect of treatment when it is applied in a new trial.[90] The idea is to reveal the potential treatment effect in a single clinical population or setting, which may be considerably different from the average. In other words, the average effect is an incomplete summary of the distribution of treatment effects, and the prediction interval aims to address this in a more interpretable way than simply reporting $\hat{\tau}^2$ or I^2.[134]

Following frequentist estimation of model (5.14) and assuming the treatment effects are normally distributed across trials, Higgins et al. propose that an approximate prediction interval can be calculated using[90]

$$\hat{\theta} \pm t_{S-2,1-\frac{\alpha}{2}} \sqrt{\hat{\tau}^2 + \text{var}(\hat{\theta})} \tag{5.19}$$

where $\text{var}(\hat{\theta})$ is the estimated variance of the summary treatment effect (equation (5.16)), S is the total number of trials in the IPD meta-analysis, and $t_{S-2,1-\frac{\alpha}{2}}$ is the critical value of the t-distribution with $S-2$ degrees of freedom, with α usually chosen as 0.05 to give a 95% prediction interval. As for the aforementioned HKSJ method for deriving confidence intervals, a t-distribution (rather than normal distribution) is used to account for uncertainty in variance estimates.

Consider Example 2 in Figure 5.2, for which the 95% prediction interval is calculated as −0.76 to 0.09. Although most of this interval is below zero, indicating the treatment will be beneficial in the majority of settings, the interval overlaps zero and so in some settings the treatment effect may be small or even slightly harmful. This finding was masked when just focusing on the average effect estimate and its confidence interval. Another example is given in Box 5.5, where there is heterogeneity in the treatment effects across trials ($\hat{\tau}^2$=0.059), and the approximate 95% prediction interval is −1.24 to −0.16. This reveals that the class of interventions are likely to be beneficial in most settings, although the magnitude of effect may vary considerably due to unexplained causes of heterogeneity.

A posterior distribution for the treatment effect in a new trial can be derived naturally following a Bayesian analysis such as model (5.18); this is also known as a predictive distribution. An example is shown in Figure 5.1(d), and it can used to make probabilistic statements. In the example of Figure 5.1(d), there is a probability of 0.77 that the odds ratio in a new trial will be less than 1 (i.e. that the intervention will be effective), and a probability of 0.46 it will be less than 0.9.

When the meta-analysis contains a small number of trials, the prediction interval will often be very wide, especially due to large uncertainty in the estimate of between-trial standard deviation. Also, a prediction interval will be most appropriate when the trials included in the meta-analysis have a low risk of bias; otherwise, it will encompass heterogeneity in treatment effects caused by these biases, in addition to that caused by genuine clinical differences. Another concern is that the closed form solution in (5.19) is only approximate, with the use of a t-distribution with $S-2$ degrees of freedom open to debate. When evaluated in a simulation study, the coverage of this prediction interval was adequate in settings with $I^2 > 30\%$ and similar trial sizes given at least five trials in the meta-analysis;[122] however, in other situations, and especially when heterogeneity is low and the trial sizes are quite varied, the coverage was far too low.

A further issue is that the prediction interval will be extremely sensitive to the assumption that true treatment effects are normally distributed across trials;[135] there is no reason why this should generally be correct.[15] To help address this, recent work has proposed alternative approaches to deriving prediction intervals, by using bootstrapping or non-parametric methods that avoid assuming a particular distribution of the true treatment effects across trials.[136,137] These appear to improve coverage performance. We anticipate further developments and comparisons to identify the best approach in the coming years.

5.4 Meta-regression and Subgroup Analyses

Sometimes meta-analysis results may be of interest for subgroups of trials defined by characteristics of the trial (and not participant-level characteristics). Trial characteristics are consistent for participants in the same trial, but may vary across trials, such as country of investigation, risk of bias classification, or the control (usual care) group type. Subgroup results can be obtained by performing a separate meta-analysis for each subgroup, and an example is shown in Box 5.6. A meta-analysis of subgroup results may yield summary estimates that are less prone to between-trial heterogeneity than the full meta-analysis (i.e. that which includes all subgroups of trials), if the subgrouping factor is associated with the magnitude of treatment effect.

Where interest lies in the actual difference in treatment effects between subgroups defined by trial characteristics, then a meta-regression can be used.[138] This extends the random treatment effects meta-analysis model (5.14) by including trial-level covariates that define the subgroups.

Box 5.6 Applied example of the second stage of a two-stage IPD meta-analysis for a binary outcome, including a meta-regression. Case study based on the IPD meta-analysis project of Rogozinska et al.[16]

The International Weight Management in Pregnancy (i-WIP) Collaborative Group (Box 5.2) undertook an IPD meta-analysis of 24 trials (8852 women, 3733 adverse maternal events) to evaluate the effect of interventions to reduce weight gain during pregnancy on composite adverse maternal outcome. The first stage produced 24 unadjusted log odds ratio estimates ($\hat{\theta}_i$) and their variances ($\text{var}(\hat{\theta}_i) = s_i^2$). The second stage combined these treatment effect estimates using meta-analysis model (5.14), which allowed treatment effects to be random. The model was fitted using REML estimation, and a 95% confidence interval for the summary effect was derived using the HKSJ approach.

The reported summary odds ratio is 0.90 (95% CI: 0.79 to 1.03), which provides some evidence of a slight reduction, on average, in the odds of adverse maternal outcome events in the intervention group compared to the control group. However, there was between-trial heterogeneity in the treatment effects ($\hat{\tau}_1^2$=0.017), with an approximate 95% prediction interval of 0.68 to 1.20 for the treatment effect in a new trial. This suggests there is considerable uncertainty about how the intervention will modify the odds of composite maternal outcome events in a new trial. When the analysis was repeated, additionally adjusting for the prognostic factor of age in the first stage, the summary results for the adjusted treatment effect were very similar to those for the unadjusted treatment effect.

Summary results were somewhat different for each intervention sub-type (diet: 0.60 (95% CI: 0.20 to 1.75); exercise: 0.81 (95% CI: 0.61 to 1.09); mixed approach: 0.97 (95% CI: 0.84 to 1.12)). To examine this formally, the following meta-regression model was fitted:

$$\hat{\theta}_i \sim N(\theta_i, s_i^2)$$
$$\theta_i \sim N(\alpha + \gamma_1 \text{EXERCISE}_i + \gamma_2 \text{MIXED}_i, \tau^2)$$

where EXERCISE is 1 for trials having an exercise (physical activity) intervention type, and 0 otherwise; and MIXED is 1 for trials having a mixed (i.e. exercise and diet) intervention type. After REML estimation, this gave parameter estimates of $\hat{\alpha} = -0.525$, $\hat{\gamma}_1 = 0.332$, and $\hat{\gamma}_2 = 0.491$. The estimated heterogeneity in treatment effect was smaller ($\hat{\tau}_1^2$=0.011) in this meta-regression than in the original meta-analysis ($\hat{\tau}_1^2$=0.015) without the intervention type covariates. However, there was insufficient evidence to conclude that summary treatment effects differed by intervention type. The ratio of odds ratios (i.e. ratio of treatment effects) for exercise and diet was exp(0.315) = 1.37 (95 % CI : 0.73 to 2.57), and for mixed and diet was exp(0.496) = 1.64 (95 % CI : 0.91 to 2.97). The wide confidence intervals highlight considerable uncertainty and the need for further research. Indeed, this particular meta-regression is a simple network meta-analysis (Chapter 14), and comparisons of the intervention sub-types are all based on indirect evidence (i.e. across trials rather than within trials).

Sources: Richard Riley; Rogozinska E, Marlin N, Jackson L, et al. Effects of antenatal diet and physical activity on maternal and fetal outcomes: individual patient data meta-analysis and health economic evaluation. *Health Technol Assess* 2017;21(41):1–158.

For example, a covariate, z_i, might be included to represent country, risk of bias, or control group type in trial i. Such a meta-regression can be written as follows:

$$\hat{\theta}_i \sim N\left(\theta_i, s_i^2\right)$$
$$\theta_i \sim N\left(\alpha + \gamma z_i, \tau^2\right) \tag{5.20}$$

As previously, parameters can be estimated using REML (with subsequent confidence intervals derived using the HKSJ approach) or a suitable Bayesian approach. Here, α represents the summary treatment effect in a trial where $z_i = 0$, and γ represents the change in the summary treatment effect for a one-unit increase in z_i. Also, τ^2 is the heterogeneity in treatment effect that remains unexplained after inclusion of z_i. An example is given in Box 5.6.

In general, meta-regression results should be viewed with great caution.[139] Firstly, with few trials (e.g. < 10), meta-regression suffers from low power to detect trial-level characteristics that are genuinely associated with changes in the overall treatment effect in a trial. Secondly, confounding across trials is likely, and so making causal statements about the impact of trial-level covariates is best avoided. For example, those trials with a higher risk of bias may also have the highest dose or be conducted in particular countries, thus making it hard to disentangle the effect of risk of bias from the effect of dose and country. Thirdly, the trial-level association of aggregated participant-level covariates (e.g. mean age, proportion male, mean biomarker value, etc) with overall treatment should not be used to make inferences about how values of participant-level covariates (e.g. age, sex, biomarker values) interact with treatment effect. Aggregation bias may lead to dramatic differences in observed relationships at the trial-level from those at the participant-level. Chapter 7 describes this issue in detail.

5.5 The *ipdmetan* Software Package

As for any statistical analysis, researchers should keep a full and annotated analysis script for their IPD meta-analyses, so that findings can be replicated quickly and transparently. The flagship package for conducting a two-stage IPD meta-analysis is *ipdmetan*, developed by Fisher for the Stata software package.[119] This package automates the calculation of trial-specific aggregate data (e.g. treatment effect estimates and their variances) from the first stage, and then produces summary meta-analysis results and a forest plot from the second stage. The package is applicable to IPD meta-analyses aiming to summarise a particular effect of interest defined by a single parameter in a regression model (such as a treatment effect, or another measure that can be estimated in a regression model, such as a prognostic effect or a treatment-covariate interaction).

To implement *ipdmetan*, IPD from all trials should be collated in a single dataset including a column identifying the trial in which each participant was included (an example is given in Box 1.1(a)). The user then specifies the trial identification variable, which regression model to use in the first stage (calling standard regression packages in Stata such as *reg*, *logit*, or *stcox*), and which meta-analysis model and estimation method(s) to use in the second stage. The package then fits a regression model to the IPD from each trial separately and stores the derived results (aggregate data) for each trial, which are then immediately used to fit a chosen meta-analysis model in the second stage. A wide variety of model and estimation options are available for the second stage, including common or random treatment effects, REML estimation, HKSJ confidence intervals and tailored

Box 5.7 Example of using Fisher's *ipdmetan* package within Stata.[119]

For the time-to-event outcome example of Box 5.4, after opening the IPD meta-analysis dataset, the following syntax was used to implement the *ipdmetan* package:

```
ipdmetan, study(trial) re(reml, hksj) forest(xtitle(hazard ratio) boxsca(30) xlab(0.2 0.5 1 2)
astext(40))  hr effect(HR) : stcox treat smk sbpi age bmi
```

The terms in the syntax are explained below:

- *study(trial)* denotes that the column called 'trial' in the dataset is the trial identification covariate
- *re(reml hksj)* denotes that the random treatment effects model (5.14) is to be fitted using REML estimation, with 95% confidence interval derived using the HKSJ method
- *forest()* includes various options for tailoring the display of the forest plot, including the size of the boxes around the trial treatment effect estimates (boxsca()), the title of the x-axis (xtitle), the values of the hazard ratio to be displayed in the x-axis (xlab()), and relative size of the text on the forest plot (astext())
- *hr* denotes that results should be displayed on the hazard ratio scale (and not the log hazard ratio scale)
- *effect(HR)* denotes that HR should be displayed above the column of trial treatment effect estimates on the right-hand side of the plot.
- The syntax after the colon denotes the method to use in the first stage to each trial separately
- *stcox treat* denotes that a Cox regression model should be fitted in each trial separately, with the treatment variable (column called 'treat' containing a value of 1 for participants in the treatment group and 0 for participants in the control group) included alongside prognostic factors of smoking ('smk'), SBP ('sbpi'), age ('age') and BMI ('bmi'). Unless told otherwise (using the *poolvar()* option before the colon), *ipdmetan* will produce meta-analysis results for the first covariate listed within the regression statement.

There are many other options are available for *ipdmetan*, and the package will be updated over time. Type 'help ipdmetan' for a comprehensive guide.

Sources: Richard Riley; Based on Fisher DJ. Two-stage individual participant data meta-analysis and generalized forest plots. *Stata Journal* 2015;15(2):369–96.

display of forest plots. An example is provided in Box 5.7. The package can be installed from within Stata, simply by typing 'ssc install ipdmetan', and then 'help ipdmetan' gives a detailed help file and range of examples.

Other meta-analysis packages may also be useful. In particular, researchers could take the dataset of treatment effect estimates and variances obtained from the first stage, and use another package to fit their meta-analysis (or meta-regression) model in the second stage. For example, available packages in Stata include *meta*, *metan*, *metaan* and *metareg*. In R, suitable packages include the exceptional *metafor*,[140] and also *rmeta* and *metaplus*, among others. Bayesian software options were mentioned previously.

Our website (www.ipdma.co.uk) provides examples of statistical code for various case studies used in this chapter.

5.6 Combining IPD with Aggregate Data from non-IPD Trials

Some eligible trials for the IPD meta-analysis project may not agree to provide their IPD. However, if suitable aggregate data (such as treatment effect estimates and their variances) can be extracted from publications or provided by trial investigators, this aggregate data can be included in the second stage of the two-stage meta-analysis. This process can be implemented as follows:

- *First stage*: The required aggregate data are either (i) calculated directly in each IPD trial using the IPD provided, or (ii) sought from publications and trial investigators for each trial not provided IPD.
- *Second stage*: Aggregate data obtained for the IPD trials and non-IPD trials are combined in a meta-analysis such as model (5.14).

The summary results can then be compared to those derived from the IPD-only meta-analysis, which should still be considered the main analysis. A detailed example of combining IPD and aggregate data in this way is provided in Chapter 9. The approach can be implemented within the *ipdmetan* package.[119] Specifically, the ad() option allows the user to call a separate file of aggregate data results for non-IPD trials, which is utilised in the second stage alongside the aggregate data derived for IPD trials by *ipdmetan* in the first stage.

The combination of IPD (from IPD trials) and aggregate data (from non-IPD trials) is best viewed as a sensitivity analysis, to ascertain if conclusions from the main IPD-only analysis are likely to be robust to the exclusion of non-IPD trials. Differences in IPD and non-IPD trials should be carefully investigated,[141,142] especially if inclusion of aggregate data from non-IPD trials appears to change or weaken conclusions. Combining IPD and non-IPD trials allows more evidence to be incorporated, and thus may reduce issues such as publication bias and data availability bias (Chapter 9). However, a major concern is that the aggregate data from non-IPD trials is not subject to the same data checking and quality standards as that from IPD trials (Chapter 4). Similarly, non-IPD trials cannot be standardised (e.g. in terms of inclusion/exclusion criteria, analysis methods, length of follow-up, adjustment for prognostic factors, etc) to the same extent of IPD trials. Hence, researchers must recognise that incorporation of non-IPD trials may lead to more heterogeneity in the meta-analysis, and less reliable or interpretable summary results than an IPD-only analysis. There may also be a lack of suitable aggregate data available for the non-IPD trials. All these reasons may simply reinforce why IPD were desired in the first place.

Occasionally, the available aggregate data for a trial might allow the missing IPD to be partially recovered; that is, IPD might be generated to match summary characteristics of a dataset in terms of the number of participants in each group, the mean outcome value or numbers of events in each group, and the distribution of some baseline covariates (prognostic factors).[8,17,143–145] The latter is the most challenging, as it requires information about the multivariate distribution of baseline covariates and outcome values, including their correlation and marginal moments such as means and variances,[143,144] which will not usually be readily available from publications. Nevertheless, if a trial investigator is prevented from sharing their IPD (for whatever reason), they might still be willing to provide details of this multivariate distribution so that a simulated version of their IPD could be utilised by the IPD meta-analysis researchers.[144] Further discussion on generating IPD is given in Section 6.4.1.

5.7 Concluding Remarks

Large proportions of IPD meta-analysis protocols and publications mention using a two-stage approach for their statistical analysis. As it utilises conventional statistical methods in each stage, the approach can be used for a wide variety of outcome types and is immediately accessible for statisticians and others with statistical expertise. Researchers can implement the approach easily via the *ipdmetan* package in Stata, and although this chapter focused on summarising treatment effects, it is also applicable to other types of IPD meta-analysis projects, such as those summarising prognostic effects or prediction model performance (Chapters 16 and 17). A potential concern, however, is that the second stage of the approach assumes treatment effect estimates in each trial are normally distributed and that their variances are known; this may be problematic when most trials in the meta-analysis are small (in terms of number of participants and/or events), and motivates rather using the one-stage approach described in the next chapter.

6

The One-stage Approach to IPD Meta-Analysis

Richard D. Riley and Thomas P.A. Debray

Summary Points

- A one-stage approach to IPD meta-analysis analyses the IPD from all trials altogether in a single statistical analysis. This typically requires a generalised linear mixed model (GLMM) or a hierarchical survival (frailty) model, which extend standard models (such as linear, logistic, Poisson and Cox) used in a single trial setting.
- A one-stage IPD meta-analysis utilises a more exact statistical likelihood than a two-stage meta-analysis approach, which is advantageous when included trials have few participants or outcome events.
- One-stage IPD meta-analysis models usually include multiple parameters and these are estimated simultaneously. For each parameter (such as the intercept, treatment effect, residual variances) the analyst must specify whether they are *common* (the same in each trial), *stratified* (different in each trial) or *random* (different in each trial and assumed drawn from a particular distribution).
- Clustering of participants within trials must be accounted for (e.g. using a stratified trial intercept or random trial intercepts for GLMMs), as otherwise summary meta-analysis results may be biased or overly precise. A stratified trial intercept is generally preferred, unless there are computational concerns. The use of random trial intercepts allows information about baseline risk to be shared across trials, which may compromise randomisation within each trial.
- Restricted maximum likelihood (REML) estimation is recommended for one-stage models with continuous outcomes, with confidence intervals derived using the approach of Kenward-Roger or Satterthwaite. For binary outcomes, unless most included trials have sparse numbers of events, REML estimation of a pseudo-likelihood is recommended.
- Where REML or a pseudo-likelihood is not available or not appropriate, maximum likelihood estimation of a one-stage model with a stratified intercept can be improved by trial-specific centering of the treatment variable, and by deriving confidence intervals using the t-distribution.
- Bayesian estimation of one-stage models is an appealing alternative to frequentist estimation methods, especially to enable direct probabilistic statements.
- The one-stage modelling framework can be extended to accomodate non-proportional hazards, trials with different designs and inclusion of aggregate data from non-IPD trials.
- Researchers must pre-specify and report their one-stage model specification and assumptions.

Individual Participant Data Meta-Analysis: A Handbook for Healthcare Research, First Edition.
Edited by Richard D. Riley, Jayne F. Tierney, and Lesley A. Stewart.

6.1 Introduction

"The last ten years have seen substantial changes in how IPD meta-analyses are performed, particularly with the growth of the use of one-stage regression models."[146]

An alternative to a two-stage IPD meta-analysis is a one-stage approach, which analyses the IPD from all trials altogether in a single step. This requires a hierarchical (multilevel) regression model, appropriate to the type of outcome data being synthesised, alongside appropriate assumptions about whether each parameter in the model (such as the intercept, treatment effect, etc.) is *common* (the same in each trial), *stratified* (different in each trial) or *random* (different in each trial and assumed drawn from a particular distribution).

The one-stage approach is growing in popularity,[146] for a number of reasons, including increased availability of software for estimating hierarchical models with random effects, and the convenience of obtaining summary results in a single step. A major driver is when trials are small (in terms of included participants or outcome events), as then one-stage meta-analysis results have better statistical properties (e.g. in terms of bias and coverage) than those from a two-stage approach.[7,14,147] In other words, one-stage analyses are deemed more *exact*,[14,147] which, statistically speaking, implies that their modelling assumptions are more likely to be correct. In particular, and in contrast to the two-stage approach, a one-stage analysis avoids synthesising trial-specific estimates that are assumed normally distributed with known variances.[15] Rather, it produces meta-analysis results whilst modelling the underlying distribution of the outcome data (e.g. normal for continuous outcomes, Bernoulli for binary outcomes, etc.) directly, which is especially important when the trials in the IPD meta-analysis have few participants or events. One-stage models are also considered to be more *flexible* than a two-stage approach,[148] which refers to the analyst being able to consider a broader set of assumptions such as whether residual variances are the same in each trial, or whether baseline hazard functions are distinct or proportional across trials. On the flipside, this flexibility can also lead to modelling mistakes and unnecessarily strong assumptions, which may produce biased or overly precise conclusions.[3,7,149]

In this chapter, we outline fundamental statistical models for one-stage IPD meta-analysis of randomised trials, within the framework of generalised linear mixed models and survival models. We focus on summarising a treatment effect, but the key principles also apply to other research topics covered in subsequent chapters of this book.

6.2 One-stage IPD Meta-Analysis Models Using Generalised Linear Mixed Models

We begin by outlining one-stage IPD meta-analysis models within the generalised linear mixed model (GLMM) statistical framework. A GLMM can be viewed as a direct extension of traditional regression models, such as linear and logistic regression, and allows the analyst to account for both clustering of participants within trials and any heterogeneity across trials. Related names for GLMMs are mixed models, multilevel models and hierarchical regression, and they are often used in other applications (outside the meta-analysis field) that involve clustering and potential heterogeneity, such as multi-centre trials (where participants are clustered within centres[74,75]) and educational research (e.g. where students clustered within classes within schools[150,151]). Complementary textbooks dedicated to the topic of GLMMs are recommended.[9,152,153]

6.2.1 Basic Statistical Framework of One-stage Models Using GLMMs

Assume that we have IPD from a total of S parallel-group randomised trials that each compares a particular treatment to a control group. As in Chapter 5, let i denote trial, j denote participant, y_{ij} denote the outcome value, x_{ij} denote treatment group allocation (initially coded as 1 for treatment and 0 for control, but Section 6.2.8.3 gives further options) and z_{1ij}, z_{2ij}, ... denote values of participant-level covariates (prognostic factors) measured at baseline (i.e. before randomisation) such as age and blood pressure.

In order to fit a one-stage model, usually the IPD from all trials needs to be stacked into a single dataset. An example with a continuous outcome is shown in Box 1.1, including columns for trial and participant identification, treatment group allocation, prognostic factors (age and baseline blood pressure) and outcome value (blood pressure at follow-up).

The basic form of GLMMs for a one-stage IPD meta-analysis of continuous, binary, ordinal, count and rate outcomes is shown in Table 6.1, where just a single covariate for treatment is included in the model equation for brevity. Extending to multiple covariates (i.e. treatment and prognostic factors), the general framework is:

$$g\left(E\left(y_{ij}\right)\right) = \alpha_i + \theta_i x_{ij} + \beta_{1i} z_{1ij} + \beta_{2i} z_{2ij} + \cdots \tag{6.1}$$

This can alternatively be written in matrix notation, containing an outcome values vector, a parameter vector, and a design matrix linking the participant-level covariate values to the corresponding parameters.[9–11] The link function, g, transforms the expected (E) value of y_{ij} to a particular scale, and takes different forms depending on the type of outcome data. For a linear regression model of continuous outcomes this is simply $g(E(y_{ij})) = E(y_{ij})$, such that no transformation (i.e. a natural link) is applied. For a logistic regression model of a binary outcome this is $\ln\left(\frac{E(y_{ij})}{1-E(y_{ij})}\right)$ or equivalently $\ln\left(\frac{p_{ij}}{1-p_{ij}}\right)$, which is a logit link function expressing the log-odds of the outcome event occurring (where p_{ij} denotes the outcome event probability). For a Poisson regression model of a count outcome, the transformation is $\ln(E(y_{ij}))$, also known as the log link function.

The parameter α_i represents the expected value of the outcome (on the transformed scale) in trial i for a participant whose covariate values are all zero; for binary outcomes, this represents a transformation of the baseline event risk. The parameters θ_i, β_{1i}, β_{2i}, ... represent the effect of a one-unit increase in the corresponding covariate x_{ij}, z_{1ij}, z_{2ij}, ... on the value of $g(E(y_{ij}))$ in trial i. The main parameter of interest is θ_i, the treatment effect in trial i; this is the mean difference in the value of $g(E(y_{ij}))$ for treatment and control groups. Note that for multinomial or ordinal outcomes, y_{ij} becomes y_{ijC} because C is additionally needed to denote category (Table 6.1).

For simplicity at this point, the GLMM framework shown in model (6.1) and Table 6.1 assumes that all unknown parameters (i.e. α_i, θ_i, β_{1i}, β_{2i}, ...) are stratified by trial; that is, a separate estimate of the parameter is defined for each trial. In practice, the user must decide whether each parameter is common, random or stratified across trials. We return to this issue in Sections 6.2.2 and 6.2.4, but for now we focus on specific details of the GLMM interpretation for each outcome type.

6.2.1.1 Continuous Outcomes

Many methodology papers consider one-stage IPD meta-analysis models for continuous outcomes.[23,108,145,150,151,155,156] The GLMM for continuous outcome data typically uses an identity link function to give a general linear regression format model (6.2), such that the treatment effect parameter, θ_i, indicates the difference in the mean outcome value for those treated compared to those for the control group, in trial i. The model's residual errors (e_{ij}) are the differences between participants' true observed outcome values and their predicted outcome values based on the fitted regression equation (e.g. $\hat{\alpha}_i + \hat{\theta}_i x_{ij}$ in model (6.2)); these are assumed normally distributed with a mean of zero and a variance of σ_i^2. An equivalent way of writing model (6.2) is:

$$
\begin{aligned}
y_{ij} &= \alpha_i + \theta_i x_{ij} + e_{ij} \\
e_{ij} &\sim N\left(0, \sigma_i^2\right)
\end{aligned}
$$

As well as being stratified by trial, residual variances might also be stratified by (i.e. allowed to be different for) treatment and control groups. Further discussion on residual variances is given in Section 6.2.5.

If the follow-up outcome of interest for analysis was also measured at baseline (e.g. depression scores may be recorded before randomisation and then at regular intervals during follow-up), we recommend modelling the final outcome value and adjusting for the baseline value (y_{0ij}) as a covariate. This is also known as an analysis of covariance (ANCOVA) model, and it is detailed as model (6.9) in Box 6.1, alongside a case study. Section 5.2.3.1 explains why ANCOVA is preferable to other approaches.[19–25]

6.2.1.2 Binary Outcomes

When modelling a binary outcome, such as developing pre-eclampsia during pregnancy, the y_{ij} value is 0 or 1, where 1 typically denotes the outcome event (e.g. onset of pre-eclampsia). Then, a logit link function (model (6.3)) can be used to form a one-stage logistic regression, which models the log-odds of the outcome event (denoted by logit(p_{ij}), where p_{ij} is the probability of having the outcome event). Here, the treatment effect of $\exp(\theta_i)$ represents the odds ratio in the ith trial, revealing how much the odds of the outcome event are reduced (or increased) for the treatment compared to the control group. Many methodology papers focus on binary outcome IPD meta-analysis.[14,157–164] A case study is given in Box 6.2. An alternative to logistic regression is to use a log-link function, so that $\exp(\theta_i)$ represents the risk ratio, which may be easier to interpret and avoids the non-collapsibility issue of the odds ratio.[55] On the other hand, using a log-link may lead to convergence problems (as probabilities are not constrained to sum to 1) and odds ratios might be preferred as they are capable of remaining constant over the entire range of baseline risks, unlike the risk ratio. An excellent discussion of the use of odds ratios or risk ratios is given by Harrell.[165]

Randomised trials often report two-by-two tables indicating the number of participants with and without the outcome event in each of the two treatment groups. Therefore, if IPD are not available and if only the treatment covariate (x_{ij}) is included in the one-stage model, then the necessary IPD can be reconstructed from these tables (Section 6.4.1) to enable the GLMM of model (6.3) to be fitted. Therefore, the main statistical advantage of obtaining IPD for meta-analysis of a binary outcome is the ability to include additional covariates (prognostic factors) in the GLMM, for example to

Table 6.1 Basic format of the GLMM for one-stage IPD meta-analysis models of a treatment effect from randomised trials with continuous, binary, ordinal, count, or time-to-event data; modified from Debray et al.,[154] where i denotes trial, j denotes participant, and y_{ij} denotes the observed outcome value. For simplicity the models only include a covariate for treatment, but inclusion of prognostic factors is recommended (Section 6.2.6).

Outcome type (y_{ij})	Model type	Basic model equation (for participant j in trial i) including a single covariate ($x_{ij}=1$ for treatment group or $x_{ij}=0$ for control group)	Equation number	Further modelling choices required*
Continuous	Linear regression	$y_{ij} \sim N\left(\mu_{ij}, \sigma_i^2\right)$ $\mu_{ij} = \alpha_i + \theta_i x_{ij}$ NB σ_i^2 specifies the residual variance is common to the control and treatment groups in trial i; alternatively it could be stratified by trial *and* treatment group by specifying σ_{ij}^2	(6.2)	α_i: stratified or random θ_i: common or random σ_i^2: common, stratified or random
Binary	Logistic regression	$y_{ij} \sim \text{Bernoulli}(p_{ij})$ $\text{logit}(p_{ij}) = \alpha_i + \theta_i x_{ij}$	(6.3)	α_i: stratified or random θ_i: common or random
Ordinal (with $C = 1$ to k ordered categories, from worst (1) to best (k))	Logistic regression (proportional odds model)	$y_{ijC} \sim \text{multinomial}\left(p_{ijC}\right)$ where $p_{ijk} = 1 - \sum_{C=1}^{k-1} p_{ijC}$ $\text{logit}(Q_{ijC}) = \alpha_{iC} + \theta_i x_{ij}$ for $C = 1$ to $(k-1)$ where $Q_{ijC} = p_{ij1} + \ldots + p_{ijC}$ and $Q_{ijk} = 1$ and $\alpha_{i1} \le \alpha_{i2} \le \ldots \le \alpha_{i(k-1)}$ NB assumes proportional odds, such that the treatment effect is common (the same) for each category 1 to $(k-1)$	(6.4)	α_{iC}: stratified or random θ_i: common or random
Multinomial (with $C = 1$ to k categories, and category k chosen as the reference)	Logistic regression	$y_{ijC} \sim \text{multinomial}\left(p_{ijC}\right)$ where $p_{ijk} = 1 - \sum_{C=1}^{k-1} p_{ijC}$ $\ln\left(\frac{p_{ijC}}{p_{ijk}}\right) = \alpha_{iC} + \theta_{iC} x_{ij}$ for $C = 1$ to $(k-1)$	(6.5)	α_{iC}: stratified or random θ_{iC}: common or random
Count	Poisson regression	$y_{ij} \sim \text{Poisson}(\mu_{ij})$ $\ln(\mu_{ij}) = \alpha_i + \theta_i x_{ij}$	(6.6)	α_i: stratified or random θ_i: common or random

(Continued)

Table 6.1 (Continued)

Outcome type (y_{ij})	Model type	Basic model equation (for participant *j* in trial *i*) including a single covariate ($x_{ij} = 1$ for treatment group or x_{ij}=0 for control group)	Equation number	Further modelling choices required*
Incidence rate	Poisson regression	$y_{ij} \sim \text{Poisson}(\mu_{ij})$ $\ln(\mu_{ij}) = \alpha_i + \theta_i x_{ij} + \ln(t_{ij})$ where $\ln(t_{ij})$ is an offset term for the log of the observed time (t_{ij}) at risk (i.e. log of the follow-up time)	(6.7)	α_i: stratified or random θ_i: common or random
Count (time-to-event)	Poisson regression** (with $C = 1$ *to* k time intervals)	$y_{ijC} \sim \text{Poisson}(\mu_{ijC})$ $\ln(\mu_{ijC}) = \alpha_i + \theta_i x_{ij} + \lambda_C + \ln(t_{ijC})$ where $\ln(t_{ijC})$ is an offset term for the length of follow-up t_{ijC} in interval C	(6.8)	α_i: stratified or random θ_i: common or random

*common: true value assumed to be the same in each trial (e.g. $\alpha_i = \alpha$)
stratified: true value allowed to be different in each trial and estimated separately (e.g. 10 α_i terms with 10 trials)
random: true value allowed to be different in each trial and assumed drawn from a distribution (e.g. $\alpha_i \sim N(\alpha, \tau_\alpha^2)$)
** equivalent to Cox proportional hazards model with the k intervals defined by each distinct event time
Source: Richard Riley, adapted from Debray et al.[154]

Box 6.1 Example of a one-stage IPD meta-analysis for a continuous outcome (systolic blood pressure, SBP). Case study based on an extension of the IPD meta-analysis project of Wang et al.,[46] as introduced in Box 5.3.

We used IPD from 10 randomised trials containing a total of 28581 participants to examine the effect of anti-hypertensive treatment on SBP at end of follow-up. We fitted the following one-stage mixed effect linear regression model using REML estimation:

$$y_{ij} = \alpha_i + \theta_i x_{ij} + \beta_{1i} y_{0ij} + e_{ij}$$
$$\theta_i \sim N(\theta, \tau_\theta^2) \qquad e_{ij} \sim N(0, \sigma_i^2) \tag{6.9}$$

Here, y_{ij} is the SBP value at end of follow-up for the jth participant in trial i, x_{ij} is 1 for treatment and 0 for control, y_{0ij} is the participant's baseline SBP value, and σ_i^2 is the residual variance in trial i. The key parameters are θ, the summary treatment effect (i.e. the mean difference in the final SBP values for treatment versus control, after adjusting for baseline values), and τ_θ^2, the between-trial variability in treatment effects. All other parameters were stratified by trial and thus (as there were 10 trials) 10 intercepts, 10 prognostic effects for baseline SBP, and 10 residual variances were included. After estimation, we derived 95% confidence intervals using the Kenward-Roger approach. Allowing separate residual variances for treatment and control groups in each trial gave very similar meta-analysis results.

We obtained a summary treatment effect of −10.16 (95% CI: −11.99 to −8.33), providing strong evidence that anti-hypertensive treatment is more effective at reducing SBP than control. The results are displayed in a forest plot below. The τ_θ^2 estimate of 7.13 suggests considerable heterogeneity in the treatment effect across trials; this is reflected by a wide 95% prediction interval of −3.76 to −16.56 for the treatment effect in a new trial. The entire interval is below zero and so even though the magnitude of treatment effect may vary considerably, anti-hypertensive treatment is expected to be beneficial in the populations and settings represented by the included trials.

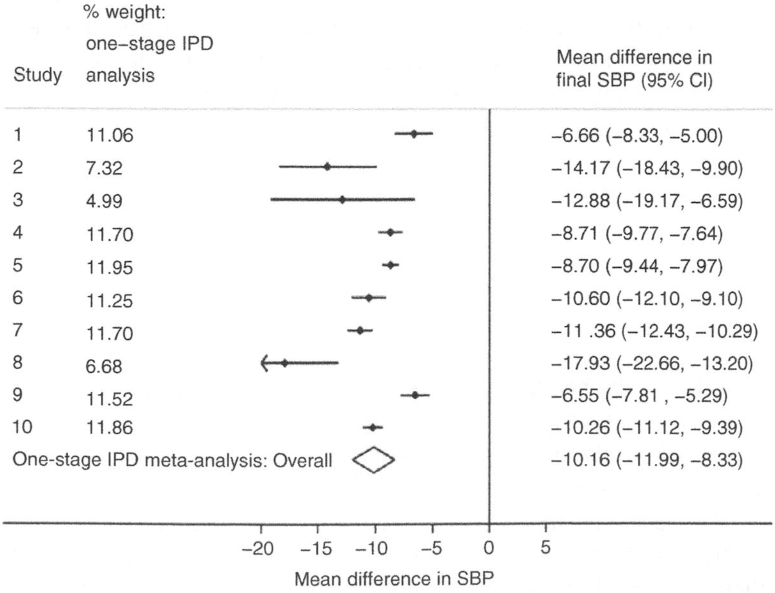

Sources: Richard Riley; Based on Wang JG, Staessen JA, Franklin SS, et al. Systolic and diastolic blood pressure lowering as determinants of cardiovascular outcome. *Hypertension* 2005;45(5):907–13.

Box 6.2 Example of a one-stage IPD meta-analysis for a binary outcome. Case study is adapted from Simmonds and Higgins.[166]

To illustrate the advantages of a one-stage IPD meta-analysis of randomised trials for binary outcomes, Simmonds and Higgins combined IPD from seven trials examining the effect of hormone replacement therapy (HRT) on the incidence of heart disease. The outcome events are sparse, and many trials have zero events in either the control or treatment group. Aggregate data derived from the IPD for each trial are provided below.

	Number of women		Number of cardiovascular events	
Trial	Control	Treatment	Control	Treatment
1	174	701	0	5
2	14	15	1	0
3	16	15	0	1
4	20	20	1	1
5	26	29	0	1
6	84	84	3	1
7	66	68	0	3

In this situation a conventional two-stage IPD meta-analysis (i.e. estimating the treatment effect and its variance in each trial separately, and then pooling these using an inverse variance weighted meta-analysis) is problematic. The treatment effect cannot be estimated in every trial unless a continuity correction is applied in those trials with a zero event; further, the assumption in the second stage that trial treatment effect estimates are normally distributed with known variances may be inappropriate. In contrast, a one-stage IPD meta-analysis directly models the binomial likelihood of the data, and so avoids deriving trial treatment effect estimates or using continuity corrections.[14] We used the data tabulated above to partially reconstruct the IPD (Section 6.4.1), with a row for each participant in the dataset denoting their trial, treatment group, and outcome event. We then used maximum likelihood (ML) estimation to fit a one-stage logistic regression model to this IPD, with the intercept stratified by trial and assuming random treatment effects:

$$y_{ij} \sim \text{Bernoulli}\left(p_{ij}\right)$$

$$\text{logit}\left(p_{ij}\right) = \alpha_i + \theta_i x_{ij}$$

$$\theta_i \sim N\left(\theta, \tau_\theta^2\right)$$

Here, y_{ij} is 1 for each participant who had the outcome event and 0 otherwise; p_{ij} is the outcome event probability for the jth participant in trial i, and α_i allows for intercepts to be stratified by trial (i.e. one intercept per trial), whilst the trial treatment effects (θ_i) are assumed normally distributed with a mean θ and between-trial variance τ_θ^2. The x_{ij} denotes the treatment group but to improve ML estimation of the between-trial variance (Section 6.2.8.3), we used trial-specific centering of x_{ij} (i.e. 1/0 for treatment/control minus the proportion of women in the treatment group for that trial). Confidence intervals were derived using the t-distribution with six degrees of freedom (Section 6.2.8.5).

Model estimation gives a summary odds ratio ($\exp(\hat{\theta})$) of 1.91 (95% CI: 0.36 to 10.15), and between-trial variance ($\hat{\tau}_\theta^2$) of 0.57. The wide confidence interval and large heterogeneity suggest the findings are inconclusive and additional trials are required to investigate the association between HRT and cardiovascular disease risk. If potentially sub-optimal or inappropriate analyses are used, notably different results are obtained:

- A Wald-based confidence interval for the summary treatment effect was much narrower (0.59 to 6.77).
- Applying a two-stage analysis, with continuity corrections of +0.5 added to zero cells, gave a much lower summary odds ratio of 1.31 and a zero estimate of between-trial heterogeneity when using REML estimation.
- Applying the one-stage model but not using trial-specific centering of the treatment variable gave a smaller summary odds ratio (1.74) and a between-trial variance estimate of zero (Section 6.2.8.3).
- Applying the one-stage model but ignoring clustering (i.e. assuming $\alpha_i = \alpha$), and without trial-specific centering of the treatment variable, gave a much lower summary odds ratio of 1.43.

Sources: Richard Riley; Adapted from Simmonds MC, Higgins JP. A general framework for the use of logistic regression models in meta-analysis. *Stat Methods Med Res* 2016;25(6):2858–77.

adjust for baseline imbalances (Section 6.2.6) or to examine treatment-covariate interactions (Chapter 7). Of course, many other advantages of IPD exist before statistical analysis, such as data checking, quality assessment, and standardisation (Chapters 3 and 4).

Compared to a two-stage approach to IPD meta-analysis (Chapter 5), a major advantage of one-stage models for binary (and multinomial, ordinal or count) outcomes is the ability to handle trials that contain a group with no participants who have the outcome event (or conversely no participants without the outcome event).[14,147,157,166] This is due to modelling the binomial likelihood directly, and avoids the need for continuity corrections, unlike the two-stage approach. Thus, one-stage models are especially important when trials contain small numbers of participants or events.[162] An example is given in Box 6.2. Including trials with double zeros (i.e. both groups have no participants with the outcome event, or conversely all participants have the outcome event) is not recommended, as they provide no information about the treatment effect unless additional assumptions are made (Section 5.2.3.2).

Where data are sparse, one-stage models for binary outcomes are prone to potential bias in summary odds ratios,[98] although any bias should be less than occurs for the two-stage approach, where data are even more sparse due to deriving trial-specific estimates separately in the first stage. Incorporating some form of penalisation during estimation of a one-stage model may help to reduce any bias in parameter estimates due to sparse data.[167] This is perhaps best implemented by adopting a Bayesian estimation framework and specifying (weakly informative) prior distributions for the unknown parameters (Section 6.2.8.8).

6.2.1.3 Ordinal and Multinomial Outcomes

The GLMM framework for logistic regression of a binary outcome can be extended to ordinal outcome data via a proportional odds model (model (6.4)),[27,38,164,168] which accounts for the multinomial and ordered nature of the data. Ordinal data relate to categories (e.g. of disease severity) that are ordered, say from worst (stage 4) to least (stage 1), with a total of $C = 1$ to k categories in each trial. Here, the outcome value, y_{ijC}, for each participant takes the value of their outcome category (C). So, for example, $y_{ijC} = 1$ if their outcome category is 1, $y_{ijC} = k$ if their outcome is category k, and so on. The underlying distribution of y_{ijC} is multinomial, with p_{ijC} denoting the probability of falling in category C. For categories $C = 1$ to $(k - 1)$, model (6.4) examines the cumulative probability (Q_{ijC}) of the outcome falling in categories 1 to C, and the proportional odds framework means that the treatment effect (θ_i) is assumed common (i.e. the same) regardless of the category, with $\exp(\theta)$ expressing the summary odds ratio (i.e. how the odds of being in a worse outcome category are changed by being in the treatment rather than the control group for participants). Detailed examples are given by Whitehead,[27] and further discussion of the proportional odds framework is given in Section 5.2.3.3.

Sometimes multinomial outcomes are not naturally ordered (e.g. living at home, with relative, at care home or in hospital), and it is not appropriate to order them from worst to best, in which case assuming proportional odds is inappropriate, and the framework of model (6.5) is preferable. Here, for categories $C = 1$ to $(k - 1)$, the probability (p_{ijC}) of being in category C is modelled relative to the probability of being in reference category (k). Now the treatment effect (θ_{iC}) is category-specific, with $\exp(\theta_C)$ expressing the summary odds ratio (i.e. how the probability of being in category C relative to the probability of being in category k are changed by being in the treatment rather than the control group). This approach can also be used for ordered outcomes, if the proportional odds assumption is considered too restrictive.

6.2.1.4 Count and Incidence Rate Outcomes

For outcome data that are counts (e.g. number of asthma events within six months), y_{ij} is the number of outcome occurrences (events) for subject j in trial i. The simplest one-stage GLMM approach for count outcome data is a Poisson regression with a log-link (model (6.6)), such that the summary treatment effect ($\exp(\theta)$) represents the ratio of expected counts in the treatment and control group. If follow-up length differs per individual, then the model can be extended to include an offset term for the log length of follow-up (model (6.7)), such that $\exp(\theta)$ is now the incidence rate ratio. An example is given in Box 6.3. Several extensions have been described that, for instance, allow for data with many zeros by introducing a discrete point mass (hierarchical zero-inflated Poisson regression).[40–42] Poisson regression can also be used to (approximately) model binary outcomes in order to estimate risk ratios.[43]

If each trial reports the total number of outcome events and total follow-up time for each group, then model (6.7) can be fitted even without the IPD.[14] So, as for binary and ordinal outcomes, a key statistical advantage of obtaining IPD is to use information on other covariates to adjust for confounding or to examine interactions. Additionally, model (6.7) assumes the rate is a constant throughout the whole follow-up period, but availability of IPD (including time of events for each individual) allows this assumption to be relaxed. Crowther et al. show that by splitting the timescale into intervals defined by distinct event times,[44] the Poisson regression approach can be adapted to fit one-stage Cox regression models for IPD meta-analysis of time-to-event data (model (6.8)), which make no assumptions about the magnitude of the baseline rate over time. Section 6.3.1.4 discusses this further.

6.2.2 Specifying Parameters as Either Common, Stratified, or Random

The word 'mixed' in GLMMs refers to the framework allowing a mixture of parameter assumptions; each parameter can either be *random* (i.e. the true parameter value is allowed to vary across trials according to a particular distribution) or *fixed*. In the IPD meta-analysis setting, fixed parameters are

Box 6.3 Example of a one-stage IPD meta-analysis for a count outcome, adapting the case study presented within Niël-Weise et al.[169] and Stijnen et al.[14]

Niël-Weise et al. conducted a meta-analysis of nine trials that examined the effect of anti-infective-treated central venous catheters in participants who used catheters long-term for parenteral nutrition or to deliver chemotherapy.[169] This treatment group is compared to a control group, in regards to the outcome of catheter-related bloodstream infection (CRBSI). Based on the IPD, the number of CRBSI events and the total number of catheter days are summarised by Stijnen et al.,[14] and given below for each trial.

	Treatment group		Control group	
Trial	Total number of CRBSI events	Total number of catheter days	Total number of CRBSI events	Total number of catheter days
1	7	1491	11	1988
2	8	1638	8	1460
3	3	11484	14	10962
4	6	1446	10	1502
5	1	370	1	482
6	1	786	8	913
7	17	6840	15	6840
8	3	1156	7	1015
9	2	400	3	440

Based on the IPD, or equivalently using the aggregate data in the above table, the following one-stage model can be fitted using maximum likelihood (ML) estimation:

$$y_{ij} \sim \text{Poisson}\left(\mu_{ij}\right)$$
$$\ln\left(\mu_{ij}\right) = \alpha_i + \theta_i x_{ij} + \ln\left(t_{ij}\right)$$
$$\theta_i \sim N\left(\theta, \tau_\theta^2\right)$$

Here, y_{ij} is the number of CRBSI events for the jth participant in trial i, and $\ln(t_{ij})$ is an offset term for their length of follow-up t_{ij}. Further, μ_{ij} is the expected number of CRBSI events for the jth participant in trial i conditional on their follow-up length and treatment group (x_{ij}). The α_i indicates that the intercept is stratified by trial (i.e. a separate intercept per trial), and the trial treatment effects (θ_i) are assumed normally distributed with a mean θ and between-trial variance τ_θ^2. The x_{ij} denotes the treatment group but, to reduce downward bias in ML estimates of between-trial variance (Section 6.2.8.3), we used trial-specific centering of x_{ij} (i.e. 1/0 for treatment/control minus the proportion of individuals in the treatment group in trial i). Confidence intervals were derived using a t-distribution with eight degrees of freedom (Section 6.2.8.5).

The estimated summary rate ratio ($\exp(\theta)$) is 0.63 (95% CI: 0.38 to 1.05) providing some evidence that, on average across trials, anti-infective-treated central venous catheters reduce the rate of CRBSI events, although the wide confidence reveals large uncertainty about the

(Continued)

Box 6.3 (Continued)

magnitude of effect on CRBSI rate. There is some heterogeneity in the treatment effect, with an estimated between-trial variance of 0.083.

Coding the treatment variable as 1/0, rather than using trial-specific centering, gives a lower estimated between-trial variance of 0. Even with trial-specific centering, there are concerns about downward bias in ML estimates of between-trial variances (Section 6.2.8.3), so we also undertook a sensitivity analysis using REML estimation of the pseudo-likelihood for this one-stage model (Section 6.2.8.4), with x_{1ij} coded as 1/0 for treatment/control. This gave a very similar summary rate ratio of 0.64, but with a slightly wider 95% confidence interval (0.38 to 1.09), due to a larger estimate of 0.14 for the between-trial variance of treatment effect.

Sources: Richard Riley; Niel-Weise BS, Stijnen T, van den Broek PJ. Anti-infective-treated central venous catheters for total parenteral nutrition or chemotherapy: a systematic review. *J Hosp Infect* 2008;69(2):114–23; Stijnen T, Hamza TH, Özdemir P. Random effects meta-analysis of event outcome in the framework of the generalized linear mixed model with applications in sparse data. *Stat Med* 2010;29:3046–67.

assumed to have either the same value in all trials (i.e. are *common*) or a distinct value for each trial (i.e. are *stratified*).[89] The meta-analysis literature traditionally uses the words *common* and *fixed* interchangeably; in particular, the phrase 'fixed-effect meta-analysis' is usually short-hand for a meta-analysis that assumes the treatment effect is common to all trials. This is unhelpful in the context of a one-stage IPD meta-analysis for various reasons. Firstly, there are multiple parameters within a one-stage model, and so loosely stating that a 'fixed-effect IPD meta-analysis was used' does not reveal which parameter (or parameters) the word 'fixed' actually refers to. Secondly, the word 'fixed' is ambiguous; it could refer to either a common or stratified parameter, even though they imply different model specifications and assumptions. Therefore, we recommend that the word 'fixed' be avoided in one-stage IPD models, and encourage researchers to use *common* or *stratified* instead. As the one-stage model produces multiple parameter estimates, is also helpful to replace vague wording such as 'common-effect meta-analysis' or 'random-effects meta-analysis' with more explicit wording about which parameters in the model are being assumed common or random (or stratified). This is especially important when the one-stage model equation is not actually provided.

The basic models shown in Table 6.1 assume all parameters are stratified by trial. Assuming a parameter is *stratified* requires a separate value of the parameter to be estimated for each trial; it allows the true value of each parameter to be trial-specific, without making any assumption about the distribution of the parameter values across trials. For example, allowing for a stratified intercept when there are 10 trials is equivalent to specifying 10 intercepts, one for each trial. This may be acceptable for so-called *nuisance parameters* (i.e. those parameters not of direct interest, such as the trial-specific intercepts, prognostic factor effects, residual variances, etc). However, stratification is unhelpful for those parameters requiring summary inferences, such as the treatment effect, and rather these must be assumed common or random. For example, allowing a common treatment effect parameter, by stratifying intercepts and prognostic factor effects, model (6.1) can be re-written as:

$$g\left(E\left(y_{ij}\right)\right) = \alpha_i + \theta x_{ij} + \beta_{1i}z_{1ij} + \beta_{2i}z_{2ij} + \cdots$$

Here, the subscript *i* term is retained for the intercept (α_i) and prognostic factor effects ($\beta_{1i}, \beta_{2i}, \ldots$) but removed for the treatment effect parameter, θ, as it is the same for every trial (i.e. $\theta_i = \theta$).

Homogeneity of treatment effect is a strong assumption, and often will be inappropriate due to unexplained between-trial heterogeneity (Section 5.3.2). To address this, the treatment effect parameter can be made random, such that the true treatment effect in each trial is assumed drawn from a particular distribution, typically a normal distribution.[15] This distribution of true treatment effects can then be summarised, for example according to the mean and variance of the normal distribution. This requires the GLMM to include random effects, which typically are denoted by the symbol u. For example, as x_{1ij} denotes the treatment group (say, x_{ij}=1 if treated and x_{ij}=0 if control), then we can place a random effect, u_i, on the treatment effect by:

$$g\left(E\left(y_{ij}\right)\right) = \alpha_i + (\theta + u_i)x_{ij} + \beta_{1i}z_{1ij} + \beta_{2i}z_{2ij} + \cdots$$
$$u_i \sim N\left(0, \tau_\theta^2\right)$$

Avoiding the u_i notation, this model can be written equivalently as:

$$g\left(E\left(y_{ij}\right)\right) = \alpha_i + \theta_i x_{ij} + \beta_{1i}z_{1ij} + \beta_{2i}z_{2ij} + \cdots$$
$$\theta_i \sim N\left(\theta, \tau_\theta^2\right)$$

This allows us to estimate θ, which denotes the average treatment effect, and τ_θ^2, which denotes the between-trial variance of treatment effects. Note that we use a subscript θ within τ_θ^2 to emphasise that this variance term relates to the treatment effect parameter, as later we discuss that random effects could also be placed on other parameters.

Importantly, even when allowing the treatment effects to be random, the nuisance parameters within the GLMM (i.e. those parameters other than the treatment effect) are still stratified by trial. This is needed to account for clustering of participants within trials, and to allow for potential between-trial heterogeneity in baseline risk and prognostic effects. An alternative option is to assume nuisance parameters are random. Section 6.2.4.2 discusses the choice between random and stratified parameters in more detail. Many researchers assume nuisance parameters are common (often because this is the default in software packages), but this is not recommended as it may lead to inappropriate conclusions, as now described.

6.2.3 Accounting for Clustering of Participants within Trials

In a one-stage IPD meta-analysis model in the GLMM framework, clustering of participants within trials should be accounted for, either by stratifying the intercept by trial ('stratified intercept') or by assuming random trial intercepts. Unfortunately, evidence suggests that many researchers are fitting one-stage models assuming a common intercept and thus ignore clustering;[1,3,146,149] that is, they fit the GLMMs in Table 6.1 but assume $\alpha_i = \alpha$. This is a very strong assumption, and essentially analyses the IPD as if it all came from a single trial. Trials are done by different investigators, in different places and settings, with different case-mix variation and lengths of follow-up, and often use different types of control treatments; thus trial differences in the control group response (also known as the baseline event risk) are expected and so trial-specific intercept values are needed.

This issue is related to whether conditional or marginal treatment effects are of interest (Section 5.2.4). Statistically speaking, ignoring clustering implies a marginal model, but accounting for clustering implies a conditional model. Marginal treatment effects are usually sought when population-level inferences are desired; then the dependence between participants from the same trial is not modelled explicitly but standard errors are adjusted for it, for example using robust standard errors (also known as sandwich estimators).[170] Summary treatment effect estimates are then interpreted as relative to participants drawn randomly from the entire target population from which analysed participants are sampled (from all trials combined). This is uncomfortable, as ignoring clustering breaks randomisation of the original trials. Further, for non-collapsible measures such as odds ratios and hazard ratios, conditional and marginal treatment effects can be very

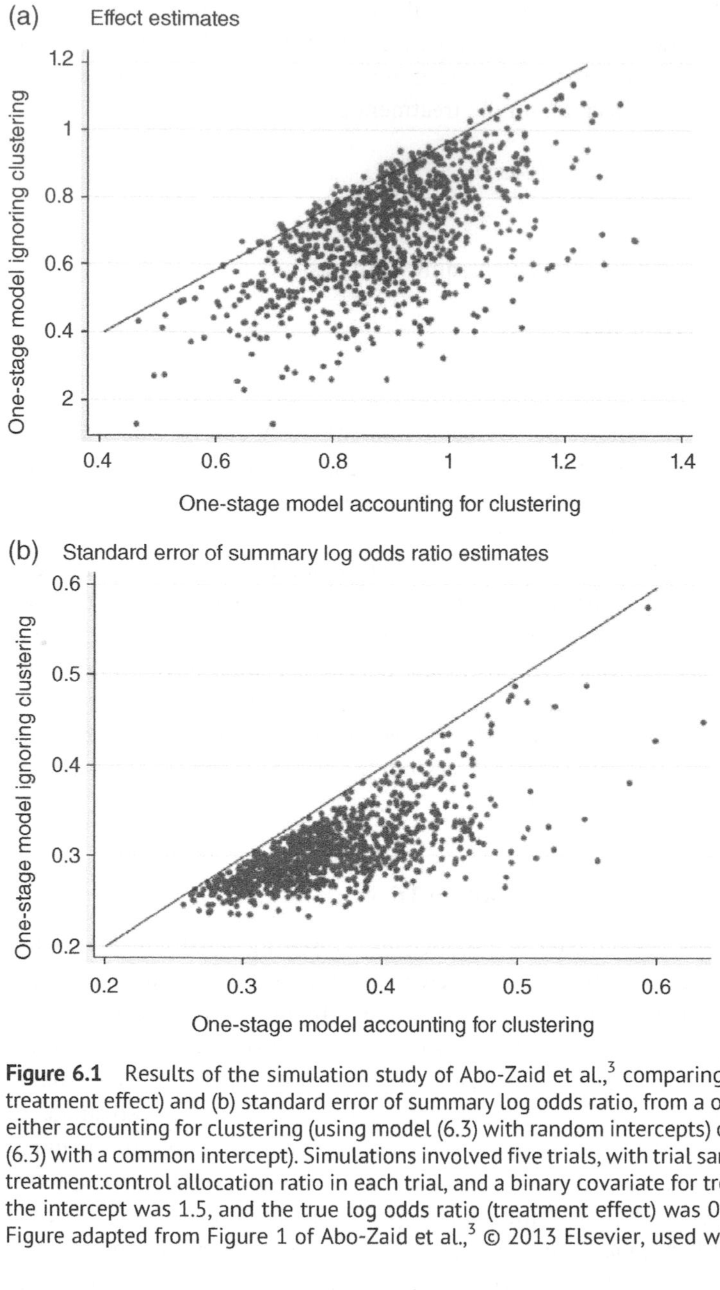

Figure 6.1 Results of the simulation study of Abo-Zaid et al.,[3] comparing (a) summary log odds ratio (i.e. treatment effect) and (b) standard error of summary log odds ratio, from a one-stage IPD meta-analysis model either accounting for clustering (using model (6.3) with random intercepts) or ignoring clustering (using model (6.3) with a common intercept). Simulations involved five trials, with trial sample sizes generated using a 20:80 treatment:control allocation ratio in each trial, and a binary covariate for treatment; the standard deviation of the intercept was 1.5, and the true log odds ratio (treatment effect) was 0.9 (common to all trials). *Source:* Figure adapted from Figure 1 of Abo-Zaid et al.,[3] © 2013 Elsevier, used with permission (CC BY 3.0).

different.[55,171,172] Thus, although not always problematic,[173] ignoring clustering can lead to spurious estimates and confidence intervals for treatment effects, especially when the proportion of participants in the treatment group varies across trials and the true effect size increases.[3,174]

Abo-Zaid et al. used simulation to compare summary treatment effects from one-stage logistic regression models that either do or do not account for clustering.[3] Results for one of their simulation settings are displayed in Figure 6.1. Across 1000 simulated IPD meta-analysis datasets, and assuming a conditional treatment effect is the estimand of interest, a one-stage model that ignores clustering produces downward bias in the summary effect estimate (Figure 6.1(a)). Also, standard errors are too small (Figure 6.1(b)), and thus subsequent confidence intervals are too precise. Outside the meta-analysis field, many others also highlight the importance of accounting for clustering, such as in cluster randomised trials[175,176] and multicentre randomised trials.[53,177–179]

6.2.3.1 Examples

To illustrate the impact of ignoring clustering, Abo Zaid et al. performed an IPD meta-analysis of two randomised trials examining whether nicotine gum increases the chances of stopping smoking,[3] building on previous work.[174,180] Assuming a common treatment effect, the summary odds ratio from a one-stage model accounting for clustering (i.e. $\text{logit}(p_{ij}) = \alpha_i + \theta x_{ij}$) is 1.80 (95% CI: 1.29 to 2.52). This is considerably larger than the unadjusted estimate of 1.40 (95% CI: 1.02 to 1.92) when ignoring clustering (i.e. $\text{logit}(p_{ij}) = \alpha + \theta x_{ij}$).

Ignoring clustering is particularly influential in this example, as the two trials had very different treatment:control allocation ratios (402:884 and 270:64), with one trial having a higher proportion in the control group, and the other trial having a higher proportion in the treatment group. Furthermore, the baseline risk of smoking cessation was very different in the control groups from the two trials. Therefore, by ignoring clustering, each trial's control group risk is compromised by that from the other trial (especially for trial 2, the smaller trial), and this impacts the summary treatment effect estimate.

Such issues are more common in IPD meta-analyses of observational studies. Abo Zaid et al. also performed an IPD meta-analysis of six cross-sectional studies of participants with suspected deep vein thrombosis (DVT),[3] where the aim was to quantify the association between a family history of thrombophilia (defined as yes or no) and the risk of truly having DVT. The proportion of participants with a family history of thrombophilia ranged from 0.03 to 0.26 in each study. A one-stage model accounting for clustering gave a summary odds ratio of 1.30 (95% CI: 1.00 to 1.70), but a one-step model ignoring clustering gave a much smaller odds ratio of 1.06 (95% CI: 0.83 to 1.37).

6.2.4 Choice of Stratified Intercept or Random Intercepts

Although the general importance of accounting for clustering is well established, how best to do this is more debatable. Specifically, should the analyst use random intercepts or a stratified intercept? The latter was assumed in model (6.1) and the basic models of Table 6.1. However, random intercepts could alternatively be specified, by adapting model (6.1) as follows:

$$
\begin{aligned}
g\left(E\left(y_{ij}\right)\right) &= \alpha_i + \theta_i x_{ij} + \beta_{1i} z_{1ij} + \beta_{2i} z_{2ij} + \cdots \\
\alpha_i &\sim N\left(\alpha, \tau_\alpha^2\right)
\end{aligned}
$$

The advantage of the stratified intercept approach is that it makes no assumptions about the distribution of intercepts across trials. The advantage of the random intercepts approach is that it requires fewer parameters to be estimated and so may reduce model convergence issues. For example, with 10 trials a stratified intercept model would estimate 10 intercept terms, but a random intercepts model reduces this to two terms, α and τ_α^2, the mean and variance of the intercepts, respectively. The impact of using a stratified intercept or random intercepts has been examined in simulation studies, as now described.

6.2.4.1 Findings from Simulation Studies

For continuous outcomes from randomised trials with a 1:1 treatment:control allocation ratio, Legha et al. performed a simulation study to compare one-stage IPD meta-analysis models using either the stratified intercept or random intercepts approach,[108] in a wide range of different simulation scenarios. Their results suggest that, as long as the restricted maximum likelihood (REML) estimation method is used, there are no important differences between one-stage models with a stratified intercept or random intercepts in terms of bias, empirical standard error, and mean-square error of the summary treatment effect estimate. The mean bias is close to zero for both approaches, and there are no important differences in their coverage performance of 95% confidence intervals. Interestingly, the random intercepts model (which assumes normality of the intercept) performs well even when trial intercepts are simulated from a highly asymmetric beta distribution. Kahan et al. also found that misspecifying the distribution of the random intercepts did not impact treatment effect results.[75]

For binary outcomes, Jackson et al. used simulation to examine one-stage IPD meta-analysis models fitted using maximum likelihood (ML) estimation, again mainly in settings with a 1:1 treatment:control allocation ratio. In contrast to the continuous outcome setting of Legha et al., when the treatment was coded as 1/0 for treatment/control Jackson et al. found important differences between summary treatment effect estimates when using a stratified intercept or random intercepts. Specifically, when there is between-trial heterogeneity in the treatment effect, ML estimation of a one-stage model with a stratified intercept substantially underestimates the between-trial variance of treatment effects; consequently 95% confidence intervals have low coverage. Coverage is much improved (i.e. closer to 95%) by using a random intercepts model. Crucially, however, when the stratified intercept model rather uses a treatment coding of +0.5/−0.5, the performance improves to be similar to that of the random intercepts model with 1/0 coding.

More generally, Riley et al. extended the Jackson simulations to settings where the treatment: control allocation was not 1:1, and found that trial-specific centering of the treatment variable is the best option when fitting a stratified intercept model with ML estimation. That is, the value of the treatment group variable for a participant in a particular trial should be coded as 1/0 (for treatment/control) minus the proportion of participants in the treatment group for that trial. For example, in a trial where 40% of participants are in the treatment group, participants in the treatment group should be coded as $1 - 0.4 = +0.6$, and participants in the control group should be coded as $0 - 0.4 = -0.4$. Then, the performance of ML estimation (in terms of bias and coverage of parameter estimates) of the stratified intercept model with trial-specific centering treatment coding is comparable to that of a random intercepts model with standard 1/0 coding. This is illustrated in Box 6.2 and Box 6.3, in which trial-specific centering of the treatment variable reduces the downward bias of ML estimates of between-trial variance compared to other treatment coding options, making it comparable to those using a random intercepts model with a standard 1/0 treatment variable coding.

6.2.4.2 Our Preference for Using a Stratified Intercept

Given these simulation findings, the choice of a stratified intercept or random intercepts might appear unimportant when fitting a one-stage IPD meta-analysis model. They will usually give very similar results when using restricted maximum likelihood (REML) estimation, and also when using ML estimation as long as variables (such as treatment) are coded using trial-specific centering in the stratified intercept model.

However, a stratified intercept model is our default approach, for a number of reasons. Stratification avoids making assumptions that the intercepts are drawn from a (normal) distribution. It also mirrors the two-stage approach (Chapter 5), where nuisance parameters are stratified naturally by analysing each trial separately in the first stage. Furthermore, and perhaps most importantly, the use of random intercepts permits sharing information across trials about control group response (baseline risk).[182,183] This is disconcerting, as it may compromise randomisation within each trial and could bias the summary treatment effect estimate. Usually any introduced bias will be small and unimportant (as in the aforementioned simulation findings),[183] especially when the treatment: control allocation ratio is similar in each trial included in the IPD meta-analysis. However, the bias could be large and important in extreme situations when included trials have an imbalance in the treatment:control allocation ratio, especially if there are few participants or events and a strong association between baseline risk and treatment effect. Accounting for correlation between the pair of random effects on the intercept and the treatment effect may introduce additional borrowing across trials (Section 6.2.4.3), but the aforementioned simulations of Jackson et al. and Riley et al. did not consider this in detail.

White et al. show an extreme meta-analysis example in which the summary treatment effect is correctly an odds ratio of 1 in a stratified model but an odds ratio of 1.35 from a random intercepts model,[184] due to the borrowing of information in the baseline risk. They conclude that "Models with random study intercepts have both appealing and unappealing properties, but their main weakness is susceptibility to bias when there are systematic differences between trials of different designs, and the evidence does not at present support their routine use".[184] The issue of random intercepts has also been highlighted in the analysis of multiple centres, and Brown and Kempton state that it "allows recovery of any between-centre treatment information which will be present when the relative sizes of the treatment groups differ between centres. The amount of extra information will depend on the degree of treatment imbalance across centres (in extreme cases, some treatments may be completely omitted from some centres) and the ratio of between-centres to treatments by centre variance components".[13]

Although our preference is to use a stratified intercept, this may not always be possible. In particular, the large number of parameters required may lead to estimation problems, including long computational times and non-convergence. In such situations assuming the intercepts are random is a sensible alternative; it will reduce model complexity (in terms of number of parameters that require estimation) whilst still allowing different values of each parameter across trials. A further option is to avoid estimating intercept parameters entirely, for example by conditioning out the trial-specific intercepts by modelling the total events,[14] or by maximizing the partial likelihood after stratifying the baseline hazard in a Cox regression model.[12] In a simulation study of binary outcomes, Jackson et al. foundthat one-stage models which condition out the trial-specific intercepts performed similarly to models that use a stratified intercept (with trial-specific centering of treatment) or random intercepts.[185]

6.2.4.3 Allowing for Correlation between Random Effects on Intercept and Treatment Effect

When a random intercepts model is chosen, there is the opportunity to account for between-trial correlation (ρ) in the random intercepts and random treatment effects; for example, when the treatment effect is larger in trials with a higher baseline risk. To allow for this correlation, the pair of random effects in each trial could be assumed drawn from a bivariate normal distribution,[186,187] essentially assuming a linear between-trial relationship between the true treatment effect and true baseline risk, as follows:

$$g\left(E\left(y_{ij}\right)\right) = \alpha_i + \theta_i x_{ij} + \beta_{1i} z_{1ij} + \beta_{2i} z_{2ij} + \cdots$$

$$\begin{pmatrix}\alpha_i\\ \theta_i\end{pmatrix} \sim N\left(\begin{pmatrix}\alpha\\ \theta\end{pmatrix}, \begin{pmatrix}\tau_\alpha^2 & \rho\tau_\alpha\tau_\theta\\ \rho\tau_\alpha\tau_\theta & \tau_\theta^2\end{pmatrix}\right)$$

Accounting for this correlation makes intuitive sense, as the true odds ratio will naturally change as the baseline risk changes.[56] It also allows the variances of responses in the control group to be smaller or larger than those in the treatment group, regardless of the treatment variable coding.[157,185] If no correlation is allowed (i.e. $\rho = 0$), then the user must be careful in coding treatment; generally +0.5/−0.5 is recommended to ensure the same variance of control and treatment group responses (otherwise with a 1/0 coding, the variation for the control group is forced to be less than or equal to the variation for intervention group).[27,157] Therefore, when fitting a one-stage model with random intercepts and random treatment effects, Turner et al. suggest the correlation should be accounted for and a 1/0 treatment variable coding used.[157] If the correlation is not estimable, then assuming it is zero and using a +0.5/−0.5 treatment variable coding is sensible.

A potential concern when allowing for between-trial correlation is that information about the baseline risk may contribute toward the summary treatment effect estimate. As an extreme example, the model could incorporate randomised trials alongside observational studies that only provide information about the control (untreated group); the latter will then – via the between-trial correlation – contribute toward the summary treatment effect. This is a similar concern to that raised in Section 6.2.4.2 about compromising within-trial randomisation by assuming random trial intercepts, and it is avoided when using the stratified intercept modelling approach. Hence, when such borrowing of information is influential, IPD meta-analysis results may be somewhat different between stratified and random approaches. To illustrate this, we re-analysed the IPD meta-analysis example of Box 6.2 by fitting the following model that assumes random intercepts and random treatment effects, and accounts for their correlation:

$$y_{ij} \sim \text{Bernoulli}\left(p_{ij}\right)$$

$$\text{logit}\left(p_{ij}\right) = \alpha_i + \theta_i x_{ij}$$

$$\begin{pmatrix}\alpha_i\\ \theta_i\end{pmatrix} \sim N\left(\begin{pmatrix}\alpha\\ \theta\end{pmatrix}, \begin{pmatrix}\tau_\alpha^2 & \rho\tau_1\tau_\alpha\\ \rho\tau_1\tau_\alpha & \tau_\theta^2\end{pmatrix}\right)$$

ML estimation (with the recommended 1/0 treatment variable coding) of this model estimates a strong negative correlation of $\hat{\rho} = -0.87$ between the pair of random effects. This leads to a smaller summary odds ratio (1.74) with a wider confidence interval (0.22 to 13.71) and a larger between-trial variance estimate ($\hat{\tau}_\theta^2 = 0.74$), as compared to those from ML estimation of the stratified intercept model with trial-specific centering coding of the treatment variable (summary odds ratio = 1.91, 95% CI: 0.36 to 10.15; $\hat{\tau}_\theta^2 = 0.57$ – see Box 6.2). The differences are due to the influence of the between-trial correlation, which allows baseline risk to contribute toward the summary treatment effect estimate.

6.2.5 Stratified or Common Residual Variances

Many researchers who apply a one-stage IPD meta-analysis model for continuous outcomes do not stratify the residual variance by trial, and rather assume it is common; for example, models (6.2) and (6.9) assume $\sigma_i^2 = \sigma^2$, which is the default option in most statistical software packages. Stratified residual variances usually need be enforced, for example by using the weights=varIdent option in the R package *lme*; the residuals(by...) option in the Stata package *mixed*; or the repeated statement within the SAS *Proc Mixed* procedure.[188]

It is possible to compare the fit of one-stage models with common or stratified residual variances,[17,189] in order to make the final choice. However, as for heterogeneity of treatment effects, there is often low power to identify genuine differences in model fit with and without trial-specific residual variances, so the decision is best made in advance. As for intercepts and treatment effects, between-trial differences in residual variances ('heteroscedasticity') is expected because trials are conducted in different populations, settings, time periods, and so forth. Hence, we recommend stratifying the residual variance per trial (and potentially by treatment group, Section 6.2.1.1).

An alternative to stratification is to place a distribution on the residual variances (sometimes referred to as double hierarchical generalised linear models[133,190]) which may be useful when all trials are small, or down-weighting smaller trials (potentially at higher risk of bias) that just happen to have a small observed residual variance. Whitehead also highlights the opportunity to model a standardised treatment difference,[27] by transforming the outcome responses to a standard N(0,1) distribution (i.e. by taking $(y_{ij} - \text{mean}(y_{ij}))/s_i$, where s_i is the standard deviation of outcome values observed in the trial), thereby ensuring that a common residual variance is more acceptable. Standardisation comes at the expense of making the treatment effect more difficult to interpret, but may be suitable when the continuous outcome scale varies across trials (Section 5.2.3.1).

6.2.6 Adjustment for Prognostic Factors

Chapter 5 recommends that two-stage IPD meta-analyses should routinely adjust (in the first stage) for key prognostic factors and, assuming the focus is on informing clinical practice at the patient level, to produce conditional treatment effects (Section 5.2.4). This recommendation remains important for one-stage models. An example is given in Box 6.1, where adjustment is made for baseline SBP in each trial.

As for the model intercept, a decision needs to be made whether prognostic factor effects are included as stratified or random in the one-stage model. Our default recommendation is to use stratified prognostic effects (i.e. estimate a separate effect of each included prognostic factor for each trial), with trial-specific centering of each prognostic factor to improve ML estimation (for the reasons explained in Section 6.2.8.3). However, if outcome data or prognostic factor categories are sparse, the stratification approach may lead to estimation difficulties, and then allowing prognostic factor effects to be random is a sensible alternative. Note that, in addition to prognostic factors, the design of a particular trial may require additional adjustment terms (e.g. to account for clustering by general practice or hospital in multi-centre trials),[74,75,191] for which stratification by trial is then sensible (as these are trial-specific).

As explained in Chapter 5, we recommend that continuous prognostic factors are kept on their continuous scale, as dichotomisation or categorisation is arbitrary and loses power,[57,63,64] and thus adjustment should at least assume a linear trend. Alternatively, trial-specific non-linear associations could be modelled, for example using a restricted cubic spline with a pre-specified number of knots[65–67] or fractional polynomials.[68–70] To deal with partially missing values of prognostic factors in a trial, trial-specific mean values could be imputed or trial-specific missing indicator variables included in the model (Section 5.2.5), which are strategies coherent with those recommended for missing covariates in a single trial.[78] Multiple imputation is a further option to deal with partially and also systematically missing variables (Chapter 18).

6.2.7 Inclusion of Trial-level Covariates

The GLMM framework shown in model (6.1) and Table 6.1 can be extended to include trial-level covariates, such as year of trial completion, country of trial, dose of treatment, and a trial's risk of bias classification. Unlike participant-level covariates such as age and biomarkers, trial-level covariates describe each trial as a whole, and thus do not change across individuals in the same trial. Thus, they cannot explain within-trial variability, but can explain between-trial heterogeneity. For example, the one-stage ANCOVA model (6.9) can be extended to include a single trial-level covariate, z_i:

$$y_{ij} = \alpha_i + \theta_i x_{ij} + \beta_{1i} y_{0ij} + e_{ij}$$
$$\theta_i \sim N\left(\gamma + \delta z_i, \tau_\theta^2\right) \qquad e_{ij} \sim N\left(0, \sigma_i^2\right) \tag{6.10}$$

Here, we have a meta-regression model ($\gamma + \delta z_i$) embedded within the one-stage IPD meta-analysis model, where γ is the mean treatment effect in trials where z_i is zero, and δ represents how the treatment effect changes across trials for a one-unit increase in z_i. By including z_i, the aim is to reduce the unexplained heterogeneity in treatment effect (τ_θ^2) compared to that from model (6.9). Inclusion of aggregated participant-level covariates (e.g. setting z_i equal to a trial's mean age) might also explain between-trial heterogeneity, but should not be used to infer relationships at the participant-level due to aggregation bias (Chapter 7).

6.2.8 Estimation of One-stage IPD Meta-Analysis Models Using GLMMs

We now discuss key estimation methods and related issues when fitting one-stage IPD meta-analysis models.

6.2.8.1 Software for Fitting One-stage Models

A detailed, though not necessarily exhaustive, summary of software available for fitting one-stage IPD meta-analysis models is given in Table 6.2. These are generic packages for fitting GLMMs, rather than IPD meta-analysis models per se, and require careful implementation to avoid modelling mistakes and estimation issues. Our website (www.ipdma.co.uk) provides code for various case studies used in this chapter.

6.2.8.2 ML Estimation and Downward Bias in Between-trial Variance Estimates

Estimation of a GLMM for a binary, ordinal or count outcome is often undertaken using ML estimation. The likelihood function of a GLMM for these outcomes cannot analytically be integrated; therefore, an approximation is often necessary. A common approach is to perform numerical integration of the likelihood using adaptive Gauss-Hermite quadrature (AGHQ). This requires a number of quadrature points to be specified, with increasing estimation accuracy as the number of points increases, but at the expense of an increased computational time and convergence problems where variances are close to zero or cluster sizes are small.[192] Five to seven quadrature points is usually adequate, in our experience, although sensitivity analysis to the choice of points is sensible. Using one quadrature point (the default in some software packages) is equivalent to using a Laplace approximation. A second approach is to construct a series of approximations to the mixed model, and to apply penalised quasi-likelihood (PQL) estimation.[193] This approach uses a weighted least-squares algorithm and is therefore straightforward to implement and computationally faster than AGHQ.

Unfortunately, when the GLMM includes random parameters to model between-trial heterogeneity, ML estimation (using AGHQ or PQL) often produces downward bias in between-trial variance estimates, and subsequently low coverage of 95% confidence intervals.[162,194–196] Riley et al. show that the problem may be substantial,[181] especially in IPD meta-analyses with small numbers of trials. For example, with a binary outcome and just three or five trials in the meta-analysis, their simulations show that the median downward bias in the estimate of between-trial variance of treatment effect is often 100% (with mean bias between 40 to 80%), and coverage of 95% confidence intervals for the summary treatment effect is around 90%. Similar results are shown for binary outcomes in a simulation study by Stijnen et al.,[14] where a one-stage IPD meta-analysis had coverage from 90.7 to 91.8% across settings, and for time-to-event outcomes by Crowther et al.,[44] with coverage often much lower than 95%, when the number of trials is 10 or less. Li et al. also show that the between-trial variance is often estimated to be zero for ML estimation of logistic and proportional odds regression models with random effects.[168] Finally, bias may also appear when trials within the IPD meta-analysis are relatively small;[162] in particular, PQL has been demonstrated to underestimate effects when modelling binary outcome data.[197]

6.2.8.3 Trial-specific Centering of Variables to Improve ML Estimation of One-stage Models with a Stratified Intercept

As previously discussed (Section 6.2.4.1), Jackson et al. and Riley et al. show that for one-stage models with a stratified intercept, ML estimation is improved when using trial-specific centering of treatment and other included variables.[181,185] Centering disentangles (i.e. makes uncorrelated) the estimation of main parameters of interest from other nuisance parameters, which leads to less downward bias in estimates of variance parameters (Figure 6.2) and thus improves coverage of 95% confidence intervals. Examples of using trial-specific centering are shown in Box 6.2 and Box 6.3.

6.2.8.4 REML Estimation

Even with trial-specific centering of included variables, downward bias in between-trial variances remains a substantial concern when using ML estimation, for either stratified intercept or random intercepts models. This is illustrated in Figure 6.2, where even the best approaches have a large downward bias in the between-trial variance estimate from ML estimation.

In the continuous outcome setting, this problem is addressed by using REML estimation,[13,105,106,198] also known as residual maximum likelihood estimation. REML separates out the estimation of the variance parameters (based on the residuals) from the estimation of the main parameters (such as the intercept and treatment effect). This typically leads to larger (approximately unbiased) between-trial variance estimates than standard ML estimation, and thereby improves coverage of 95% confidence intervals for the main parameters such as the treatment effect.[108,181] Therefore, REML is our recommended estimation method for GLMMs of continuous outcomes, for which a 1/0 coding of the treatment variable is adequate.[108,181] An example is given in Box 6.1.

Unfortunately, there is no natural extension from ML to REML estimation for the exact likelihood defined by a GLMM of a binary, ordinal or count outcome, as the model residuals cannot be estimated separately from the main parameters. Thus ML estimation is generally the default estimation choice for GLMMs of non-continuous outcomes, for which downward bias in between-trial variance estimates and low coverage of confidence intervals is a strong concern, especially with a small number of trials in the IPD meta-analysis. To address this issue, Wolfinger and O'Connell suggest using a pseudo-likelihood approximation of the exact likelihood,[199] where the outcome response variable is transformed to an approximately linear scale. This allows REML to be used for GLMMs of non-continuous outcomes, but at the expense of an approximate likelihood. This may be an acceptable trade-off in some situations, to improve between-trial variance estimates and confidence interval coverage. For example, when there are, say, 15 or fewer trials in the IPD meta-analysis, and most have reasonable numbers of participants and events, REML estimation of

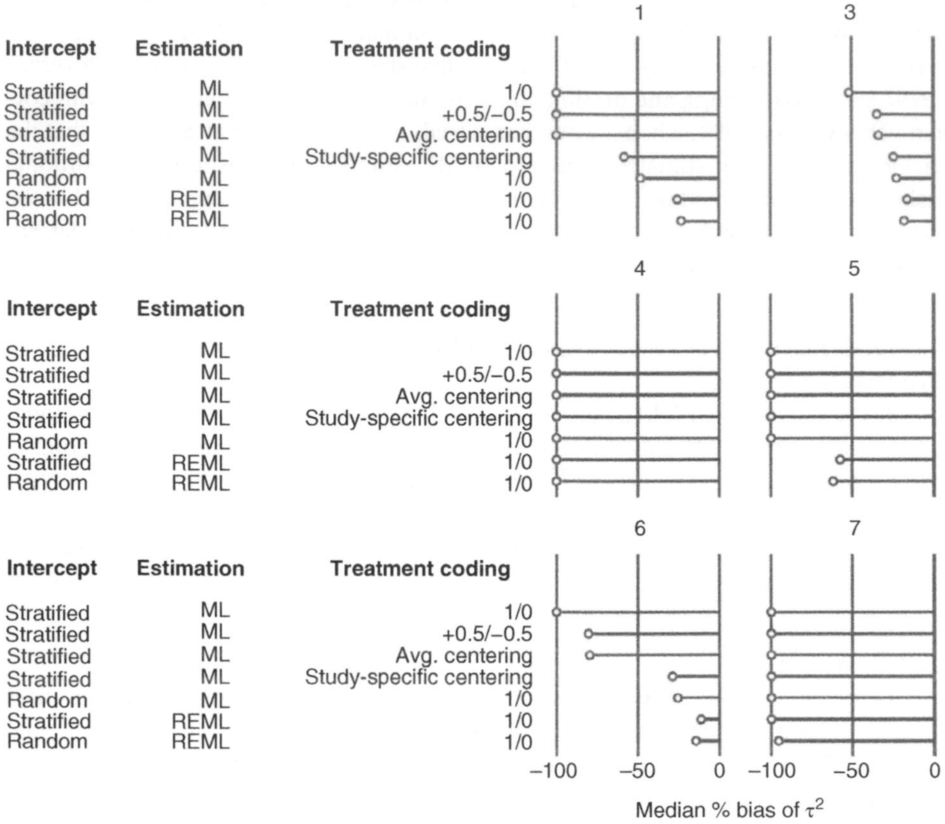

∗ Numbers above each graph relate to the scenario settings of Riley et al.[181]; see the article for full details about each setting. True value for τ_θ^2 was 0.024, except in scenario 3 where τ_θ^2 was 0.168. 'Avg. centering' is equivalent to 1/0 minus

Figure 6.2 Simulation results for binary outcomes from Riley et al.[181] for six scenarios (labelled 1, 3, 4, 5, 6, and 7∗) where the mean treatment effect was an odds ratio of 1, and each trial in the IPD meta-analysis had a random treatment prevalence from 10 to 90%. The median percentage bias of the estimates of between-trial variance of treatment effects (τ_θ^2) are shown for models with a stratified intercept or random intercepts, fitted using either ML estimation of the exact likelihood or REML estimation of the pseudo-likelihood, for different treatment variable coding options. *Source:* Figure taken from Figure 2 of Riley et al.[181], reproduced with permission, © 2020 Wiley.

the pseudo-likelihood may be a good approximation and perform much better than ML estimation of the exact likelihood.[200] REML also allows the Kenward-Roger or Satterthwaite corrections to the confidence interval (Section 6.2.8.5).

An example is given in Box 6.3, which shows that the REML pseudo-likelihood approach gave a larger between-trial variance estimate and a wider confidence interval for the summary treatment effect, compared to ML estimation of the exact likelihood. The approach can be applied in specialist software such as MLwiN, or by using the *Proc GLIMMIX* package in SAS or the *runmlwin* package in Stata.[201] These packages allow the user to choose first- and second-order linearisations of the likelihood. For example, in MLwiN the first-order marginal quasi-likelihood linearisation of the likelihood ('mql1' option) is noted in the accompanying help files as the most stable and fastest to converge, but an accurate (though potentially less stable) estimation option is a second-order penalised quasi-likelihood linearisation ('pql2' option), with the estimates from the first-order approach used as initial values.

Riley et al. used simulation to compare one-stage IPD meta-analyses of a binary outcome fitted using ML estimation of the exact likelihood or REML estimation of the pseudo-likelihood.[181] Their findings are summarised in Figure 6.2, and suggest that REML estimation of the pseudo-likelihood generally has less downward bias in between-trial variance estimates than ML estimation of the exact likelihood. However, this REML approach may not be appropriate when data are sparse (i.e. most trials are small and have few or even zero events), as other work indicates the pseudo-likelihood is not accurate in sparse data situations.[153] Problems with REML estimation of the pseudo-likelihood are revealed when parameter estimates are unstable. Instability is evident when first-order and second-order linearisation of the likelihood lead to very different parameter estimates, or when different parameterisations that should not affect REML (such as centering of covariates) change parameter estimates importantly. In such situations, ML estimation of the exact likelihood is preferred. To illustrate this, consider again the applied example of Box 6.2, which had sparse data (most trials had a zero event for either the treatment or control group). When REML estimation of the pseudo-likelihood is applied, the estimates are hugely unstable, with first- and second-order linearisations giving widely different results. Hence, the ML estimates with trial-specific centering shown in Box 6.2 are more reliable in this example. A Bayesian approach could also be considered in this case, which would retain the exact likelihood during parameter estimation and could be combined with empirically based prior distributions for the between-trial variance (Section 6.2.8.8).[130,202]

6.2.8.5 Deriving Confidence Intervals for Parameters Post-estimation

After ML or REML estimation of a one-stage IPD meta-analysis model, standard confidence intervals can be derived for each parameter based on large-sample inference that assumes estimates are approximately normally distributed. For example, a standard ('Wald-based') confidence interval for the summary treatment effect (θ) can be calculated using

$$\hat{\theta} \pm z_{1-\frac{\alpha}{2}}\sqrt{\text{var}(\hat{\theta})} \tag{6.11}$$

where $\hat{\theta}$ is the estimated summary treatment effect, $\text{var}(\hat{\theta})$ is its variance, and $z_{1-\frac{\alpha}{2}}$ is the critical value of the standard normal distribution, which equals 1.96 when α is 0.05 (i.e. a 95% confidence interval is desired).

For continuous outcomes, Legha et al. show that this standard approach produces confidence intervals that are too narrow when there is heterogeneity in the treatment effect,[108] as it does not account for the uncertainty in estimated variances in the one-stage model, in particular the between-trial variance of the treatment effect. To address this, confidence intervals based on small-sample inference can be used, notably the Kenward–Roger and Satterthwaite corrections.[203,204] These methods are also known as denominator-degrees-of-freedom (DDF) adjustments, and derive confidence intervals based on values from a t-distribution (rather than 1.96 based on a normal distribution). Further, the Kenward-Roger approach also modifies (inflates) the estimated variance of parameters post-estimation.[198] For example, the Kenward-Roger (KR) corrected $(1-\alpha)100\%$ CI for the summary treatment effect is given by:

$$\hat{\theta} \pm t_{v;1-\frac{\alpha}{2}}\sqrt{\text{var}_{\text{KR}}(\hat{\theta})} \tag{6.12}$$

where $\hat{\theta}$ is as before, but now a bias-adjusted (inflated) variance $\left(\mathrm{Var}_{\mathrm{KR}}(\hat{\theta})\right)$ is used, and $t_{\upsilon;1-\frac{\alpha}{2}}$ (the critical value of the t-distribution with an adjusted degrees of freedom, υ) instead of $z_{1-\frac{\alpha}{2}}$. The Satterthwaite corrected $(1-\alpha)100\%$ CI is given by:

$$\hat{\theta} \pm t_{\upsilon;1-\frac{\alpha}{2}}\sqrt{\mathrm{var}(\hat{\theta})} \tag{6.13}$$

where $t_{\upsilon;1-\frac{\alpha}{2}}$ is as in the Kenward-Roger correction, but the original (unadjusted) variance of $\hat{\theta}$ is used.

Legha et al. compared the coverage of standard, Kenward-Roger and Satterthwaite 95% confidence intervals for the summary treatment effect,[108] after fitting the one-stage IPD meta-analysis model (6.2) with a random treatment effect with either stratified intercept or random intercepts. They found that the Kenward-Roger and Satterthwaite methods have similar coverage that is mostly close to 95% (though sometimes overly conservative), which substantially improves upon the Wald-based approach, whose coverage is typically less than 95%, and often around 90%. Given their similarity in coverage, the main role of both Kenward-Roger and Satterthwaite corrections appears to be their use of the t-distribution to derive confidence intervals, and the use of Kenward-Roger's adjusted variance seems to have relatively less impact.

Riley et al. show that Wald-based confidence intervals were often too narrow after ML estimation of one-stage models of binary outcomes,[181] and suggested replacing 1.96 with the value of a t-distribution with $S-1$ degrees of freedom, where S is the number of trials in the IPD meta-analysis. Their simulations suggest this generally improves coverage of 95% confidence intervals to be closer to 95%. However, as for the Kenward-Roger and Satterthwaite approaches for continuous outcomes, the approach can lead to over-coverage (> 95%) in some scenarios. Other options include using the profile likelihood[205] and bootstrapping.[206]

6.2.8.6 Prediction Intervals

Post estimation of a one-stage IPD meta-analysis, approximate 95% prediction intervals can be derived for the treatment effect in a new trial using the same options outlined in Section 5.3.10 of Chapter 5.[90,136,137]

6.2.8.7 Derivation of Percentage Trial Weights

In a one-stage IPD meta-analysis the contribution of each trial is hidden, as summary parameter estimates are derived directly, without the need to calculate trial-specific estimates and weights. Furthermore, a one-stage model estimates multiple parameters, and so percentage trial weights can be derived for each parameter estimate (and indeed may differ for each). Riley et al. show how to derive percentage trial weights for one-stage IPD meta-analysis models post estimation,[207] by decomposing the total variance matrix of parameter estimates into trial-specific contributions, via a decomposition of Fisher's observed information matrix into independent trial-specific contributions. The approach requires an appreciation of matrix algebra, and so we refer to the original publication for further details.[207] An example of percentage weights derived by the method is provided in the forest plot within Box 6.1.

Kontopantelis and Reeves suggested that "*patient weights are uniform and therefore each study's weight is the ratio of its participants over the total number of participants across all trials*".[208] However, this will not usually be correct.[207] Consider trial 3 in the meta-analysis of Box 6.1. Based on Kontopantelis and Reeves the percentage weight for trial 3 is 0.60%, but it is actually 4.99% using the more exact calculation based on decomposition of the variance matrix.[207]

6.2.8.8 Bayesian Estimation for One-stage Models

Estimation of one-stage IPD meta-analysis models can also be undertaken using a Bayesian approach, which combines the likelihood function (which represents the observed data) with prior information (e.g. based on evidence external to the data), to form a joint posterior distribution for the unknown parameters. Detailed discussion of the advantages of Bayesian methods for IPD meta-analysis is provided in Section 5.3.8, including accounting for all parameter uncertainty when making inferences, and making probabilistic statements about treatment efficacy and clinical benefit. Conclusions may be sensitive to the choice of prior distributions, especially with few trials.[127]

As a brief example, we applied a Bayesian framework to the one-stage IPD meta-analysis of Box 6.1, to examine the effect of anti-hypertensive treatment on SBP. The likelihood is as shown in Box 6.1, which is a linear regression including adjustment for baseline. Additionally for the Bayesian approach, a vague prior was chosen for θ and a realistically vague prior for τ, as follows,

Likelihood:	$y_{ij} = \alpha_i + \theta_i x_{ij} + \beta_{1i} y_{0ij} + e_{ij}$	
	$\theta_i \sim N(\theta, \tau_\theta^2)\ e_{ij} \sim N(0, \sigma_i^2)$	(6.14)
Prior distributions:	$\tau_\theta \sim N(0,5)I(0,\ )$	
	$\theta \sim N(0, 1000000)$	

where the I(0,) notation denotes that the distribution is truncated at 0, so that non-negative values are avoided. We used Gibbs sampling in WinBUGS, with a burn-in of 10,000 samples and inferences made from a further 10,000. This gave a posterior mean for the summary treatment effect of −10.11 (95% CrI: −12.15 to −8.31), a median between-trial variance of 6.51, and a 95% prediction interval for the treatment effect in a single setting of −16.15 to −4.44; these are all similar results to those from the frequentist analysis using REML estimation (Box 6.1). The Bayesian approach additionally allows probabilistic statements, which are clinically helpful. For example, there is a 96% probability that the reduction in SBP in a single population will be at least 5mmHG more than control.

6.2.9 A Summary of Recommendations

Based on the evidence and examples described in the previous sections, Box 6.4 summarises our key recommendations for conducting a one-stage IPD meta-analysis of randomised trials to estimate a summary treatment effect. Some of the recommendations focus on a frequentist estimation approach, but a Bayesian framework is also suitable.

6.3 One-stage Models for Time-to-event Outcomes

Now we consider one-stage IPD meta-analysis models for time-to-event outcomes, within a Cox proportional hazards framework. The content draws on existing reviews and methodological articles for IPD meta-analyses and multilevel survival models.[5,44,209–214]

6.3.1 Cox Proportional Hazard Framework

Consider that IPD from multiple randomised trials with a parallel-group design are available, with participants in treatment and control groups followed from randomisation until their subsequent time of outcome event (e.g. death) or censoring (i.e. end of follow-up). Similar to the issue of trial-specific intercepts in GLMMs, it is fundamental to account for clustering within one-stage models for time-to-event outcomes, using either stratified or frailty models.[210]

Box 6.4 Recommendations for one-stage IPD meta-analysis models using GLMMs

- **Use a random treatment effect.**
Justification: Typically the included trials are conducted in different settings, populations and time periods. Therefore, some heterogeneity of treatment effect is expected. Heterogeneity might be reduced by inclusion of prognostic factors (Section 6.2.6) or trial-level covariates (6.2.7), but usually unexplained heterogeneity remains and so should be acknowledged.

- **Stratify by trial the intercept and parameters for other non-treatment variables (such as prognostic factors and residual variances). If convergence issues arise, then consider making the intercept (and other non-treatment variables) random.**
Justification: Although a random intercept will usually give similar results to a stratified intercept, in some situations it may compromise randomisation (as it allows baseline risk information to be shared across trials). If a stratified intercept model fails to converge (e.g. with rare events or many parameters), assuming random intercepts is a sensible compromise, in which case accounting for the correlation between the random effects on intercept and treatment effect may be important. Another option is to entirely condition out the trial intercepts (Section 6.2.4.2).

- **Use trial-specific centering of the treatment variable (and any other included variables, such as prognostic factors) when using ML estimation of a one-stage model with a stratified intercept.**
Justification: Simulation studies and mathematical reasoning show that this improves ML estimation of between-trial variances and the coverage of confidence intervals for the summary treatment effect (Section 6.2.8.3).

- **For continuous outcomes, allow a separate residual variance per trial.**
Justification: As heteroscedasticity of residual variances is likely across trials, allowing a separate residual variance per trial (i.e. stratifying the residual variance) is a sensible default approach. Only if convergence or computational issues arise do we recommend using a common residual variance (Section 6.2.5). Stratifying residual variances by trial *and* by treatment group may also be important.

- **For frequentist estimation of one-stage models for continuous outcomes, use REML estimation and derive confidence intervals for the summary treatment effect using the approach of either Kenward-Roger or Satterthwaite.**
Justification: REML estimation provides better estimates of between-trial variances, and simulation studies show that coverage of 95% confidence intervals for the summary treatment is improved when using Kenward-Roger or Satterthwaite corrections based on the *t*-distribution (Sections 6.2.8.4 and 5.3.7). A Bayesian approach is an appealing alternative.

- **For frequentist estimation of one-stage models for binary, ordinal or count outcomes, use REML estimation of the pseudo-likelihood approach unless most trials in the meta-analysis are small (in terms of participants or outcome events), which then warrants ML estimation of the exact likelihood.**
Justification: Although estimation of the exact likelihood is preferred, ML estimation is known to produce downwardly biased estimates of between-trial variances. Therefore, unless most included trials are small, REML estimation of an approximate pseudo-likelihood specification may improve estimation of between-trial variances and coverage of confidence intervals (Section 6.2.8.4). When either REML or ML estimation is used, coverage is improved using confidence intervals based on the *t*-distribution (Section 6.2.8.5). A Bayesian approach is an appealing alternative.

ML = maximum likelihood, REML = restricted maximum likelihood.

Source: Richard Riley.

6.3.1.1 Stratifying Using Proportional Baseline Hazards and Frailty Models

If we assume that trial baseline hazards are proportional to each other, and there is potential for between-trial heterogeneity in the treatment effect, the corresponding one-stage Cox model can be written as:

$$\begin{aligned} h_{ij}(t) &= h_0(t)\exp(\alpha_{0i} + \theta_i x_{ij}) \\ \theta_i &\sim N(\theta, \tau_\theta^2) \end{aligned} \tag{6.15}$$

Here, $h_0(t)$ is the baseline hazard function in the reference trial (say $i = 1$) and each intercept (α_{0i}) represents the proportional effect on the baseline hazard function due to the ith trial (with α_{01} constrained to be zero). The average treatment effect is the log hazard ratio, θ, and the between-trial variance in treatment effect is τ_θ^2. The summary hazard ratio is $\exp(\theta)$. Additional covariates might be included after the $\theta_i x_{ij}$ term, for example to account for clustering by centre within trials, or to adjust for a pre-specified set of prognostic factors (Section 6.2.6); the effects of such covariates must either be stratified by trial or assumed random. Trial-level covariates (e.g. year of completion, risk of bias) can also be included to help explain heterogeneity in treatment effect, by replacing the θ term with a meta-regression such as $\gamma + \delta z_i$ (Section 6.2.7).

Rather than using a separate intercept per trial, a frailty term can be added to the baseline hazard. In the survival analysis literature, the word *frailty* is essentially the name for random effects being added to a parameter (e.g. intercept) within the baseline hazard. This allows the baseline hazards in each trial to have the same shape but a different magnitude, as drawn from a particular distribution. The estimated treatment effect is then to be interpreted relative to other participants in the same trial with the same frailty (and values of any included prognostic factors). If the baseline hazard of this model is left unspecified, this leads to the Cox proportional hazards model with random trial intercept and random treatment effect. Extension to allow for the correlation of this pair of random effects is possible and may be sensible (akin to the discussion in Section 6.2.4.3). It is common to assume a gamma distribution for the frailty (e.g. via the 'shared' option within the *stcox* module within Stata[215]), for mathematical or computational reasons, or a normal distribution for the log-frailty, as this has similarities to the generalised linear mixed effects model,[216,217] though many other distributions are possible.[216,218] Previous studies have demonstrated that the gamma frailty model appears to be fairly robust to misspecification of the frailty distribution,[219,220] and that it describes the frailty of survivors for a large class of hazard models.[221]

6.3.1.2 Stratifying Baseline Hazards without Assuming Proportionality

Presuming that the hazard functions are proportional across trials may be a strong assumption. Therefore, in general we prefer to allow a unique baseline hazard function for each trial,[222] as follows:

$$\begin{aligned} h_{ij}(t) &= h_{0i}(t)\exp(\theta_i x_{ij}) \\ \theta_i &\sim N(\theta, \tau_\theta^2) \end{aligned} \tag{6.16}$$

Here, $h_{0i}(t)$ is the unique baseline hazard function in the ith trial, and other terms are as previously defined. As before, the model can be extended to include additional participant-level covariates (e.g. prognostic factors stratified by trial), and also trial-level covariates.

6.3.1.3 Comparison of Approaches

In general, where the focus is on the treatment effect, assuming proportional or stratified baseline hazards will usually produce similar results. However, model (6.16) makes fewer assumptions than model (6.15) or frailty models, and also avoids sharing information about control group rates across trials. Thus, model (6.16) is our default recommendation for one-stage IPD meta-analysis models of time-to-event outcomes. Of course, if the assumption of proportional baseline hazards and frailty models are correct, then this may improve power and estimation precision,[218,220,223] but this is difficult to justify in advance. Frailty models are perhaps best when the number of participants and outcome events per trial is relatively low, given that estimation issues may arise with separate baseline hazards per trial.

6.3.1.4 Estimation Methods

A summary of available software for fitting one-stage Cox and related models is shown in Table 6.2. Frequentist estimation of one-stage Cox models and frailty models is generally done via ML estimation (of the partial likelihood). As discussed for ML estimation of GLMMs, we recommend trial-specific centering of the treatment and other variables to improve between-trial variance estimates and coverage of confidence intervals (Section 6.2.8.3 and Box 6.3). For example, for each trial we recommend using a treatment variable coding of 1/0 (treatment/control) minus the proportion of trial participants in the treatment group.[181]

Crowther et al. show how to fit one-stage time-to-event models in a GLMM framework, using Poisson mixed effects regression and ML estimation.[44] Essentially, a one-stage Cox model can be fitted using a Poisson GLM due to the shared form of the contribution to the partial log-likelihood, by splitting follow-up time into as many intervals as there are events (Table 6.1). This may be computationally intensive, and so sometimes a smaller number of time intervals are chosen (e.g. defined by every six months or year), which still closely approximate the Cox model. An illustrative example is given in Figure 6.4.

Rondeau et al. suggest using penalised maximum likelihood to investigate between-trial heterogeneity of baseline rates and treatment effects, and their potential correlation.[224] As discussed for GLMMs (Section 6.2.8.2), ML estimation of survival models is prone to downward bias in between-trial variance estimates (even with trial-specific centering of variables), as shown in one-stage Cox models by Crowther et al.[44] Bowden suggested using the EM algorithm to enable REML estimation of a one-stage model,[5] and Bayesian approaches are an appealing alternative.[222] Summary treatment effects should be presented alongside 95% confidence (credible) intervals, together with between-trial variance estimates and, ideally, 95% prediction intervals.[90,222]

6.3.1.5 Example

Extending the IPD meta-analysis described in Box 6.1, we evaluated whether anti-hypertensive treatment reduces all-cause mortality compared to control.[44] Fitting a one-stage Cox model using ML estimation to the 10 randomised trials (and with trial-specific centering of the treatment variable), the summary hazard ratio is 0.88 (95% CI: 0.79 to 0.97) either when assuming proportional model (6.15) or unique model (6.16) baseline hazards for each trial, or when using a frailty model (assuming a gamma distribution). Results are also similar when using a Bayesian framework, though with slightly wider 95% credible intervals.[44] All approaches suggest that anti-hypertensive treatment reduces mortality rate in hypertension patients.

6.3.2 Fully Parametric Approaches

The Cox model framework is semi-parametric, as the form of the baseline hazard (either for the reference trial in model (6.15) or for all trials in model (6.16)) is left unspecified. Sometimes the baseline hazards (or related measures, such as the baseline survival function) are themselves of interest; in

Table 6.2 Software for fitting one-stage IPD meta-analysis via the GLMM or survival modelling frameworks described in this chapter

Software	Package	Brief summary of the software and package
R	ecoreg	Estimation of participant-level covariate-outcome associations at the aggregate level using AD ("ecological inference") or a combination of AD and IPD ("hierarchical-related regression").
	glmmML	Fitting of binomial and Poisson regression models with random intercepts. Estimation is performed using ML or using the Gauss-Hermite approximation to the likelihood. Allows for non-normal distributions in the specification of random intercepts.
	hglm	Fitting of GLMM where the random effects may come from a conjugate exponential-family distribution.
	lme4	Fitting of GLMM using ML or REML (for mixed linear models only).
	rstanarm	Fitting of GLMM using Bayesian Markov chain Monte Carlo.
	MASS	Fitting of GLMM using penalised quasi-likelihood (PQL) with the function glmmPQL.
	nlme	Fitting of linear mixed effect models using ML or REML.
	survival	Fitting of Cox PH and mixed effect survival models using penalised partial likelihood estimation (PPL). Stratified, frailty and marginal specifications are possible.
	frailtypack	Fitting of Cox and parametric random effects and stratified models. Estimation of joint nested frailty models.
	coxme	Fitting of mixed effects Cox PH models.
	SemiCompRisks	Bayesian and frequentist random effects parametric and semi-parametric models for competing events.
	parfm	Estimation of parametric frailty models.
	PenCoxFrail	Estimation of regularised Cox frailty models.
	mexhaz	Flexible (excess) hazard regression models, non-proportional effects, and random effects.
	dynfrail	Semi-parametric dynamic frailty models.
	frailtyEM	Frailty models with a semi-parametric baseline hazard, recurrent events.
	joineR	Joint random effects modelling of repeated measurements and time-to-event.
	joint.Cox	Joint frailty-copula models with smoothing splines.
	JointModel	Joint model for longitudinal and time-to-event outcomes.
	joineRML	Joint time-to-event and multiple continuous longitudinal outcomes.
SAS	PROC GLIMMIX	Fitting of GLMM using ML or REML estimation of the (pseudo) likelihood.
	PROC GLM	Fitting of GLMM using MOM.
	PROC LOGISTIC	Fitting of mixed nonlinear models (binary/ordinal/nominal responses) using ML.

(Continued)

Table 6.2 (Continued)

Software	Package	Brief summary of the software and package
	PROC MIXED, HPMIXED	Fitting of mixed linear models using ML, REML, or MOM. The HPMIXED allows higher performance.
	PROC NLMIXED	Fitting of mixed nonlinear models using (approximated) ML. Fitting of mixed effects parametric survival models.
	PROC PHREG	Fitting of Cox models, including stratification or frailty.
	PROC GENMOD	Fitting of Poisson regression, marginal models.
Stata	gllamm	Fitting of GLMM using ML.
	REGOPROB2	Fitting of random effects generalised-ordered probit models.
	stmixed	Fitting of (flexible) parametric survival models with mixed effects.
	XT	Fitting of GLMM.
	stcox	Fitting of Cox models, with stratified and frailty specifications.
	mixed	Fitting of mixed effects linear regression models.
	xtlogit	Fitting of mixed effects logistic regression models using adaptive or non-adaptive Gaussian-Hermite approximation of the likelihood.
	melogit	Fitting of mixed effects logistic regression models.
	mestreg	Fitting of parametric survival models with mixed effects.
	mepoisson	Fitting of mixed effects Poisson regression models.
MLwiN, MLn		Fitting of GLMM and mixed effects survival models using ML, REML, EM and Bayesian approaches.
NONNEM		General package for fitting of GLMM.
HLM		Fitting of two- and three-level GLMM using first-order penalised quasi-likelihood.
WinBUGS, JAGS, Stan, OpenBUGS		General packages to fit Bayesian models using Markov chain Monte Carlo estimation.
The Survival Kit		Fitting of Bayesian mixed effects survival models.

GLMM, generalised linear mixed model; AD, aggregate data: PH, proportional hazards; REML, restricted (or residual) maximum likelihood; ML, maximum likelihood; EM, expectation maximization, MoM, methods of moments.
Source: Thomas Debray.

particular, when developing a prognostic model,[225,226] or translating treatment effects back to the absolute risk scale. In this situation, a one-stage parametric survival model might be preferred, to give a smooth estimate of the baseline survival or (cumulative) hazard. Standard parametric distributions (e.g. exponential, Weibull or gamma) or accelerated failure time (AFT) models could be used.[222]

For more flexibility to model complex hazard functions, Crowther et al. propose a one-stage IPD meta-analysis model akin to model (6.16), but modelling the baseline cumulative hazard ($\ln(H_0(t))$ in each trial via restricted cubic splines.[222,227] This is done by fitting a series of cubic functions and forcing them to join (and be smoothed) at certain points (called internal knots), whilst constraining the function to be linear in the tails (i.e. before the first internal knot and after the last internal knot). If there are zero internal knots, $\ln(H_0(t))$ becomes the baseline hazard for a Weibull model.[228] Crowther implemented the framework using *stmixed* in Stata, which extends the framework of

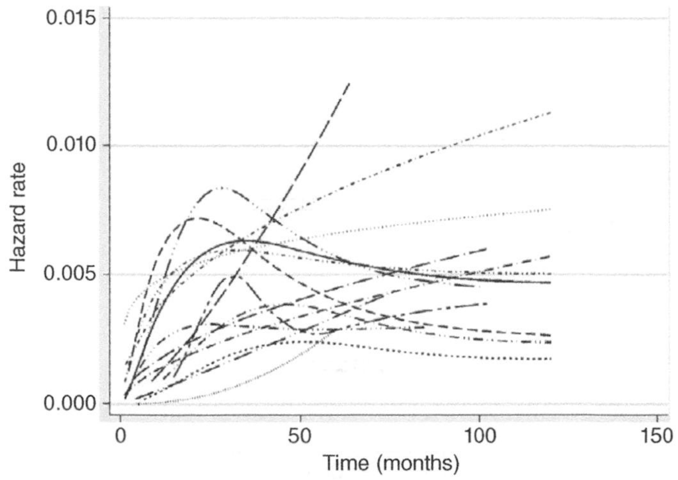

Figure 6.3 Baseline hazard functions from ML estimation of a one-stage IPD meta-analysis of 15 breast cancer studies of mortality rate,[222] where the cumulative baseline hazard functions are stratified by study, allowed to be non-proportional, and modelled using restricted cubic splines. *Source:* Figure taken from Figure 3 of Crowther et al.,[222] used with permission, © 2014 Wiley.

Royston-Parmar to allow mixed effects, such as random treatment effects. The degrees of freedom (*df*) for the baseline hazard function are calculated as $df = m + 1$, where m is the number of internal knots. Royston and Lambert suggest that 2–3 *df* are usually adequate to model the baseline hazard function in small datasets and 4–5 *df* in larger datasets.[228,229] The approach provides very similar hazard ratio estimates to those from a one-stage Cox model,[228,230] but additionally provides the baseline hazard and cumulative hazard ($H_0(t)$) functions. An example is shown in Figure 6.3, where a baseline hazard function is estimated for each of 15 breast cancer studies.

6.3.3 Extension to Time-varying Hazard Ratios and Joint Models

So far, our one-stage survival models have assumed that the hazard ratios for each included covariate are constant over time; in particular, that the treatment effect is the same at all time points. However, non-proportional hazards (i.e. non-constant, time-varying hazard ratios) should always be examined, for example by including a (non-linear) interaction between each covariate and time, or by comparing hazard ratios within relevant time periods. For example, let us return to the example in Section 6.3.1.5 where we evaluated the effect of anti-hypertensive treatment on all-cause mortality. In the first year of treatment the summary hazard ratio is 0.66 (95% CI: 0.52 to 0.84), but this reduces to 0.94 (95% CI: 0.84 to 1.05) from year 1 onwards.[44] This is illustrated in Figure 6.4.

When a frailty is applied to the baseline hazard, the median hazard ratio can also be used to evaluate the meaning of this frailty in the context of the different trials.[231,232] The median hazard ratio is the median relative difference in the hazard of outcome event occurrence when comparing identical participants from two randomly selected trials ordered by hazard. An example in the IPD meta-analysis setting is provided by de Jong et al.[214]

Non-proportional hazards can sometimes be handled more naturally with models that assume proportionality on another scale.[228,233] For instance, a treatment might temporarily reduce the hazards, but as time progresses and the effect wears off, hazards converge and thereby violate the proportional hazards assumption. This can be modelled with a proportional odds regression

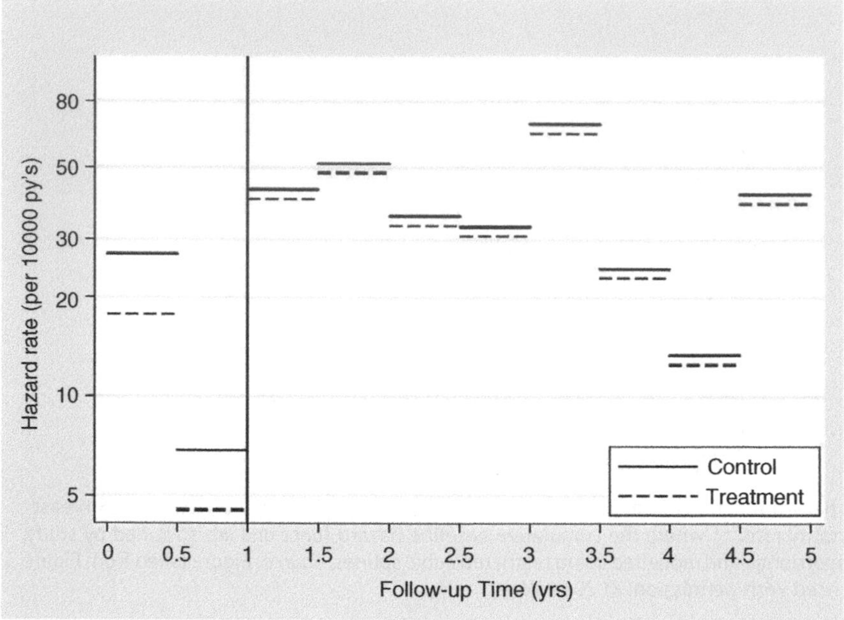

Figure 6.4 Estimated baseline hazard rate for one of the 10 trials included in the one-stage Cox regression model of Crowther et al.,[44] as estimated using Poisson regression and applied to an IPD meta-analysis to examine the effect of anti-hypertensive treatment on all-cause mortality. The model used 10 time-intervals defined by every six months of follow-up, assumed constant hazard rate in each interval stratified by trial, with non-proportional hazards for treatment (hazard ratio assumed different before and after one year). *Source:* Figure taken from Figure 5 of Crowther et al.,[44] reproduced with permission, © 2012 Springer Nature (CC-BY 2.0).

model such as the log-logistic, which assumes that covariates have a constant additive effect on the log odds of survival.[227,234,235] In this model, the hazard ratio naturally approaches 1 over time, whereas the odds remain proportional.

The implementation of one-stage IPD meta-analysis models with non-proportional hazards (e.g. with non-linear trends modelled using splines) may complicate the interpretation of regression parameters, and so alternative measures have been proposed to summarise treatment effects. For instance, the restricted mean survival time represents the area under the survival curve until a particular time.[236–239] Thus, it can be calculated for treatment and control groups, and their difference quantifies the treatment effect, which represents the expected gain (or loss) in survival until the chosen time for the treatment group, as compared to the control group. The percentile ratio is another effect measure suggested to make the interpretation of survival models more straightforward.[240] Briefly, the percentile ratio is defined as the expected ratio for the time at which a certain fraction of the participants will have an event in the treatment group as compared to the control group. The percentile ratio is easiest to interpret for accelerate failure time models, as the percentile ratio does not depend on the percentile chosen in such models and always equals the acceleration factor.

Another important extension is the joint modelling of longitudinal and time-to-event data, for example to model the trend in a patient's SBP over time whilst simultaneously modelling their risk of death. As described by Ibrahim et al,[241] this approach may provide more efficient and less biased estimates of the treatment effect. In a one-stage IPD meta-analysis framework, this requires specifying a one-stage IPD meta-analysis for the longitudinal sub-model and a one-stage IPD meta-analyses for the time-to-event sub-models, as shown by Suddell et al.[242] These multiple sub-models are fitted simultaneously and the key aspect is that they involve shared parameters across the sub-models, and so have much synergy with the next section on simultaneously combining different sources of evidence.

6.4 One-stage Models Combining Different Sources of Evidence

The previous one-stage models assumed IPD are available from multiple randomised trials with a parallel-group design. Sometimes IPD are not available for all trials, or the IPD comes from trials with different designs. In such situations, the one-stage modelling framework needs to be refined or extended, and some examples are now described.

6.4.1 Combining IPD Trials with Partially Reconstructed IPD from Non-IPD Trials

When IPD are not available, it may be possible to partially reconstruct the IPD using aggregate data available within trial publications, such as two-by-two tables, means and standard deviations, or even Kaplan-Meier curves. The general premise is that the reconstructed IPD should match the known summary characteristics of the IPD, in terms of the sample size, number of events, mean values, and correlation amongst covariates, and so forth.[8,144] Then, the previously described one-stage IPD meta-analysis models can be used to synthesise the actual and reconstructed IPD, and thus combine IPD and non-IPD trials. This is especially appealing if most trials are small, as it allows the more exact likelihood of a one-stage model to be fitted (rather than the two-stage approach described in Chapter 5).

For continuous outcomes, Papadimitropoulou et al. propose a method to generate pseudo-IPD from aggregate data using the reported final score mean and standard deviation, and sample size, for each treatment group.[17] They showed that a one-stage meta-analysis of the pseudo-IPD (akin to the linear mixed model (6.2) with a random treatment effect) leads to identical results had the true IPD been available. Further, it allowed them to examine how conclusions change according to the use of a stratified intercept or random intercepts, and stratified or common residual variances.

For binary outcome data, IPD can be partly reconstructed from the aggregated information in published two-by-two tables.[8] For example, if the number of participants who were dead and alive for each of the treatment and control groups is known, IPD can be re-created in a binary data format, where control/treatment group and alive/dead are represented by a series of zeros and ones. This is illustrated in Box 6.5. Similarly, for multinomial (including ordinal) outcome data IPD may be reconstructed given information on the number of responses falling into each category for each treatment group. For survival data, methods existing for reconstructed IPD from published Kaplan-Meier curves are implemented in software such as the *ipdfc* package in Stata.[243,244]

Reconstruction of IPD including participant-level covariates is difficult, as information about the multivariate distributions (e.g. means, variances and correlations) would be needed for outcomes and covariates in order to recreate covariate values reliably (Section 5.6).[144] Thus adjustment for prognostic factors will be difficult for trials only enabling reconstructed IPD to be included. Key exceptions are for categorical covariates, as two-by-two tables might be available for each category, and for baseline values of a continuous outcome, as the correlation between baseline and follow-up values might be more readily obtainable.[143] Of course, re-creating IPD loses many of the advantages of having the real IPD, in particular examining quality, checking eligibility of participants, and obtaining values of participant-level covariates and outcomes that were not reported in trial publications (Chapter 4).

Box 6.5 Example of pseudo-IPD reconstructed from reported aggregate data, to enable a one-stage IPD meta-analysis for a binary outcome such as model (6.3), albeit without adjustment for prognostic factors

- Say trial 1 only provides aggregate data in the form of a two-by-two table:

	Dead	Alive
Treatment	3	7
Control	5	5

- This can be converted to pseudo-IPD, where the number of those in the treatment and control groups, together with the number of deaths therein, correspond to the values observed in the two-by-two table.

Trial	Participant	Treatment	Control	Dead
1	1	1	0	1
1	2	1	0	1
1	3	1	0	1
1	4	1	0	0
1	5	1	0	0
1	6	1	0	0
1	7	1	0	0
1	8	1	0	0
1	9	1	0	0
1	10	1	0	0
1	11	0	1	1
1	12	0	1	1
1	13	0	1	1
1	14	0	1	1
1	15	0	1	1
1	16	0	1	0
1	17	0	1	0
1	18	0	1	0
1	19	0	1	0
1	20	0	1	0

Source: Richard Riley.

6.4.2 Combining IPD and Aggregate Data Using Hierarchical Related Regression

When IPD are not available for a particular trial, and cannot be reconstructed, then it is possible to incorporate aggregate data from that trial in the one-stage meta-analysis framework. This requires the specification of two (or more) regression models with shared parameters, also known as hierarchical related regression.[8,156,245] For example, if we assume that a treatment effect estimate ($\hat{\theta}_i$) and its variance (s_i^2) can be extracted for non-IPD trials, then for a continuous outcome situation we could write the following one-stage model:

IPD trials:	$y_{ij} = \alpha_i + \theta_i x_{ij} + \beta_{1i} y_{0ij} + \varepsilon_{ij}$
	$\varepsilon_{ij} \sim \mathrm{N}(0, \sigma_i^2)$
Non-IPD trials:	$\hat{\theta}_i \sim N(\theta_i, s_i^2)$
All trials:	$\theta_i \sim N(\theta, \tau_\theta^2)$

Here, IPD and non-IPD trials have different models but two shared parameters: the average treatment effect (θ) and the between-trial heterogeneity (τ_θ^2). In IPD trials we model the continuous outcomes of the included participants, with a stratified intercept, stratified residual variance, and stratified prognostic effect for baseline value (y_{0ij}), whereas for non-IPD trials we model the estimated treatment effect ($\hat{\theta}_i$) and its variance (s_i^2) in each trial. A similar framework is possible for other outcomes, such as binary or time-to-event outcomes, except the IPD trials then have a one-stage logistic or survival model specification.[8,159,246]

To specify such hierarchical related regression models, the analyst requires software that allows a likelihood function to be written directly by the user, for each of the IPD and non-IPD trials, which are then jointly maximised (e.g. using ML or REML estimation) or utilised within a Bayesian estimation. For continuous outcomes, we can 'trick' existing general linear mixed model software to do this for us, through the use of a dummy variable ($D_i = 1$ for IPD trials, and $D_i = 0$ for non-IPD trials) and a transformed response variable, y_{ij}^*. This was proposed by Riley et al.,[156] building on work by Goldstein et al.[151] Using the previous model as an example, we can write:

$$y_{ij}^* = D_i\alpha_i + \theta_i x_{ij}^* + D_i\beta_{1i}y_{0ij} + \varepsilon_{ij}^*$$

where

$$y_{ij}^* = y_{ij} \text{ if } D_i = 1 \text{ and } y_{ij}^* = \hat{\theta}_i \text{ if } D_i = 0$$
$$x_{ij}^* = x_{ij} \text{ if } D_i = 1 \text{ and } x_{ij}^* = 1 \text{ if } D_i = 0$$
$$\varepsilon_{ij}^* \sim N(0, \sigma_i^2) \text{ if } D_i = 1 \text{ and } \varepsilon_{ij}^* \sim N(0, \mathrm{var}(\hat{\theta}_i)) \text{ if } D_i = 0$$
$$\theta_i \sim N(\theta, \tau_\theta^2)$$

This dummy variable approach requires frequentist (such as SAS Proc Mixed) or Bayesian software that allows us to hold fixed (i.e. at user-specified values) variances estimates (s_i^2) for the non-IPD trials. As before, all trials will contribute toward the summary treatment effect, but only the IPD trials are able to estimate other parameter estimates. Further discussion on including non-IPD trials is given in Section 5.6.

6.4.3 Combining IPD from Parallel-group, Cluster and Cross-over Trials

It is important to reflect the design of each trial in the one-stage IPD meta-analysis model. So far we have considered one-stage models for synthesising randomised trials with a parallel-group design. However, hierarchical related regression can also be used to handle trials with different designs. Essentially, a different likelihood (model) is allowed for each design type, but they contained shared parameters such as the treatment effect and between-trial variance in treatment effect. For example, Sutton et al. considered the combination of IPD from a mixture of cluster trials and parallel-group trials,[163] for evaluating the treatment effect on a binary outcome. For the parallel-group trials they specified model (6.3) with random treatment effects, but for the cluster trials they specified a slightly different model to account for participants nested within clusters in each trial, as follows:

parallel-group trials:	$y_{ij} \sim \text{Bernoulli}(p_{ij})$
	$\text{logit}(p_{ij}) = \alpha_i + \theta_i x_{ij}$
Cluster trials:	$y_{ikj} \sim \text{Bernoulli}(p_{ikj})$
	$\text{logit}(p_{ikj}) = \alpha_{ik} + \theta_i x_{ikj}$
	$\alpha_{ik} \sim N(\alpha_i, \tau_k^2)$
All trials:	$\theta_i \sim N(\theta, \tau_\theta^2)$

As before, i denotes trial, j denotes participant, and y_{ij} denotes the binary outcome value. Additionally for cluster trials, k denotes the cluster within trial i. The parallel-group and cluster trial models are similar, except that the cluster trial model assumes that the log-odds of the outcome in the control group clusters are drawn from a distribution with mean α_i (the average control group log-odds across clusters in trial i) and between-trial variance τ_k^2. Thus the design of the cluster trial (i.e. participants nested within clusters receiving the same treatment) is accounted for. The two models are estimated simultaneously (Sutton et al. suggest a Bayesian framework for this[163]) and, as they both assume $\theta_i \sim N(\theta, \tau_\theta^2)$, the parallel-group and cluster trials contribute together toward estimates of the overall summary treatment effect (θ) and between-trial variance (τ_θ^2).

The hierarchical regression modelling framework can be adapted to other types of trial design (such as cross-over trials or multi-centre trials), and extended to include trial-level covariates and treatment-covariate interactions (Chapter 7).

6.5 Reporting of One-stage Models in Protocols and Publications

One-stage models are often poorly reported upon publication,[1,146,161,247] with assumptions hidden like a black box. The exact model specification and assumptions should be clearly detailed in both the protocol and the trial publication, including information about which model parameters are assumed common, stratified, or random (and if any multiple random effects are correlated). Results can still be presented as forest plots. These are usually produced following a two-stage IPD meta-analysis approach; but the plot can be forced to display summary results from a one-stage analysis (for example, using the option 'first' within the Stata package metan[248]), whilst still displaying trial-specific estimates as derived from a separate analysis in each trial or by calculating the empirical Bayes trial estimates after fitting the one-stage model.[207,249] Adherence to PRISMA-IPD is recommended (see Chapter 10).[247]

6.6 Concluding Remarks

One-stage IPD meta-analysis models fall within the framework of GLMMs and hierarchical survival models, and are an important tool for IPD meta-analyses, especially when data are sparse. Whilst this makes them appealing to statisticians used to analysing multilevel structures and fitting mixed effects models, their complexity can also lead to errors (e.g. ignoring clustering) and challenges for estimation and coding. Lots of researchers will also find the one-stage approach more technical than the two-stage approach outlined in Chapter 5. It is, therefore, reassuring that one-stage and two-stage analyses usually give similar results,[7] and Chapter 8 provides a detailed comparison with recommendations. Extension of the approaches to examine how participant-level characteristics modify (interact with) treatment effect is considered in the next chapter.

7

Using IPD Meta-Analysis to Examine Interactions between Treatment Effect and Participant-level Covariates

Richard D. Riley and David J. Fisher

Summary Points

- A key component of stratified and precision medicine research is to identify participant-level characteristics (covariates) that are associated with changes in a treatment's effect. These are known as treatment-covariate interactions.
- When IPD from multiple randomised trials are available, an IPD meta-analysis provides the opportunity to increase power to detect true treatment-covariate interactions.
- When done properly, an IPD meta-analysis avoids using *across*-trial information from a meta-regression of the observed treatment effects (based on all trial participants) and *aggregated* values of participant-level covariates (such as mean age, proportion male). Such analyses are prone to aggregation bias and may not reflect actual interactions at the participant level.
- A two-stage IPD approach to estimating treatment-covariate interactions avoids aggregation bias by estimating treatment-covariate interactions in each trial separately, and then synthesising them in the second stage. This ensures that only within-trial information is used.
- A one-stage IPD meta-analysis to the estimation of treatment-covariate interactions must ensure that within-trial and across-trial information are separated out, by either (i) stratifying all nuisance parameters by trial, or (ii) centering the covariate by its mean and allowing the mean covariate value to explain between-trial heterogeneity.
- Many current IPD meta-analysis projects apply a one-stage model that amalgamates within-trial and across-trial information; this is not recommended.
- If interactions do exist, they are more likely to be detected when continuous covariates and outcomes are analysed on their continuous scale.
- Treatment-covariate interactions may be non-linear (e.g. U- or J-shaped), and should be investigated, for example using a two-stage multivariate IPD meta-analysis summarising interactions defined by a restricted cubic spline function.
- Treatment-covariate interactions may depend on the scale of analysis; for example, they may arise on the odds ratio scale, even when there is no interaction on the risk ratio scale.
- Predicting an individual's treatment effect conditional on their covariate values requires the combination of risk prediction models and treatment-covariate interactions.

Individual Participant Data Meta-Analysis: A Handbook for Healthcare Research, First Edition.
Edited by Richard D. Riley, Jayne F. Tierney, and Lesley A. Stewart.

7.1 Introduction

There is an increasing interest in precision medicine, where the aim is to select treatments for individual patients, or groups of similar patients, based on their particular characteristics such as stage of disease or particular gene mutations.[250] This concept is also known as personalised medicine or stratified care,[251] and aims to optimise treatment decisions (maximise benefits, reduce harms) and reduce unnecessary costs. For example, generally trastuzumab is only given to the subgroup (stratum) of breast cancer patients who are human epidermal growth factor receptor 2 (HER-2) positive, as it is known to lock on to the HER-2 protein, block the receptor and stop the cells from dividing and growing,[252] and so is inappropriate for women who are HER-2 negative.

A key component of precision medicine research is exploring whether particular participant-level characteristics (covariates) are associated with a differential treatment effect.[250] In other words, the goal is to identify *treatment-covariate interactions* that can be used to identify types of patients who are expected to gain the most from receiving particular treatments, and thus may warrant different clinical decisions than other types of patients. Other names given to covariates that interact with treatment effect include effect moderators, predictors of treatment effect and, mainly in the cancer literature, predictive markers. Types of covariates that may interact with treatment effect include standard clinical characteristics (e.g. tumour grade, symptoms) and patient demographics (e.g. age, sex), and also genetic information and biomarker measurements, such as HER-2. Covariates may even reflect a combination of factors (e.g. disease stage and BMI are based on values of two or more other variables).

Though some treatment-covariate interactions (such as trastuzumab and HER-2) are suspected in advance due to strong biological rationale, others are only identified following secondary investigations of existing data. Single randomised trials are typically powered on the treatment effect averaged across all participants recruited from the population of interest, and so do not have sufficient power to detect more granular differences in treatment effect across subgroups of participants. Powering a single trial to detect a genuine treatment-covariate interaction will typically require at least four times the sample size needed to evaluate the overall treatment effect, and often substantially more,[253] making it expensive and usually infeasible. When IPD from multiple randomised trials are available, meta-analysis provides the opportunity to increase power to detect genuine treatment-covariate interactions.[254] For this reason, many IPD meta-analyses of randomised trials are initiated specifically to examine one or more treatment-covariate interactions. A well-known example is given in Box 7.1, where the collation of IPD from 55 randomised trials and about 37000 women suggests that the effect of adjuvant tamoxifen therapy in early-stage breast cancer patients is largest in those who are oestrogen reception (ER) positive.

In this chapter, we outline the importance of IPD meta-analysis projects for examining treatment-covariate interactions at the participant level, and describe why a traditional meta-regression based on published aggregate data is severely flawed. Using illustrated examples, and building on earlier work,[255] we describe statistical methods to summarise a treatment-covariate interaction in an IPD meta-analysis, extending the two-stage and one-stage frameworks introduced in Chapters 5 and 6. We emphasise that genuine treatment-covariate interactions are rare, and much care is

Box 7.1 Example of an IPD meta-analysis that identified a treatment-covariate interaction in breast cancer.[268]

The Early Breast Cancer Trialists' Collaborative Group obtained IPD from 55 trials,[268] including 37000 women with early-stage breast cancer, and examined whether the benefit of adjuvant tamoxifen varied according to oestrogen receptor (ER) status. The summary meta-analysis results (hazard ratios comparing the risk of cancer recurrence after five years, for treatment versus control) are shown below, for each ER group and overall. There is strong evidence of a larger treatment effect for the ER positive group, and it is unclear whether there is any benefit in those classed as ER negative.

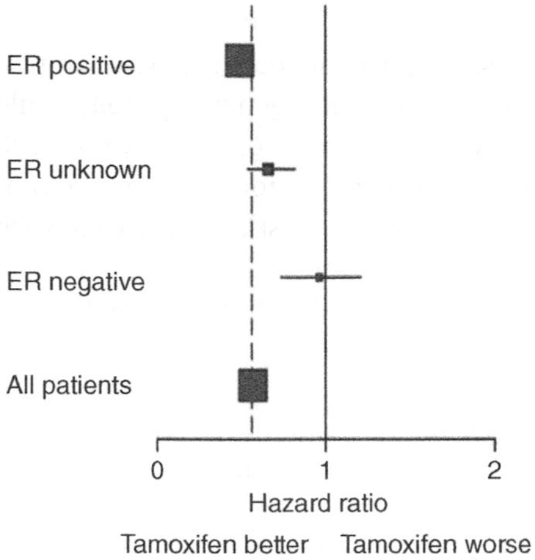

Source: Richard Riley; forest plot reproduced using data extracted from Figure 1 of the article published by the Early Breast Cancer Trialists' Collaborative Group in *The Lancet*.[268]

needed before concluding they exist. In particular, meta-analysts must separate out within-trial and across-trial variation, and appropriately handle continuous covariates, including consideration of non-linear relationships. We also highlight some common misconceptions, building on previous work in both IPD meta-analysis and single trial settings.[156,253,256–265] We note that treatment-covariate interactions are sometimes described within research labelled 'heterogeneous treatment effects' or 'treatment effect heterogeneity', where heterogeneity refers to participant-level variability.[266,267] However, in this book – and indeed the meta-analysis literature in general – we reserve the word heterogeneity for variability between trials.

7.2 Meta-regression and Its Limitations

In this section, we describe the use of meta-regression to estimate treatment-covariate interactions based solely on across-trial information, and explain why this is potentially misleading and generally not recommended due to *low power* and *aggregation bias*.

7.2.1 Meta-regression of Aggregated Participant-level Covariates

Consider an IPD meta-analysis of $i = 1$ to S parallel-group randomised trials, each comparing a treatment to a control. The two-stage framework of Chapter 5 uses, in the first stage, the IPD for each trial separately to derive (using all participants) the treatment effect estimate ($\hat{\theta}_i$) and its variance ($\text{var}(\hat{\theta}_i) = s_i^2$). Then, assuming the s_i^2 are known and that there is between-trial heterogeneity in the treatment effects, the second stage fits a meta-analysis model with random treatment effects:

$$\begin{aligned} \hat{\theta}_i &\sim N(\theta_i, s_i^2) \\ \theta_i &\sim N(\theta, \tau^2) \end{aligned} \tag{7.1}$$

Here, θ denotes the average treatment effect across trials, and τ^2 denotes the between-trial heterogeneity in treatment effect. We may wish to investigate whether any heterogeneity could be explained (and thus the magnitude of τ^2 reduced) by the inclusion of trial-level covariates.[139] This requires a *meta-regression*, which was introduced in Section 5.4, and extends model (7.1) to incorporate covariates that reflect the design or characteristics of the trial, such as the intended dose of treatment, year of trial completion, or country of recruitment. Such trial-level covariates do not vary across participants in the same trial, but are characteristics of the trial itself.

Although hugely problematic (Section 7.2.2), researchers sometimes use meta-regression to investigate aggregated participant-level covariates (such as mean age and proportion male), which summarise characteristics (such as age and sex) which usually do vary between participants in the same trial. Then the aim of meta-regression is to examine whether the value of such aggregated participant-level covariates is associated with the size of the treatment effect (θ_i) across trials. For instance, the treatment effect might be larger in trials with a younger mean age or a greater proportion of females. Consider a meta-regression with the inclusion of one covariate, $\bar{z}_i$, which denotes the mean of a particular participant-level covariate (e.g. mean age) in trial i. Then, the meta-regression is written as:

$$\begin{aligned} \hat{\theta}_i &\sim N(\theta_i, s_i^2) \\ \theta_i &\sim N(\alpha + \gamma_A \bar{z}_i, \tau^2) \end{aligned} \tag{7.2}$$

In model (7.2), α denotes the expected treatment effect for a trial where $\bar{z}_i = 0$, and τ^2 denotes the unexplained between-trial heterogeneity after accounting for $\bar{z}_i$. Of key interest is γ_A, which denotes how the expected treatment effect changes across trials for a one-unit increase in the mean covariate value, $\bar{z}_i$. The A denotes that the estimate of γ_A is based solely on *across-trial* information, which is an important concept that we will tackle throughout this chapter. Estimation methods for fitting model (7.2) are as discussed in Chapter 5; for example, in a frequentist framework, restricted maximum likelihood (REML) estimation can be used and subsequent confidence intervals derived using the Hartung-Knapp Sidik-Jonkman (HKSJ) approach.[111]

7.2.2 Low Power and Aggregation Bias

To best inform precision medicine, an IPD meta-analysis should aim to estimate the interaction between treatment effect and a covariate measured at the participant-level; let us denote this interaction as γ_W, where W emphasises this is based on *within-trial* information at the participant-level. For example, if the covariate is age (measured in years) then an estimate of the treatment-age interaction (γ_W) would reveal how much the treatment effect changes for each one-year increase in age. Fisher et al. label such interactions as 'deft'.[258]

Meta-regression model (7.2) does not use actual values of participant-level covariates, but rather uses aggregated values (e.g. mean age in each trial); nevertheless, the premise is that $\hat{\gamma}_A$ may provide an unbiased estimate of γ_W. For example, if $\bar{z}_i$ represents the trial mean age, then the assumption is that γ_A will reflect the interaction between treatment effect and age at the participant level. Unfortunately, even when this premise is correct, a meta-regression usually has low power to identify genuine treatment-covariate interactions;[269] typically there are only a small number of trials (e.g. < 15) available for meta-analysis, and there needs to be large variation in the mean covariate value across trials to have sufficient power to detect a genuine interaction at the participant level.[259] For example, Berlin et al. examined the effect of elevated panel reactive antibodies on the effectiveness of anti-lymphocyte antibody induction.[270] Applying meta-regression model (7.2), and thus examining the association of a trial's treatment effect (as derived using all participants) and the proportion of trial participants with elevated antibodies, they found no evidence of an association (difference in log odds ratio $= 0.01$, $p = 0.68$). However, when IPD were obtained and the treatment-covariate interaction investigated at the participant level using within-trial information (using methods described in subsequent sections), they found a substantial difference in the treatment effect (log odds ratio) between elevated and non-elevated participants (difference in log odds ratio $= -1.33$, $p = 0.01$).

A further, and more critical, problem is that meta-regression of trial-level covariates is prone to trial-level confounding, such that observed across-trial associations do not properly reflect the participant-level relationships within trials. This is generally known as *aggregation bias*, and sometimes referred to as *ecological bias* or the *ecological fallacy*.[270–272] For example, meta-regression may identify that trials with a larger mean age have a larger treatment effect; however, those trials with a higher mean age might also have a higher intended dose of the treatment, and therefore the larger effect in such trials could be due to a higher dose rather than having older participants.[156] Trial-level confounding (and thus aggregation bias) is avoided when examining interactions at the participant level (i.e. based on *within-trial* information); for example, even though the intended dose of a drug may vary across trials, it is typically fixed within a particular treatment group within a trial.

For these reasons, using a meta-regression of across-trial information to estimate treatment-covariate interactions at the participant-level has been labelled as 'daft',[258] and we recommend it be avoided. At best it serves only as an exploratory analysis, but even this is questionable given the discrepancy of across-trial and within-trial estimates observed in real applications.

7.2.3 Empirical Evidence of the Difference Between Using Across-trial and Within-trial Information to Estimate Treatment-covariate Interactions

Fisher et al. provide empirical evidence, across a range of settings in 31 re-analyses, of the difference between treatment-covariate interactions estimated using across-trial information (a 'daft' analysis using aggregated data) or within-trial information (a 'deft' analysis using participant-level information).[258] Their findings show that the discrepancy can be dramatic (Figure 7.1). In 13 (42%) of the 31 re-analyses the estimate of γ_W (which is based on participant-level information) is in a different direction to the estimate of γ_A (from a meta-regression of aggregated data). For example, in one application $\hat{\gamma}_A$ from meta-regression is 18.43 (95% CI: 8.16 to 28.69), in the opposing direction to

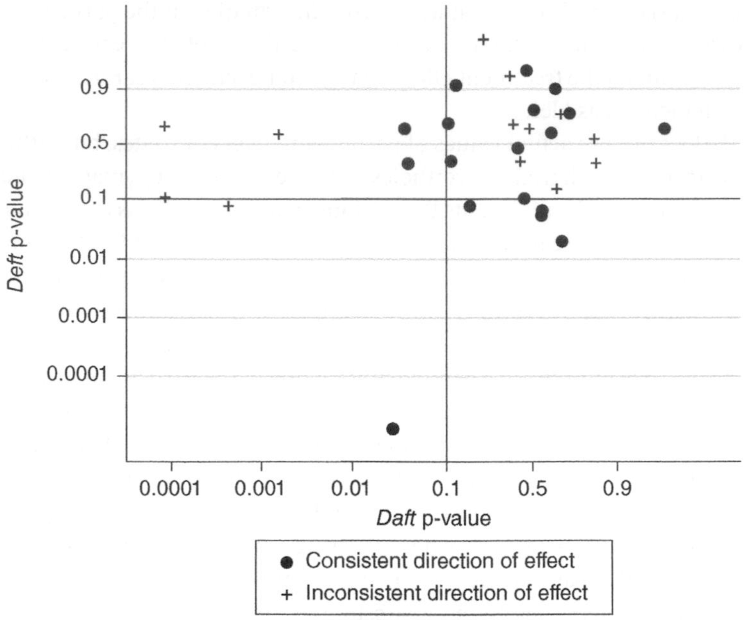

NB: Added lines are at $p = 0.1$, which is an arbitrary level of statistical significance, but sometimes used for an interaction test within trials that were not powered to detect interactions.

Figure 7.1 Scatter plot (on logit scale) of p-values from 31 re-analyses of treatment-covariate interactions, based on $\hat{\gamma}_W$ from using within-trial information (labelled as 'deft') or $\hat{\gamma}_A$ using across-trial information (labelled as 'daft'), as shown by Fisher et al.[258] *Source:* Figure taken from Figure 3 of Fisher et al.,[258] reproduced with permission,

the estimated treatment-covariate interaction ($\hat{\gamma}_W$) of −6.47 (95% CI: −13.65 to 0.71) when using participant-level information. Across the 31 re-analyses there are seven $\hat{\gamma}_A$ with a p-value of < 0.1, but only two of the corresponding $\hat{\gamma}_W$ also have a p-value of < 0.1 (Figure 7.1). Of the six $\hat{\gamma}_W$ with a p-value of < 0.1, only two of the corresponding $\hat{\gamma}_A$ have a p-value of < 0.1.

7.3 Two-stage IPD Meta-Analysis to Estimate Treatment-covariate Interactions

As outlined in Section 7.2.2, the meta-regression problems of low power and aggregation bias can be addressed by estimating treatment-covariate interactions using participant-level information. This can be achieved in an IPD meta-analysis using either a two-stage or a one-stage approach. In this section we describe these approaches in the context of IPD from randomised trials with a parallel-group design. The key principles also apply to other trials designs, such as cluster trials, but the equations need to be modified appropriately for the design (Section 5.2.5).

7.3.1 The Two-stage Approach

A two-stage IPD meta-analysis for summarising treatment-covariate interactions is a straight-forward extension of the two-stage methods introduced in Chapter 5. In the first stage, the treatment-covariate interactions are estimated using the IPD in each trial separately; in the second stage, these interaction estimates are pooled using a chosen meta-analysis model.[259] By only pooling interaction estimates derived from within-trial information (i.e. based at the participant level), this approach automatically avoids trial-level confounding and aggregation bias that may occur in meta-regression model (7.2) based on across-trial information.[212,256] The approach can be implemented using the *ipdmetan* software package.[119] Our website (www.ipdma.co.uk) provides examples of statistical code for various case studies used in this chapter.

Consider IPD from a parallel-group trial, comparing a treatment ($x_{ij} = 1$) to a control ($x_{ij} = 0$). Let z_{ij} be a participant-level covariate (e.g. the age of participant j in trial i), observed for all participants in each trial, and consider a continuous outcome, such as SBP (y_{ij}). Then the first stage is to apply a linear regression *in each trial separately*, adjusting for the baseline SBP (y_{0ij}) and the covariate (z_{ij}), whilst including the treatment (x_{ij}) and the treatment-covariate interaction ($x_{ij}z_{ij}$):

$$\begin{aligned} y_{ij} &= \alpha_i + \beta_{1i}z_{ij} + \beta_{2i}x_{ij} + \beta_{3i}y_{0ij} + \gamma_{Wi}x_{ij}z_{ij} + e_{ij} \\ e_{ij} &\sim N\left(0, \sigma_i^2\right) \end{aligned} \tag{7.3}$$

If a binary outcome was of interest (i.e. $y_{ij}= 0$ or 1), then alternatively a binomial regression could be fitted in each trial separately, such as a logistic regression:

$$\begin{aligned} y_{ij} &\sim \text{Bernoulli}(p_i) \\ \ln\left(\frac{p_i}{1-p_i}\right) &= \alpha_i + \beta_{1i}z_{ij} + \beta_{2i}x_{ij} + \gamma_{Wi}x_{ij}z_{ij} \end{aligned} \tag{7.4}$$

If a time-to-event outcome was of interest, then a Cox proportional hazards regression model might be fitted in each trial separately:

$$\lambda_{ij}(t) = \lambda_{0i}(t)\exp\left(\beta_{1i}z_{ij} + \beta_{2i}x_{ij} + \gamma_{Wi}x_{ij}z_{ij}\right) \tag{7.5}$$

These models examine the treatment-covariate interaction (γ_{Wi}) after adjusting for the prognostic effect (β_{2i}) of the covariate of interest (x_{ij}); additionally model (7.3) adjusts for the prognostic effect (β_{3i}) of y_{0ij}. Models (7.3) to (7.5) should also adjust for other (ideally pre-defined) prognostic factors where possible, as recommended in Section 5.2.4.[273] Model (7.5) could also be extended to include interactions with time to model non-proportional hazards (Sections 5.2.3.5 and 6.3.3).

In each model, the key parameter of interest is the treatment-covariate interaction term, γ_{Wi}, which indicates the expected change in treatment effect for a one-unit increase in z_{ij} for trial i. For a continuous covariate, this assumes the effect of the interaction is linear (although extension to non-linear trends is important, Section 7.6.2). Incorporation of β_{1i} adjusts for the prognostic effect of the covariate of interest (and β_{3i} in model (7.3) adjusts for the baseline value), whilst β_{2i} provides the expected treatment effect for participants with a value of $z_{ij} = 0$. As mentioned, the W is used to emphasise that the interaction, γ_{Wi}, is based solely on *within*-trial information.

Estimation of the appropriate model in each trial, for example using maximum likelihood estimation (potentially with Firth's correction or another penalisation method if sparse data bias is a concern[98,167]) produces a treatment-covariate interaction estimate, $\hat{\gamma}_{Wi}$, and its variance, $\text{var}(\hat{\gamma}_{Wi})$. Then, in the second stage the $\hat{\gamma}_{Wi}$ values are combined across trials in either a common-effect model (i.e. the true interaction is assumed the same in all trials),

$$\hat{\gamma}_{Wi} \sim N(\gamma_W, \text{var}(\hat{\gamma}_{Wi})) \tag{7.6}$$

or a random-effects model (i.e. the true interactions are assumed random across trials):

$$\hat{\gamma}_{Wi} \sim N(\gamma_{Wi}, \text{var}(\hat{\gamma}_{Wi}))$$
$$\gamma_{Wi} \sim N(\gamma_W, \tau^2) \tag{7.7}$$

Estimation methods are as described in Chapter 5; for example, model (7.7) can be estimated using REML with subsequent confidence intervals derived using the HKSL approach or, if wider, the standard approach (Section 5.3.7).[111] The estimate of γ_W summarises the difference in the expected treatment effect for two participants who differ in z_{ij} by one unit. For a continuous outcome modelled using the linear regression of model (7.3) in the first stage, γ_W represents a difference in mean difference; for a binary outcome modelled using the logistic regression of model (7.4) in the first stage, γ_W represents a difference in log odds ratios (i.e. $\exp(\hat{\gamma}_W)$ gives a ratio of odds ratios); and for a time-to-event outcome modelled using Cox regression model (7.5) in the first stage, γ_W represents a difference in log hazard ratios (i.e. $\exp(\hat{\gamma}_W)$ is a ratio of hazard ratios).

Note that model (7.7) allows for between-trial heterogeneity in the true treatment-covariate interaction. It may arise due to differences across trials in, for example, the dose of the treatment, the length of follow-up, the measurement of the covariate, and the magnitude of any interaction. It may also be due to case-mix differences in the trial populations, for example leading to between-trial differences in the distribution of within-trial confounders and even the covariate itself. For instance, if a treatment-covariate interaction is non-linear, and the covariate distribution is narrow in some trials and wide in others, then this will induce between-trial heterogeneity in the treatment-covariate interaction, unless the non-linear association is modelled directly (Section 7.6.2). The magnitude and impact of heterogeneity can be summarised as described in Chapter 5, for example by providing estimates of between-trial variances and using 95% prediction intervals (Sections 5.3.4 and 5.3.10).

7.3.2 Applied Example: Is the Effect of Anti-hypertensive Treatment Different for Males and Females?

Using IPD from 10 randomised trials of anti-hypertensive treatment (introduced in Box 6.1), we examined whether the treatment effect on SBP is different for males compared to females.[46,156] In the first stage, model (7.3) was fitted with final blood pressure as the outcome, and sex (males = 1, females = 0) as the covariate, z_{ij}, of interest. Figure 7.2 provides a forest plot of the treatment-sex interaction estimates, $\hat{\gamma}_{Wi}$, plotted as circles. Circles are recommended by Fisher et al. to help distinguish a forest plot of interaction estimates from a standard forest plot of treatment effect estimates, for which squares are typically used.[119,256,258] In the second stage, model (7.7) was estimated using REML, and this gave a summary interaction estimate of $\hat{\gamma}_W =$ 0.77 (95% CI: −0.52 to 2.07). Hence, there is no evidence of an important difference in treatment effect for males compared to females; the summary interaction estimate is close to zero and clinically unimportant, whilst the confidence interval overlaps zero, and there is also between-trial heterogeneity.

If IPD had not been available in this example, researchers may have been tempted to extract aggregate data and fit meta-regression model (7.2) to examine the across-trial association between the trial treatment effect estimates and the proportion male in each trial. This trial-level relationship is depicted in Figure 7.3 by the steep solid line, suggesting a strong association, where trials with a greater proportion of males have a lower treatment effect ($\hat{\gamma}_A = 15.10$ mmHg (95% CI: 8.78 to 21.41)). This contrasts with the small and unimportant within-trial interaction estimates given in Figure 7.2 and depicted by the generally flat dashed lines in Figure 7.3.

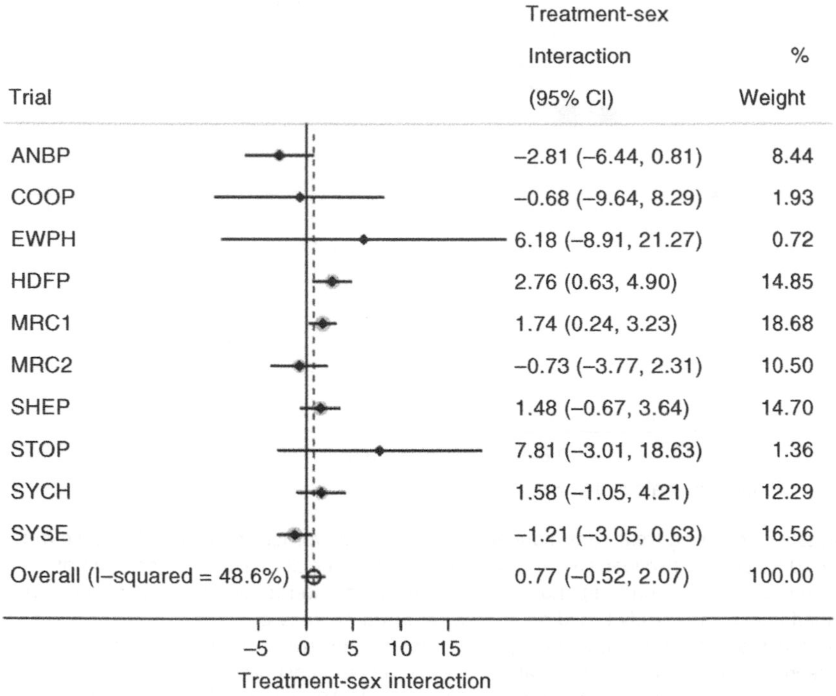

*Model (7.3) was used in the first stage, and model (7.7) in the second stage; estimation used REML in both stages, and the confidence interval for the summary interaction was derived using the Hartung-Knapp Sidik-Jonkman approach.The interactions refer to the difference between males and females in the treatment effect (i.e. their difference in the mean difference in final SBP for treatment versus control, after adjusting for baseline).

Figure 7.2 A two-stage IPD meta-analysis of treatment-sex interactions, summarising the difference in the effect of anti-hypertensive treatment for males compared to females*. Case study based on an extension of IPD meta-analysis project of Wang et al.[46] as reported by Riley et al.[156] *Source:* Figure taken from Figure 1 of Riley et al.,[255] reproduced with permission, © 2020 Wiley.

The discrepancy is due to the across-trial association being affected by aggregation bias and trial-level confounding; those trials with a higher proportion male also are systematically different in other characteristics such as age, comorbidities, and treatment dose. Only by using the within-trial information via the IPD is the treatment-covariate interaction restricted to the participant level (Figure 7.2).

7.3.3 Do Not Quantify Interactions by Comparing Meta-Analysis Results for Subgroups

It may be tempting to perform a two-stage IPD meta-analysis of the treatment effect in each subgroup separately (e.g. men, women; smokers, non-smokers), and then compare them via a statistical test or by calculating their difference. This is a common approach as it is apparently simple and leads to nice graphical displays for each subgroup, as illustrated for the effect of tamoxifen in ER positive and negative subgroups in Box 7.1. However, the approach is flawed, as it amalgamates within-trial and across-trial information; Fisher et al. thus call it a 'deluded' analysis.[258] Because subgroup results are being compared at the meta-analysis level (rather than solely within trials), the approach allows across-trial information and thus aggregation bias to seep through, and

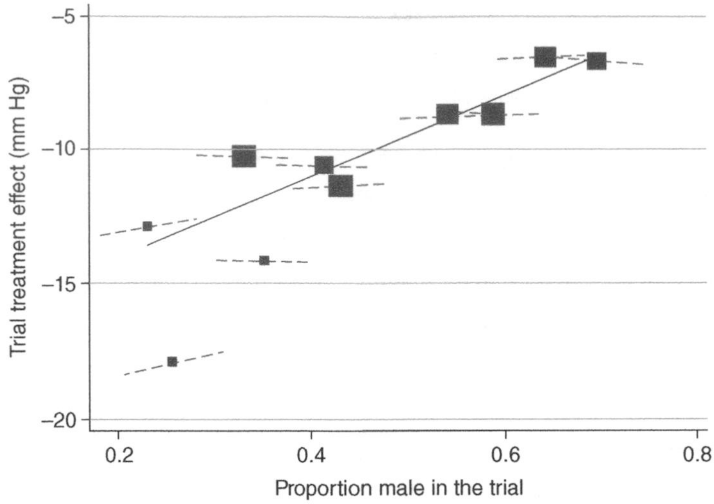

Figure 7.3 Is blood pressure-lowering treatment more effective amongst women than men? Evidence from an IPD meta-analysis of 10 trials of anti-hypertensive treatment showing the across-trial association of treatment effect and proportion male (solid line) and the participant-level interaction of sex and treatment effect in each trial (dashed lines). Case study based on an that reported by Riley et al.[156]

Each block represents one trial, and the block size is proportional to the size of the trial. Across-trial association (from meta-regression model (7.2) of the trial treatment effects against proportion male) is denoted by gradient of solid line (–); this suggests a large improved effect of a 15.10 mmHg (95% CI: 8.78 to 21.41) greater reduction in SBP in trials with only females compared to only males. Participant-level treatment-sex interaction within each trial (as derived from model (7.3)) is denoted by gradient of dashed lines (- - -), which on average suggests a 0.77 mmHg (95% CI: −0.52 to 2.07) greater treatment effect for females than males, which is neither clinically or statistically significant. *Source:* Figure adapted from Figure 1 in Riley et al., with permission, © 2007 Wiley.

potentially distort the true difference between subgroups. Although Fisher et al. show that, across all meta-analyses in their sample, the *average* difference of interaction estimates from 'deluded' analyses compared to their 'deft' equivalents is close to zero,[258] in any particular meta-analysis the percentage difference could be large (between about −20% to 20%; Figure 7.4).

This approach was used by the Early Breast Cancer Trialists' Collaboration to examine the differential effect of adjuvant tamoxifen treatment according to ER status (Box 7.1).[268] They provided separate meta-analysis results for the ER positive and ER negative subgroups, and then performed a chi-square test of whether they are equal, which is strongly rejected ($p < 0.00001$) at five years. Even though each subgroup result is itself based only on within-trial information, the comparison between subgroups is made at the trial level (aggregated level), and therefore introduces across-trial information arising from changes in the proportion of participants who are ER positive across trials.

The larger the differences in mean covariate values across trials, the larger the potential contribution of the across-trial information in this flawed analysis. One way to understand this is to consider an extreme situation, where one of the trials contains only those who are ER negative. Such a trial cannot contribute any within-trial information about the interaction between ER status and treatment effect at the participant level, as there are no ER positive participants. However, the trial would still contribute toward the subgroup result for ER negative participants, and thus subsequently will contribute toward the difference between meta-analysis results for ER positive and ER negative subgroups. This issue is avoided by meta-analysing the treatment-covariate interaction estimates observed within trials (i.e. by using the two-stage approach outlined in Section 7.3.1).

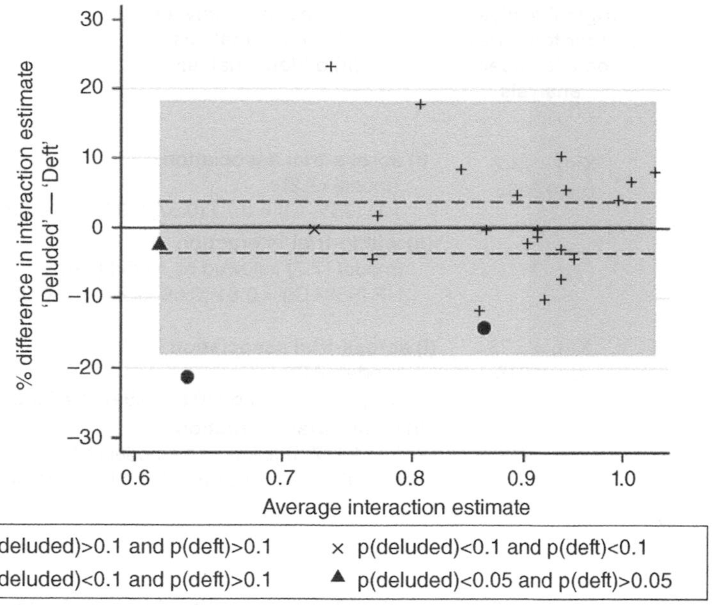

Figure 7.4 Bland-Altman plot showing level of agreement between treatment-covariate interactions based on $\hat{\gamma}_W$ from using within-trial information (labelled as 'deft') or $\hat{\gamma}_{WA}$ amalgamating within-trial and across-trial information (labelled as 'deluded'), as reported by Fisher et al.[258]

Shaded area = Bland-Altman 95% limits of agreement;[274] solid line represents mean difference (bias); dashed lines are 95% confidence intervals around the mean difference. Average interaction is the unweighted average of the interaction estimates from 'deluded' and 'deft' analyses. Treatment-covariate interactions (as measured on the log scale) might have a positive or a negative sign, but in this plot they have all been set to negative. Hence, differences in interaction effects below the zero line represent cases where a 'deluded' analysis gives a result in the same direction as, but more extreme than, the equivalent 'deft' analysis, and vice versa. *Source:* Figure adapted from Figure 4 of Fisher et al.[258] (where 31 interactions were re-analysed, but only the 26 with treatment effects measured by hazard ratios or odds ratios are plotted); adapted with permission,

Had this preferred analysis be done, would the apparent treatment-ER interaction remain the same? Given the strong biological rationale (tamoxifen is an oestrogen receptor antagonist, and so targeted specifically for ER positive patients), we envisage so, but this warrants further investigation.

Another example is that of the PORT Meta-Analysis Trialists' Group, who examined whether there is an interaction between stage of disease or nodal status with the effect of postoperative radiotherapy for non-small cell lung cancer.[275] They calculated meta-analysis results for each subgroup, and then tested for differences in these meta-analysis results, which was highly significant for both stage and nodal status. Figure 7.5 shows a re-analysis of this data using the two-stage IPD meta-analysis approach described in Section 7.3.1. It is clear that the original conclusions are strongly influenced by across-trial information, as the summary interactions are closer to 1 based on just the within-trial information, and there is no longer clear evidence that nodal status interacts with treatment effect. For such reasons, the PORT Meta-Analysis Trialists' Group later updated their work with additional trials and updated disease staging data,[276] with interactions correctly examined using within-trial information.

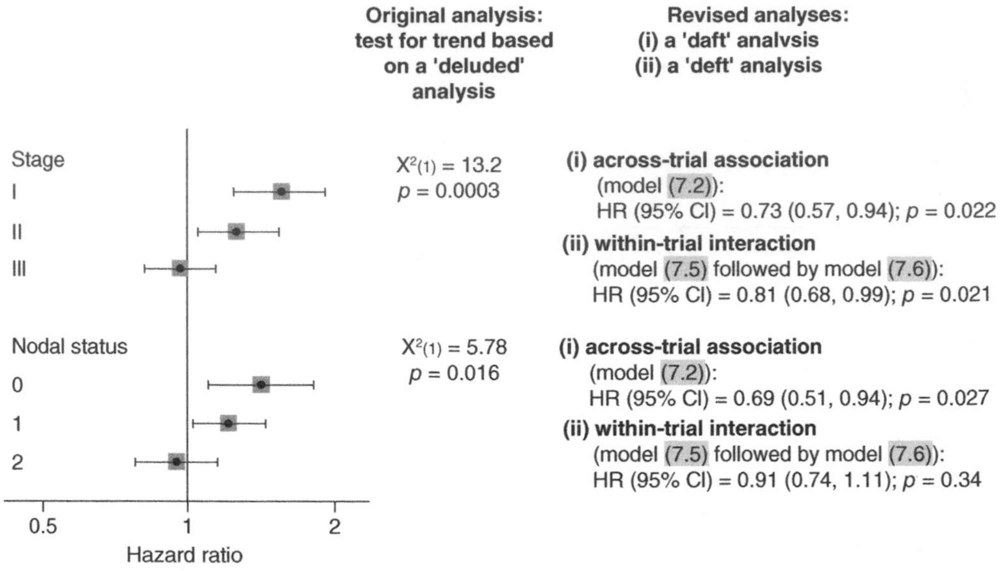

Figure 7.5 PORT meta-analysis results for the interaction between treatment effect and each of stage of disease and nodal status. The original analysis is as reported in 1998 and used a 'deluded' analysis approach that amalgamates within-trial and across-trial information;[275] the revised analysis shows corrected results when separating out across-trial and within-trial information. All analyses assume the interaction is common across trials and can be modelled by linear trend across categories to be consistent with the original analysis. *Source:* David Fisher.

7.4 The One-stage Approach

A one-stage IPD meta-analysis can also be used to summarise treatment-covariate interactions, by extending the framework introduced in Chapter 6. However, this is not straightforward. Simply including a treatment-covariate interaction term may introduce aggregation bias, as it allows across-trial information to contribute toward the summary interaction estimate, in combination with within-trial information.[155,156,159] To avoid aggregation bias, within-trial and across-trial information must be disentangled,[156,212,246,256,277] a principle which is also recognised outside the IPD meta-analysis field in other areas that contain clustering,[278–281] such as multicentre trials.

The following sub-sections explain these issues in detail, still focusing on an IPD meta-analysis of randomised trials with a parallel-group design. We begin by specifying one-stage Cox regression models for a time-to-event outcome, and always allow a *separate* (i.e. not necessarily proportional) baseline hazard specification per trial, and assume proportional hazards for included covariates (i.e. constant hazard ratios over time). Chapter 6 discusses other potential specifications of a one-stage Cox model.[5,44,210,224,282–284] Also, we assume that for a continuous covariate z_{ij}, the treatment-covariate interaction is a linear effect; that is, a one-unit increase in z_{ij} has the same interaction with the treatment effect across the entire distribution of z_{ij} values. Extension to non-linear trends is considered in Section 7.6.2.

7.4.1 Merging Within-trial and Across-trial Information

Simply including a treatment-covariate interaction term within a one-stage model is often flawed, as it potentially merges within-trial and across-trial information. For example, the following one-stage Cox regression model allows within-trial and across-trial information to contribute toward the treatment-covariate interaction estimate:

$$\lambda_{ij}(t) = \lambda_{0i}(t)\exp\left(\beta_1 z_{ij} + \beta_2 x_{ij} + \gamma_{WAi} x_{ij} z_{ij}\right)$$
$$\gamma_{WAi} \sim N\left(\gamma_{WA}, \tau^2\right) \tag{7.8}$$

Here $\lambda_{0i}(t)$ denotes the unique baseline hazard function in trial i, which ensures that the clustering of participants within trials is accounted for; $x_{ij}z_{ij}$ represents the interaction term between the treatment (x_{ij}, typically coded as 1 for treatment and 0 for control, though this may be sub-optimal, Section 6.2.8.3) and covariate (z_{ij}) of interest, and τ^2 allows for between-trial variability in this interaction across trials. Also, β_1 is the change in the log hazard for a one-unit increase in z_{ij} (i.e. the prognostic effect of z_{ij}) and β_2 is the treatment effect for participants with $z_{ij} = 0$.

As written, β_1 and β_2 are assumed common across all trials, but to allow for between-trial heterogeneity, random effects could be placed on them. Nevertheless, whether common or random, the fact that these parameters are *not* stratified by trial has the direct consequence that the included interaction parameter, γ_{WA}, represents an amalgamation of within-trial information and across-trial information (hence the label *WA*), and so is inappropriate.

As discussed in Section 7.3.3, merging within-trial and across-trial information is undesirable when estimating treatment-covariate interactions. We do not recommend it, as the influence of the across-trial information may bias results, and lead to misleading conclusions about whether a particular treatment-covariate interaction truly exists at the participant-level. Unfortunately, many IPD meta-analysis researchers adopt this approach,[148,257,258] often unknowingly. More appropriate one-stage methods that separate within-trial and across-trial information should be used, as now described.

7.4.2 Separating Within-trial and Across-trial Information

There are two main ways of preventing amalgamation of within-trial and across-trial information when estimating the treatment-covariate interaction in a one-stage IPD meta-analysis model:[255]

1) Center the covariate z_{ij} about its trial-specific mean, $\bar{z}_i$, and add an additional term which allows the covariate means ($\bar{z}_i$) to explain between-trial heterogeneity in the treatment effect;[255,257,277,280] or
2) Stratify by trial each of the other parameters outside the interaction term,[255] including the parameter representing the reference treatment effect (i.e. the treatment effect at the covariate's reference value, typically $z_{ij} = 0$ or, if the covariate is centered, $z_{ij} = \bar{z}_i$).

Let us consider these two approaches in relation to a one-stage survival model. Our website (www.ipdma.co.uk) provides examples of statistical code to implement the approaches.

7.4.2.1 Approach (i) for a One-stage Survival Model: Center the Covariate and Include the Covariate Mean

For time-to-event outcomes, approach (i) leads to a one-stage Cox regression model of:[255,257]

$$\lambda_{ij}(t) = \lambda_{0i}(t)\exp\left(\beta_{1i} z_{ij} + \beta_{2i} x_{ij} + \gamma_{Wi} x_{ij}\left(z_{ij} - \bar{z}_i\right)\right)$$
$$\beta_{2i} \sim N(\varphi + \gamma_A \bar{z}_i, \tau_1^2)$$
$$\gamma_{Wi} \sim N\left(\gamma_W, \tau_2^2\right) \tag{7.9}$$

In this model, τ_2^2 is the between-trial variance of the within-trial interaction, and τ_1^2 is the residual between-trial variance in the treatment effect (i.e. that not explained by $\bar{z}_i$). Inclusion of the $\gamma_A \bar{z}_i$

term, together with the centering of z_{ij} within the interaction term, disentangles γ_W (the within-trial interaction of interest) and γ_A (the across-trial association) such that they are uncorrelated with each other, and thus $\hat{\gamma}_W$ will be based solely on within-trial information.[156,280] By contrast, model (7.8) provides an interaction estimate ($\hat{\gamma}_{WA}$) that is a weighted average of $\hat{\gamma}_W$ and $\hat{\gamma}_A$, which may increase precision but confuses interpretation and introduces potential for aggregation bias.

If the $\gamma_A\bar{z}_i$ term is not included in model (7.9), then the interaction term will represent some weighted average of $\hat{\gamma}_W$ and the magnitude of aggregation bias ($\hat{\gamma}_{bias} = \hat{\gamma}_A - \hat{\gamma}_W$; Section 7.4.5). This is less of a concern than when amalgamating $\hat{\gamma}_W$ and $\hat{\gamma}_A$ (the 'deluded' analysis), as $\hat{\gamma}_{bias}$ will usually have much larger variance than $\hat{\gamma}_W$, and thus have very little weight in the amalgamation of $\hat{\gamma}_W$ and $\hat{\gamma}_{bias}$. Nevertheless, including the $\gamma_A\bar{z}_i$ term avoids this concern entirely and is therefore recommended, as shown in model (7.9).

7.4.2.2 Approach (ii) for a One-stage Survival Model: Stratify All Nuisance Parameters by Trial

Approach (ii) leads to a one-stage Cox regression model such as:[255]

$$\begin{aligned} &\lambda_{ij}(t) = \lambda_{0i}(t)\exp\left(\beta_{1i}z_{ij} + \beta_{2i}x_{ij} + \gamma_{Wi}x_{ij}z_{ij}\right) \\ &\gamma_{Wi} \sim N\left(\gamma_W, \tau^2\right) \end{aligned} \tag{7.10}$$

In this model, each of the nuisance parameters (i.e. the $\lambda_{0i}(t)$, β_{1i} and β_{2i} parameters which are not of primary interest) are stratified by trial, and random effects are placed only on the within-trial interaction. This stratification of nuisance parameters by trial, in particular β_{2i} representing the treatment effect at the covariate's reference value, ensures that γ_W only contains within-trial information. It also closely reflects the two-stage approach, where all nuisance parameters are naturally stratified by trial as they are estimated in each trial separately in the first stage. Note that if one-stage model (7.10) was extended to adjust for other covariates (e.g. prognostic factors), ideally they should also be stratified by trial. Further, although no longer needed to remove aggregation bias, centering all covariates (including the treatment covariate x_{ij}) in model (7.10) may still be sensible, for example to improve maximum likelihood estimation (Sections 6.2.8.3 and 7.4.4).[181]

7.4.2.3 Approaches (i) and (ii) for Continuous and Binary Outcomes

Approaches (i) and (ii) can be used to remove aggregation bias for other model types, such as linear and logistic regression. For example, using approach (i) and thus trial-specific covariate centering, a one-stage model to estimate the treatment-covariate interaction for a continuous outcome is[156,255]

$$\begin{aligned} &y_{ij} = \alpha_i + \beta_{1i}z_{ij} + \beta_{2i}x_{ij} + \beta_{3i}y_{0ij} + \gamma_{Wi}x_{ij}\left(z_{ij} - \bar{z}_i\right) + \varepsilon_{ij} \\ &\beta_{2i} \sim N\left(\varphi + \gamma_A\bar{z}_i, \tau_1^2\right) \\ &\gamma_{Wi} \sim N\left(\gamma_W, \tau_2^2\right) \end{aligned} \tag{7.11}$$

and for a binary outcome is:[159,255]

$$\begin{aligned} &y_{ij} \sim \text{Bernoulli}\left(p_{ij}\right) \\ &\text{logit}\left(p_{ij}\right) = \alpha_i + \beta_{1i}z_{ij} + \beta_{2i}x_{ij} + \gamma_{Wi}x_{ij}\left(z_{ij} - \bar{z}_i\right) \\ &\beta_{2i} \sim N\left(\varphi + \gamma_A\bar{z}_i, \tau_1^2\right) \\ &\gamma_{Wi} \sim N\left(\gamma_W, \tau_2^2\right) \end{aligned} \tag{7.12}$$

Rather using approach (ii) and so stratifying nuisance parameters by trial, we can write the model for a continuous outcome as

$$y_{ij} = \alpha_i + \beta_{1i}z_{ij} + \beta_{2i}x_{ij} + \beta_{3i}y_{0ij} + \gamma_{Wi}x_{ij}z_{ij} + \varepsilon_{ij}$$
$$\gamma_{Wi} \sim N(\gamma_W, \tau^2) \tag{7.13}$$

and for a binary outcome as:

$$y_{ij} \sim \text{Bernoulli}\left(p_{ij}\right)$$
$$\text{logit}\left(p_{ij}\right) = \alpha_i + \beta_{1i}z_{ij} + \beta_{2i}x_{ij} + \gamma_{Wi}x_{ij}z_{ij}$$
$$\gamma_{Wi} \sim N(\gamma_W, \tau^2) \tag{7.14}$$

7.4.2.4 Comparison of Approaches (i) and (ii)

In all these models outlined for approaches (i) and (ii), the key parameter of interest is the treatment-covariate interaction, γ_W, which denotes the expected change in the treatment effect (e.g. log hazard ratio for models (7.9) and (7.10)) for each one-unit increase in z_{ij}, and is based solely on within-trial information. Additionally, models (7.9), (7.11) and (7.12) provide γ_A, which represents the expected change in a trial's treatment effect for every one-unit increase in $\bar{z}_j$, and is based only on across-trial information (essentially from a meta-regression).

The estimate of γ_W should usually be very similar regardless of whether approach (i) or (ii) is taken. However, models (7.9), (7.11) and (7.12) assume the β_{2i} have a mean of $\alpha + \gamma_A\bar{z}_i$, and so the γ_A represents the slope of an assumed *linear* across-trial relationship of the treatment effect and the covariate mean $\bar{z}_j$. Further research is needed to establish whether any consequences arise (e.g. in terms of aggregation bias toward γ_W using approach (i)) when the true relationship across trials is non-linear. Usually the across-trial relationship will not be of interest, in which case approach (ii) should be used as it avoids making any such assumptions. Section 7.6.2 describes how to extend the models to allow non-linear trends for continuous covariates.

7.4.3 Applied Examples

We now consider two examples that illustrate the potential differences between interaction estimates based on within-trial information (γ_W) or amalgamated information (γ_{WA}).

7.4.3.1 Is Age an Effect Modifier for Epilepsy Treatment?

Epilepsy is one of the most common neurological disorders. Researchers conducted an IPD meta-analysis of five randomised trials to compare the effects of two antiepileptic drugs, sodium valproate (SV, treatment = 1) and carbamazepine (CBZ, treatment = 0), when used as monotherapy in 1225 participants with partial onset seizures or generalised onset seizures.[210,285,286] Hua et al. extended previous work,[210,257] to examine the treatment effect (SV versus CBZ) on the outcome of time to 12-month remission, and whether age at randomisation (in years) interacts with the treatment effect. ML estimation was used to fit the one-stage Cox models (7.8) and (7.9), but initially assuming no between-trial heterogeneity in the interaction term.

The findings revealed the potential impact of aggregation bias, and the importance of separating out within-trial and across-trial information. The estimated treatment-covariate interaction from model (7.8), which amalgamates within-trial and across-trial information, appears important ($\hat{\gamma}_{WA}$ = −0.009, 95% CI: −0.016 to −0.002, p = 0.014); it suggests that for every 10-year increase in age the hazard ratio (comparing SV to CBZ) reduces by about 9% (exp(−0.009 × 10) = 0.91). However, when fitting model (7.9) and only using within-trial information, the summary treatment-covariate interaction was smaller and no longer statistically significant ($\hat{\gamma}_W = -0.006$, 95% CI: −0.018 to 0.006, $p = 0.33$). The difference was due to the impact of aggregation bias; $\hat{\gamma}_W$ is smaller than $\hat{\gamma}_A$ (= −0.012, 95% CI: −0.021 to −0.002, $p = 0.022$), and the estimate of aggregation bias is −0.006 (95% CI: −0.021 to 0.102).

The one-stage analysis of age was extended to adjust for the prognostic factors of epilepsy type and log number of seizures. The findings are similar: there is no strong evidence that age interacts with treatment effect ($\hat{\gamma}_W = -0.006$, 95% CI: −0.017 to 0.006, $p = 0.35$). The confidence interval for γ_W is wide, and so further research is still warranted about whether age is a genuine treatment-covariate interaction.[210,285,286] For comparison, a two-stage IPD meta-analysis was fitted by applying Cox model (7.5) in the first stage and common-effect model (7.6) in the second stage. This gave almost identical results ($\hat{\gamma}_W = -0.007$, 95% CI: −0.018 to 0.005, $p = 0.28$), as did one-stage model (7.10) that stratifies the reference treatment effect by trial ($\hat{\gamma}_W = -0.007$, 95% CI: −0.018 to 0.005, $p = 0.28$). Results were similar when additionally centering the treatment covariate or allowing for between-trial heterogeneity in the treatment-age interaction.

7.4.3.2 Is the Effect of an Early Support Hospital Discharge Modified by Having a Carer Present?

Fisher et al. re-examined a published meta-analysis evaluating the efficacy of a strategy of early supported hospital discharge (ESD) compared to conventional hospital services and discharge arrangements for the care of patients with acute stroke.[258,287] The main outcome was mortality, but intermediate outcomes such as duration of hospital stay were also reported. Perhaps unsurprisingly, overall the ESD strategy reduces the mean duration of stay, but an exploratory subgroup analysis suggests that this effect is modified by the presence or absence of a carer to give additional support to the patient. Fisher et al. identified that this subgroup analysis was undertaken using the flawed approach described in Section 7.3.3, with a random-effects model fitted within each subgroup. To address this, they re-analysed the data separating out within-trial and across-trial interactions (Section 7.5.1 gives more details on their approach).[258] Figure 7.6 shows the surprising result that the summary interaction estimates based solely on either within-trial or across-trial information are in completely opposite directions, and their confidence intervals do not even overlap. As a consequence, the interaction estimate based on amalgamated information falls in between and appears (clinically and statistically) non-significant, thus masking the potentially important finding (based on within-trial information) that participants with a carer may have a slightly better treatment effect than those without a carer. Further research is needed to confirm whether this exploratory finding is genuine.

This is an extreme example. It is driven mainly by a single trial (Montreal), in which *all* participants had a carer present but whose overall effect was relatively small. In the amalgamated ('deluded') analysis, this large trial pulls the interaction estimates toward the null, reversing the direction of the interaction estimate based solely on within-trial information. Nonetheless, the value of this example is twofold: firstly, to warn against using across-trial information to summarise treatment-covariate interactions in meta-analysis; and, secondly, to emphasise the specific point that trials without participant-level variation in a covariate of interest should not contribute to the estimation of within-trial interaction. Note that for simplicity the analyses of Fisher et al. assumed the treatment-covariate interaction is common (i.e. the same) in all trials. This makes extreme results like this more likely to be observed, and may not be entirely appropriate.[258]

7.4.4 Coding of the Treatment Covariate and Adjustment for Other Covariates

So far, our one-stage models have coded the treatment variable, x_{ij}, as 1 for treatment group and 0 for control. However, ML estimation of one-stage IPD meta-analysis models can be improved when

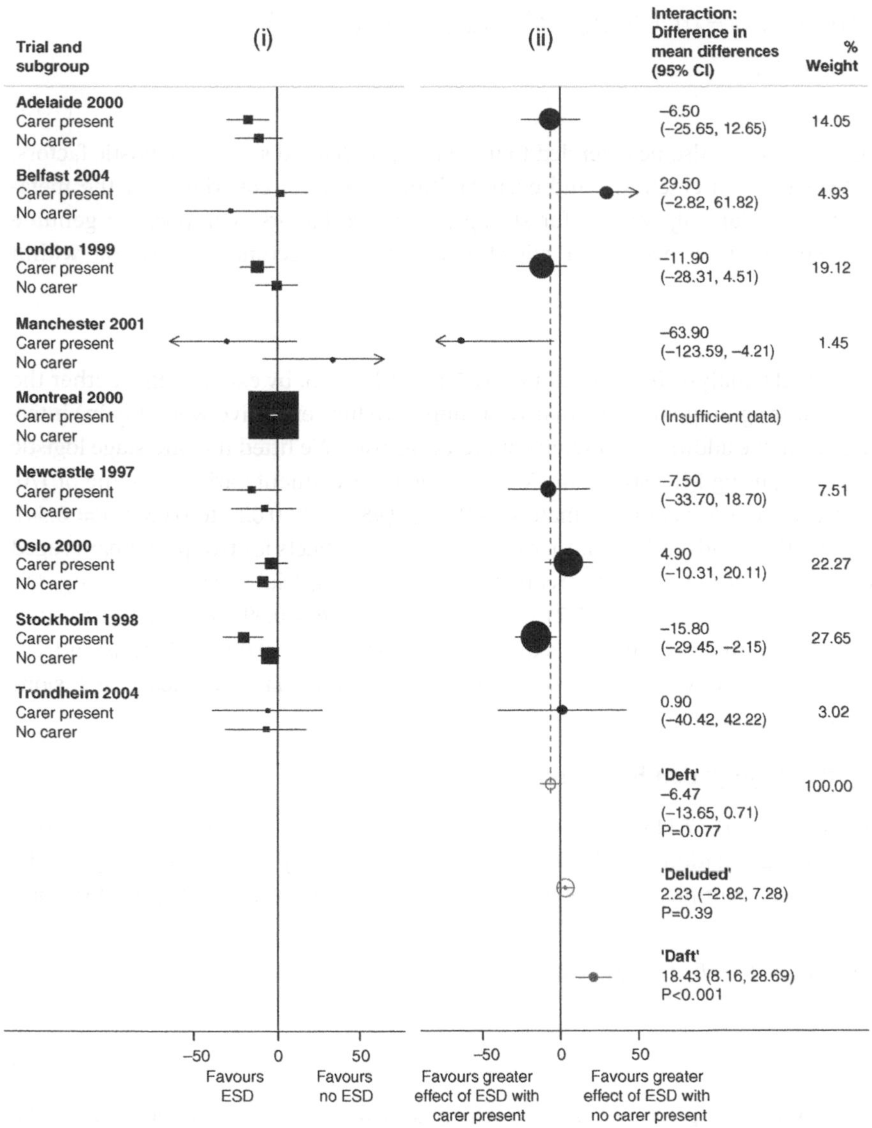

Figure 7.6 Representations of how the effect of an early supported hospital discharge (ESD) strategy on hospital stay duration may vary by whether participants had a carer present or not. Sizing of squares and circles are in proportion to the inverse of the variance of the estimates. In column (i) results are presented by trial first, then by subgroup; in column (ii) the treatment-covariate interaction estimates are shown for each trial and then from various meta-analyses (where 'deft' indicates it is based solely on within-trial interactions; 'daft' indicates it is based solely on across-trial information; and 'deluded' indicates it uses both within-trial and across-trial information). Percentage weights are from the 'deft' analysis. *Source:* Figure adapted from Figure 2 of Fisher et al.[258] with permission, © 2017 BMJ Publishing Group Ltd. (CC-BY 4.0).

using trial-specific centering of the treatment variable and indeed other covariates (Section 6.2.8.3).[181] This is most relevant for one-stage models for non-continuous outcomes, for which ML estimation is typically the default in mixed model software packages (NB this is not a concern when REML estimation is used, for example for continuous outcomes as discussed in Section 6.2.8.4[108,181]). For example, extending the one-stage Cox regression of model (7.9) with all covariates centered by their trial-specific means, we have:

$$\lambda_{ij}(t) = \lambda_{0i}(t)\exp\left(\beta_{1i}(z_{ij} - \bar{z}_i) + \beta_{2i}(x_{ij} - \bar{x}_i) + \gamma_{Wi}(x_{ij} - \bar{x}_i)(z_{ij} - \bar{z}_i)\right)$$
$$\beta_{2i} \sim N(\varphi + \gamma_A \bar{z}_i, \tau_1^2)$$
$$\gamma_{Wi} \sim N(\gamma_W, \tau_2^2) \tag{7.15}$$

All our one-stage models can also be extended to include a pre-defined set of prognostic factors, multiple treatment-covariate interactions, and even multiple trial-level covariates (at the meta-regression level). In particular, adjustment for strong prognostic factors is important; genuine interactions should be identified even after adjustment for other factors (see criteria within Section 7.9).

7.4.4.1 Example

We extended the IPD meta-analysis introduced in Box 5.1 and Box 5.5, by examining whether the effect of interventions during pregnancy (primarily aiming to reduce excessive weight gain) interacts with age in regards to the additional outcome of pre-eclampsia. We fitted the one-stage logistic regression of model (7.12) using ML estimation. When using the treatment variable coding of 1/0, the summary treatment-age interaction estimate was 0.0092 (95% CI: –0.020 to 0.038; $p = 0.54$), which is the log of the ratio of odds ratios, comparing the treatment effects for two participants aged one year apart. However, when coding the treatment variable using trial-specific centering, the summary interaction estimate was –0.0002 (95% CI: –0.041 to 0.041; $p = 0.99$). The change in summary estimate and wider confidence interval is due to the τ_2^2 estimate of 0.0013 when using trial-specific centering compared to 0 when using 1/0 coding. This does not change clinical conclusions here, but it might in other situations.

7.4.5 Estimating the Aggregation Bias Directly

After estimation of models (7.9), (7.11) and (7.12) the difference in $\hat{\gamma}_W$ and $\hat{\gamma}_A$ may be interpreted as the estimated amount of aggregation bias. It can be calculated directly by fitting a one-stage model including $x_{ij}z_{ij}$ and $\bar{z}_j$. For example, a one-stage Cox model that estimates the aggregation bias directly is:

$$\lambda_{ij}(t) = \lambda_{0j}(t)\exp\left(\beta_{1i}x_{ij} + \beta_{2i}z_{ij} + \gamma_{Wi}x_{ij}z_{ij}\right)$$
$$\beta_{1i} \sim N(\varphi + \gamma_{bias}\bar{z}_i, \tau_1^2)$$
$$\gamma_{Wi} \sim N(\gamma_W, \tau_2^2) \tag{7.16}$$

Here, the aggregation bias is represented by γ_{bias}, which is akin to $\gamma_A - \gamma_W$ in model (7.9).[159] An estimate of γ_{bias} may be of interest to methodologists examining the magnitude of aggregation bias empirically. However, we do not recommend using $\hat{\gamma}_{bias}$ to decide whether aggregation bias exists in a particular application. There is usually low power to identify or statistically test for aggregation bias (i.e. $\gamma_{bias} \neq 0$), due to typically imprecise estimates of γ_A. More importantly, we have described how γ_A and γ_W have different interpretations, and so it is questionable whether combining them can genuinely improve inference.

7.4.6 Reporting Summary Treatment Effects for Subgroups after Adjusting for Aggregation Bias

In previous sections we have discussed the importance of using $\hat{\gamma}_W$ as an estimate of the treatment-covariate interaction effect free from aggregation bias. In Section 7.3.3 we cautioned against quantifying the interaction by comparing pooled subgroup-specific treatment effects. However, it may be desirable – particularly from a clinical perspective – to also present meta-analytic results in the form of subgroup-specific treatment effects. So, how might this be achieved?

One simple approach might be to display the summary treatment effect results from a meta-analysis of each subgroup, but also accompany them with meta-analysis results for $\hat{\gamma}_W$ to quantify the actual difference between them. However, if aggregation bias exists there remains a concern that readers will over-interpret the visual plot and, for example, decide that there is a difference between subgroups if their summary treatment effects differ and corresponding confidence intervals do not overlap. As discussed in Section 7.3.3, this comparison is wrong because it is not based solely on within-trial information. Instead, it may be preferable to report subgroup-specific summary treatment effects as derived following a one-stage model by estimating *marginal* effects (White et al., personal communication). A similar approach, requiring a few additional assumptions and approximations, may be used to obtain summary treatment effects for subgroups within a two-stage framework (White et al., personal communication), thus also allowing inclusion of "recovered" interactions from non-IPD trials as described in Section 7.5.1. An application of this approach is presented in Burdett et al.[288] A related concept is the prediction of treatment effects in new patients (Section 7.11).[266,267]

7.5 Combining IPD and non-IPD Trials

We now discuss how to handle non-IPD trials when summarising treatment-covariate interactions in an IPD meta-analysis project.

7.5.1 Can We Recover Interaction Estimates from non-IPD Trials?

Without IPD, the available trial information is usually the treatment effect estimate (as derived based on all participants), alongside summary characteristics such as the proportion male and the mean age. Unfortunately, treatment-covariate interactions are not commonly reported, or at least not reported in full, as they are usually secondary objectives or exploratory analyses. A major concern is selective reporting, such that significant interactions are reported in more detail than those non-significant. Often only a p-value for the interaction test may be available, rather than an actual estimate of the interaction. Different trials will also handle continuous covariates differently, such as assuming a linear trend or categorisation; if the latter, different cut-points (e.g. age < 55 versus age ≥ 55 in some trials, and age < 70 versus age ≥ 70 in others) are usual across trials. The adjustment variables may also differ across trials.

All these issues reinforce why IPD are advantageous. However, sometimes it is possible to recover interaction estimates from non-IPD trials, and these could then be included in the second stage of the two-stage approach outlined in Section 7.3.1. The best scenario for recovering interaction estimates is with a binary outcome and a binary covariate. If, for each trial, the numbers of participants and outcome events are presented by treatment arm and by covariate subgroup, then the original IPD dataset can be reconstructed exactly, as described in Section 6.4.1. Then, the IPD meta-analysis models specified within Sections 7.3.1 and 7.4.2 can be applied.

If those numbers are not known, and/or the outcome is not binary (but the covariate still is), then a within-trial interaction can still be estimated from other information. Consider the example introduced in Section 7.4.3.2 and Figure 7.6. Fisher et al. extracted treatment effect estimates for each "carer" subgroup for eight trials (excluding the Montreal trial; Section 7.4.3.2).[258] Since participant subgroups within a trial are independent, the within-trial interaction in each trial ($\hat{\gamma}_{Wi}$) can be estimated by taking the difference in these subgroup-specific treatment effect estimates (on the scale of analysis, i.e. log odds ratio, log hazard ratio, mean difference, etc), with variance equal to the sum of the estimated subgroup-specific variances. For example, letting $\hat{\theta}_{1i}$ and $\hat{\theta}_{2i}$ be treatment effect estimates in trial i for subgroup 1 and 2, respectively, we can write

$$\hat{\gamma}_{Wi} = \hat{\theta}_{2i} - \hat{\theta}_{1i}$$
$$\text{var}(\hat{\gamma}_{Wi}) = \text{var}(\hat{\theta}_{2i}) + \text{var}(\hat{\theta}_{1i}) \tag{7.17}$$

where $\text{var}(\hat{\theta}_{2i})$ and $\text{var}(\hat{\theta}_{1i})$ are the estimated variances of the treatment effect estimates of subgroups 2 and 1, respectively, in trial i. Such $\hat{\gamma}_{Wi}$ derived from non-IPD trials can then be combined with IPD trials, as described in Section 7.5.2.

This approach may be generalised for covariates grouped into $C = 1$ to k ordered categories ($k > 2$), subject to the assumption of a linear trend across the categories, using variance-weighted least squares estimation in each of the non-IPD trials:

$$\hat{\theta}_{Ci} = \hat{\theta}_{1i} + (C-1)\gamma_{Wi} + \varepsilon_{Ci}$$
$$\varepsilon_{Ci} \sim N(0, \text{var}(\hat{\theta}_{Ci})) \tag{7.18}$$

Fitting this model (e.g. in Stata using the *vwls* command) gives $\hat{\gamma}_{Wi}$, an estimate of the expected difference in treatment effect for those in category C compared to category $C - 1$. For simplicity, it is assumed that the categories are evenly spaced, such that the index C may be used directly as the independent variable, but this does not have to be the case.

In the example of Figure 7.6, for which IPD were not available, relevant data were available for a large number of eligible trials and enabled calculation of within-trial treatment-covariate interactions using these approaches. This will often be the case for large randomised trials of non-rare diseases, such as the common cancers or heart disease, which will often pre-specify a core set of subgroups of particular interest. The advent of online publication including extensive supplementary material has led to more complete subgroup (and other secondary) analyses being available, particularly for subgroups defined by binary or categorical covariates. It is more problematic for continuous covariates, especially when interest is in non-linear interactions (Section 7.6.2). However, extending previous work,[17] Papadimitropoulou et al. show how to generate pseudo-IPD for randomised trials of continuous outcomes reported at baseline and follow-up,[143] which allows the interaction between baseline values and treatment effect to be examined at the participant level, using either the two-stage or one-stage approach described in Sections 7.3.1 and 7.4.2. The approach requires aggregate data of means, standard deviations and sample sizes to be available per group within each trial, at baseline and follow-up, together with the correlation of the baseline and follow-up measurements. In an applied example, Papadimitropoulou et al. found that results were practically identical to when the actual IPD were available.[143]

Of course, it is also fundamental to ask trial investigators to provide treatment-covariate interactions directly.[258] At the very least, subgroup-specific treatment effects may be obtainable (it could be that these are readily available but were simply omitted from the publication), or perhaps the multivariate distribution of outcomes and covariates of interest can be obtained (e.g. in terms of means, variances, and correlations) so that IPD can be reconstructed as described by Bonofiglio et al.[144]

7.5.2 How to Incorporate Interaction Estimates from Non-IPD Trials in an IPD Meta-Analysis

When a treatment-covariate interaction estimate, $\hat{\gamma}_{Wi}$, and its variance, $\text{var}(\hat{\gamma}_{Wi})$, are available for non-IPD trials, they can be combined with IPD trials in either the two-stage or one-stage approach.

The two-stage approach is straightforward and usually will suffice. In the second stage, the $\hat{\gamma}_{Wi}$ derived directly from the IPD in IPD trials are combined with the $\hat{\gamma}_{Wi}$ extracted (or derived from the aggregate data) from non-IPD trials, for example using model (7.7).

A one-stage approach is more complex, as it requires the specification of two regression models with shared parameters, also known as hierarchical related regression.[8,156,245] For example, for a continuous outcome situation we could use the following model:

$$\begin{aligned}
&\text{IPD trials:} && y_{ij} = \alpha_i + \beta_{1i} z_{ij} + \beta_{2i} x_{ij} + \beta_{3i} y_{0ij} + \gamma_{Wi} x_{ij}\left(z_{ij} - \bar{z}_i\right) + \varepsilon_{ij} \\
& && \varepsilon_{ij} \sim \mathrm{N}\left(0, \sigma_i^2\right) \\
&\text{Non-IPD trials:} && \hat{\gamma}_{Wi} \sim N(\gamma_W, \mathrm{var}(\hat{\gamma}_{Wi})) \\
&\text{All trials:} && \gamma_{Wi} \sim N(\gamma_W, \tau^2)
\end{aligned} \tag{7.19}$$

The IPD and non-IPD trials have different models, but have two shared parameters: the mean treatment-covariate interaction (γ_W) and the between-trial heterogeneity in the interaction (τ^2). In IPD trials all nuisance parameters are stratified by trial and we model the continuous outcomes of the included participants (y_{ij}), whereas for non-IPD trials we model the treatment-covariate interaction estimates ($\hat{\gamma}_{Wi}$). A similar framework is possible for binary and time-to-event outcomes, with the non-IPD as written, but with the IPD trials having a logistic or Cox regression model specification, for example.[8,159,246]

To specify related regression models, the analyst requires software (either frequentist or Bayesian) that allows a likelihood function to be written directly by the user, comprising the likelihoods for each of the IPD and non-IPD trials. However, for continuous outcomes, we can trick existing general linear mixed model software to do this for us, through the use of a dummy variable ($D_i = 1$ for IPD trials, and $D_i = 0$ for non-IPD trials) and a transformed response variable, y_{ij}^*. This was proposed by Riley et al.,[156] building on work by Goldstein et al.,[151] and is written as follows:

$$\begin{aligned}
&\text{All trials:} && y_{ij}^* = D_i\alpha_i + D_i\beta_{1i} z_{ij} + D_i\beta_{2i} x_{ij} + \gamma_{Wi} I_{ij} + D_i\beta_{3i} y_{0ij} + \varepsilon_{ij}^* \\
& && y_{ij}^* = y_{ij} \text{ if } D_i = 1 \text{ and } y_{ij}^* = \hat{\gamma}_{Wi} \text{ if } D_i = 0 \\
& && I_{ij} = x_{ij}\left(z_{ij} - \bar{z}_i\right) \text{ if } D_i = 1 \text{ and } I_{ij} = 1 \text{ if } D_i = 0 \\
& && \varepsilon_{ij}^* \sim \mathrm{N}\left(0, \sigma_i^2\right) \text{ if } D_i = 1 \text{ and } \varepsilon_{ij}^* \sim \mathrm{N}(0, \mathrm{var}(\hat{\gamma}_{Wi})) \text{ if } D_i = 0 \\
& && \gamma_{Wi} \sim N(\gamma_W, \tau^2)
\end{aligned} \tag{7.20}$$

This requires software such as SAS Proc Mixed that allows us to hold fixed variances estimates (i.e. the $\mathrm{var}(\hat{\gamma}_{Wi})$) for the non-IPD trials. As before, all trials will contribute toward the summary treatment-covariate interaction, but only the IPD trials are able to estimate other parameter estimates.

Riley et al. also modified this framework to accommodate non-IPD trials that only provide a treatment effect estimate (as based on all participants) and its variance, alongside mean covariate values;[156] such aggregate data can contribute toward meta-regression results, but not within-trial interactions. This approach has been applied in the context of network meta-analysis,[289] to improve consistency in the network (Chapter 14). An extended idea is suggested by Yamaguchi et al.,[145] who simulate the missing IPD in non-IPD trials based on their reported aggregate data, assuming exchangeability between IPD and non-IPD trials. A simulation study examining the performance of the methods suggests it improves the estimation of within-trial interactions, compared to when just using IPD trials, when the IPD trials represent only 10% to 40% of the available evidence. However, the method is computationally advanced and makes strong assumptions that the treatment effect and the residual variance are common (i.e. the same) in all trials.

7.6 Handling of Continuous Covariates

In this section we explain why categorisation, and in particular dichotomisation, of continuous covariates is inappropriate, and encourage modelling of non-linear treatment-covariate interactions.

7.6.1 Do Not Categorise Continuous Covariates

Let us return to the tamoxifen example of Box 7.1. The findings appear to strongly suggest that breast-cancer patients benefit from tamoxifen if they are ER positive, but may not if they are ER negative. However, this is misleading as ER is actually a continuous biomarker, and the researchers have categorised ER into negative, positive and unclear groups. This means that cut-points were used in the IPD meta-analysis project to subgroup participants into one of these categories; indeed, the project's publication states, "ER-positive was defined as at least 10 fmol ER per mg cytosol protein where quantitative measurements were available, but was otherwise accepted as reported."[268]

Categorisation can be avoided by analysing continuous covariates such as ER on their continuous scale, and thereby allowing estimates of treatment effect conditional on a participant's actual ER value. The usual argument for categorisation, and in particular dichotomisation, of continuous variables is to aid clinical interpretation and maintain simplicity. However, it can rarely, if ever, be justified that an individual patient whose value is just below the cut-point is completely different from a patient whose value is just above it. Arbitrary categorisation also makes interpretation difficult. The Early Breast Cancer Collaboration themselves recognise this when stating: "The definition used to distinguish ER-positive from ER-negative tumours may also be important because some studies suggest that even women with tumours that contain very low but still detectable amounts of the receptor protein may still benefit from tamoxifen." In some trials the categorisation may be embedded in the IPD provided (i.e. the original value has been lost), and this issue may have impeded the Early Breast Cancer Trialists' Collaborative Group.

The use of cut-points for continuous covariates can also lead to data-dredging, in particular when 'optimal' cut-points are sought that minimise the corresponding p-value of the predictor.[63] For example, Mistry et al. propose a tree-based recursive partitioning algorithm (called IPD-SIDES) to identify subgroup effects in an IPD meta-analysis,[290] when there are many covariates of interest (i.e. in an exploratory analysis). However, a limitation is that the tree-based approach requires the use of cut-points to dichotomise continuous covariates, rather than leaving them as continuous. It is well-known that dichotomisation loses statistical power to detect a genuine interaction.[57,63,64,264,291,292] One example, described more fully in Section 12.5.2, shows that the loss of information by dichotomising BMI (rather than keeping as continuous) is similar to throwing away IPD from about 10 of 24 trials containing 1761 participants (about 60% of the total participants).[293] Why spend one or two years painstakingly obtaining, cleaning and harmonising IPD from multiple trials only to throw 60% of the data just before the analysis? This is a bad idea![57]

Consider again the IPD meta-analysis of interventions aimed at reducing excessive weight gain in pregnancy.[16] One outcome of interest was caesarean section. A two-stage IPD meta-analysis of 32 trials shows that the intervention reduced the odds of caesarean section by about 10% (summary OR = 0.91; 95% CI: 0.83 to 0.99). It is of interest whether the mother's age interacts with this treatment effect. If we arbitrarily dichotomise age at 35 years, so that it becomes a binary covariate (i.e. 0 if age $\leq$35, and 1 if age $>$35), then a two-stage IPD meta-analysis assuming the intervention effect is random (i.e. model (7.4) followed by model (7.7)) shows no clear evidence of an interaction between age and treatment effect (summary ratio of ORs = 1.14, 95% CI: 0.90 to 1.45). However, if we keep age as a continuous variable, then there is stronger evidence that the intervention becomes less effective in reducing the odds of caesarean section as a woman's age increases. For every five-year increase in age the odds ratio increases by about 10% (summary ratio of ORs = 1.10, 95% CI: 1.00 to 1.20), and the risk ratio increases by about 6% (summary ratio of RRs = 1.06, 95% CI: 0.98 to 1.15).

7.6.2 Interactions May Be Non-linear

7.6.2.1 Rationale and an Example

All the models and examples provided so far in this chapter have assumed a linear trend for the interaction of treatment and a continuous covariate. However, sometimes the interaction may be non-linear, as emphasised by Royston and Sauerbrei,[264] and considered in detail by Kasenda et al.[294,295] A non-linear relationship implies that the change in treatment effect for every one-unit increase in the covariate may vary across the distribution of the covariate. Therefore, non-linear interactions should routinely be evaluated when the interaction of continuous covariates and treatment effect is of interest, for example using cubic splines (Box 7.2) or fractional polynomials (Box 7.3).

For example, Wang et al. consider whether there is an interaction between age and the effect of hypertensive treatment, and identify a non-linear relationship, with older participants between 60 and 80 years old seeming to benefit more than younger participants and those older than 80.[46] Their original analysis categorised age, but we update their analysis to examine the expected change in treatment effect as a smooth, non-linear function of age (Figure 7.7),[255] with the reference group being the treatment effect for 55-year-old participants. A J-shaped relationship is visible; in particular, there is strong evidence that younger participants have the smallest treatment effect. For instance, when compared to 40-year-old participants, 55-year-old participants have about a

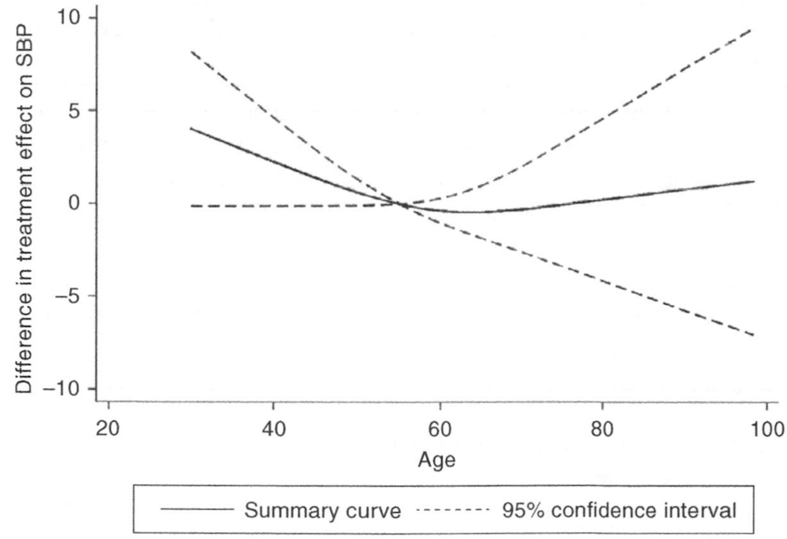

Figure 7.7 Evidence for a potential non-linear interaction between age and the effect of anti-hypertensive treatment on final SBP value, as shown by Riley et al.[255] The reference group is the treatment effect for participants aged 55 years old.

Figure created by fitting an analysis of covariance model in each trial separately, with the interaction between age and treatment modelled via a restricted cubic spline function (with knot positions of 39, 60 and 75), and then the trial-specific parameter estimates (relating to the interaction) pooled in a multivariate meta-analysis with random effects to allow for between-trial heterogeneity in all parameters. *Source:* Figure taken from Figure 3 of Riley et al.,[255] reproduced with permission, © 2020 Wiley.

3 mmHg greater mean reduction in SBP from using the treatment (compared to control). In very old ages the treatment effect also appears to reduce slightly (Figure 7.7), but there is large uncertainty (wide confidence intervals) in the older age range. Further, although evidence supports the J-shaped interaction, treatment effect differences across ages are clinically quite small, and all participants still benefit from treatment regardless of their age (Section 7.11).

Interestingly, when just assuming a linear interaction term between treatment and age, there is no clear evidence of an interaction; the expected change in treatment effect for each year increase of age is −0.05 (95% CI: −0.19 to 0.12). Hence, the linear assumption hides the more J-shaped interaction revealed by the non-linear modelling approach.

7.6.2.2 Two-stage Multivariate IPD Meta-Analysis for Summarising Non-linear Interactions

Figure 7.7 was obtained by modelling the effect of age and its interaction with treatment via a restricted cubic spline function, which is a flexible way of modelling smooth non-linear relationships.[66] Briefly, a restricted cubic spline is obtained by fitting a series of cubic functions and forcing them to join (and be smoothed) at certain points (called internal knots), whilst constraining the function to be linear in the tails (i.e. before the first internal knot and after the last internal knot). The magnitude and shape of the curve are defined by multiple parameters depending on the number of knots chosen. Rather than using a reference group whose covariate value is 0, it helps to center the spline variables at a meaningful value (for example, 55 years was chosen as the reference group in Figure 7.7, as it was approximately the average age across trials). Further details of restricted cubic spline functions are given in Box 7.2.

In a two-stage approach to IPD meta-analysis of a non-linear interaction, this restricted cubic spline is fitted in each trial separately (first stage, Box 7.4) and the parameter estimates defining

Box 7.2 Brief introduction to modelling non-linear relationships for a continuous covariate using restricted cubic splines

Let the original continuous covariate (e.g. age) be denoted by z. Rather than simply assuming a linear association with the outcome of interest (e.g. $Y = \delta_0 + \delta_1 z$), a restricted spline function, denoted by $f(z)$, allows for a potential non-linear association.[66] It is obtained by fitting a series of cubic functions and forcing them to join (and be smoothed) at certain points (called internal knots), whilst constraining the function to be linear in the tails (i.e. before the first internal knot and after the last internal knot). The magnitude and shape of the curve is defined by multiple parameters depending on the number of knots chosen. If we assume there are k internal knots in total at locations $t_1, t_2, \ldots, t_k$, then the restricted cubic spline is:

$$f(z) = \delta_0 + \delta_1 z_1 + \delta_2 z_2 + \ldots + \delta_{k-1} z_{k-1}$$

where $z_1 = z$ and thus there is an assumed linear association between z and the outcome before the first internal knot (i.e. when $z < t_1$), and for $c = 1, \ldots, k-2$,

$$z_{c+1} = (z - t_c)^3_+ - (z - t_{k-1})^3_+ \frac{(t_k - t_c)}{(t_k - t_{k-1})} + (z - t_k)^3_+ \frac{(t_{k-1} - t_c)}{(t_k - t_{k-1})}$$

where the A_+ notation means that $A = A$ if $A > 0$, and $A = 0$ if $A \leq 0$. This specification of z_{c+1} also forces the trend to there be a linear association between z and the outcome after the last internal knot (i.e. when $z \geq t_k$).

Therefore, using a restricted cubic spline in a regression analysis will include the original covariate (z) as linear and $k-2$ piecewise cubic variables. So with k internal knots, there are $k-1$ parameters to estimate which define the spline function, plus an intercept term, δ_0. We can examine whether the use of the spline function (i.e. $f(z)$) adds value over and above assuming a linear trend by comparing the change in the model fit (e.g. the likelihood ratio statistic).

In terms of how to choose the number of knots, Harrell states that "for many datasets, $k = 4$ offers an adequate fit of the model and is a good compromise between flexibility and loss of precision caused by overfitting a small sample".[66] If the sample size is small, three knots should be used in order to have enough observations in between the knots to be able to fit each polynomial. The location of the knots are best pre-specified, based on the quantiles of the continuous variable, with the following suggested by Harrell:[66]

Number of internal knots, k	Knot location in terms of quantiles of the z variable						
3	0.1	0.5	0.9				
4	0.05	0.35	0.65	0.95			
5	0.05	0.275	0.5	0.725	0.95		
6	0.05	0.23	0.41	0.59	0.77	0.95	
7	0.025	0.1833	0.3417	0.5	0.6583	0.8167	0.975

Source: Box taken from Figure 4 of Riley et al.,[255] reproduced with permission, © 2020 Wiley.

Box 7.3 Brief introduction to allowing for non-linear relationships using fractional polynomials

Fractional polynomials offer a limited but flexible set of transformations to describe the potentially non-linear association between a continuous covariate, z, and a particular outcome.[68–70] Instead of assuming a linear trend (e.g. $Y = \alpha + \delta_1 z$), a fractional polynomial function of degree $m \geqslant 1$ is allowed, of the form $Y = \alpha + \sum_{k=1}^{m} \delta_k z^{p_k}$, where the fractional powers $p_1, \ldots, p_m$ are selected from a small predefined set. Royston and Sauerbrei recommend choosing powers from among {−2, −1, −0.5, 0, 0.5, 1, 2, 3}, with zx^0 corresponding to $\ln(z)$.[69] Powers are allowed to repeat in fractional polynomials; each time a power repeats, it is multiplied by another $\ln(z)$. For example, if power 3 is selected twice, z^3 and $z^3\ln(z)$ are used. Automated procedures in statistical software test all possible transformations of degree m to select the most appropriate transformation(s) for the data. Usually an m of 1 or 2 will suffice.

the interaction of this function with treatment are then combined in a multivariate meta-analysis (second stage, Box 7.5). For instance, in the first stage of our example, we pre-defined three internal knots (at the same location in each trial) for the restricted cubic function of the association between age and final SBP in the control group, which led to three parameters per trial defining the spline function in each trial (an intercept and two slope terms). The interaction of this spline function with the treatment effect was then estimated, leading to a within-trial treatment-covariate interaction for each slope in each trial ($\hat{\gamma}_{W1i}$ and $\hat{\gamma}_{W2i}$, Box 7.4). These slope terms define the expected change (difference) in treatment effect across covariate values, relative to the chosen reference group of participants (here, 55 years old).

Box 7.4 Overview of the first stage of a two-stage multivariate IPD meta-analysis to summarise a non-linear treatment-covariate interaction using a restricted cubic spline

To summarise a treatment-covariate interaction across multiple trials where the covariate (z) is continuous and has a potentially non-linear association with the outcome, we can apply a two-stage multivariate IPD meta-analysis utilising restricted cubic splines. The key steps are now described, in relation to the hypertension example of Figure 7.7 which examined a treatment-age interaction.

- ***Create the restricted spline transformation of z, which requires choosing the number of knots and their location.*** The number and location of the knots must be identical for each trial. Usually three or four knots will suffice. Their location could be defined by quantiles of the covariate distribution observed within the entire IPD from all trials, as explained in Box 7.2. However, if the distribution of the covariate varies considerably across trials, then knot locations might be modified so that they fall at relevant places.

  For example, in the hypertension example, some trials included only older participants (>60 years). Hence, we considered it important that one of the knots for age was located at 60. We chose three knots, and placed these at 39 (the 0.1 quantile value), 60 (the 0.48 quantile value) and 75 (the 0.9 quantile value).
- ***Estimate the treatment-covariate interaction in each trial.*** This requires the specification and estimation of a suitable regression model, followed by storing the parameter estimates (and corresponding variance matrix) that define the treatment-covariate interaction. The module *mvmeta* in Stata allows the user to perform a particular regression analysis in each trial, and automatically stores the relevant estimates and corresponding variance matrix.[302,303]

  For example, in the hypertension example we fitted the following model in each trial separately:

$$y_{ij} = \alpha_i + f\left(\text{age}_{ij}\right) + \beta_{2i}x_{ij} + \beta_{3i}y_{0ij} + f\left(x_{ij}\text{age}_{ij}\right) + e_{ij}$$
$$e_{ij} \sim N\left(0, \sigma_i^2\right)$$

  with the restricted cubic spline function defined by

$$f\left(\text{age}_{ij}\right) = \delta_{1i}\text{age}_{1ij} + \delta_{2i}\text{age}_{2ij}$$

  and age_{1ij} and age_{2ij} denoting the first and second spline transformations of age (Box 7.2), respectively. The interaction between the spline function and treatment is defined by

$$f\left(x_{ij}\text{age}_{ij}\right) = \gamma_{W1i}x_{ij}\text{age}_{1ij} + \gamma_{W2i}x_{ij}\text{age}_{2ij}$$

  Of key interest were estimates of γ_{W1i} and γ_{W2i}, as these defined the treatment-covariate interaction in trial i, together with their variances ($\text{var}(\gamma_{W1i})$ and $\text{var}(\gamma_{W2i})$) and covariance ($\text{cov}(\hat{\gamma}_{W1i}, \hat{\gamma}_{W2i})$).

  To aid interpretation, before model estimation it may be helpful to center the spline transformations by a useful reference value. For example, in the hypertension examine we repeated the above analysis in each trial after centering age_{1ij} and age_{2ij} by values that corresponded to an age of 55 years. These led to (age_{1ij} − 55) and (age_{2ij} − 3.16).

Note that if some parameters cannot be estimated in some trials (e.g. due to a narrow distribution of z_{ij}, or perfect prediction), then data augmentation can be used (for example, via the *mvmeta_make* package by White[302]). Essentially this adds just a few individuals to the problematic groups, and leads to an arbitrary parameter estimate but with a very large variance (e.g. 1000000000) and any associated covariances set to zero, such that the estimates will receive barely any weighting in the subsequent multivariate meta-analysis.

Source: Box taken from Figure 5A of Riley et al.,[255] reproduced with permission, © 2020 Wiley.

Box 7.5 Overview of the second stage of a two-stage multivariate IPD meta-analysis to summarise a non-linear treatment-covariate interaction using a restricted cubic spline

After the first stage described in Box 7.4, the second stage involves pooling the non-linear interaction terms, as follows:

- ***Perform a multivariate meta-analysis of the treatment-covariate interaction estimates, to produce a summary of the treatment-covariate interaction.*** The multivariate approach allows the joint synthesis of multiple parameter estimates, whilst accounting for their correlation.[304,305] It can be fitted, for example, using REML estimation and is described in detail in Chapter 13.

  In the hypertension example of Figure 7.7 we fitted a bivariate meta-analysis with random effects allowing for between-trial heterogeneity,

$$\begin{pmatrix}\hat{\gamma}_{W1i}\\ \hat{\gamma}_{W2i}\end{pmatrix}\tilde{N}\left(\begin{pmatrix}\gamma_{W1i}\\ \gamma_{W2i}\end{pmatrix},\begin{pmatrix}\mathrm{var}(\hat{\gamma}_{W1i}) & \mathrm{cov}(\hat{\gamma}_{W1i},\hat{\gamma}_{W2i})\\ \mathrm{cov}(\hat{\gamma}_{W1i},\hat{\gamma}_{W2i}) & \mathrm{var}(\hat{\gamma}_{W2i})\end{pmatrix}\right)$$
$$\begin{pmatrix}\gamma_{W1i}\\ \gamma_{W2i}\end{pmatrix}\tilde{N}\left(\begin{pmatrix}\gamma_{W1}\\ \gamma_{W2}\end{pmatrix},\begin{pmatrix}\tau_1^2 & \tau_{12}\\ \tau_{12} & \tau_2^2\end{pmatrix}\right)$$

  where τ_1^2 and τ_2^2 define the between-trial variances of γ_{W1i} and γ_{W2i}, respectively, and τ_{12} defines their between-trial covariance.

  The summary estimates of $\hat{\gamma}_{W1}$ and $\hat{\gamma}_{W2}$ define the summary treatment-age interaction of $\gamma_{W1}x_{ij}\mathrm{age}_{1ij} + \gamma_{W2}x_{ij}\mathrm{age}_{2ij}$.
- ***Plot the summary treatment-covariate interaction and its confidence interval across the distribution of covariate values.*** After estimation of the multivariate model, the summary treatment-covariate interaction function can be applied (e.g. via the *predict* post-estimation command in Stata) to each participant in the original IPD, to obtain their predicted treatment-covariate interaction; i.e. the difference in their treatment effect compared to that for the reference participants (in our example, this was 55-year-olds). This predicted value can then be plotted (on the *y*-axis) against the original covariate value (on the *x*-axis). The standard error (s.e.) of the predicted value can also be estimated, and then a confidence interval calculated (e.g. using predicted estimate ± 1.96 × s.e.). The upper and lower values of the confidence interval can then be plotted (Figure 7.7).

Source: Box taken from Figure 5B of Riley et al.,[255] reproduced with permission, © 2020 Wiley.

A multivariate meta-analysis can synthesise these multiple slope estimates, whilst accounting for their correlation (both within trials and between trials), as described in Box 7.5 (and more fully in Chapter 13).[296] It produces a summary estimate for each term, from which the summary (pooled) spline function can be derived, to summarise the expected change in treatment effect for covariate values relative to the chosen reference value. This summary curve can then be plotted graphically to visualise the non-linearity and aid clinical interpretation. The trial-specific estimated curves from the first stage (or trial-specific empirical Bayes curves obtained post-estimation from the second stage) might also be presented, as shown by Gasparrini et al.[296] Other graphical displays have been proposed.[297,298]

A similar approach is a two-stage multivariate IPD meta-analysis of a polynomial function.[299] In the first stage, the within-trial interaction defined by the chosen polynomial function is estimated in each trial (e.g. based on a quadratic shape, calculated using $\gamma_{W1}x_{ij}z_{ij} + \gamma_{W2}x_{ij}z_{ij}^2$); in the second stage, the parameter estimates of this function ($\hat{\gamma}_{W1}$ and $\hat{\gamma}_{W2}$) are jointly synthesised accounting for their correlation, which produces a summary function. In particular, fractional polynomial functions provide a limited but flexible set of power transformations to describe a potentially non-linear association.[69,265] These are described further in Box 7.3.

In a single trial, restricted cubic splines and fractional polynomials usually give similar results,[300] though in some situations fractional polynomials better recover simpler non-linear trends, whereas splines better recover more complex trends.[300] However, to allow a multivariate meta-analysis a limitation of fractional polynomials is that the same powers must be specified in each trial (i.e. the shape of the non-linear association is fixed across trials) in order for the parameters of the function to be combinable across trials. In contrast, as long as the same number and location of knots are used in each trial, a restricted cubic spline function is more flexible as the shape of the non-linear association can vary across trials. Therefore, we generally prefer a multivariate IPD meta-analysis of a restricted cubic spline function. A summary of how to use multivariate meta-analysis to model non-linear treatment-covariate interactions is given in Box 7.4 and Box 7.5. Sauerbrei and Royston show that it is possible to combine different fractional polynomial power transformations across trials if the predicted values of the function are pooled (rather than the parameters defining the function),[301] with the pooling of predictions done at each value of the covariate separately.

7.6.2.3 One-stage IPD Meta-Analysis for Summarising Non-linear Interactions

A one-stage IPD meta-analysis model might also be used to examine non-linear treatment-covariate interactions. This might initially seem more intuitive, as it allows all model parameters (including the non-linear function) to be obtained in a single framework. However, in practice it is very difficult to undertake coherently. First, by modelling non-linear functions, we add further parameters to be estimated alongside the trial-specific intercepts and adjustment factors. There are also potentially multiple (correlated) random effects (e.g. one for each of the parameters of the spline function). These issues may cause estimation and convergence problems. Secondly, when centering covariates by their trial-specific means to avoid aggregation bias (i.e. building on models (7.9), (7.11) and (7.12)), the interpretation of the spline function becomes problematic. Unless all trials have the same mean covariate value, the change in treatment effect for a one-unit increase in a covariate from its mean will have a different interpretation in each trial; this will make the summary spline function uninterpretable. For these reasons, we prefer the two-stage approach for examining non-linear treatment-covariate interactions, or a one-stage approach that avoids centering by stratifying trial parameters outside the interaction term (i.e. build on models (7.10), (7.13) and (7.14)).

7.7 Handling of Categorical or Ordinal Covariates

In this section we use 'categorical' to imply a lack of ordering among categories, whereas 'ordinal' implies that an order exists, whether or not categories are separated by fixed intervals. Note that if there are only two categories, these definitions coincide, and such binary covariates can be handled using the methods already described, and therefore are not considered further in this section.

With an ordinal covariate, the simplest model conceptually is to assume a linear trend in the treatment effect across the categories. This can be done by simply applying the methods previously described, treating the categorical covariate exactly as if it were continuous. In this case, covariates will usually be coded using constant intervals, that is, 1, 2, 3 or similar. However, non-constant intervals could also be used with sufficient justification; for example, if one of the extreme categories were to be considered as being very different from the others. As before, to avoid the potential for aggregation bias, a two-stage approach can be used to estimate and then combine interactions between treatment effect and the ordinal variable. Alternatively, a one-stage approach should stratify the treatment variable and other nuisance parameters by trial, and/or the covariate should be centered around its trial-level mean – which in this context will be dependent upon the chosen coding system.

The alternative, applicable to either categorical or ordinal covariates, is to analyse the difference in treatment effect between each category and a single reference category. This involves meta-analysing multiple effects simultaneously, and is therefore handled by a one-stage model with the treatment variable and the covariate each interacted with the trial identifier, or a two-stage approach with multivariate meta-analysis in the second stage.

As described for continuous covariates in Section 7.6.1, it is preferable to analyse categorical and ordinal covariates without further categorisation. However, in some circumstances it may be unavoidable. For example, if data are sparse in certain categories, it may be necessary to make a decision either to remove those categories from the analysis, or to collapse them with adjacent categories, in order to obtain interpretable results.

7.8 Misconceptions and Cautions

Precision medicine based on treatment-covariate interactions is often heralded as the new standard for clinical practice and research. However, some realism is needed and we must be cautious before concluding one genuinely exists.[306] In this section we draw attention to some important misconceptions and cautions when considering treatment-covariate interactions in an IPD meta-analysis, which complement the general statistical pitfalls for personalised medicine discussed by Senn.[307]

7.8.1 Genuine Treatment-covariate Interactions Are Rare

> "*Given the large body of literature documenting research into potential predictive biomarkers and extensive investment into stratified medicine, we identified relatively few predictive biomarkers included in licensing. These were also limited to a small number of clinical areas.*"[308]

The actual identification, validation, and successful implementation of treatment-covariate interactions within clinical practice is rare,[251,260] especially outside of targeted cancer drugs. A sensible starting point – for funders, researchers, health professionals, and patients – is that the relative effect of treatment is very similar for all patients, unless there is strong justification otherwise (e.g. from previous findings, biological rationale). For example, in 2013 a review of the European Medicines Agency (EMA) found that the proportion of licensed drugs for which biomarkers were used to predict benefit (an indication) or harm (a contra-indication) was still very small relative to the total number of drugs licensed.[308] The evidence for the biomarkers recommended was also often weak.

Inappropriate statistical analyses may also lead to wrong conclusions about treatment-covariate interactions in an IPD meta-analysis. We have discussed many of these already, including the aggregation bias problem of meta-regression; the danger of amalgamating within-trial and across-trial information in an IPD meta-analysis; and the dichotomisation of continuous covariates. Another common problem is categorisation of continuous *outcomes*, which can mislead researchers into thinking there are differential responses to treatment. Classifying participants as either responders or non-responders, based on an arbitrary threshold (cut-point) value for a continuous outcome (e.g. SBP < 120 mmHg at follow-up), will lead to those just above the threshold being classed differently from those just below it, which is nonsense. It also leads to misclassification when there is measurement error.[306] If we assume that there is random error of observed outcome values about a true value, then participants with true outcome value close to the threshold may be observed above or below it due to error. For example, if we define participants with an SBP < 120 mmHg at follow-up as responders, then two participants with the same underlying mean blood pressure of 125 mmHg may be classed differently (i.e. one responder and one non-responder), due to random error. Therefore continuous outcomes should be analysed on their continuous scale, in addition to continuous covariates (Section 7.6.1).

Even genuine interactions might not be large enough or sufficient to implement precision medicine. For example, in a review of 279 published IPD meta-analyses that reported at least one subgroup analysis, 102 articles (36.6%) reported a statistically significant subgroup-treatment interaction for the main outcome. However, only "a modest number of these interactions may offer opportunities for stratified medicine decisions".[309]

7.8.2 Interactions May Depend on the Scale of Analysis

Further caution is needed when examining changes of odds ratios across subgroups to identify treatment-covariate interactions. The treatment effect as defined by a risk ratio may be a constant across subgroups, but the odds ratio can still differ when the covariate of interest is a prognostic factor. The reason for this is that the magnitude of the odds ratio depends on the baseline risk, and the difference between the odds ratio and the risk ratio becomes more pronounced as the baseline risk becomes larger (i.e. it moves away from 0 toward 1). Therefore, if the covariate under consideration is a prognostic factor, the baseline risk of participants will depend on their value of this factor (regardless of treatment). This will lead to an interaction between the covariate and the treatment effect as measured by an odds ratio, even when there is no interaction on the risk ratio scale. This is superbly illustrated by Shrier and Pang.[56] Therefore, when examining treatment-covariate interactions within a logistic regression, there needs to be consideration of this phenomenon, especially when the outcome is not rare for particular subgroups. The issue may also arise when comparing hazard (rate) ratios across subgroups, as these too depend on the baseline risk in each subgroup. Therefore, alternative or additional analyses that examine changes in the risk ratio across subgroups are warranted, to check if differences remain on that scale.

The risk ratio scale may also be problematic in some situations as, unlike the odds ratio, its value may be bounded.[66] For example, the risk ratio in a trial can only be > 2 when the baseline risk is <0.5. If the baseline risk is above 0.5, then the risk ratio is bounded below 2. Therefore, substantial changes in the baseline risk across subgroups (e.g. much less than 0.5 in some and much higher than 0.5 in others), may lead to differences in treatment effects across the subgroups due to the bounding issue. For time-to-event outcomes, a further issue is that allowing for non-proportional hazards (e.g. with a treatment by log(time) interaction) rather than proportional hazards may lead to different conclusions about the treatment-covariate interaction, and therefore it is important to examine this.

7.8.3 Measurement Error May Impact Treatment-covariate Interactions

Measurement error may also lead to observed treatment-covariate interactions, when they actually do not exist.[60] For example, assume there is no interaction between an effective treatment and a particular biomarker, but that the biomarker is measured with error, with the error increasing as the true biomarker value increases. Measurement error sometimes (though certainly not always[310]) dilutes effect estimates, such that they are attenuated toward the null. If that occurs in this particular example, we would observe larger treatment effect estimates at lower covariate values, as those treatment effect estimates at higher covariate values have more measurement error and thus are more diluted. This will lead to an observed treatment-covariate interaction, even though it does not exist. The converse may also happen; that is, differential measurement error across covariate values may mask a genuine treatment-covariate interaction. Therefore, if measurement error is a concern, methods are needed to incorporate it whilst examining treatment-covariate interactions.[311] Keogh and White provide an excellent tutorial.[312] IPD meta-analysis may help address measurement error concerns if trials provide IPD with multiple measurements per participant, as then the measurement error could be explicitly modelled (an example is given in Chapter 16).[312] Note that measurement error is a further reason why categorisation of continuous variables should be avoided,[310] as it can lead to misclassification and other issues.

7.8.4 Even without Treatment-covariate Interactions, the Treatment Effect on Absolute Risk May Differ across Participants

For binary or time-to-event outcomes, treatment-covariate interactions correspond to changes across individual participants in the treatment effect as measured on the relative scale (e.g. risk ratio, odds ratio, hazard ratio). However, another approach to personalising or stratifying the use of treatments is to consider their impact on *absolute* risks. Those patients with the highest absolute risk will derive the largest absolute benefit from a treatment (e.g. greatest reduction in probability of the outcome event) when the treatment effect expressed in relative terms is the same for all patients. For example, if the relative treatment effect on mortality risk is estimated as a risk ratio of 0.5 for all patients, then a patient whose mortality risk is 0.5 will have it reduced to 0.25, but a patient whose mortality risk is 0.1 will have it reduced to 0.05. Therefore, the *absolute* reduction in risk is larger for the higher-risk patient (0.25 absolute reduction) than the lower-risk patient (0.05 reduction). If the treatment is expensive or has side effects, it might be restricted to those at highest risk, as they have the most to gain. Therefore, even in the absence of treatment-covariate interactions, treatment decisions might be tailored conditional on absolute outcome risk. For this purpose, prognostic models are important, as these predict absolute outcome risk for a new patient conditional on their values of multiple predictors (Chapter 17).[251,313]

7.8.5 Between-trial Heterogeneity in Treatment Effect Should Not Be Used to Guide Whether Treatment-covariate Interactions Exist at the Participant Level

Consider a meta-analysis for which there is no evidence of between-trial heterogeneity in trial treatment effects. In this situation, it may be tempting to conclude that the treatment effect is the same for all participants. However, the absence of between-trial heterogeneity does not confirm that there are no interactions at the participant-level. Firstly, if there is a genuine treatment-covariate interaction at the participant level, but the distribution of the covariate is very similar across trials, then (assuming no other participant-level or trial-level effect modifiers differ across trials) the treatment effect will be the same in each trial (i.e. there will be no heterogeneity). Secondly, even if the distribution of the covariate does change across trials, the trial treatment effects may still be homogenous; for example, this may arise due to chance, or because the covariate has a non-linear (e.g. U-shaped) interaction with treatment (so that the treatment effect may still be the same in two trials with very different mean covariate values), or even due to multiple effect modifiers acting in combination and different directions.

To illustrate this issue, we extended the IPD meta-analysis of 10 trials of anti-hypertensive treatment in Box 5.4, to evaluate the treatment effect (based on all participants) on the rate of cardiovascular disease.[82,255] This gave a summary hazard ratio of 0.74 (95% CI: 0.67 to 0.81) and no observed between-trial heterogeneity ($\hat{\tau}^2 = 0$). However, when applying a two-stage IPD meta-analysis to examine the interaction between baseline SBP and treatment effect (as described in Box 7.4 and Box 7.5), there is some suggestion of a non-linear interaction, with the treatment effect gradually reducing as the baseline SBP moves from about 170 mmHg toward 120 mmHG (Figure 7.8). Hence, despite the lack of observed between-trial heterogeneity in treatment effects, the IPD meta-analysis has revealed some evidence of a potentially important interaction at the participant-level.

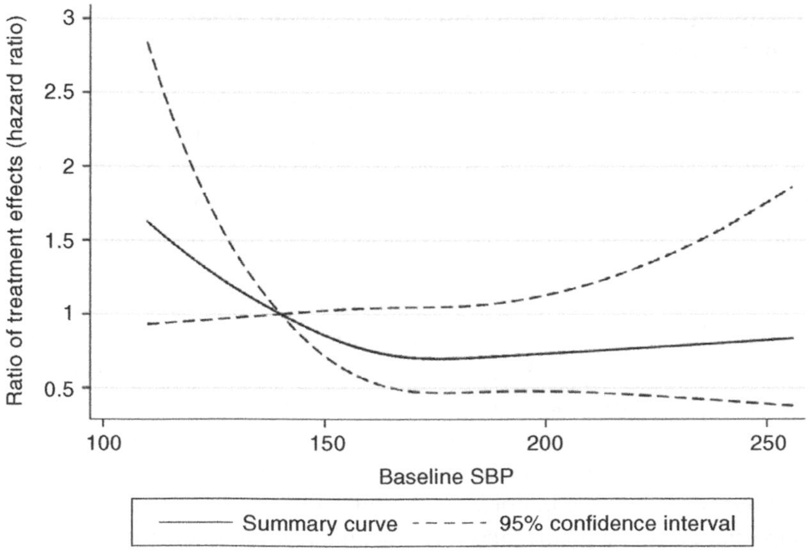

Figure 7.8 Evidence of a potential non-linear interaction between baseline SBP and the effect of anti-hypertensive treatment on the rate of CVD, even though there was no observed between-trial heterogeneity in treatment effects. *Source:* Figure taken from Figure 7 of Riley et al.,[255] reproduced with permission, © 2020 Wiley.

Conversely, heterogeneity in the overall treatment effect does not imply that an interaction must exist at the participant level. Heterogeneity can arise due to changes in trial-level characteristics such as intended dose, follow-up length, and setting, even when there is no interaction at the participant level. Hence, the decision to investigate treatment-covariate interactions should not be driven by the presence of between-trial heterogeneity in treatment effect, and should be rather motivated by the supposed (biological) mechanism of treatment response.

7.9 Is My Identified Treatment-covariate Interaction Genuine?

Existing guidance for the analysis of subgroup effects in randomised trials also holds for IPD meta-analyses examining treatment-covariate interactions.[261] In particular, aside from the aforementioned analysis issues, the identification of genuine treatment-covariate interactions should be guided (or justified) by sound, often biological, reasoning and hypotheses regarding the expected working (causal) mechanism of the treatment.[261,314] Box 7.6 provides suggested criteria of Sun et al. for checking the credibility of a treatment-covariate interaction (which they call a subgroup effect),[261] including an item about the need for evidence to be based on within-trial information, rather than across-trial information. We also recommend two excellent tutorials which discuss intricate issues such as dose-response relationships, measurement error, adjusting for confounders, dealing with multiple covariates, and multiplicative versus additive scales.[60,61]

Box 7.6 Criteria for examining the credibility of a treatment-covariate interaction (termed 'subgroup effect'), as proposed by Sun et al.[261]

Design

- Is the subgroup variable a characteristic measured at baseline or after randomisation?
- Is the effect suggested by comparisons within rather than between studies?
- Was the hypothesis specified a priori?
- Was the direction of the subgroup effect specified a priori?
- Was the subgroup effect one of a small number of hypothesised effects tested?

Analysis

- Does the interaction test* suggest a low likelihood that chance explains the apparent subgroup effect?
- Is the significant subgroup effect independent?

Context

- Is the size of the subgroup effect large?
- Is the interaction consistent across studies?
- Is the interaction consistent across closely related outcomes within the study?
- Is there indirect evidence that supports the hypothesised interaction (biological rationale)?

---

* We suggest focusing on the interaction estimate and its 95% confidence interval, rather than a test.

7.10 Reporting of Analyses of Treatment-covariate Interactions

Many IPD meta-analysis publications do not specify clearly enough how they examined interactions. Fisher et al. reviewed 82 meta-analyses that examined treatment-covariate interactions,[258] and found that 54 (66%) did not explain sufficiently their analysis method, in terms of whether within-trial and across-trial information was separated. Reporting bias is also a concern, such that interactions and subgroups considered significant are more likely to be reported. To resolve such concerns, the use (by researchers) and enforcement (by journals) of the PRISMA-IPD reporting guideline is recommended.[247] This guideline contains specific items about reporting statistical methods used, how interactions were modelled and full reporting of all analysis results. PRISMA-IPD is covered in detail in Chapter 10.

7.11 Can We Predict a New Patient's Treatment Effect?

Once an interaction has been identified as genuine and clinically relevant, the next step is to establish how best to predict an individual patient's treatment effect. This is a complex issue, especially when there are different sources of heterogeneity,[266,267,315–317] and has received relatively little attention in the IPD meta-analysis setting, in which aggregation bias is again a concern. We now briefly illustrate some possible approaches for predicting treatment effects for individual patients based on IPD meta-analysis, but stress that these are initial suggestions.

Let us return to the IPD meta-analysis described in Section 7.6.2, which suggests a potential non-linear interaction between age and the magnitude of the anti-hypertensive effect, with younger participants (below about 55) having gradually less benefit (in terms of reduction in SBP) than older participants. This treatment-age interaction is shown by the smooth curve in Figure 7.7; it reveals the summary estimate of the *difference* in treatment effect for participants with a particular age compared to participants aged 55. However, the curve does not tell us the predicted (expected) treatment effect for a newly diagnosed hypertension patient with a particular age. To obtain this, we might perform a multivariate IPD meta-analysis, where we estimate and then meta-analyse the two slopes (γ_{W1i} and γ_{W2i}) of the spline function (as defined in Box 7.4), and the trial-specific treatment effect for participants aged 55 (β_{2i}), which is our reference group. Then, using the obtained summary estimates ($\hat{\beta}_2, \hat{\gamma}_{W1}, \hat{\gamma}_{W2}$) from the multivariate meta-analysis, we can predict an individual patient's treatment effect conditional on their age:

$$\begin{aligned}&\text{Predicted treatment effect for a new patient } j\\ &= \hat{\beta}_2 + \hat{\gamma}_{W1}\left(\text{age}_{1j} - 55\right) + \hat{\gamma}_{W2}\left(\text{age}_{2j} - 3.16\right)\\ &= -10.66 - \left(0.251 \times \left(\text{age}_{1j} - 55\right)\right) + \left(0.156 \times \left(\text{age}_{2j} - 3.16\right)\right)\end{aligned} \tag{7.21}$$

Here, −10.66 is the summary treatment effect (averaged across all trials) for participants aged 55, and age_{1j} and age_{2j} represent, respectively, the new patient's values of the first and second spline transformation of their age. Applying the prediction equation to a patient aged 40 years old, their corresponding age_{1j} is 40 and age_{2j} is 0.00077, and thus their predicted treatment effect is

$$-10.66 - (0.251 \times (40 - 55)) + (0.15 \times (0.00077 - 3.16)) = -7.39\text{mmHg}$$

The predicted treatment effect across a range of ages is summarised in Figure 7.9.

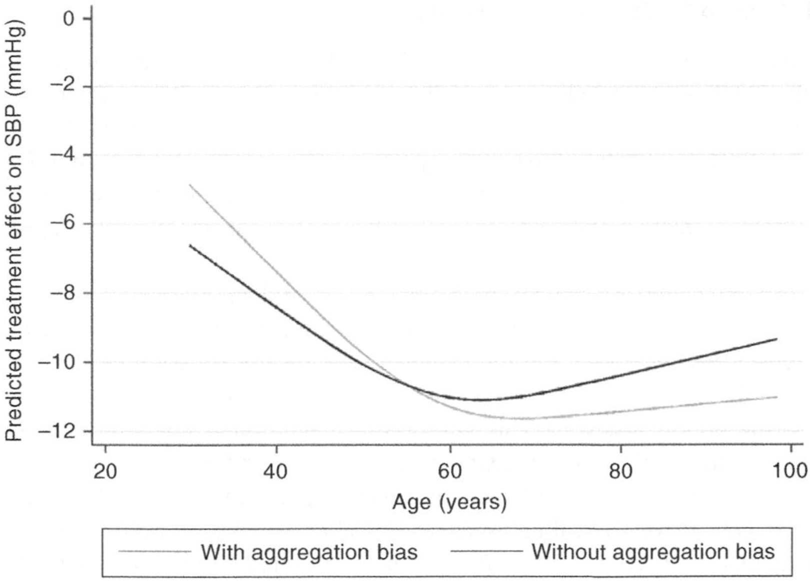

Figure 7.9 The predicted effect of anti-hypertensive treatment on SBP conditional on an a new patient's age, based on a multivariate meta-analysis either with (model (7.21)) or without (model (7.22)) aggregation bias in the summary treatment-age interactions. *Source:* Figure taken from Figure 6 of Riley et al.,[255] reproduced with permission, © 2020 Wiley.

A concern is that applying a multivariate meta-analysis of $\hat{\beta}_{2i}, \hat{\gamma}_{W1i}$ and $\hat{\gamma}_{W2i}$ from each trial will account for the correlation amongst these parameters, both within and between trials. Yet again this allows the potential for aggregation bias to influence the summary interaction terms, $\hat{\gamma}_{W1}$ and $\hat{\gamma}_{W2}$, as their correlation with $\hat{\beta}_2$ allows the borrowing of across-trial information. Though it is perhaps sensible for $\hat{\beta}_2$ (as it is our reference treatment effect averaged across trials), we should want our summary interactions terms to be based solely on within-trial information, as previously argued. To address this, we might replace the summary $\hat{\gamma}_{W1}$ and $\hat{\gamma}_{W2}$ estimates shown in equation (7.21) with −0.178 and 0.133, their respective estimates from a multivariate meta-analysis ignoring any correlation with $\hat{\beta}_{2i}$ terms (Box 7.5). Then the modified prediction equation is:

$$\text{Predicted treatment effect for new patient } j = \hat{\beta}_2 + \hat{\gamma}_{W1}\left(\text{age}_{1j} - 55\right) + \hat{\gamma}_{W2}\left(\text{age}_{2j} - 3.16\right)$$

$$= -10.66 - \left(0.178 \times \left(\text{age}_{1j} - 55\right)\right) + \left(0.133 \times \left(\text{age}_{2j} - 3.16\right)\right) \qquad (7.22)$$

This allows us to produce predicted treatment effects conditional on age, summarised across all trials and removing aggregation bias (and thus has synergy with the ideas discussed in Section 7.4.6). Using model (7.22) for a new patient aged 40 years old, their predicted treatment effect is

$$-10.66 - (0.178 \times (40 - 55)) + (0.133 \times (0.00077 - 3.16)) = -8.41 \text{ mmHg}$$

which is larger that the −7.39 predicted previously. Importantly, the predicted curve across the entire age range is noticeably shallower after removing aggregation bias (Figure 7.9), because the aggregation bias (arising from incorporating across-trial information) made the interaction estimate more extreme than when based solely on within-trial information.

7.11.1 Linking Predictions to Clinical Decision Making

Predictions such as from equation (7.22) can be linked to clinical decision making. For example, treatment might be limited to those predicted to have a (clinically relevant) benefit from the treatment. In our example, across all ages the predicted effect of anti-hypertensive treatment is at least 5 mmHg, and so all new patients are predicted to benefit by a clinically useful amount, even if the magnitude varies due to the treatment-age interaction. This is an important message. Even when there is a treatment-covariate interaction, the treatment may still work usefully for all patients, just with a different magnitude.

However, treatment effect prediction is a complex problem,[266,267,317] and our example is an over-simplification. Firstly, personalised decisions need to be placed in the context of the scale use to measure the treatment effect (Section 7.8.2), and the patient's baseline risk (or baseline starting value). The combination of these sources of information allows the translation of a patient's predicted treatment effects to the absolute risk scale. This requires the integration of prognostic models (for baseline risk prediction conditional on each patient's covariate values) and predicted treatment effects (again conditional on covariate values if interactions exist). Prognostic models are discussed further in Chapter 17. Secondly, if we are willing to make clinical decisions (and even withhold treatment) based on a patient's predicted treatment effect, then there should be a firm understanding of the causal mechanism and pathway (in addition to other considerations, such as the cost-effectiveness of the approach). When predicting treatment effects conditional on covariate values, it would be reassuring to know that the covariates are directly interacting with the treatment (i.e. they are causal), and not due to merely being associated with the actual causal factor(s).[61]

Thirdly, after fitting a regression model to predict treatment effect conditional on multiple covariates, there is potential for overfitting. This refers to when outcome predictions from the model are too extreme, and can be addressed by using penalisation (shrinkage) estimation approaches,[315,318–320] rather than traditional estimation methods (e.g. unpenalised maximum likelihood estimation). Options for penalisation include a global (uniform) shrinkage, ridge regression, the lasso, and elastic net.[321,322] In our hypertension example, which predicts a treatment effect conditional on age, overfitting is potentially of limited concern, as we only estimated two parameters (excluding the intercept), pre-defined our knots values in the spline function and had a large sample size.

7.12 Concluding Remarks

Researchers often embark on an IPD meta-analysis project to examine treatment-covariate interactions at the participant level. Although such interactions are rare, IPD meta-analyses can help find any genuine interactions, as they circumvent the problems of low power and aggregation bias facing meta-regression of across-trial information. In this chapter we outlined key statistical methods, misconceptions and pitfalls in the context of IPD meta-analyses of randomised trials, but the key points are also applicable to interactions in IPD meta-analyses of observational studies.[60]

New research methods are likely to emerge on this topic in the coming years. One key challenge is to disentangle different sources of variation,[323] and Senn recommends we need more of *N*-of-1 trials,[307] to repeatedly test multiple treatments in the same person, including the same treatment multiple times. When discussing the role of interactions in practice, researchers must consider IPD meta-analysis results alongside other information, such as causal and biological reasoning, baseline risk, and predicted treatment effect sizes (Sections 7.8.4 and 7.11).

8

One-stage versus Two-stage Approach to IPD Meta-Analysis: Differences and Recommendations

Richard D. Riley, Danielle L. Burke, and Tim Morris

Summary Points

- An IPD meta-analysis may be conducted using either a one-stage or a two-stage approach.
- The one-stage approach analyses the IPD from all trials simultaneously, for example in a generalised linear mixed model. The two-stage approach firstly uses the IPD to derive aggregate data (such as treatment effect estimates) in each trial separately, and secondly combines this aggregate data in a meta-analysis model.
- Many published articles have compared the one-stage and two-stage approaches via theory, simulation and empirical examples.
- Crucially, differences in one-stage and two-stage summary results will usually be small when the same assumptions and estimation methods are used.
- When notable differences do arise, generally they are caused by a change in modelling assumptions and/or estimation methods, and not due to using a one-stage or two-stage process *per se*. Thus, the choice of model assumptions and estimation methods is more important than selection of a one-stage or two-stage approach.
- An important exception is when most trials in the meta-analysis are small (in terms of numbers of participants or outcome events). In this case a one-stage approach is recommended, as it uses a more exact statistical likelihood than that assumed in the second stage of the two-stage approach.
- In other situations, researchers can feel free to choose either a one-stage or a two-stage approach, with due care given to their choice of modelling assumptions, parameter specification, and estimation methods as guided by Chapters 5 to 7.
- Unless most trials in the IPD meta-analysis are small, generally the two-stage approach will suffice. It is also more accessible (especially for those familiar with conventional aggregate data meta-analysis approaches), and more easily enables visual summaries (e.g. forest plots). It is also more convenient for including trials that only provide remote access to their IPD (so cannot be merged with other IPD), and trials that only provide aggregate data.
- It may be helpful to do both a one-stage and a two-stage analysis (and report both), to check whether conclusions are robust to the choice of approach.

Individual Participant Data Meta-Analysis: A Handbook for Healthcare Research, First Edition.
Edited by Richard D. Riley, Jayne F. Tierney, and Lesley A. Stewart.

8.1 Introduction

Two-stage, or not two-stage, that is the question.

Chapters 5 to 7 describe two-stage and one-stage statistical approaches to IPD meta-analysis of randomised trials.[324] In the two-stage approach, firstly the IPD are used to obtain aggregate data for each trial separately, and secondly these aggregate data are combined using a meta-analysis model. The one-stage approach analyses the IPD from all trials in a single step, for example using a generalised linear mixed model that accounts for the clustering of participants within trials.[3] Historically, meta-analysis has been understood, taught and conducted using a two-stage approach.[4–6] However, one-stage methods more conveniently produce meta-analysis results in a single step,[147,325] which may be especially important when the IPD meta-analysis contains trials that are small (i.e. have few participants or outcome events). Yet, one-stage methods are also criticised for being computationally intensive and prone to estimation problems.[212,325] This can be confusing for those planning an IPD meta-analysis project. Should they choose a one-stage or a two-stage approach? Meta-Analysis results and conclusions may depend on the choice,[325] and so the decision could be crucial.

In this chapter we summarise when and why differences can arise between one-stage and two-stage IPD meta-analyses, using real examples. We focus on the setting in which the IPD meta-analysis aims to summarise a particular effect of interest. We stress that, when the same assumptions and estimation methods are used, one-stage and two-stage approaches usually give very similar results. In other words, any differences usually arise because of changes in modelling assumptions and estimation procedures, and not due to the choice of one-stage or two-stage *per se*. An important exception is when most trials in the IPD meta-analysis have few participants or outcome events, as then a one-stage approach is more exact. Recommendations are provided for choosing between one-stage and two-stage approaches in practice, extending previously published guidance.[7,120] This chapter is intended for a broader audience than the previous three chapters. Equations are presented mostly within tables, and the main text focuses on illustrative examples to reinforce the key messages.

8.2 One-stage and Two-stage Approaches Usually Give Similar Results

8.2.1 Evidence to Support Similarity of One-stage and Two-stage IPD Meta-Analysis Results

Several articles have investigated the difference between one-stage and two-stage IPD meta-analysis results,[4,5,120,148,154,211,262,325–327] either empirically, theoretically or via simulation. Where the aim is to summarise a particular effect, most of these articles suggest that one-stage and two-stage approaches give very similar results. For IPD meta-analyses of binary outcomes, Stewart et al. conclude that "one-stage statistical analyses may not add much value to simpler two-stage approaches".[4] Debray et al. also investigated binary outcomes,[325] and agree that one-stage and two-stage approaches give similar results in general, but each has potential estimation challenges. Senn explains the theoretical equivalence of one-stage and two-stage likelihood specifications for binary outcome meta-analyses without covariates and assuming a common treatment effect.[183] Similarly, for time-to-event outcomes, Bowden et al. conclude: "if the aim of a meta-analysis is to estimate the treatment effect under a random effects model, there appears to be only a very small gain in fitting more complex and computationally intensive one-stage models".[5] For continuous outcomes, Mathew and Nördstrom extend previous theoretical work to suggest that, asymptotically, one-stage and two-stage summary estimates coincide exactly when the treatment effect and the intercept term are assumed common to all trials,[328–330] albeit an unrealistic modelling situation (Section 8.3.2). Two overviews of IPD meta-analysis also note that one-stage and two-stage approaches usually give very similar results.[325,331]

A conventional two-stage IPD meta-analysis only summarises a single parameter in the second stage (i.e. a 'univariate' meta-analysis model is used); in contrast, a one-stage analysis summarises multiple parameters simultaneously. For example, consider an IPD meta-analysis of randomised trials to summarise a treatment effect. A two-stage analysis produces a summary treatment effect by synthesising a single estimate of treatment effect from each trial. In contrast, a one-stage approach produces a summary treatment effect alongside other parameter estimates (such as intercepts, prognostic factor effects, etc). Therefore, statisticians might envisage that a one-stage analysis is automatically more powerful; that is, by estimating all parameters simultaneously, it should incorporate more information. However, in situations where the main parameter of interest can be estimated in every trial, accounting for its correlation with other parameters has surprisingly little impact on the summary result[332–333].* For example, based on analytic reasoning, Lin and Zeng conclude that for all commonly used parametric and semiparametric models, there is no asymptotic efficiency gain by a one-stage IPD meta-analysis if the parameter of main interest has a common value across trials and the nuisance parameters (e.g. intercepts, adjustment terms, residual variances) are stratified by trial (i.e. a separate term is estimated for each trial).[327]

Morris et al.[120] also found that one-stage and two-stage analyses have similar efficiency. Their article evaluates IPD meta-analysis models for continuous outcomes from randomised trials and concludes that the number of stages used is irrelevant, as the precision of the summary treatment effect will be approximately equal when the approaches make the same assumptions about the treatment effect (i.e. common or random) and other nuisance parameters. For example, when assuming a common treatment effect and that intercepts are stratified by trial, one-stage and two-stage approaches provide practically identical parameter estimates and standard errors, when they also make the same assumption about the trial residual variances; either (i) they both assume the residual variances are the same (common) for all trials, or (ii) they both assume the residual variances are distinct (different) for each trial. By default, most software that fits a one-stage approach will assume trial residual variances are the same, whilst a two-stage approach will usually assume they are distinct. But these default assumptions can be changed[183] so that the assumptions about residual variances agree for one-stage and two-stage; then, their meta-analysis results will be practically identical. An example is shown in Figure 8.1, and we discuss this further in Section 8.3.6.

* For further details see Chapter 13, where we describe how univariate meta-analysis of a single parameter and multivariate meta-analysis of multiple parameters usually give similar results when all trials estimate all parameters.

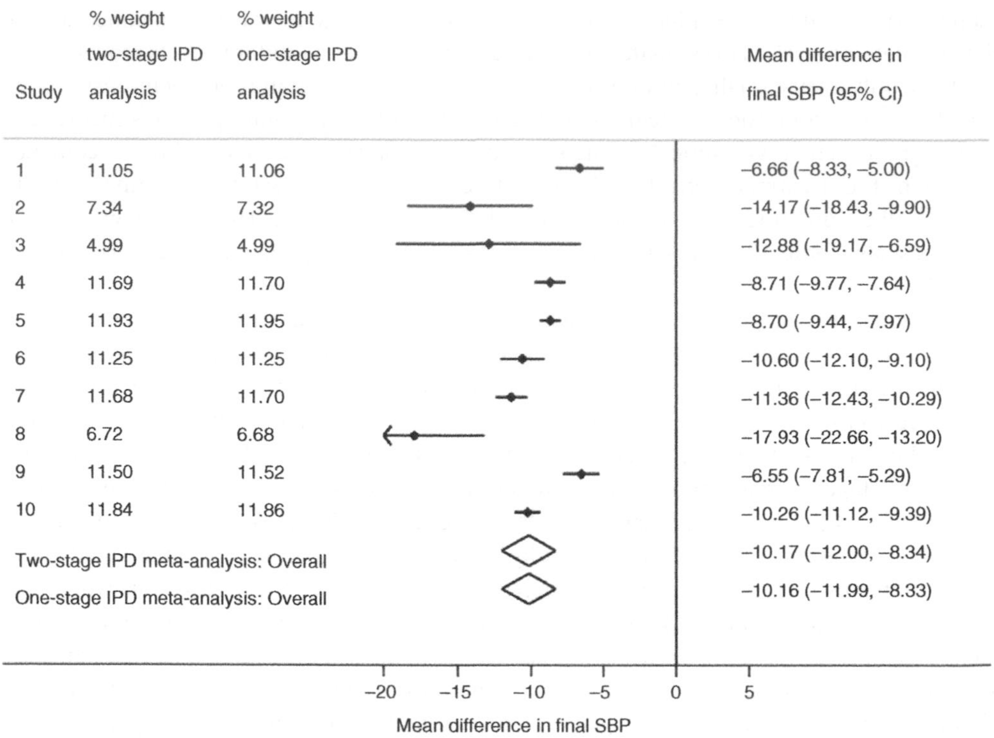
Study
% weight two-stage IPD analysis
% weight one-stage IPD analysis
Mean difference in final SBP (95% CI)
1 11.05 11.06 −6.66 (−8.33, −5.00)
2 7.34 7.32 −14.17 (−18.43, −9.90)
3 4.99 4.99 −12.88 (−19.17, −6.59)
4 11.69 11.70 −8.71 (−9.77, −7.64)
5 11.93 11.95 −8.70 (−9.44, −7.97)
6 11.25 11.25 −10.60 (−12.10, −9.10)
7 11.68 11.70 −11.36 (−12.43, −10.29)
8 6.72 6.68 −17.93 (−22.66, −13.20)
9 11.50 11.52 −6.55 (−7.81, −5.29)
10 11.84 11.86 −10.26 (−11.12, −9.39)
Two-stage IPD meta-analysis: Overall −10.17 (−12.00, −8.34)
One-stage IPD meta-analysis: Overall −10.16 (−11.99, −8.33)
−20
−15
−10
−5
0
5
Mean difference in final SBP

Figure 8.1 One-stage and two-stage IPD meta-analysis summary results from 10 randomised trials to evaluate the effect of anti-hypertensive treatment on SBP.[82] The treatment effect is measured by the mean difference (treatment versus control) in final SBP after adjusting for baseline SBP. Both one-stage and two-stage approaches assume a random treatment effect and stratify all other nuisance parameters (i.e. intercepts, adjustment terms, and residual variances) by trial. REML estimation was applied and Wald-based confidence intervals derived (Section 8.3.8). One-stage weights were derived using the approach of Riley et al.[207] *Source:* Figure taken from Figure 1 of Riley et al.,[207] reproduced with permission, © 2017 Sage Journals (CC-BY 3.0).

8.2.2 Examples

We now provide examples that illustrate the general similarity between one-stage and two-stage IPD meta-analysis results. Figure 8.1 shows a continuous outcome example, where IPD are available from 10 randomised trials to evaluate the effect of anti-hypertensive treatment on SBP,[82,207] as introduced in Box 6.1. We applied one-stage and two-stage approaches to IPD meta-analysis, allowing for between-trial heterogeneity in the treatment effect and stratifying all other parameters by trial (i.e. intercepts, adjustment for baseline, residual variances). For both approaches, we used restricted maximum likelihood (REML) estimation and derived confidence intervals using the standard (Wald-based) approach. The summary results obtained are practically identical regardless of whether the one-stage or two-stage approach was used, with negligible differences in their summary treatment effect estimates and 95% confidence intervals.

One-stage and two-stage results are also similar for an IPD meta-analysis of a time-to-event outcome for the same 10 hypertension trials.[44] We used maximum likelihood (ML) estimation and assumed a common treatment effect in both one-stage and two-stage approaches, whilst stratifying the baseline hazard by trial. The summary treatment effect and 95% confidence interval from the two-stage approach (hazard ratio = 0.74; 95% CI: 0.68 to 0.81) are almost identical to those from the one-stage approach (hazard ratio = 0.74; 95% CI: 0.67 to 0.81),[7] and the findings suggest that the treatment reduces the rate of cardiovascular disease compared to control.

Lastly, consider the binary outcome example of Debray et al.,[325] who used an IPD meta-analysis of three observational studies to examine whether erythema (a binary variable: yes/no) is a risk factor for having a deep vein thrombosis (DVT). The three studies were moderate to large (containing 153, 541 and 1028 participants), and the outcome prevalence of DVT in each erythema category ranged from 10 to 29%, with no zero events in any study. Assuming a common erythema effect in all models, and stratifying all nuisance parameters by study, the summary results from ML estimation are identical for the two-stage and one-stage analyses (odds ratio = 1.35, 95% CI: 1.03 to 1.77), and suggest that participants with erythema have an increase in the odds of DVT compared to without erythema.

8.2.3 Some Claims in Favour of the One-stage Approach Are Misleading

Later in this chapter, Section 8.3.1 describes certain situations where a one-stage approach to IPD meta-analysis is theoretically preferable to a two-stage approach.[14,147] However, it is important to emphasise that such situations are rare. Furthermore, some previous claims of superiority for the one-stage approach are unfair, and simply arise from the comparison allowing stronger assumptions in the one-stage approach than in the two-stage approach. For example, Mathew and Nördstrom suggest that in some conditions "significant loss of precision may result from using the two-step IPD meta-analysis estimator".[329] However, their main example of an inequality was when the intercept term was assumed common to all trials, which is of no practical interest and indeed dangerous as a one-stage model with a common intercept ignores clustering of participants within trials (Section 6.2.3).[3] Similarly, based on a laudable simulation study, Kontopantelis conclude that "a fully specified one-stage model should be preferred, especially when investigating interactions" because it leads to more precise interaction estimates.[148] However, his one-stage models allowed both within-trial and across-trial information to contribute toward the summary interaction estimate. As discussed in Chapter 7, this is not recommended as the incorporation of across-trial information may introduce aggregation bias due to trial-level confounding.[257,258] However, in the very specific setting investigated by Kontopantelis there was no trial-level confounding, and so it is no surprise that his one-stage model (which combines within-trial and across-trial information) gives more precise interaction estimates than the two-stage approach (which solely uses within-trial information). In real applications trial-level confounding is a genuine threat,[258] and so his recommendation to favour a one-stage approach is inappropriate, and rather we draw attention to his more general finding that "a fully specified one-stage model that accounts for study-varying intercepts and a two-stage approach are very close in terms of performance, irrespective of heterogeneity levels and IPD sizes".[148]

8.3 Ten Key Reasons Why One-stage and Two-stage Approaches May Give Different Results

Section 8.2.2 reflects our view that one-stage and two-stage IPD meta-analysis results are usually very similar. However, occasionally notable differences can arise in practice.[329] For example, Box 8.1 and Figure 8.2 show an IPD meta-analysis published in the *BMJ*,[334] with quite large differences in the results from a one-stage analysis (summary odds ratio = 0.88, 95% CI: 0.81 to 0.96) and

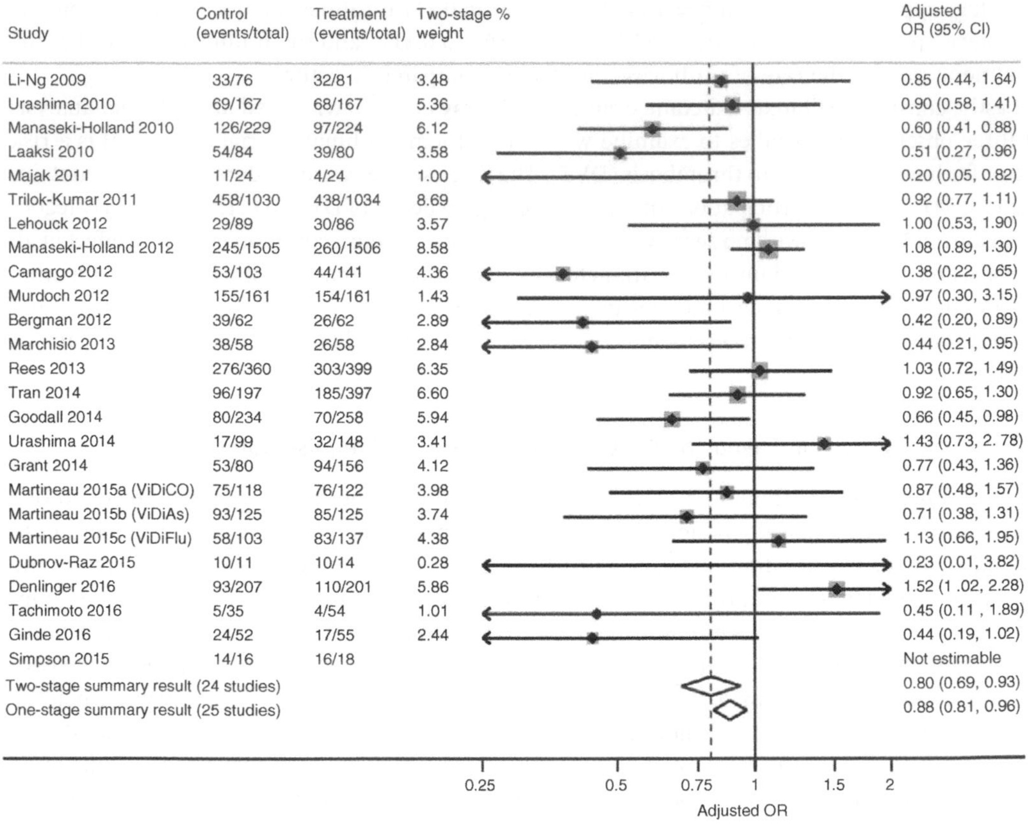
Study | Control (events/total) | Treatment (events/total) | Two-stage % weight | Adjusted OR (95% CI)
Li-Ng 2009 | 33/76 | 32/81 | 3.48 | 0.85 (0.44, 1.64)
Urashima 2010 | 69/167 | 68/167 | 5.36 | 0.90 (0.58, 1.41)
Manaseki-Holland 2010 | 126/229 | 97/224 | 6.12 | 0.60 (0.41, 0.88)
Laaksi 2010 | 54/84 | 39/80 | 3.58 | 0.51 (0.27, 0.96)
Majak 2011 | 11/24 | 4/24 | 1.00 | 0.20 (0.05, 0.82)
Trilok-Kumar 2011 | 458/1030 | 438/1034 | 8.69 | 0.92 (0.77, 1.11)
Lehouck 2012 | 29/89 | 30/86 | 3.57 | 1.00 (0.53, 1.90)
Manaseki-Holland 2012 | 245/1505 | 260/1506 | 8.58 | 1.08 (0.89, 1.30)
Camargo 2012 | 53/103 | 44/141 | 4.36 | 0.38 (0.22, 0.65)
Murdoch 2012 | 155/161 | 154/161 | 1.43 | 0.97 (0.30, 3.15)
Bergman 2012 | 39/62 | 26/62 | 2.89 | 0.42 (0.20, 0.89)
Marchisio 2013 | 38/58 | 26/58 | 2.84 | 0.44 (0.21, 0.95)
Rees 2013 | 276/360 | 303/399 | 6.35 | 1.03 (0.72, 1.49)
Tran 2014 | 96/197 | 185/397 | 6.60 | 0.92 (0.65, 1.30)
Goodall 2014 | 80/234 | 70/258 | 5.94 | 0.66 (0.45, 0.98)
Urashima 2014 | 17/99 | 32/148 | 3.41 | 1.43 (0.73, 2. 78)
Grant 2014 | 53/80 | 94/156 | 4.12 | 0.77 (0.43, 1.36)
Martineau 2015a (ViDiCO) | 75/118 | 76/122 | 3.98 | 0.87 (0.48, 1.57)
Martineau 2015b (ViDiAs) | 93/125 | 85/125 | 3.74 | 0.71 (0.38, 1.31)
Martineau 2015c (ViDiFlu) | 58/103 | 83/137 | 4.38 | 1.13 (0.66, 1.95)
Dubnov-Raz 2015 | 10/11 | 10/14 | 0.28 | 0.23 (0.01, 3.82)
Denlinger 2016 | 93/207 | 110/201 | 5.86 | 1.52 (1 .02, 2.28)
Tachimoto 2016 | 5/35 | 4/54 | 1.01 | 0.45 (0.11 , 1.89)
Ginde 2016 | 24/52 | 17/55 | 2.44 | 0.44 (0.19, 1.02)
Simpson 2015 | 14/16 | 16/18 | | Not estimable
Two-stage summary result (24 studies) | 0.80 (0.69, 0.93)
One-stage summary result (25 studies) | 0.88 (0.81, 0.96)
0.25
0.5
0.75
1
1.5
2
Adjusted OR

Figure 8.2 Forest plot showing the one-stage and two-stage IPD meta-analysis results that correspond to the case study of Box 8.1 *Source:* Richard Riley, produced using data extracted from the original publication.[334]

a two-stage analysis (summary odds ratio = 0.80, 95% CI: 0.69 to 0.93). In such situations, researchers need to understand why this discrepancy occurs, and which approach is more reliable. Examining the reason for the difference may even help to identify errors because, as stated, usually one-stage and two-stage results should be very similar.

Differences in summary results from one-stage and two-stage approaches typically arise when they weight trials differently in the meta-analysis.[207] We now describe 10 potential reasons why this may occur. Some of these are inter-related but are presented separately for clarity. Expanding on reasons published by Burke et al.,[7] these cover changes in model assumptions, parameter specifications, and estimation methods. In each example used to illustrate our arguments, we ensure that exactly the same trials and IPD are used for both one-stage and two-stage analyses, and thus any differences cannot be attributed to discrepant data. We focus mainly on IPD meta-analyses of randomised trials and the use of frequentist estimation methods, although the additional implications of a Bayesian approach are mentioned.

8.3.1 Reason I: Exact One-stage Likelihood When Most Trials Are Small

In a two-stage IPD meta-analysis, the effect estimates derived for each trial in the first stage are assumed in the second stage to have a normal sampling distribution with a known

Box 8.1 Case study of an IPD meta-analysis with a notable difference between one-stage and two-stage IPD meta-analysis results, which most likely arises due to a change in the estimation method, and not the use of one-stage or two-stage *per se*.

Background: Martineau et al. synthesised IPD from 25 randomised controlled trials (10933 participants) to examine whether Vitamin D supplementation prevented acute respiratory tract infections.[334] The main outcome was incidence of at least one acute respiratory tract infection during follow-up.

Methods: Both one-stage and two-stage IPD meta-analyses were applied for each outcome separately "using a random effects model adjusted for age, sex, and trial duration to obtain the pooled intervention effect with a 95% confidence interval". In the one-stage approach they "modelled IPD from all studies simultaneously whilst accounting for the clustering of participants within studies" and, as the treatment effect was summarised by an adjusted odds ratio (OR), it is likely that a logistic regression framework was used.

Results: The one-stage and two-stage results are notably different, as shown in the forest plot of Figure 8.2. Though both provide evidence that vitamin D supplementation is effective on average (i.e. summary OR is < 1), the effect is larger (20% compared to 12% reduction in odds of infection) and the confidence interval substantially wider (e.g. lower bound of 0.69 compared to 0.81) in the two-stage analysis compared to the one-stage analysis.

What is causing the difference? Initially the difference might be presumed due to the two-stage analysis excluding the Simpson trial, because an adjusted odds ratio estimate was not estimable in that trial. This trial can still be included in the one-stage analysis, as it models the exact binomial likelihood and avoids deriving trial-specific estimates (Reason I, Section 8.3.1). However, the omission of the Simpson trial is unlikely to be the main cause of the difference here, as it corresponds to excluding just 34 participants from the 10933 included in the one-stage analysis. Also, the two-stage approach itself is not a concern, as assuming normality of trial-specific estimates and known variances is likely to be a good approximation in this example (Section 8.3.1), because the event is not rare and many trials are large.

Rather, the difference in one-stage and two-stage results is probably caused by different estimation methods (Reason IV, Section 8.3.4), and not the use of one-stage or two-stage *per se*. The one-stage method most likely used ML estimation, which leads to downward bias in estimates of between-trial variance (τ^2) (Reason III, Section 8.3.3). However, the second stage of the two-stage approach used DerSimonian and Laird (methods of moments) estimation, which generally has better (larger) estimates of τ^2 than maximum likelihood estimation. This difference in estimates of τ^2 causes different trial weights in the two-stage analysis compared to the one-stage analysis, and subsequently the different summary results shown on the forest plot.

Had $\hat{\tau}^2$ been the same in one-stage and two-stage analyses, the meta-analysis results would have been practically identical. To illustrate this, we repeated the two-stage IPD meta-analysis but forced $\hat{\tau}^2$ to be zero; this gave a summary OR of 0.88 (95% CI: 0.81 to 0.96), which is exactly the same as that reported for the one-stage analysis in the forest plot in Figure 8.2. Hence, although not stated in the original article, it is likely that the one-stage IPD meta-analysis actually estimated τ^2 to be zero. So we conclude that the differences in the summary results shown in the forest plot arise due to a $\hat{\tau}^2$ of 0 in the one-stage analysis (from maximum likelihood estimation) and 0.061 in the two-stage analysis (from DerSimonian and Laird estimation), and not due to the choice of one-stage or two-stage itself.

Sources: Richard Riley; Based on Martineau AR, Jolliffe DA, Hooper RL, et al. Vitamin D supplementation to prevent acute respiratory tract infections: systematic review and meta-analysis of individual participant data. *BMJ* 2017;356:i6583.

variance.[14,15,147,157,325] These assumptions are reasonable if most trials have moderate to large sample sizes, as normality is justified by the Central Limit Theorem and the variance will then be estimated with reasonable accuracy.[15] This is the situation in Box 8.1, where most trials have more than 30 participants and 10 outcome events per group. However, the assumptions are unreliable when most of the included trials are small (e.g. <20–30 participants in each group) or, specifically for binary, count and time-to-event outcomes, when most trials have few (e.g. <10) or even no outcome events in one or more groups.[14] Furthermore, effect estimates (e.g. odds ratios, rate ratios) in generalised linear models such as logistic and Poisson regression are upwardly biased in situations where outcome events are sparse,[98,167] unless penalised estimation methods are used such as Firth's approach.[167]

In contrast, a one-stage IPD meta-analysis approach obtains summary results whilst more exactly modelling the distribution of the IPD at the participant level;[14] for example, a Bernoulli likelihood can be used within trials to model binary outcome data and summarise odds ratios, whilst a Poisson likelihood can be used within trials to model time-to-event data and summarise incidence rate (hazard) ratios.[14,44] This avoids making assumptions of normality and known variances of treatment effect estimates in each trial. Even more crucial, a two-stage approach that weights effect estimates by inverse variances (in the second stage) will require a continuity correction to be applied (in the first stage) to any trial that has zero outcome events in one of the treatment groups; for example, convention is to add +0.5 to all cells in the trial's two-by-two table, although other options have been proposed (Section 5.2.3.2).[32,33,335] In contrast, a one-stage approach does not require the use of continuity corrections in such situations, as the exact likelihood naturally accommodates any trial with zero outcome events in one of the groups, and avoids calculating trial-specific variances.

Therefore, in situations where most of the included trials are small (either in terms of the number of participants or the number of outcome events), a one-stage approach is recommended. The benefit of one-stage models with sparse data is shown by Hamza et al. and Stijnen et al.[14,147] They performed simulation studies in a range of settings, and found substantial bias in the summary treatment effect estimates and serious under-coverage of confidence intervals (even as low as 50% rather than 95% coverage in some settings). Box 6.2 shows an IPD meta-analysis of seven randomised trials with sparse outcome events in most trials, and applying a two-stage analysis (with continuity corrections of +0.5) gives a summary odds ratio of 1.31 (95% CI: 0.22 to 5.16) and a between-trial variance estimate of zero, whilst a more appropriate one-stage analysis gives a larger summary odds ratio of 1.91 (95% CI: 0.36 to 10.15) and a larger between-trial variance estimate of 0.57. Clearly, the choice of one-stage or two-stage approach has a big impact in this example.

To illustrate this issue beyond randomised trials, Figure 8.3 illustrates an IPD meta-analysis of nine studies that assessed the test accuracy of positron emission tomography in the diagnosis of Alzheimer's disease.[147] Each of the nine studies has a small number of participants (range: 19 to 50) with a combined total of 254 diseased participants and 218 true positive test results; three studies contained zero false positives (observed sensitivity of 100%). The IPD meta-analysis results show large differences in the summary logit sensitivity estimate between the one-stage (2.20) and two-stage (1.70) approaches, relating to a summary sensitivity of 0.90 and 0.85, respectively (Figure 8.3). The estimated τ^2 was also different (0.97 in one-stage analysis, 0.37 in two-stage analysis), which may be especially important for making predictive inferences about test sensitivity in a new population (Chapter 15).[336] The differences were reflected by notable changes in the percentage trial weights, especially for those trials with zero false negatives (Figure 8.3).[249] For example, the percentage weight of trial 8 was larger (7.6%) in the one-stage analysis compared to the two-stage analysis (3.6%).

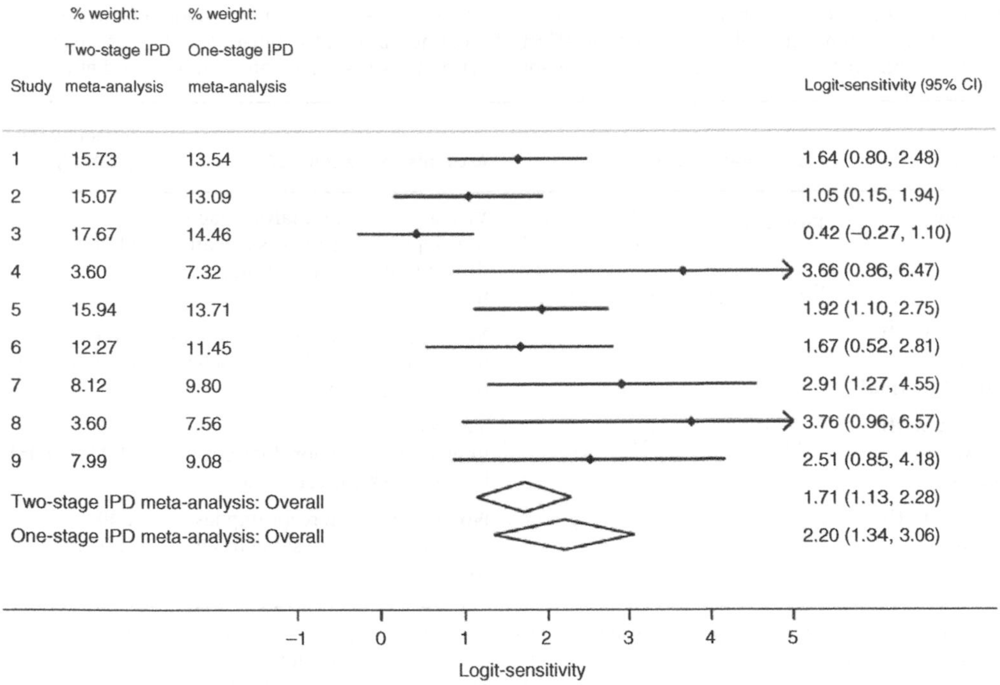
% weight: Two-stage IPD meta-analysis
% weight: One-stage IPD meta-analysis
Study
Logit-sensitivity (95% CI)
1 15.73 13.54 1.64 (0.80, 2.48)
2 15.07 13.09 1.05 (0.15, 1.94)
3 17.67 14.46 0.42 (–0.27, 1.10)
4 3.60 7.32 3.66 (0.86, 6.47)
5 15.94 13.71 1.92 (1.10, 2.75)
6 12.27 11.45 1.67 (0.52, 2.81)
7 8.12 9.80 2.91 (1.27, 4.55)
8 3.60 7.56 3.76 (0.96, 6.57)
9 7.99 9.08 2.51 (0.85, 4.18)
Two-stage IPD meta-analysis: Overall 1.71 (1.13, 2.28)
One-stage IPD meta-analysis: Overall 2.20 (1.34, 3.06)
–1
0
1
2
3
4
5
Logit-sensitivity

Figure 8.3 Forest plot showing one-stage and two-stage IPD meta-analysis results of the sensitivity of the positron emission tomography (PET) test in diagnosing Alzheimer's disease. For both one-stage and two-stage analyses ML estimation was used, and random effects were included to allow for between-study heterogeneity in the true logit sensitivity. The two-stage approach used continuity corrections (+0.5 added to both the number of true positives and the number of false positives) in the first stage to derive logit sensitivity estimates and their variances in each study. Sensitivity of the PET test is the probability of being PET positive for participants who truly have Alzheimer's disease. Results correspond to a summary sensitivity of 0.85 (two-stage) and 0.90 (one-stage). *Source:* Figure taken from Figure 2 of Burke et al.,[7] reproduced with permission, © 2016 Wiley.

8.3.2 Reason II: How Clustering of Participants Within Trials Is Modelled

A two-stage IPD meta-analysis automatically accounts for clustering of participants within trials by analysing the data from each trial separately in the first stage. However, a one-stage IPD meta-analysis models all data simultaneously, and therefore the analyst must account for the clustering of participants in the model as described in Sections 6.2.3 and 6.2.4. When researchers ignore the clustering of participants within trials in a one-stage approach, this may cause differences to the two-stage approach. To illustrate this, Abo-Zaid et al. used an IPD meta-analysis of two randomised controlled trials that involved a total of 1,620 participants to investigate whether nicotine gum increases the odds of smoking cessation.[3] Assuming a common treatment effect, the summary odds ratio estimate was considerably smaller when ignoring clustering within a one-stage approach (1.40) than when accounting for clustering by using either a two-stage approach (1.77) or a one-stage approach (1.80) that stratified intercepts (baseline risks) by trial (Table 8.1). When ignoring clustering, participants are essentially assumed to come from the same trial and thus have the same baseline risk. If this assumption is wrong then, due to non-collapsibility of the odds ratio,[55] it can severely influence the summary meta-analysis results, as in the nicotine gum example.

There are different options to account for the clustering in a one-stage IPD meta-analysis, as shown in the model specifications within Table 8.1. Section 6.2.4.2 recommends that, ideally,

Table 8.1 Comparison of summary results from ML estimation of one-stage and two-stage IPD meta-analyses of two randomised trials examining the effect of nicotine gum on the binary outcome of smoking cessation. All approaches assume a common treatment effect and results are taken from Abo-Zaid et al.[174]

Approach	Model specification	Accounts for clustering?	Summary OR (95% CI)
Two-stage	First stage: $\ln\left(\frac{p_{ij}}{1-p_{ij}}\right) = \alpha_i + \theta_i x_{ij}$ Second stage: $\hat{\theta}_i \sim N\left(\theta, s_i^2\right)$	**Yes,** as approach analyses each trial separately in first stage and thus intercepts are stratified by trial	1.77 (1.26 to 2.49)
One-stage with intercept stratified by trial	$\ln\left(\frac{p_{ij}}{1-p_{ij}}\right) = \alpha_i + \theta x_{ij}$	**Yes,** as stratifying the intercept by trial allows for different baseline risk for each trial	1.80 (1.29 to 2.52)
One-stage with random intercept	$\ln\left(\frac{p_{ij}}{1-p_{ij}}\right) = \alpha_i + \theta x_{ij}$ $\alpha_i \sim N(\alpha, \delta^2)$	**Yes,** as assuming random intercepts allows for different baseline risk for each trial	1.75 (1.25 to 2.45)
One-stage with common intercept	$\ln\left(\frac{p_{ij}}{1-p_{ij}}\right) = \alpha + \theta x_{ij}$	**No,** as single intercept implies baseline risk is the same in all trials	1.40 (1.02 to 1.92)

OR, odds ratio; CI, confidence interval; p_{ij} is the outcome probability for participant j in trial i; θ_i is the treatment effect (ln odds ratio) in trial i; θ is the summary treatment effect; x_{ij} is 1 if in the nicotine gum group and 0 if in the control group; α_i is the trial-specific intercept; δ^2 is the between-trial heterogeneity in the intercepts; α is the average trial intercept; s_i^2 is the variance of $\hat{\theta}_i$ in trial i and is assumed known.
Sources: Richard Riley; Based on Altman DG, Deeks JJ. Meta-analysis, Simpson's paradox, and the number needed to treat. *BMC Med Res Methodol* 2002;2:3.

one-stage models should stratify by trial, such that intercepts (e.g. in one-stage generalised linear mixed models) or baseline hazard functions (e.g. in one-stage Cox regression or parametric survival models) are estimated separately for each trial. This is comparable to the two-stage approach, where nuisance parameters such as intercepts or baseline hazards are generally estimated separately in each trial. So when one-stage models do not stratify by trial, this may cause different results to those from the two-stage approach. For example, if the one-stage model assumes random intercepts (such that trial intercepts are assumed drawn from a normal distribution) or that the baseline hazard functions are proportional across trials (such that their shape is assumed the same), a stronger assumption is made and this may influence parameter estimates, standard errors and confidence intervals. This is evident in Table 8.1, where the one-stage analysis with random intercepts has a slightly smaller odds ratio and a narrower confidence interval than that for either the two-stage approach or the one-stage model stratifying intercepts by trial.

8.3.3 Reason III: Coding of the Treatment Variable in One-stage Models Fitting with ML Estimation

> *"... we have seen that apparently innocuous changes in the model form can have serious consequences for maximum likelihood estimation."*[185]

It is well-recognised that standard ML estimation tends to underestimate variances, such as the between-trial variance of true treatment effects (τ^2).[108,337–342] However, it is less well-known that the downward bias in the ML estimate of τ^2 increases as the number of parameters in the model increases. In the second stage of the two-stage approach, τ^2 is estimated together with just one parameter (the summary treatment effect). However, in a one-stage approach, τ^2 is estimated alongside many other nuisance parameters, such as trial-specific intercepts and adjustment terms. Therefore, the downward bias in the estimate of τ^2 can be considerably worse in a one-stage model fitted using ML estimation,[185] compared to a two-stage analysis that uses ML estimation in the second stage. As explained in Section 6.2.8.4, this can be addressed by using REML estimation in the one-stage model, which for non-continuous outcomes requires the use of a pseudo-likelihood (an approximation to the exact likelihood, which is suitable when most trials in the meta-analysis are not small). In situations where ML estimation is used to fit one-stage models with stratified nuisance parameter, downward bias in the estimate of τ^2 can be reduced by using trial-specific centering of included variables (Section 6.2.8.3). For example, when using ML estimation, a one-stage model stratifying the intercept by trial and including a treatment variable should code each participant as 1/0 (for treatment/control) minus the proportion treated in their trial. This centering improves estimation performance, such that ML estimates from the one-stage model should agree closely with ML estimates from a two-stage analysis (unless most trials are small, Reason I).

For example, Table 8.2 shows summary results from ML estimation of one-stage IPD meta-analyses of the 10 trials of anti-hypertensive treatment introduced in Figure 8.1. When coding the treatment variable using trial-specific centering the estimate of τ^2 is 5.87, which is very similar

Table 8.2 Summary results from an IPD meta-analysis of 10 randomised trials evaluating the effect of anti-hypertensive treatment versus control on reduction in SBP. Results are for illustration, to show differences in summary results when ML estimation is used for different one-stage model specification and treatment coding options.

Approach	Model specification	Coding of treatment variable	Summary mean difference (95% CI)	$\hat{\tau}^2$
One-stage with intercept and baseline adjustment terms stratified by trial	$y_{ij} = \alpha_i + \beta_{1i} y_{0ij} + \theta_i x_{ij} + e_{ij}$ $\theta_i \sim N(\theta, \tau^2)$	1/0 for treatment/control	−10.03 (−11.58 to −8.47)	4.94
		Trial-specific centering	−10.09 (−11.77 to −8.41)	5.87
Two-stage	First stage: $y_{ij} = \alpha_i + \beta_{1i} y_{0ij} + \theta_i x_{ij} + e_{ij}$ Second stage: $\hat{\theta}_i \sim N(\theta_i, s_i^2)$ $\theta_i \sim N(\theta, \tau^2)$	Either coding	−10.09 (−11.78 to −8.41)	5.90

CI, confidence interval; τ^2, between-trial heterogeneity in the treatment effect; y_{ij} is the final SBP value for participant j in trial i; θ_i is the treatment effect (mean difference) in trial i; θ is the summary treatment effect; s_i^2 is the variance of the treatment effect estimate ($\hat{\theta}_i$) in trial i; x_{ij} denotes treatment group (anti-hypertensive treatment or control); α_i is the intercept in trial i; β_{1i} denotes the prognostic effect of baseline blood pressure (y_{0ij}) in trial i; e_{ij} is the residual error; trial-specific centering = 1/0 minus proportion treated in that trial.
Source: Richard Riley.

to the estimate of 5.90 from the two-stage approach. In contrast, the traditional 1/0 coding estimates τ^2 to be 4.94, which leads to narrower confidence intervals for the summary treatment effect.

8.3.4 Reason IV: Different Estimation Methods for τ^2

Following on from Reason III, differences in one-stage and two-stage results may also be due to the analyst using different estimation methods. This is the likely reason for the difference in one-stage and two-stage meta-analysis results in Box 8.1. In particular, mainly for historical reasons, the default estimation method in most software packages is usually REML or ML estimation for a one-stage approach, but the DerSimonian and Laird method for the second stage of a two-stage approach.[96] For example, in the aforementioned IPD meta-analysis of 10 trials of anti-hypertensive treatment, the value of $\hat{\tau}^2$ is much smaller when using a two-stage approach via DerSimonian and Laird ($\hat{\tau}^2$=3.07) compared to using REML estimation for either a one-stage ($\hat{\tau}^2$=7.13) or a two-stage approach ($\hat{\tau}^2$=7.18) (Table 8.3). This larger value of $\hat{\tau}^2$ leads to a larger summary treatment effect with a wider 95% confidence interval (Table 8.3), and would have even more impact upon predictive inferences, such as 95% prediction intervals.[134]

A related reason for a difference would be if a two-stage approach used a frequentist estimation framework (e.g. REML) and a one-stage approach used a Bayesian framework (or vice-versa). In a Bayesian approach, the likelihood is combined with prior distributions for unknown parameters (Section 5.3.8). The larger the weight of the prior distributions, the more potential there is for Bayesian analysis results to differ from frequentist analysis results.

8.3.5 Reason V: Specification of Prognostic Factor and Adjustment Terms

How prognostic (adjustment) factors are handled in a one-stage analysis may impact results and create differences to the two-stage approach. This is a similar issue to the specification of trial

Table 8.3 Summary treatment effect results for the hypertension data to illustrate the differences in summary results according to the estimation method

Approach	Model specification	Estimation method	Summary mean difference (95% CI)	$\hat{\tau}^2$
Two-stage	First stage: $y_{ij} = \alpha_i + \beta_{1i}y_{0ij} + \theta_i x_{ij} + e_{ij}$ Second stage:	REML first stage; DerSimonian and Laird second stage	−9.84 (−11.13 to −8.56)	3.09
	$\hat{\theta}_i \sim N(\theta_i, s_i^2)$ $\theta_i \sim N(\theta, \tau^2)$	REML first and second stages	−10.17 (−12.00 to −8.34)	7.18
One-stage with intercept and baseline adjustment term stratified by trial	$y_{ij} = \alpha_i + \beta_{1i}y_{0ij} + \theta_i x_{ij} + e_{ij}$ $\theta_i \sim N(\theta, \tau^2)$	REML	−10.16 (−11.99 to −8.34)	7.13

CI, confidence interval; REML, restricted maximum likelihood estimation; τ^2, between-trial heterogeneity in the treatment effect. y_{ij} is the final SBP value for participant j in trial i; θ_i is the treatment effect (mean difference) in trial i; θ is the summary treatment effect; s_i^2 is the variance of the treatment effect estimate ($\hat{\theta}_i$) in trial i; x_{ij} denotes treatment group (anti-hypertensive treatment or control); α_i is the intercept in trial i; β_{1i} denotes the prognostic effect of baseline blood pressure (y_{0ij}) in trial i; e_{ij} is the residual error.
Source: Richard Riley.

intercepts to account for clustering (Reason II). Many researchers fit a one-stage model that assumes the effect of prognostic factors is common (i.e. the same in all trials). However, by analysing each trial separately in the first stage, a two-stage approach naturally stratifies by trial, and so allows a separate effect of each prognostic factor in each trial. The equivalent stratification approach in a one-stage model is to include a distinct prognostic factor effect for each trial; so for example with 10 trials, the one-stage model would estimate 10 effects for each prognostic factor (one for each trial). If this is implemented in a one-stage model (perhaps with trial-specific centering to improve ML estimation; Reason III), then the one-stage and two-stage analyses should give similar results as they now make the same assumptions (other things being equal, like choice of estimation method).

To illustrate this we used the IPD from the 10 trials of anti-hypertensive treatment to examine whether smoking (binary variable: yes/no) is a prognostic factor for high SBP at follow-up, after adjusting for baseline blood pressure and treatment group. We compared one-stage REML results when including baseline blood pressure and treatment group as either common or stratified adjustment terms. All models stratified the intercept by trial and assume random trial effects for smoking. The summary adjusted odds ratio for smoking and its 95% confidence interval are very similar for the one-stage approach with stratified adjustment terms and a two-stage approach, as expected (Table 8.4). However, the one-stage approach that assumes the adjustment factor effects are common gives a lower prognostic effect of smoking and a wider confidence interval.

A related reason for differences between two-stage and one-stage results is when the one-stage model places random effects on the adjustment factor effects; this allows borrowing of information across trials, which can lead to potentially different summary results than those from a two-stage approach, or indeed a one-stage approach that stratifies by trial.[7]

Table 8.4 One-stage and two-stage REML results for the prognostic effect of smoking on blood pressure at follow-up, for different specifications of the adjustment for baseline blood pressure and treatment group, using an IPD meta-analysis of 10 randomised trials of anti-hypertensive treatment.

Approach	Model specification	Specification of effect of adjustment factors	Summary mean difference (smokers versus non-smokers), 95% CI	$\hat{\tau}^2$
Two-stage	First stage: $y_{ij} = \alpha_i + \beta_{1i} y_{0ij} + \beta_{2i} x_{ij} + \theta_i \text{smoke}_{ij} + e_{ij}$ Second stage: $\hat{\theta}_i \sim N(\theta_i, s_i^2)$ $\theta_i \sim N(\theta, \tau^2)$	Stratified by trial	1.76 (1.04 to 2.47)	0.23
One-stage with intercepts stratified by trial	$y_{ij} = \alpha_i + \beta_{1i} y_{0ij} + \beta_{2i} x_{ij} + \theta_i \text{smoke}_{ij} + e_{ij}$ $\theta_i \sim N(\theta, \tau^2)$	Stratified by trial	1.76 (1.04 to 2.47)	0.23
One-stage with intercept stratified by trial	$y_{ij} = \alpha_i + \beta_1 y_{0ij} + \beta_2 x_{ij} + \theta_i \text{smoke}_{ij} + e_{ij}$ $\theta_i \sim N(\theta, \tau^2)$	Common	1.69 (0.95 to 2.43)	0.27

τ^2 is the between-trial heterogeneity in the prognostic effect of smoking; y_{ij} is the final SBP value for participant j in trial i; smoke$_{ij}$ denotes smoking status (smokers or non-smokers); θ_i is the prognostic effect (mean difference) of smoking in trial i; θ is the summary prognostic effect of smoking; s_i^2 is the variance of the prognostic effect estimate ($\hat{\theta}_i$) in trial i; x_{ij} denotes treatment group (anti-hypertensive treatment or control); α_i is the intercept in trial i; β_{1i} denotes the prognostic effect of baseline blood pressure (y_{0ij}) in trial i; β_{1i} denotes the treatment effect (y_{0ij}) in trial i; e_{ij} is the residual error.

Source: Richard Riley.

8.3.6 Reason VI: Specification of the Residual Variances

Fitting a linear regression involves estimating the variance of residuals. In a two-stage IPD meta-analysis of randomised trials with a continuous outcome, the residual variance is automatically stratified by trial because, in the first stage, each trial is analysed separately. This can be replicated in a one-stage IPD meta-analysis by estimating a separate residual variance for each trial, which is sometimes referred to as allowing for heteroscedasticity. However, we suspect most one-stage applications assume homoscedasticity (the default in most software packages), which implies all trials have the same residual variance. Senn shows that homoscedasticity can also be replicated in a two-stage approach.[183]

Therefore, both one-stage and two-stage approaches allow the choice of either homoscedasticity or heteroscedasticity. We recommend the latter (Section 6.2.5), but clearly if one-stage and two-stage approaches make different choices, their summary results may disagree. This is illustrated again using the IPD meta-analysis of 10 hypertension trials to summarise the effect of anti-hypertensive treatment. When we assume heteroscedasticity, the one-stage and two-stage results are almost identical (Table 8.5). However, a one-stage analysis assuming homoscedasticity gives a slightly larger summary result, a larger estimate of τ^2, and wider confidence intervals.

Another option is for one-stage models to allow the residual variances to be drawn from a distribution (essentially placing random effects on the residual variance), which could be achieved

Table 8.5 Summary results from one-stage and two-stage IPD meta-analyses of 10 randomised trials examining the effect of anti-hypertensive treatment on SBP, using different specifications of the residual variances. REML estimation was used in all analyses.

Approach	Model specification	Specification of residual variances	Summary mean difference (95% CI)	$\hat{\tau}^2$
One-stage with intercepts stratified by trial	$y_{ij} = \alpha_i + \beta_{1i} y_{0ij} + \theta_i x_{ij} + e_{ij}$ $e_{ij} \sim N\left(0, \sigma_j^2\right)$ $\theta_i \sim N(\theta, \tau^2)$	Common	−10.34 (−12.25 to −8.43)	8.19
One-stage with intercepts stratified by trial	$y_{ij} = \alpha_i + \beta_{1i} y_{0ij} + \theta_i x_{ij} + e_{ij}$ $e_{ij} \sim N\left(0, \sigma_{ij}^2\right)$ $\theta_i \sim N(\theta, \tau^2)$	Stratified by trial	−10.16 (−11.99 to −8.34)	7.13
Two-stage	First stage: $y_{ij} = \alpha_i + \beta_{1i} y_{0ij} + \theta_i x_{ij} + e_{ij}$ $e_{ij} \sim N\left(0, \sigma_{ij}^2\right)$ Second stage: $\hat{\theta}_i \sim N(\theta_i, s_i^2)$ $\theta_i \sim N(\theta, \tau^2)$	Stratified by trial	−10.17 (−12.00 to −8.34)	7.18

CI, confidence interval; τ^2, between-trial heterogeneity in the treatment effect. All models assume a random treatment effect. Both one-stage models included stratified intercept and adjustment for baseline. y_{ij} is the final SBP value for participant j in trial i; θ_i is the treatment effect (mean difference) in trial i; θ is the summary treatment effect; s_i^2 is the variance of the treatment effect estimate ($\hat{\theta}_i$) in trial i; x_{ij} denotes treatment group (anti-hypertensive treatment or control); α_i is the intercept in trial i; β_{1i} denotes the prognostic effect of baseline blood pressure (y_{0ij}) in trial i; e_{ij} is the residual error.
Source: Richard Riley.

using double hierarchical generalized linear models or within a Bayesian framework.[190,343] This may also lead to differences to the two-stage approach, as it allows the residual variances in one trial to learn (borrow strength) from those in other trials. Another related issue is when a two-stage analysis stratifies residual variances by trial *and* treatment group but a one-stage model does not, or vice versa (Sections 5.2.3.1 and 6.2.1.1).

8.3.7 Reason VI: Choice of Common Effect or Random Effects for the Parameter of Interest

Perhaps the most obvious explanation for differences between one-stage and two-stage results is that, for the parameter of interest (e.g. treatment effect), inadvertently the meta-analyst might assume a common effect in one approach but random effects in the other. For example, using the hypertension dataset, we summarised the effect of treatment on SBP using a one-stage IPD meta-analysis assuming a common treatment effect, and compared it to a two-stage IPD meta-analysis assuming (in the second stage) a random treatment effect. Unsurprisingly the summary treatment effects are notably different: the one-stage approach gives −9.31 (95% CI: −9.70 to −8.92) and the two-stage approach gives −10.17 (95% CI: −12.00 to −8.34).

When fitting one-stage models, care is needed to ensure that the implemented random effects are on the parameter(s) desired. In particular, a potential confusion is that statistical software packages that fit generalised linear mixed models will, by default, assume a random intercept term but a common treatment effect term, unless otherwise specified by the user. In contrast, software packages that fits a random-effects model in the second stage of a two-stage IPD meta-analysis will usually assume random treatment effects by default.

8.3.8 Reason VIII: Derivation of Confidence Intervals

Another potential reason for differences between one-stage and two-stage results is the method for deriving confidence intervals. Estimation of an IPD meta-analysis model will produce a summary treatment effect estimate ($\hat{\theta}$) and its standard error ($\text{SE}(\hat{\theta})$). Conventionally, a standard (also known as z-based or Wald-based) $100(1-\alpha)\%$ confidence interval for the summary treatment effect is then calculated using

$$\hat{\theta} \pm \left(z_{1-(\alpha/2)} \times \text{SE}\left(\hat{\theta}\right)\right)$$

where θ is on the same scale as in the fitted meta-analysis model (e.g. log odds ratio, log risk ratio, log hazard ratio, or (standardised) mean difference), and z is the standard normal deviate. For example, if $\alpha = 0.05$ then $z_{1-(\alpha/2)} = 1.96$ and the standard 95% confidence interval is given by $\hat{\theta} \pm \left(1.96 \times \text{SE}\left(\hat{\theta}\right)\right)$.

Such confidence intervals are often too narrow, as no account is taken of the uncertainty in $\hat{\tau}^2$ [121–344] or potentially other variance terms estimated during the one-stage or two-stage approach. To address this, Chapters 5 and 6 discuss alternative methods for deriving confidence intervals, which are generally considered preferable,[110] such as the Hartung-Knapp-Sidik-Jonkman (HKSJ) method for use after a two-stage meta-analysis,[111–113,345,346] and Satterthwaite and Kenward-Roger methods for use after a one-stage meta-analysis.[203,204] Also a Bayesian approach could be used, to more naturally propagate uncertainty in all parameter estimates when deriving credible intervals (Sections 5.3.8 and 6.2.8.8).

Hence, various options for deriving confidence intervals exist for one-stage and two-stage IPD meta-analyses, which may lead to differences in their results. For example, following REML estimation of the one-stage and two-stage analyses presented in Figure 8.1, confidences interval for both approaches are very similar (−11.99 to −8.34) because they were both derived using $\hat{\theta} \pm \left(z_{1-(\alpha/2)} \times \mathrm{SE}(\hat{\theta})\right)$. However, using the HKSJ approach following the two-stage meta-analysis, the 95% confidence interval is slightly wider (−12.45 to −7.89).

8.3.9 Reason IX: Accounting for Correlation Amongst Multiple Outcomes or Time-points

The way that multiple outcomes or time-points are handled may cause differences between one-stage and two-stage IPD meta-analysis results. In a one-stage approach, it is more usual to model all outcomes or time-points simultaneously, for example using a multilevel model where multiple responses (due to the multiple outcomes or time-points) are nested within participants who are themselves nested within trials.[347] In such models, the correlation between all outcomes or time-points is accounted for when deriving the summary treatment effects for each outcome or time-point. This can be replicated in a two-stage IPD meta-analysis but requires a multivariate model in the second stage, to synthesise the treatment effects for the multiple outcomes or time-points simultaneously whilst accounting for their correlation.[82,305] As such multivariate models are non-standard in the meta-analysis field, most researchers opt to perform a separate ('univariate') meta-analysis for each outcome or time-point independently. This may lead to differences between one-stage and two-stage results, as accounting for correlation can lead to more precise and potentially different summary estimates.[348] This is most pertinent in situations where some outcomes or time-points are missing in some trials (Chapter 13).[304]

An example of the difference between a standard two-stage approach that ignores correlation and a one-stage approach that accounts for correlation is shown in Figure 8.4, for an IPD meta-analysis of five trials that evaluated the effect of selegiline versus placebo on the mini-mental state

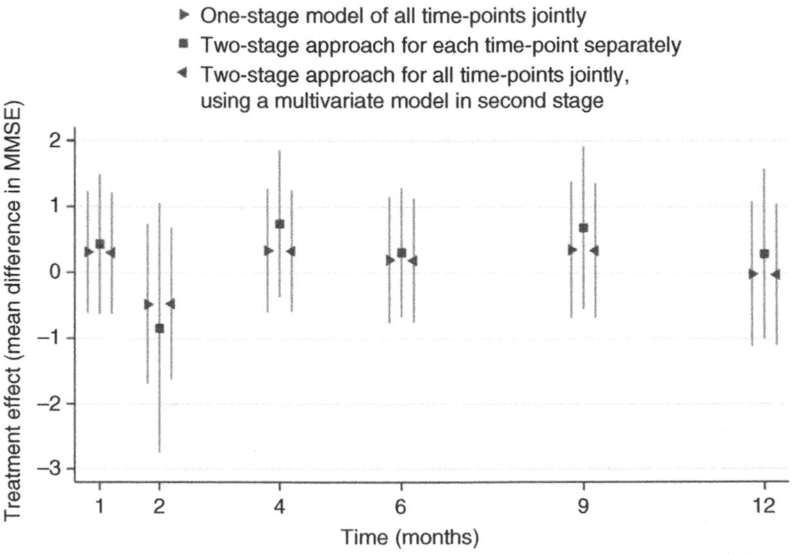

Figure 8.4 Summary treatment effect estimates and 95% confidence intervals from one-stage and two-stage IPD meta-analyses of five trials examining the difference in the mini-mental score examination (MMSE) at various time-points.[347] Treatment effect gives the mean difference in MMSE between Selegiline and Placebo after adjusting for baseline MMSE. *Sources:* Tim Morris; Jones AP, Riley RD, Williamson PR, et al. Meta-analysis of individual patient data versus aggregate data from longitudinal clinical trials. *Clin Trials 2009*;6(1):16–27.

examination score (MMSE) at multiple time-points.[27,347] There are large differences in the summary treatment effects and their standard errors for one-stage and two-stage approaches (Figure 8.4). For example, at four months, the treatment effect is 0.34 for the one-stage model, compared to 0.75 for the two-stage model. Differences are due to the one-stage approach utilising the correlation amongst time-points, which allows the 'borrowing of strength' from the available data to increase precision compared to analysing time-points separately.[349] Such correlation is ignored in the standard two-stage approach applied. However, when we did account for this correlation using a multivariate model in the second stage of the two-stage approach, the differences with the one-stage approach are resolved (Figure 8.4). Thus, yet again, we observe that when the same assumptions are made, the one-stage and two-stage summary results closely agree.

8.3.10 Reason X: Aggregation Bias for Treatment Covariate Interactions

Chapter 7 emphasises that interactions between a treatment effect and participant-level covariates are best estimated using only within-trial information (i.e. at the participant level). Otherwise, when also using across-trial information (i.e. about the association of trial treatment effects and mean participant-level covariate values), aggregation bias can occur because across-trial associations often do not reflect the true within-trial relationships at the participant level.[256,270]

A two-stage approach to the estimation of treatment-covariate interactions automatically avoids aggregation bias by fitting a separate model in each trial to obtain within-trial interaction estimates, which are then synthesised in the second stage.[259] Section 7.4.2 describes how this can be achieved in a one-stage approach, by separating out within-trial and across-trial information in the modelling framework.[156,256–258,277,280] Many researchers rather fit one-stage models that amalgamate within-trial and across-trial information, which is inappropriate and can lead to substantial differences from the two-stage approach.

Riley et al. examined a treatment-age interaction within the IPD meta-analysis of 10 trials of antihypertensive treatment, for the outcome of systolic blood pressure.[156] A one-stage model with an amalgamated interaction term gave strong evidence of an association between age and treatment effect (interaction = –0.067, 95% CI: –0.094 to –0.040, $p <$ <0.001), suggesting that at an older age the treatment gives a larger reduction in blood pressure compared to control. However, when using a one-stage model that correctly separates the within-trial and across-trial interactions there was much weaker evidence of an association (interaction = –0.050, 95% CI: –0.116 to 0.017; p = 0.14), and the results were almost identical to the two-stage approach (interaction = –0.049, 95% CI: –0.115 to 0.017, p = 0.14). Thus, in the original one-stage analysis the across-trial information was having a substantial impact on both the estimate and precision of the summary interaction, which was causing the difference to the results from a two-stage approach. Section 7.6.2 considers extension to non-linear interactions for age and treatment.

8.3.11 Other Potential Causes

The reasons for differences described in Sections 8.3.1 to 8.3.10 are not exhaustive, as differences can also occur for other reasons. For example, different sets of trials and/or participants may be included in the one-stage and two-stage approaches; the analyst may make unintentional errors such as pooling odds ratios (rather than log odds ratios) in the second stage of the two-stage approach; or different sets of adjustment factors may be used in the two-stage and one-stage approaches. Differences may also arise owing to differences in how missing outcome or covariate data are handled (Section 5.2.5; Chapter 18), how automated selection procedures are employed, and how (non-linear) trends are modelled (Chapter 16).[301]

8.4 Recommendations and Guidance

So, two-stage or not two-stage? There is not a blanket answer that covers all IPD meta-analysis projects. The choice between one-stage and two-stage approaches depends on many factors, including the clinical question, the parameter(s) of interest, the desired specification of the model, the desired estimation method, the assumptions researchers are willing to make, the potential for non-convergence and missing data, and whether trials are small and/or have few events. It may also depend on the skill sets and experience in the research team. Where expertise allows, conducting a simulation study in advance of data analysis may be helpful, to compare the statistical performance of one-stage and two-stage approaches in simulated settings that reflect the number and size of trials in the planned IPD meta-analysis.

Nevertheless, two general recommendations can be made (Box 8.2). Firstly, unless most trials are small (in terms of number of participants or outcome events), researchers can feel free to choose either a one-stage or a two-stage approach. We generally prefer the two-stage approach, as it automatically stratifies parameter estimates by trial (in the first stage); utilises (in the second stage) well-known meta-analysis methods that offer familiarity and transparency to researchers (e.g. inverse variance methods); and easily enables visual summaries (e.g. forest plots). It is also more

Box 8.2 Two general recommendations about choosing between one-stage and two-stage IPD meta-analyses

i) Unless most trials in the IPD meta-analysis are small (in terms of the number of participants or outcome events), researchers can feel free to choose either a one-stage or a two-stage approach.

Justification: In most situations, any differences in one-stage and two-stage results can be attributed to the use of different assumptions or estimation methods, and when they are made consistent any differences should be negligible (Section 8.2). Usually, the choice of modelling assumptions (e.g. common or random treatment effects) and estimation methods (e.g. ML or REML) is more important than whether one or two stages are employed. Chapters 5 to 7 provide detailed guidance on how to undertake two-stage and one-stage approaches.

ii) When most trials in the IPD meta-analysis are small (in terms of number of participants or outcome events), a one-stage approach is recommended.

Justification: a one-stage approach enables a more exact statistical likelihood than that assumed in the second stage of the two-stage approach, which is most important when data are sparse (Reason I). For example, if most trials have fewer than 30 participants per group, or fewer than 10 events per group, then sparse data is a concern and a one-stage approach should be preferred. The one-stage approach is, however, not necessarily a panacea in this situation. For example, there may be estimation difficulties due to large numbers of parameters; the best method for deriving confidence intervals may be unclear; and perhaps only ML estimation is available, such that there is a strong concern about downward bias in between-trial variance estimates. Many of these issues can be addressed by taking a Bayesian approach to a one-stage IPD meta-analysis, perhaps with empirically based prior distributions for the between-trial variance. The advantages of a Bayesian framework are discussed in Section 5.3.8.

Source: Richard Riley.

convenient for including trials that only provide remote access to their IPD (so cannot be merged with other IPD), and trials for which only aggregate data (and not IPD) are available.

Secondly, if most trials in the IPD meta-analysis are small, a one-stage approach is recommended due to using a more exact likelihood, although it is still not a panacea in this situation (Box 8.2). Where feasible, it can be helpful to do both one-stage and two-stage analyses (and report both) to check whether conclusions are robust to the choice of approach. If they differ importantly, then the 10 reasons outlined in this chapter should help identify the cause of the difference.

8.5 Concluding Remarks

Appropriate statistical methods are an essential component of IPD meta-analysis projects. Chapters within Part 2 of this book have detailed and compared two-stage and one-stage methods for synthesising IPD from randomised trials, where the aim is to summarise treatment effects and treatment-covariate interactions. Extension to other areas will be considered in Parts 4 and 5 (including IPD meta-analysis projects examining multiple outcomes, multiple treatments, diagnostic tests, prognostic factors, and clinical prediction models), but firstly Part 3 focuses on critical appraisal and dissemination, which is a crucial yet often neglected component of IPD meta-analysis research.

Part II References

1 Simmonds MC, Higgins JPT, Stewart LA, et al. Meta-analysis of individual patient data from randomized trials: a review of methods used in practice. *Clinical Trials* 2005;2:209–217.

2 Riley RD, Lambert PC, Abo-Zaid G. Meta-analysis of individual participant data: rationale, conduct, and reporting. *BMJ* 2010;340:c221.

3 Abo-Zaid G, Guo B, Deeks JJ, et al. Individual participant data meta-analyses should not ignore clustering. *J Clin Epidemiol* 2013;66(8):865–873 e4.

4 Stewart GB, Altman DG, Askie LM, et al. Statistical analysis of individual participant data meta-analyses: a comparison of methods and recommendations for practice. *PLoS One* 2012;7(10):e46042.

5 Bowden J, Tierney JF, Simmonds M, et al. Individual patient data meta-analysis of time-to-event outcomes: one-stage versus two-stage approaches for estimating the hazard ratio under a random effects model. *Res Synth Methods* 2011;2(3):150–162.

6 Higgins JPT, Green SB. Cochrane Handbook for Systematic Reviews of Interventions Version 5.1.0 [updated March 2011]: The Cochrane Collaboration (Available from www.handbook.cochrane.org) 2011.

7 Burke DL, Ensor J, Riley RD. Meta-analysis using individual participant data: one-stage and two-stage approaches, and why they may differ. *Stat Med* 2017;36(5):855–875.

8 Riley RD, Simmonds MC, Look MP. Evidence synthesis combining individual patient data and aggregate data: a systematic review identified current practice and possible methods. *J Clin Epidemiol* 2007;60(5):431–439.

9 Brown H, Prescott R. *Applied Mixed Models in Medicine* (3rd edition). Chichester, UK: Wiley 2015.

10 McCulloch CE, Searle SR, Neuhaus JM. Generalized, *Linear, and Mixed Models* (2nd edition). Hoboken, NJ: Wiley 2008.

11 Littell RC, Milliken GA, Stroup WW, et al. *SAS System for Mixed Models*. SAS Institute Inc. 1996.

12 Cox DR. Regression models and life-tables. *JRoyal Stat Soc Series B* 1972;34(2):187–220.

13 Brown HK, Kempton RA. The application of REML in clinical trials. *Stat Med* 1994;13(16):1601–1617.

14 Stijnen T, Hamza TH, Özdemir P. Random effects meta-analysis of event outcome in the framework of the generalized linear mixed model with applications in sparse data. *Stat Med* 2010;29:3046–3067.

15 Jackson D, White IR. When should meta-analysis avoid making hidden normality assumptions? *Biom J* 2018;60(6):1040–1058.

16 Rogozinska E, Marlin N, Jackson L, et al. Effects of antenatal diet and physical activity on maternal and fetal outcomes: individual patient data meta-analysis and health economic evaluation. *Health Technol Assess* 2017;21(41):1–158.

17 Papadimitropoulou K, Stijnen T, Dekkers OM, et al. One-stage random effects meta-analysis using linear mixed models for aggregate continuous outcome data. *Res Synth Methods* 2019;10(3):360–375.

Individual Participant Data Meta-Analysis: A Handbook for Healthcare Research, First Edition.
Edited by Richard D. Riley, Jayne F. Tierney, and Lesley A. Stewart.

18 Shieh G. Power and sample size calculations for comparison of two regression lines with heterogeneous variances. *PLoS One* 2018;13(12):e0207745.

19 Vickers AJ, Altman DG. Statistics notes: analysing controlled trials with baseline and follow up measurements. *BMJ* 2001;323(7321):1123–1124.

20 Deeks JJ, Higgins JP, Altman DG. Analysing data and undertaking meta-analyses. In: Higgins JP, Green S, eds. *Cochrane Handbook for Systematic Reviews of Interventions: Cochrane Book Series.* Chichester, UK: Wiley 2008.

21 Senn S. Change from baseline and analysis of covariance revisited. *Stat Med* 2006;30:4334–4344.

22 McKenzie JE, Herbison GP, Deeks JJ. Impact of analysing continuous outcomes using final values, change scores and analysis of covariance on the performance of meta-analytic methods: a simulation study. *Res Synth Methods* 2016;7(4):371–386.

23 Riley RD, Kauser I, Bland M, et al. Meta-analysis of randomised trials with a continuous outcome according to baseline imbalance and availability of individual participant data. *Stat Med* 2013;32 (16):2747–2766.

24 Frison LJ, Pocock SJ. Linearly divergent treatment effects in clinical trials with repeated measures: efficient analysis using summary statistics. *Stat Med* 1997 16:2855–2872.

25 Van Breukelen GJ. ANCOVA versus change from baseline: more power in randomized studies, more bias in nonrandomized studies. *J Clin Epidemiol* 2006;59:920–925.

26 White IR, Thompson SG. Adjusting for partially missing baseline measurements in randomized trials. *Stat Med* 2005;24(7):993–1007.

27 Whitehead A. *Meta-analysis of Controlled Clinical Trials*. West Sussex, UK: Wiley 2002.

28 White IR, Thomas J. Standardized mean differences in individually-randomized and cluster-randomized trials, with applications to meta-analysis. *Clin Trials* 2005;2(2):141–151.

29 Murad MH, Wang Z, Chu H, et al. When continuous outcomes are measured using different scales: guide for meta-analysis and interpretation. *BMJ* 2019;364:k4817.

30 Borenstein M. *Introduction to Meta-analysis*. Chichester, UK: Wiley 2009.

31 Cummings P. The relative merits of risk ratios and odds ratios. *Arch Pediatr Adolesc Med* 2009;163 (5):438–445.

32 Bradburn MJ, Deeks JJ, Berlin JA, et al. Much ado about nothing: a comparison of the performance of meta-analytical methods with rare events. *Stat Med* 2007;26(1):53–77.

33 Sweeting MJ, Sutton AJ, Lambert PC. What to add to nothing? Use and avoidance of continuity corrections in meta-analysis of sparse data. *Stat Med* 2004;23(9):1351–1375.

34 Spittal MJ, Pirkis J, Gurrin LC. Meta-analysis of incidence rate data in the presence of zero events. *BMC Med Res Methodol* 2015;15:42.

35 Cox DR, Snell EJ. *The Analysis of Binary Data* (2nd edition). London: Chapman & Hall 1989.

36 Heinze G, Schemper M. A solution to the problem of separation in logistic regression. *Stat Med* 2002;21(16):2409–2419.

37 Kuss O. Statistical methods for meta-analyses including information from studies without any events—add nothing to nothing and succeed nevertheless. *Stat Med* 2015;34(7):1097–1116.

38 Whitehead A, Omar RZ, Higgins JP, et al. Meta-analysis of ordinal outcomes using individual patient data. *Stat Med* 2001;20(15):2243–2260.

39 Ananth CV, Kleinbaum DG. Regression models for ordinal responses: a review of methods and applications. *Int J Epidemiol* 1997;26(6):1323–1333.

40 Hall DB. Zero-inflated Poisson and binomial regression with random effects: a case study. *Biometrics* 2000;56(4):1030–1039.

41 Yau KK, Lee AH. Zero-inflated Poisson regression with random effects to evaluate an occupational injury prevention programme. *Stat Med* 2001;20(19):2907–2920.

42 Lee AH, Wang K, Scott JA, et al. Multi-level zero-inflated poisson regression modelling of correlated count data with excess zeros. *Stat Methods Med Res* 2006;15(1):47–61.

43 Zou G. A modified Poisson regression approach to prospective studies with binary data. *Am J Epidemiol* 2004;159(7):702–706.

44 Crowther MJ, Riley RD, Staessen JA, et al. Individual patient data meta-analysis of survival data using Poisson regression models. *BMC Med Res Methodol* 2012;12:34.

45 Heinze G, Schemper M. A solution to the problem of monotone likelihood in Cox regression. *Biometrics* 2001;57(1):114–119.

46 Wang JG, Staessen JA, Franklin SS, et al. Systolic and diastolic blood pressure lowering as determinants of cardiovascular outcome. *Hypertension* 2005;45(5):907–913.

47 Senn SJ. Covariate imbalance and random allocation in clinical trials. *Stat Med* 1989;8(4):467–475.

48 Senn S. *Statistical Issues in Drug Development* (2nd edition). Chichester, UK and Hoboken, NJ: Wiley 2007.

49 Senn S. Seven myths of randomisation in clinical trials. *Stat Med* 2013;32(9):1439–1450.

50 Hernandez AV, Eijkemans MJ, Steyerberg EW. Randomized controlled trials with time-to-event outcomes: how much does prespecified covariate adjustment increase power? *Ann Epidemiol* 2006;16:41–48.

51 Maas AI, Steyerberg EW, Marmarou A, et al. IMPACT recommendations for improving the design and analysis of clinical trials in moderate to severe traumatic brain injury. *Neurotherapeutics* 2010;7(1):127–134.

52 Roozenbeek B, Maas AI, Lingsma HF, et al. Baseline characteristics and statistical power in randomized controlled trials: selection, prognostic targeting, or covariate adjustment? *Crit Care Med* 2009;37(10):2683–2690.

53 Hernández AV, Steyerberg EW, Habbema JD. Covariate adjustment in randomized controlled trials with dichotomous outcomes increases statistical power and reduces sample size requirements. *J Clin Epidemiol* 2004;57(5):454–460.

54 Burgess S. Estimating and contextualizing the attenuation of odds ratios due to non collapsibility. *Commun Stat Theory and Methods* 2017;46(2):786–804.

55 Greenland S, Robins MR, Pearl J. Confounding and collapsibility in causal inference. *Statistical Science* 1999;14:29–46.

56 Shrier I, Pang M. Confounding, effect modification, and the odds ratio: common misinterpretations. *J Clin Epidemiol* 2015;68(4):470–474.

57 Royston P, Altman DG, Sauerbrei W. Dichotomizing continuous predictors in multiple regression: a bad idea. *Stat Med* 2006;25(1):127–141.

58 Harrell Jr. FE. https://twitter.com/f2harrell/status/1008090230438744069, 2018.

59 Huitfeldt A, Goldstein A, Swanson SA. The choice of effect measure for binary outcomes: introducing counterfactual outcome state transition parameters. *Epidemiol Methods* 2018;7(1):20160014.

60 Greenland S. Basic problems in interaction assessment. *Environ Health Perspect* 1993;101 Suppl 4:59–66.

61 VanderWeele Tyler J, Knol Mirjam J. A tutorial on Interaction. *Epidemiol Methods* 2014;3(1):33.

62 Riley RD, Moons KGM, Snell KIE, et al. A guide to systematic review and meta-analysis of prognostic factor studies. *BMJ* 2019;364:k4597.

63 Altman DG, Lausen B, Sauerbrei W, et al. Dangers of using "optimal" cutpoints in the evaluation of prognostic factors. *J Natl Cancer Inst* 1994;86(11):829–835.

64 Altman DG, Royston P. Statistics notes: the cost of dichotomising continuous variables. *BMJ* 2006;332:1080.

65 Durrleman S, Simon R. Flexible regression models with cubic splines. *Stat Med* 1989;8:551–561.

66 Harrell FE, Jr. *Regression Modeling Strategies: With Applications to Linear Models, Logistic and Ordinal Regression, and Survival Analysis* (2nd edition). New York: Springer 2015.

67 Nieboer D, Vergouwe Y, Roobol MJ, et al. Nonlinear modeling was applied thoughtfully for risk prediction: the Prostate Biopsy Collaborative Group. *J Clin Epidemiol* 2015;68(4):426–434.

68 Sauerbrei W, Royston P. Building multivariable prognostic and diagnostic models: transformation of the predictors by using fractional polynomials. *J Royal Stat SocSeries A* 1999;162:71–94.

69 Royston P, Sauerbrei W. *Multivariable model-building – A pragmatic approach to regression analysis based on fractional polynomials for modelling continuous variables.* Chichester, UK: Wiley 2008.

70 Royston P, Altman DG. Regression using fractional polynomials of continuous covariates: parsimonious parametric modelling. *J Royal Stat Soc Series C* 1994;43(3):429–467.

71 Donner A, Klar N. Issues in the meta-analysis of cluster randomized trials. *Stat Med* 2002;21 (19):2971–2980.

72 Eldridge S, Kerry S. *A Practical Guide to Cluster Randomised Trials in Health Services Research.* Chichester, UK: Wiley 2012.

73 Bland JM, Kerry SM. Statistics notes. *Trials randomised in clusters. BMJ* 1997;315(7108):600.

74 Kahan BC. Accounting for centre-effects in multicentre trials with a binary outcome – when, why, and how? *BMC Med Res Methodol* 2014;14:20.

75 Kahan BC, Morris TP. Analysis of multicentre trials with continuous outcomes: when and how should we account for centre effects? *Stat Med* 2013;32(7):1136–1149.

76 Jones B, Teather D, Wang J, et al. A comparison of various estimators of a treatment difference for a multi-centre clinical trial. *Stat Med* 1998;17(15–16):1767–1777.

77 Localio AR, Berlin JA, Ten Have TR, et al. Adjustments for center in multicenter studies: an overview. *Ann Intern Med* 2001;135(2):112–123.

78 Sullivan TR, White IR, Salter AB, et al. Should multiple imputation be the method of choice for handling missing data in randomized trials? *Stat Methods Med Res* 2018;27(9):2610–2626.

79 Groenwold RH, Donders AR, Roes KC, et al. Dealing with missing outcome data in randomized trials and observational studies. *Am J Epidemiol* 2012;175(3):210–217.

80 Jackson D, White IR, Seaman S, et al. Relaxing the independent censoring assumption in the Cox proportional hazards model using multiple imputation. *Stat Med* 2014;33(27):4681–4694.

81 Cro S, Morris TP, Kenward MG, et al. Sensitivity analysis for clinical trials with missing continuous outcome data using controlled multiple imputation: a practical guide. *Stat Med* 2020;39(21):2815–2842.

82 Riley RD, Price MJ, Jackson D, et al. Multivariate meta-analysis using individual participant data. *Res Synth Method* 2015;6:157–174.

83 Fibrinogen Studies Collaboration. Systematically missing confounders in individual participant data meta-analysis of observational cohort studies. *Stat Med* 2009;28(8):1218–1237.

84 Audigier V, White IR, Jolani S, et al. Multiple imputation for multilevel data with continuous and binary variables. *Statist Sci* 2018;33(2):160–83.

85 Jolani S, Debray TP, Koffijberg H, et al. Imputation of systematically missing predictors in an individual participant data meta-analysis: a generalized approach using MICE. *Stat Med* 2015;34(11):1841–1863.

86 Quartagno M, Grund S, Carpenter J. jomo: a flexible package for two-level joint modelling multiple imputation. *R Journal* 2019;11(2):205–228.

87 Groenwold RH, White IR, Donders AR, et al. Missing covariate data in clinical research: when and when not to use the missing-indicator method for analysis. *CMAJ* 2012;184(11):1265–1269.

88 Whitehead A, Whitehead J. A general parametric approach to the meta-analysis of randomized clinical trials. *Stat Med* 1991;10(11):1665–1677.

89 Rice K, Higgins JPT, Lumley T. A re-evaluation of fixed effect(s) meta-analysis. *J RoyalStat Soc Series A StatSoc* 2018;181(1):205–227.

90 Higgins JP, Thompson SG, Spiegelhalter DJ. A re-evaluation of random-effects meta-analysis. *J Royal Stat Soc Series A* 2009;172:137–159.

91 Jackson D, Turner R, Rhodes K, et al. Methods for calculating confidence and credible intervals for the residual between-study variance in random effects meta-regression models. *BMC Med Res Methodol* 2014;14:103.

92 Jackson D, Bowden J, Baker R. Approximate confidence intervals for moment-based estimators of the between-study variance in random effects meta-analysis. *Res Synths Methods* 2015;6 (4):372–382.

93 Jackson D, Bowden J. Confidence intervals for the between-study variance in random-effects meta-analysis using generalised heterogeneity statistics: should we use unequal tails? *BMC Med Res Methodol* 2016;16:118.

94 Jackson D. Confidence intervals for the between-study variance in random effects meta-analysis using generalised Cochran heterogeneity statistics. *Res Synth Methods* 2013;4(3):220–229.

95 Langan D, Higgins JPT, Jackson D, et al. A comparison of heterogeneity variance estimators in simulated random-effects meta-analyses. *Res Synth Methods* 2019;10(1):83–98.

96 DerSimonian R, Laird N. Meta-analysis in clinical trials. *Control Clin Trials* 1986;7:177–188.

97 Rucker G, Schwarzer G, Carpenter JR, et al. Undue reliance on I(2) in assessing heterogeneity may mislead. *BMC Med Res Methodol* 2008;8:79.

98 Greenland S, Mansournia MA, Altman DG. Sparse data bias: a problem hiding in plain sight. *BMJ* 2016;352:i1981.

99 Yusuf S, Peto R, Lewis J, et al. Beta blockade during and after myocardial infarction: an overview of the randomized trials. *Progr Cardiovasc Dis* 1985;17:335–371.

100 Mantel N, Haenszel W. Statistical aspects of the analysis of data from retrospective studies of disease. *J Nat Cancer Inst* 1959;22:719–748.

101 Langan D, Higgins JP, Simmonds M. An empirical comparison of heterogeneity variance estimators in 12 894 meta-analyses. *Res Synth Methods* 2015;6(2):195–205.

102 Review Manager (RevMan). Version 5.3 [program]. Copenhagen: The Nordic Cochrane Centre, The Cochrane Collaboration, 2014.

103 Kontopantelis E, Reeves D. Performance of statistical methods for meta-analysis when true study effects are non-normally distributed: a comparison between DerSimonian-Laird and restricted maximum likelihood. *Stat Methods Med Res* 2012;21(6):657–659.

104 DerSimonian R, Kacker R. Random-effects model for meta-analysis of clinical trials: an update. *Contemp Clin Trials* 2007;28(2):105–114.

105 Patterson HD, Thompson R. Recovery of inter-block information when block sizes are unequal. *Biometrika* 1971;58(3):545–554.

106 Harville DA. Maximum Likelihood approaches to variance component estimation and to related problems. *J Am Stat Assoc* 1977;72(358):320–338.

107 Veroniki AA, Jackson D, Viechtbauer W, et al. Methods to estimate the between-study variance and its uncertainty in meta-analysis. *Res Synth Methods* 2016;7(1):55–79.

108 Legha A, Riley RD, Ensor J, et al. Individual participant data meta-analysis of continuous outcomes: a comparison of approaches for specifying and estimating one-stage models. *Stat Med* 2018;37 (29):4404–4420.

109 Paule RC, Mandel J. Consensus values and weighting factors. *J Res Natl Bur Stand* 1982;87:377–385.

110 Cornell JE, Mulrow CD, Localio R, et al. Random-effects meta-analysis of inconsistent effects: a time for change. *Ann Intern Med* 2014;160(4):267–270.

111 Hartung J, Knapp G. A refined method for the meta-analysis of controlled clinical trials with binary outcome. *Stat Med* 2001;20(24):3875–3889.

112 Hartung J, Knapp G. On tests of the overall treatment effect in meta-analysis with normally distributed responses. *Stat Med* 2001;20(12):1771–1782.

113 Sidik K, Jonkman JN. A simple confidence interval for meta-analysis. *Stat Med* 2002;21 (21):3153–3159.

114 Wiksten A, Rucker G, Schwarzer G. Hartung-Knapp method is not always conservative compared with fixed-effect meta-analysis. *Stat Med* 2016;35(15):2503–2515.

115 Jackson D, Law M, Rucker G, et al. The Hartung-Knapp modification for random-effects meta-analysis: a useful refinement but are there any residual concerns? *Stat Med* 2017;36(25):3923–3934.

116 Rover C, Knapp G, Friede T. Hartung-Knapp-Sidik-Jonkman approach and its modification for random-effects meta-analysis with few studies. *BMC Med Res Methodol* 2015;15(1):99.

117 van Aert RCM, Jackson D. A new justification of the Hartung-Knapp method for random-effects meta-analysis based on weighted least squares regression. *Res Synth Methods* 2019;10(4):515–527.

118 Sidik K, Jonkman JN. Robust variance estimation for random effects meta-analysis. *Comput Stat Data Anal* 2006;50(12):3681–3701.

119 Fisher DJ. Two-stage individual participant data meta-analysis and generalized forest plots. *Stata J* 2015;15(2):369–396.

120 Morris TP, Fisher DJ, Kenward MG, et al. Meta-analysis of Gaussian individual patient data: Two-stage or not two-stage? *Stat Med* 2018;37(9):1419–1438.

121 IntHout J, Ioannidis JP, Borm GF. The Hartung-Knapp-Sidik-Jonkman method for random effects meta-analysis is straightforward and considerably outperforms the standard DerSimonian-Laird method. *BMC Med Res Methodol* 2014;14:25.

122 Partlett C, Riley RD. Random effects meta-analysis: coverage performance of 95% confidence and prediction intervals following REML estimation. *Stat Med* 2017;36(2):301–317.

123 Bayes T. An essay toward solving a problem in the doctrine of chances. *Philos Trans R Soc* 1764;53:418.

124 Sutton AJ, Abrams KR. Bayesian methods in meta-analysis and evidence synthesis. *Stat Methods Med Res* 2001;10(4):277–303.

125 Bodnar O, Link A, Arendacka B, et al. Bayesian estimation in random effects meta-analysis using a non-informative prior. *Stat Med* 2017;36(2):378–399.

126 Dias S, Sutton AJ, Ades AE, et al. Evidence synthesis for decision making 2: a generalized linear modeling framework for pairwise and network meta-analysis of randomized controlled trials. *Med Decis Making* 2013;33(5):607–617.

127 Lambert PC, Sutton AJ, Burton PR, et al. How vague is vague? A simulation study of the impact of the use of vague prior distributions in MCMC. *Stat Med* 2005;24:2401–2428.

128 Turner RM, Dominguez-Islas CP, Jackson D, et al. Incorporating external evidence on between-trial heterogeneity in network meta-analysis. *Stat Med* 2019;38(8):1321–1335.

129 Rhodes KM, Turner RM, White IR, et al. Implementing informative priors for heterogeneity in meta-analysis using meta-regression and pseudo data. *Stat Med* 2016;35(29):5495–5511.

130 Turner RM, Davey J, Clarke MJ, et al. Predicting the extent of heterogeneity in meta-analysis, using empirical data from the Cochrane Database of Systematic Reviews. *Int J Epidemiol* 2012;41 (3):818–827.

131 Spiegelhalter DJ, Abrams KR, Myles JP. *Bayesian Approaches to Clinical Trials & Health-Care Evaluation*. Chichester, UK: Wiley 2004.

132 Burke DL, Bujkiewicz S, Riley RD. Bayesian bivariate meta-analysis of correlated effects: impact of the prior distributions on the between-study correlation, borrowing of strength, and joint inferences. *Stat Methods Med Res* 2018;27(2):428–450.

133 Senn S, Schmitz S, Schritz A, et al. Random main effects of treatment: a case study with a network meta-analysis. *Biom J* 2019;61(2):379–390.

134 Riley RD, Higgins JP, Deeks JJ. Interpretation of random effects meta-analyses. *BMJ* 2011;342:d549.

135 Lee KJ, Thompson SG. Flexible parametric models for random-effects distributions. *Stat Med* 2008;27(3):418–434.

136 Wang CC, Lee WC. A simple method to estimate prediction intervals and predictive distributions: summarizing meta-analyses beyond means and confidence intervals. *Res Synth Methods* 2019;10 (2):255–266.

137 Nagashima K, Noma H, Furukawa TA. Prediction intervals for random-effects meta-analysis: a confidence distribution approach. *Stat Methods Med Res* 2019;28(6):1689–1702.

138 Berkey CS, Hoaglin DC, Antczak-Bouckoms A, et al. Meta-analysis of multiple outcomes by regression with random effects. *Stat Med* 1998;17(22):2537–2550.

139 Thompson SG, Higgins JPT. How should meta-regression analyses be undertaken and interpreted? *Stat Med* 2002;21:1559–1574.

140 Viechtbauer W. Conducting meta-analyses in R with the metafor Package. *J Stat Softw* 2010;36(3):48.

141 McCormack K, Scott N, Grant A. Are trials with individual patient data available different from trials without individual patient data available? 9th Annual Cochrane Colloquium Abstracts, Lyon, France, 2001.

142 Scott NW, McCormack K, Graham P, et al. Open mesh versus non-mesh for repair of femoral and inguinal hernia. *Cochrane Database Syst Rev* 2002(4):CD002197.

143 Papadimitropoulou K, Stijnen T, Riley RD, et al. Meta-analysis of continuous outcomes: using pseudo IPD created from aggregate data to adjust for baseline imbalance and assess treatment-by-baseline modification. *Res Synth Methods* 2020;11(6):780–794.

144 Bonofiglio F, Schumacher M, Binder H. Recovery of original individual person data (IPD) inferences from empirical IPD summaries only: applications to distributed computing under disclosure constraints. *Stat Med* 2020;39(8):1183–1198.

145 Yamaguchi Y, Sakamoto W, Goto M, et al. Meta-analysis of a continuous outcome combining individual patient data and aggregate data: a method based on simulated individual patient data. *Res Synth Methods* 2014;5(4):322–351.

146 Simmonds M, Stewart G, Stewart L. A decade of individual participant data meta-analyses: a review of current practice. *Contemp Clin Trials* 2015;45(Pt A):76–83.

147 Hamza TH, van Houwelingen HC, Stijnen T. The binomial distribution of meta-analysis was preferred to model within-study variability. *J Clin Epidemiol* 2008;61(1):41–51.

148 Kontopantelis E. A comparison of one-stage vs two-stage individual patient data meta-analysis methods: a simulation study. *Res Synth Methods* 2018;9(3):417–430.

149 Abo-Zaid G, Sauerbrei W, Riley RD. Individual participant data meta-analysis of prognostic factor studies: state of the art? *BMC Med Res Methodol* 2012;12:56.

150 Goldstein H, Browne W, Rasbash J. Multilevel modelling of medical data. *Stat Med* 2002;21 (21):3291–3315.

151 Goldstein H, Yang M, Omar RZ, et al. Meta-analysis using multilevel models with an application to the study of class size effects. *J Royal Stat Soc Series C ApplStat2000*;49:399–412.

152 McCullagh P, Nelder JA. *Generalized Linear Models* (2nd Edition). *Taylor & Francis* 1989.

153 Stroup WW. *Generalized Linear Mixed Models: Modern Concepts, Methods and Applications*. Boca Raton, FL: CRC Press 2012.

154 Debray TP, Moons KG, van Valkenhoef G, et al. Get real in individual participant data (IPD) meta-analysis: a review of the methodology. *Res Synth Methods* 2015;6(4):293–309.

155 Higgins JP, Whitehead A, Turner RM, et al. Meta-analysis of continuous outcome data from individual patients. *Stat Med* 2001;20(15):2219–2241.

156 Riley RD, Lambert PC, Staessen JA, et al. Meta-analysis of continuous outcomes combining individual patient data and aggregate data. *Stat Med* 2008;27(11):1870–1893.

157 Turner RM, Omar RZ, Yang M, et al. A multilevel model framework for meta-analysis of clinical trials with binary outcomes. *Stat Med* 2000;19(24):3417–3432.

158 Warn DE, Thompson SG, Spiegelhalter DJ. Bayesian random effects meta-analysis of trials with binary outcomes: methods for the absolute risk difference and relative risk scales. *Stat Med* 2002;21 (11):1601–1623.

159 Riley RD, Steyerberg EW. Meta-analysis of a binary outcome using individual participant data and aggregate data. *Res Synth Methods* 2010;1:2–9.

160 Debray TPA, Moons KGM, Abo-Zaid GMA. Individual participant data meta-analysis for a binary outcome: one-stage or two-stage? *PLoS ONE* 2013;8(4):e60650.

161 Thomas D, Radji S, Benedetti A. Systematic review of methods for individual patient data meta-analysis with binary outcomes. *BMC Med Res Methodol* 2014;14:79.

162 Thomas D, Platt R, Benedetti A. A comparison of analytic approaches for individual patient data meta-analyses with binary outcomes. *BMC Med Res Methodol* 2017;17(1):28.

163 Sutton AJ, Kendrick D, Coupland CA. Meta-analysis of individual- and aggregate-level data. *Stat Med* 2008;27:651–669.

164 Thompson SG, Turner RM, Warn DE. Multilevel models for meta-analysis, and their application to absolute risk differences. *Stat Methods Med Res* 2001;10(6):375–392.

165 Harrell Jr. FE. Assessing heterogeneity of treatment effect, estimating patient-specific efficacy, and studying variation in odds ratios, risk ratios, and risk differences. *Statistical Thinking* (http://www.fharrell.com/post/varyor/), 2019.

166 Simmonds MC, Higgins JP. A general framework for the use of logistic regression models in meta-analysis. *Stat Methods Med Res* 2016;25(6):2858–2877.

167 Firth D. Bias reduction of maximum likelihood estimates. *Biometrika* 1993;80(1):27–38.

168 Li B, Lingsma HF, Steyerberg EW, et al. Logistic random effects regression models: a comparison of statistical packages for binary and ordinal outcomes. *BMC Med Res Methodol* 2011;11(1):77.

169 Niel-Weise BS, Stijnen T, van den Broek PJ. Anti-infective-treated central venous catheters for total parenteral nutrition or chemotherapy: a systematic review. *J Hosp Infect* 2008;69(2):114–123.

170 Gardiner JC, Luo Z, Roman LA. Fixed effects, random effects and GEE: what are the differences? *Stat Med* 2009;28(2):221–239.

171 Robinson LD, Jewell NP. Some surprising results about covariate adjustment in logistic regression models. *Int Stat Rev* 1991;58:227–240.

172 Gail MH, Wieand S, Piantadosi S. Biased estimates of treatment effect in randomized experiments with nonlinear regressions and omitted covariates. *Biometrika* 1984;71:431–444.

173 Parzen M, Lipsitz SR, Dear KBG. Does clustering affect the usual test statistics of no treatment effect in a randomized clinical trial? *Biom J* 1998;40(4):385–402.

174 Altman DG, Deeks JJ. Meta-analysis, Simpson's paradox, and the number needed to treat. *BMC Med Res Methodol* 2002;2:3.

175 Peters TJ, Richards SH, Bankhead CR, et al. Comparison of methods for analysing cluster randomized trials: an example involving a factorial design. *Int J Epidemiol* 2003;32(5):840–846.

176 Bland JM. Cluster randomised trials in the medical literature: two bibliometric surveys. *BMC Med Res Methodol* 2004;4:21.

177 Lee KJ, Thompson SG. The use of random effects models to allow for clustering in individually randomized trials. *Clin Trials* 2005;2(2):163–173.

178 Steyerberg EW, Bossuyt PM, Lee KL. Clinical trials in acute myocardial infarction: should we adjust for baseline characteristics? *Am Heart J* 2000;139(5) 745–751.

179 Turner EL, Perel P, Clayton T, et al. Covariate adjustment increased power in randomized controlled trials: an example in traumatic brain injury. *J Clin Epidemiol* 2012;65(5):474–481.

180 Rice VH, Stead LF. Nursing interventions for smoking cessation. *The Cochrane Database of Systematic Reviews (Complete Reviews)* 2001;CD001188

181 Riley RD, Legha A, Jackson D, et al. One-stage individual participant data meta-analysis models for continuous and binary outcomes: comparison of treatment coding options and estimation methods. *Stat Med* 2020;39(19):2536–2355.

182 Senn S. The many modes of meta. *Drug Inf J* 2000;34(2):535–549.

183 Senn S. Hans van Houwelingen and the art of summing up. *Biom J* 2010;52(1):85–94.

184 White IR, Turner RM, Karahalios A, et al. A comparison of arm-based and contrast-based models for network meta-analysis. *Stat Med* 2019;38(27):5197–5213.

185 Jackson D, Law M, Stijnen T, et al. A comparison of seven random-effects models for meta-analyses that estimate the summary odds ratio. *Stat Med* 2018;37(7):1059–1085.

186 Van Houwelingen HC, Arends LR, Stijnen T. Advanced methods in meta-analysis: multivariate approach and meta-regression. *Stat Med* 2002;21(4):589–624.

187 Van Houwelingen HC, Zwinderman KH, Stijnen T. A bivariate approach to meta-analysis. *Stat Med* 1993;12(24):2273–2284.

188 Ehrenberg AS. The unbiased estimation of heterogeneous error variances. *Biometrika* 1950;37 (3-4):347–357.

189 Bartlett MS, Fowler RH. Properties of sufficiency and statistical tests. *Proc RSocLondon Ser A – Math Phy Sci* 1937;160(901):268–282.

190 Lee Y, Noh M. Modelling random effect variance with double hierarchical generalized linear models. *Statistical Modelling* 2012;12(6):487–502.

191 Kahan BC, Morris TP. Adjusting for multiple prognostic factors in the analysis of randomised trials. *BMC Med Res Methodol* 2013;13:99.

192 Pinheiro JC, Bates DM. Approximations to the log-likelihood function in the nonlinear mixed-effects model. *J Comput Graph Stat* 1995;4(1):12–35.

193 Dean CB, Ugarte MD, Militino AF. Penalized quasi-likelihood with spatially correlated data. *Comput Stat Data Anals* 2004;45(2):235–248.

194 Paccagnella O. Sample size and accuracy of estimates in multilevel models. *Methodology* 2011;7 (3):111–120.

195 Moineddin R, Matheson FI, Glazier RH. A simulation study of sample size for multilevel logistic regression models. *BMC Med Res Methodol* 2007;7(1):34.

196 McNeish DM, Stapleton LM. The effect of small sample size on two-level model estimates: a review and illustration. *Educ Psychol Rev* 2016;28(2):295–314.

197 Breslow NE, Clayton DG. Approximate inference in generalized linear mixed models. *J Am Stat Assoc* 1993;88:9–25.

198 McNeish D. Small sample methods for multilevel modeling: a colloquial elucidation of REML and the Kenward-Roger correction. *Multivariate Behav Res* 2017;52(5):661–670.

199 Wolfinger R, O'Connell M. Generalized linear mixed models: a pseudo-likelihood approach. *J Stat Comput Simul* 1993;48:233–243.

200 Piepho HP, Madden LV, Roger J, et al. Estimating the variance for heterogeneity in arm-based network meta-analysis. *Pharm Stat* 2018;17(3):264–277.

201 Leckie G, Charlton C. runmlwin: Stata module for fitting multilevel models in the MLwiN software package. Centre for Multilevel Modelling, University of Bristol, 2011.

202 Rhodes KM, Turner RM, Higgins JP. Predictive distributions were developed for the extent of heterogeneity in meta-analyses of continuous outcome data. *J Clin Epidemiol* 2015;68(1):52–60.

203 Kenward MG, Roger JH. Small sample inference for fixed effects from restricted maximum likelihood. *Biometrics* 1997;53(3):983–997.

204 Satterthwaite FE. An approximate distribution of estimates of variance components. *Biometrics* 1946;2(6):110–114.

205 Hardy RJ, Thompson SG. A likelihood approach to meta-analysis with random effects. *Stat Med* 1996;15:619–629.

206 Charlton C, Rasbash J, Browne WJ, et al. MLwiN Version 3.03. Centre for Multilevel Modelling, University of Bristol, 2019.

207 Riley RD, Ensor J, Jackson D, et al. Deriving percentage study weights in multi-parameter meta-analysis models: with application to meta-regression, network meta-analysis and one-stage individual participant data models. *Stat Methods Med Res* 2018;27(10):2885–2905.

208 Kontopantelis E, Reeves D. A short guide and a forest plot command (ipdforest) for one-stage meta-analysis. *Stata J* 2014;13(3):574–587.

209 Austin PC. A tutorial on multilevel survival analysis: methods, models and applications. *Int Stat Rev* 2017;85(2):185–203.

210 Tudur-Smith C, Williamson PR, Marson AG. Investigating heterogeneity in an individual patient data meta-analysis of time to event outcomes. *Statn Med* 2005;24(9):1307–1319.

211 Tudur Smith C, Williamson PR. A comparison of methods for fixed effects meta-analysis of individual patient data with time to event outcomes. *Clin Trials* 2007;4(6):621–630.

212 Thompson SG, Kaptoge S, White I, et al. Statistical methods for the time-to-event analysis of individual participant data from multiple epidemiological studies. *Int J Epidemiol* 2010;39 (5):1345–1359.

213 Smith CT, Williamson PR, Marson AG. An overview of methods and empirical comparison of aggregate data and individual patient data results for investigating heterogeneity in meta-analysis of time-to-event outcomes. *J Eval Clin Pract* 2005;11(5):468–478.

214 de Jong VMT, Moons KGM, Riley RD, et al. Individual participant data meta-analysis of intervention studies with time-to-event outcomes: a review of the methodology and an applied example. *Res Synth Methods* 2020;11(2):148–168.

215 Statistical Software: *Release 14.0. Stata Corporation [program]: College Station*, TX: StataCorp LP, 2015.

216 Wienke A. *Frailty Models in Survival Analysis*. Boca Raton, FL: Chapman & Hall/CRC 2010.

217 Vaida F, Donohue MC, Overholser R, et al. Conditional Akaike information under generalized linear and proportional hazards mixed models. *Biometrika* 2011;98(3):685–700.

218 Duchateau L, Janssen P. *The Frailty Model*. New York: Springer 2008.

219 Glidden DV, Vittinghoff E. Modelling clustered survival data from multicentre clinical trials. *Stat Med* 2004;23(3):369–388.

220 Munda M, Legrand C. Adjusting for centre heterogeneity in multicentre clinical trials with a time-to-event outcome. *Pharm Stat* 2014;13(2):145–152.

221 Abbring JH, Van Den Berg GJ. The unobserved heterogeneity distribution in duration analysis. *Biometrika* 2007;94(1):87–99.

222 Crowther MJ, Look MP, Riley RD. Multilevel mixed effects parametric survival models using adaptive Gauss-Hermite quadrature with application to recurrent events and individual participant data meta-analysis. *Stat Med* 2014;33(22):3844–3858.

223 Carlin BP, Hodges JS. Hierarchical proportional hazards regression models for highly stratified data. *Biometrics* 1999;55(4):1162–1170.

224 Rondeau V, Michiels S, Liquet B. Investigating trial and treatment heterogeneity in an individual patient data meta-analysis of survival data by means of the penalized maximum likelihood approach. *Stat Med* 2008;27(11):1894–1910.

225 Debray TP, Moons KG, Ahmed I, et al. A framework for developing, implementing, and evaluating clinical prediction models in an individual participant data meta-analysis. *Stat Med* 2013;32 (18):3158–3180.

226 Royston P, Parmar MKB, Sylvester R. Construction and validation of a prognostic model across several studies, with an application in superficial bladder cancer. *Stat Med* 2004;23:907–926.

227 Royston P, Parmar MKB. Flexible parametric proportional-hazards and proportional-odds models for censored survival data, with application to prognostic modelling and estimation of treatment effects. *Statistics in Medicine* 2002;21:2175–2197.

228 Royston P, Lambert PC. *Flexible Parametric Survival Analysis Using Stata: Beyond the Cox Model.* College Station, TX: CRC Press 2011.

229 Rutherford MJ, Crowther MJ, Lambert PC. The use of restricted cubic splines to approximate complex hazard functions in the analysis of time-to-event data: a simulation study. *JStat Comput Simul* 2015;85(4):777–793.

230 Lambert PC, Royston P. Further developments of flexible parametric models for survival analysis. *Stata J* 2009;9:265–290.

231 Bengtsson T, Dribe M. Quantifying the family frailty effect in infant and child mortality by using median hazard ratio (MHR). *Historical Methods: A Journal of Quantitative and Interdisciplinary History* 2010;43(1):15–27.

232 Austin PC, Wagner P, Merlo J. The median hazard ratio: a useful measure of variance and general contextual effects in multilevel survival analysis. *Stat Med* 2017;36(6):928–938.

233 Kay R, Kinnersley N. On the use of the accelerated failure time model as an alternative to the proportional hazards model in the treatment of time to event data: a case study in influenza. *Drug Information Journal* 2002;36(3):571–579.

234 Bennett S. Log-logistic regression models for survival data. *J Royal StatSoc Series C Appl Stat* 1983;32 (2):165–171.

235 Bennett S. Analysis of survival data by the proportional odds model. *Stat Med* 1983;2(2):273–277.

236 Royston P, Parmar MK. The use of restricted mean survival time to estimate the treatment effect in randomized clinical trials when the proportional hazards assumption is in doubt. *Stat Med* 2011;30 (19):2409–2421.

237 Wei Y, Royston P, Tierney JF, et al. Meta-analysis of time-to-event outcomes from randomized trials using restricted mean survival time: application to individual participant data. *Stat Med* 2015;34 (21):2881–2898.

238 Royston P, Parmar MK. Restricted mean survival time: an alternative to the hazard ratio for the design and analysis of randomized trials with a time-to-event outcome. *BMC Med Res Methodol* 2013;13:152.

239 Lueza B, Rotolo F, Bonastre J, et al. Bias and precision of methods for estimating the difference in restricted mean survival time from an individual patient data meta-analysis. *BMC Med Res Methodol* 2016;16:37.

240 Siannis F, Barrett JK, Farewell VT, et al. One-stage parametric meta-analysis of time-to-event outcomes. *Stat Med* 2010;29(29):3030–45.

241 Ibrahim JG, Chu H, Chen LM. Basic concepts and methods for joint models of longitudinal and survival data. *J Clin Oncoly* 2010;28(16):2796–2801.

242 Sudell M, Kolamunnage-Dona R, Gueyffier F, et al. Investigation of one-stage meta-analysis methods for joint longitudinal and time-to-event data through simulation and real data application. *Stat Med* 2019;38(2):247–268.

243 Wei Y, Royston P. Reconstructing time-to-event data from published Kaplan-Meier curves. *Stata J* 2017;17(4):786–802.

244 Guyot P, Ades AE, Ouwens MJ, et al. Enhanced secondary analysis of survival data: reconstructing the data from published Kaplan-Meier survival curves. *BMC Med Res Methodol* 2012;12:9.

245 Jackson C, Best N, Richardson S. Hierarchical related regression for combining aggregate and individual data in studies of socio-economic disease risk factors. *J Royal Stat Soc Series A* 2008;171:159–178.

246 Riley RD, Dodd SR, Craig JV, et al. Meta-analysis of diagnostic test studies using individual patient data and aggregate data. *Stat Med* 2008;27(29):6111–6136.

247 Stewart LA, Clarke M, Rovers M, et al. Preferred reporting items for systematic review and meta-analyses of individual participant data: the PRISMA-IPD Statement. *JAMA* 2015;313(16):1657–1665.

248 Harris R, Bradburn M, Deeks J, et al. metan: fixed- and random-effects meta-analysis. *Stata J* 2008;8 (1):3–28.

249 Burke DL, Ensor J, Snell KIE, et al. Guidance for deriving and presenting percentage study weights in meta-analysis of test accuracy studies. *Res Synth Methods* 2018;9(2):163–178.

250 Hingorani AD, Windt DA, Riley RD, et al. Prognosis research strategy (PROGRESS) 4: stratified medicine research. *BMJ* 2013;346:e5793.

251 Riley RD, van der Windt D, Croft P, et al., editors. *Prognosis Research in Healthcare: Concepts, Methods and Impact*. Oxford, UK: Oxford University Press, 2019.

252 Hudis CA. Trastuzumab – mechanism of action and use in clinical practice. *N Engl J Med* 2007;357 (1):39–51.

253 Brookes ST, Whitely E, Egger M, et al. Subgroup analyses in randomized trials: risks of subgroup-specific analyses; power and sample size for the interaction test. *J Clin Epidemiol* 2004;57 (3):229–236.

254 Thompson SG, Higgins JP. Treating individuals 4: can meta-analysis help target interventions at individuals most likely to benefit? *Lancet* 2005;365(9456):341–346.

255 Riley RD, Debray TPA, Fisher D, et al. Individual participant data meta-analysis to examine interactions between treatment effect and participant-level covariates: statistical recommendations for conduct and planning. *Stat Med* 2020;39(15):2115–2137.

256 Fisher DJ, Copas AJ, Tierney JF, et al. A critical review of methods for the assessment of patient-level interactions in individual participant data meta-analysis of randomized trials, and guidance for practitioners. *J Clin Epidemiol* 2011;64(9):949–967.

257 Hua H, Burke DL, Crowther MJ, et al. One-stage individual participant data meta-analysis models: estimation of treatment-covariate interactions must avoid ecological bias by separating out within-trial and across-trial information. *Stat Med* 2017;36(5):772–789.

258 Fisher DJ, Carpenter JR, Morris TP, et al. Meta-analytical methods to identify who benefits most from treatments: daft, deluded, or deft approach? *BMJ* 2017;356:j573.

259 Simmonds MC, Higgins JP. Covariate heterogeneity in meta-analysis: criteria for deciding between meta-regression and individual patient data. *Stat Med* 2007;26(15):2982–2999.

260 Wallach JD, Sullivan PG, Trepanowski JF, et al. Evaluation of evidence of statistical support and corroboration of subgroup claims in randomized clinical trials. *JAMA Intern Med* 2017;177 (4):554–560.

261 Sun X, Briel M, Walter SD, et al. Is a subgroup effect believable? Updating criteria to evaluate the credibility of subgroup analyses. *BMJ* 2010;340:c117.

262 Koopman L, van der Heijden GJ, Hoes AW, et al. Empirical comparison of subgroup effects in conventional and individual patient data meta-analyses. *Int J Technol Assess Health Care* 2008;24 (3):358–361.

263 Koopman L, van der Heijden GJ, Glasziou PP, et al. A systematic review of analytical methods used to study subgroups in (individual patient data) meta-analyses. *J Clin Epidemiol* 2007;60 (10):1002–1009.

264 Royston P, Sauerbrei W. Interactions between treatment and continuous covariates: a step toward individualizing therapy. *J Clin Oncol* 2008;26(9):1397–1399.

265 Royston P, Sauerbrei W. A new approach to modelling interactions between treatment and continuous covariates in clinical trials by using fractional polynomials. *Stat Med* 2004;23 (16):2509–2525.

266 Kent DM, Paulus JK, van Klaveren D, et al. The Predictive Approaches to Treatment effect Heterogeneity (PATH) statement. *Ann Intern Med* 2019;172(1):35–45.

267 Kent DM, Steyerberg E, van Klaveren D. Personalized evidence based medicine: predictive approaches to heterogeneous treatment effects. *BMJ* 2018;363:k4245.

268 Early Breast Cancer Trialists' Collaborative Group. Tamoxifen for early breast cancer: an overview of the randomised trials. *Lancet* 1998 351:1451–1467.

269 Lambert PC, Sutton AJ, Abrams KR, et al. A comparison of summary patient-level covariates in meta-regression with individual patient data meta-analysis. *J Clin Epidemiol* 2002;55(1):86–94.

270 Berlin JA, Santanna J, Schmid CH, et al. Individual patient- versus group-level data meta-regressions for the investigation of treatment effect modifiers: ecological bias rears its ugly head. *Stat Med* 2002;21(3):371–387.

271 Robinson WS. Ecological correlations and the behavior of individuals. *American Sociological Review* 1950;15(3):351–357.

272 Selvin HC. Durkheim's suicide and problems of empirical research. *Am J Sociol* 1958;63(6):607–619.

273 VanderWeele TJ, Knol MJ. Interpretation of subgroup analyses in randomized trials: heterogeneity versus secondary interventions. *Ann Intern Med* 2011;154(10):680–683.

274 Bland JM, Altman DG. Statistical methods for assessing agreement between two methods of clinical measurement. *Lancet* 1986;1(8476):307–310.

275 Group PM-aT. Postoperative radiotherapy in non-small-cell lung cancer: systematic review and meta-analysis of individual patient data from nine randomised controlled trials. *Lancet* 1998;352 (9124):257–263.

276 Burdett S, Rydzewska L, Tierney JF, et al. A closer look at the effects of postoperative radiotherapy by stage and nodal status: updated results of an individual participant data meta-analysis in non-small-cell lung cancer. *Lung Cancer* 2013;80(3):350–352.

277 Simmonds MC. *Statistical methodology for individual patient data meta-analysis*. PhD Thesis, University of Cambridge 2006

278 Neuhaus JM, Kalbfleisch JD. Between- and within-cluster covariate effects in the analysis of clustered data. *Biometrics* 1998;54(2):638–645.

279 Mancl LA, Leroux BG, DeRouen TA. Between-subject and within-subject statistical information in dental research. *J Dent Res* 2000;79(10):1778–1781.

280 Begg MD, Parides MK. Separation of individual-level and cluster-level covariate effects in regression analysis of correlated data. *Stat Med* 2003;22(16):2591–2602.

281 Dwyer T, Blizzard L. A discussion of some statistical methods for separating within-pair associations from associations among all twins in research on fetal origins of disease. *Paediatr Perinat Epidemiol* 2005;19 Suppl 1:48–53.

282 Sargent DJ. A general framework for random effects survival analysis in the Cox proportional hazards setting. *Biometrics* 1998;54(4):1486–1497.

283 Katsahian S, Latouche A, Mary JY, et al. Practical methodology of meta-analysis of individual patient data using a survival outcome. *Contemp Clin Trials* 2008;29(2):220–230.

284 Simmonds MC, Higgins JP, Stewart LA. Random-effects meta-analysis of time-to-event data using the expectation-maximisation algorithm and shrinkage estimators. *Res Synth Methods* 2013;4 (2):144–155.

285 Williamson PR, Clough HE, Hutton JL, et al. Statistical issues in the assessment of the evidence for an interaction between factors in epilepsy trials. *Stat Med* 2002;21(18):2613–2622.

286 Marson AG, Williamson PR, Hutton JL, et al. Carbamazepine versus valproate monotherapy for epilepsy. *Cochrane Database Syst Rev* 2000(3):CD001030.

287 Fearon P, Langhorne P, Early Supported Discharge T. *Services for reducing duration of hospital care for acute stroke patients. Cochrane Database Syst Rev* 2012(9):CD000443.

288 Burdett S, Boevé LM, Ingleby FC, et al. Prostate radiotherapy for metastatic hormone-sensitive prostate cancer: A STOPCAP Systematic Review and Meta-analysis. *European Urology* 2019;76 (1):115–124.

289 Donegan S, Williamson P, D'Alessandro U, et al. Combining individual patient data and aggregate data in mixed treatment comparison meta-analysis: individual patient data may be beneficial if only for a subset of trials. *Stat Med* 2013;32(6):914–930.

290 Mistry D, Stallard N, Underwood M. A recursive partitioning approach for subgroup identification in individual patient data meta-analysis. *Stat Med* 2018;37(9):1550–1561.

291 Cox DR. Note on grouping. *JAMA* 1957;52(280):543–547.

292 Cohen J. The cost of dichotomization. *Appl Psychol Meas* 1983;7:249–253.

293 Ensor J, Burke DL, Snell KIE, et al. Simulation-based power calculations for planning a two-stage individual participant data meta-analysis. *BMC Med Res Methodol* 2018;18(1):41.

294 Kasenda B, Sauerbrei W, Royston P, et al. Multivariable fractional polynomial interaction to investigate continuous effect modifiers in a meta-analysis on higher versus lower PEEP for patients with ARDS. *BMJ Open* 2016;6(9):e011148.

295 Kasenda B, Sauerbrei W, Royston P, et al. Investigation of continuous effect modifiers in a meta-analysis on higher versus lower PEEP in patients requiring mechanical ventilation – protocol of the ICEM study. *Systematic Reviews* 2014;3:46.

296 Gasparrini A, Armstrong B, Kenward MG. Multivariate meta-analysis for non-linear and other multi-parameter associations. *Stat Med* 2012;31:3821–3839.

297 Wang XV, Cole B, Bonetti M, et al. Meta-STEPP with random effects. *Res Synth Methods* 2018;9 (2):312–317.

298 Wang XV, Cole B, Bonetti M, et al. Meta-STEPP: subpopulation treatment effect pattern plot for individual patient data meta-analysis. *Stat Med* 2016;35(21):3704–3716.

299 White IR, Kaptoge S, Royston P, et al. Meta-analysis of non-linear exposure-outcome relationships using individual participant data: a comparison of two methods. *Stat Med* 2019;38(3):326–338.

300 Binder H, Sauerbrei W, Royston P. Comparison between splines and fractional polynomials for multivariable model building with continuous covariates: a simulation study with continuous response. *Stat Med* 2013;32(13):2262–2277.

301 Sauerbrei W, Royston P. A new strategy for meta-analysis of continuous covariates in observational studies. *Stat Med* 2011;30(28):3341–3360.
302 White IR. Multivariate random-effects meta-regression: updates to mvmeta. *Stata Jl* 2011;11:255–270.
303 White IR. Multivariate meta-analysis. *Stata J* 2009;9:40–56.
304 Riley RD, Jackson D, Salanti G, et al. Multivariate and network meta-analysis of multiple outcomes and multiple treatments: rationale, concepts, and examples. *BMJ* 2017;358:j3932.
305 Jackson D, Riley RD, White IR. Multivariate meta-analysis: potential and promise. *Stat Med* 2011;30:2481–2498.
306 Senn S. Individual response to treatment: is it a valid assumption? *BMJ* 2004;329(7472):966–968.
307 Senn S. Statistical pitfalls of personalized medicine. *Nature* 2018;563(7733):619–621.
308 Malottki K, Biswas M, Deeks JJ, et al. Stratified medicine in European Medicines Agency licensing: a systematic review of predictive biomarkers. *BMJ Open* 2014;4(1):e004188.
309 Schuit E, Li AH, Ioannidis JPA. How often can meta-analyses of individual-level data individualize treatment? A meta-epidemiologic study. *Int J Epidemiol* 2019;48(2):596–608.
310 van Smeden M, Lash TL, Groenwold RHH. Reflection on modern methods: five myths about measurement error in epidemiological research. *Int J Epidemiol* 2020;49(1):338–347.
311 Carroll RJ, Ruppert D, Stefanski LA, et al. *Measurement Error in Nonlinear Models: A Modern Perspective* (2nd edition). CRC Press 2006.
312 Keogh RH, White IR. A toolkit for measurement error correction, with a focus on nutritional epidemiology. *Stat Med* 2014;33(12):2137–2155.
313 Steyerberg EW, Moons KG, van der Windt DA, et al. Prognosis Research Strategy (PROGRESS) 3: prognostic model research. *PLoS Med* 2013;10(2):e1001381.
314 Pincus T, Miles C, Froud R, et al. Methodological criteria for the assessment of moderators in systematic reviews of randomised controlled trials: a consensus study. *BMC Med Res Methodol* 2011;11:14.
315 van Klaveren D, Balan TA, Steyerberg EW, et al. Models with interactions overestimated heterogeneity of treatment effects and were prone to treatment mistargeting. *J Clin Epidemiol* 2019;114:72–83.
316 Kent DM, Nelson J, Dahabreh IJ, et al. Risk and treatment effect heterogeneity: re-analysis of individual participant data from 32 large clinical trials. *Int J Epidemiol* 2016;45(6):2075–2088.
317 Kent DM, van Klaveren D, Paulus JK, et al. The Predictive Approaches to Treatment effect Heterogeneity (PATH) statement: explanation and elaboration. *Ann Intern Med* 2020;172(1): W1–W25.
318 Copas JB. Using regression models for prediction: shrinkage and regression to the mean. *Stat Methods Med Res* 1997;6(2):167–183.
319 Steyerberg EW, Harrell FEJ, Borsboom GJ, et al. Internal validation of predictive models: efficiency of some procedures for logistic regression analysis. *J Clin Epidemiol* 2001;54:774–781.
320 Steyerberg EW, Borsboom GJ, van Houwelingen HC, et al. Validation and updating of predictive logistic regression models: a study on sample size and shrinkage. *Stat Med* 2004;23 (16):2567–2586.
321 Copas JB. Regression, prediction and shrinkage. *J Royal Stat Soc Series B Methodol* 1983;45 (3):311–354.
322 Tibshirani R. Regression shrinkage and selection via the lasso. *J Royal Stat Soc Series B* 1996;58:267–288.
323 Senn S. Mastering variation: variance components and personalised medicine. *Stat Med* 2016;35 (7):966–977.

324 Gasparrini A, Armstrong B. Reducing and meta-analysing estimates from distributed lag non-linear models. *BMC Med Res Methodol* 2013;13:1.

325 Debray TP, Moons KG, Abo-Zaid GM, et al. Individual participant data meta-analysis for a binary outcome: one-stage or two-stage? *PLoS One* 2013;8(4):e60650.

326 Steinberg KK, Smith SJ, Stroup DF, et al. Comparison of effect estimates from a meta-analysis of summary data from published studies and from a meta-analysis using individual patient data for ovarian cancer studies. *Am J Epidemiol* 1997;145(10):917–925.

327 Lin DY, Zeng D. On the relative efficiency of using summary statistics versus individual-level data in meta-analysis. *Biometrika* 2010;97(2):321–332.

328 Mathew T, Nordstrom K. On the equivalence of meta-analysis using literature and using individual patient data. *Biometrics* 1999;55(4):1221–1223.

329 Mathew T, Nordström K. Comparison of one-step and two-step meta-analysis models using individual patient data. *Biom J* 2010;52(2):271–287.

330 Olkin I, Sampson A. Comparison of meta-analysis versus analysis of variance of individual patient data. *Biometrics* 1998;54(1):317–322.

331 Tierney JF, Vale C, Riley R, et al. Individual participant data (IPD) meta-analyses of randomised controlled trials: guidance on their use. *PLoS Med* 2015;12(7):e1001855.

332 Riley RD, Abrams KR, Lambert PC, et al. An evaluation of bivariate random-effects meta-analysis for the joint synthesis of two correlated outcomes. *Stat Med* 2007;26(1):78–97.

333 Sohn SY. Multivariate meta-analysis with potentially correlated marketing study results. *Nav Res Logist* 2000;47:500–510.

334 Martineau AR, Jolliffe DA, Hooper RL, et al. Vitamin D supplementation to prevent acute respiratory tract infections: systematic review and meta-analysis of individual participant data. *BMJ* 2017;356:i6583.

335 Rucker G, Schwarzer G, Carpenter J, et al. Why add anything to nothing? The arcsine difference as a measure of treatment effect in meta-analysis with zero cells. *Stat Med* 2009;28(5):721738.

336 Riley RD, Ahmed I, Debray TP, et al. Summarising and validating test accuracy results across multiple studies for use in clinical practice. *Stat Med* 2015;34(13):2081–2103.

337 Sidik K, Jonkman JN. A comparison of heterogeneity variance estimators in combining results of studies. *Stat Med* 2007;26(9):1964–1981.

338 Thompson SG, Sharp SJ. Explaining heterogeneity in meta-analysis: a comparison of methods. *Stat Med* 1999;18(20):2693–2708.

339 Berkey CS, Hoaglin DC, Mosteller F, et al. A random-effects regression model for meta-analysis. *Stat Med* 1995;14(4):395–411.

340 Austin PC. Estimating multilevel logistic regression models when the number of clusters is low: a comparison of different statistical software procedures. *The International Journal of Biostatistics* 2010;6(1):Article 16.

341 Noh M, Lee Y. REML estimation for binary data in GLMMs. *J Multivar Anal* 2007;98(5):896–915.

342 Broström G, Holmberg H. Generalized linear models with clustered data: fixed and random effects models. *Computl Stat Data Anal* 2011;55:3123–3134.

343 Lee Y, Nelder JA. Double hierarchical generalized linear models (with discussion). *J Royal Stat Soc Series C Appl Stat* 2006;55(2):139–185.

344 Knapp G, Hartung J. Improved tests for a random effects meta-regression with a single covariate. *Stat Med* 2003;22(17):26932710.

345 Hartung J. An alternative method for meta-analysis. *Biom J* 1999;41(8):901–916.

346 Sidik K, Jonkman JN. On constructing confidence intervals for a standardized mean difference in meta-analysis. *Commun Stat – Simul Comput*2003;32(4):1191–203.

347 Jones AP, Riley RD, Williamson PR, et al. Meta-analysis of individual patient data versus aggregate data from longitudinal clinical trials. *Clin Trials* 2009;6(1):16–27.

348 Riley RD. Multivariate meta-analysis: the effect of ignoring within-study correlation. *J Royal Stat Soc Series A Stat Soc* 2009;172.

349 Jackson D, White IR, Price M, et al. Borrowing of strength and study weights in multivariate and network meta-analysis. *Stat Methods Med Res* 2017;26(6):2853–2868.

Part III

Critical Appraisal and Dissemination

9

Examining the Potential for Bias in IPD Meta-Analysis Results

Richard D. Riley, Jayne F. Tierney, and Lesley A. Stewart

Summary Points

- An important part of an IPD meta-analysis project is to examine the robustness of IPD meta-analysis results to potential biases that could occur.
- Publication-related biases hide relevant trials and data, often those with 'negative' findings (e.g. statistically non-significant results). As for any type of review, this could lead to IPD meta-analysis results being biased toward favourable effects.
- Availability bias is a concern if IPD are obtained from only a subset of the trials from which requested, and the provision of IPD is linked to trial findings. This may also make the IPD meta-analysis results biased, although the direction of bias is hard to predict.
- These issues may lead to small-study effects in the IPD meta-analysis, where smaller trials exhibit different (often greater) effect estimates than larger trials.
- Small-study effects may be examined visually using a funnel plot, which displays study effect estimates (x-axis) against some measure of their precision (y-axis), e.g. standard error of the treatment effect. Small-study effects are revealed by asymmetry in the plot.
- Small-study effects may also be due to factors that cause between-trial heterogeneity; for example, if smaller trials are conducted in populations and settings that genuinely lead to larger effect estimates. So evidence of asymmetry does not prove that publication, availability and/or selective reporting biases exist.
- The impact of availability bias can be investigated by utilising aggregate data from non-IPD trials in sensitivity analyses. IPD and aggregate data are then combined and the obtained results compared with the main IPD meta-analysis results. However, obtaining suitable aggregate data may be problematic, and the process may simply reinforce why IPD were required in the first place.
- Other sensitivity analyses may be needed to examine bias concerns. In particular, analyses restricted to trials at low risk of bias investigate whether the meta-analysis conclusions are influenced by trial quality.
- Selective outcome availability may also occur, if trials that provide their IPD do not give all the outcomes that were actually recorded, potentially leading to biased IPD meta-analysis results for some outcomes. Multivariate meta-analysis may help reduce this issue.

Individual Participant Data Meta-Analysis: A Handbook for Healthcare Research, First Edition.
Edited by Richard D. Riley, Jayne F. Tierney, and Lesley A. Stewart.

9.1 Introduction

Obtaining IPD can reduce many of the potential biases facing conventional meta-analyses of published aggregate data. Previous chapters, for example, outline how IPD meta-analysis projects usually attempt to obtain and include unpublished trials, unreported outcomes, and wrongly omitted participants, and IPD enables the use of improved and standardised statistical analysis methods across trials. Nevertheless, an IPD meta-analysis project is not necessarily bias-free, and so results may be at risk from multiple sources of bias arising from IPD retrieval to synthesis methods. In particular, researchers should be vigilant in ensuring that the IPD obtained is of good quality (low risk of bias) and representative of the existing evidence base for the target population(s) of interest, and that appropriate meta-analysis methods are used.

Fundamentally, researchers should minimise the potential for bias in their IPD meta-analysis results by adopting appropriate standards throughout the whole project. Chapters 3 and 4 describe techniques and approaches to minimise bias when identifying relevant trials, selecting which IPD to obtain, and cleaning and checking the IPD received. Initiation of, and regular communication with, a collaborative group including the original trial investigators can mitigate concerns, for example by identifying unpublished trials, obtaining missing outcomes and resolving errors in the IPD provided. Establishing an IPD meta-analysis project team with expertise in specialist areas is critical, for example, in ensuring that high-quality methods are applied when searching for relevant trials, setting up and maintaining databases to house IPD, and performing meta-analysis.

Nevertheless, as in all research projects, biases may still arise even when best practice is applied. Therefore, in this chapter we describe how researchers can examine the potential impact of biases on IPD meta-analysis results by using sensitivity analyses, funnel plots, and a combination of IPD and aggregate data. We begin by outlining key bias threats and how they may impact IPD meta-analysis findings.

9.2 Publication and Reporting Biases of Trials

Publication bias is a well-known threat to the validity of traditional meta-analyses based on aggregate data. It occurs when trials with statistically significant or clinically favourable results are more likely to be published than trials with non-significant or unfavourable results.[1–4] This leads to meta-analyses which synthesise an incomplete set of the evidence and produce summary results that are potentially biased toward favourable treatment effects.[5] Other related reporting biases exist on the continuum toward publication,[6] such as time-lag bias where trials with unfavourable findings take longer to be published.[7,8]

9.2.1 Impact on IPD Meta-Analysis Results

IPD meta-analysis projects have strong potential to reduce publication bias in meta-analysis by obtaining data for unpublished trials.[9] As described in Chapter 3, inclusive and collaborative group approaches to data sharing can draw on collaborators' knowledge to identify completed but unpublished trials. Unpublished IPD may also be available in a data repository, where researchers house their published and unpublished IPD to support initiatives such as IPD meta-analyses. Lists of ongoing and recently completed trials can also be gathered from trial registries, and discussions started with those trial investigators in order to obtain IPD as soon as possible after completion (reducing the potential impact of time-lag bias). Further, after a trial's IPD are obtained, the actual handling and analysis of that IPD is unaffected by whether the trial was published or what aggregate data could be obtained for it.

Nevertheless, publication and related biases may still impact IPD meta-analysis projects.[9–12] Publication bias hides eligible trials and thus their IPD may not be sought if collaborators are unaware of it. Burdett et al. found that 11 IPD meta-analyses in cancer tended to give more favourable treatment effects when excluding IPD from trials in the grey literature (i.e. unpublished trials, trials published in non-English language journals, and trials reported as meeting abstracts, book chapters, and letters).[13] Most differences were modest, but in one IPD meta-analysis there was stronger evidence that post-operative radiotherapy was detrimental to the survival of patients with non-small-cell lung cancer when all trials (hazard ratio = 1.21, 95% CI: 1.05 to 1.39, $p = 0.001$) rather than only fully published trials were included (hazard ratio = 1.13, 95% CI: 0.95 to 1.34, $p = 0.066$).

9.2.2 Examining Small-study Effects Using Funnel Plots

After performing an IPD meta-analysis, the potential for publication-related biases can be examined statistically, for example by using a (contour-enhanced) funnel plot and a statistical test for asymmetry.[2,4,14–17] A funnel plot displays trial treatment effect estimates (x-axis) against some measure of their precision (y-axis), such as the standard error of the treatment effect. Where no publication bias is present, the premise is that the plot should show a funnel-like shape, with estimates spanning down from the larger trials symmetrically in both directions with increasing variability.

Asymmetry in a funnel plot is also known as small-study effects,[18] and may be a consequence of publication-related biases, especially when smaller trials have more positive effects (i.e. in favour of treatment being effective) than larger trials. If there is asymmetry, then a *contour-enhanced* funnel plot is helpful in revealing whether those (perceived to be) missing trials are likely to fall in regions where trial results are not statistically significant;[17] if so, this adds credence to the concern that asymmetry is due to publication bias, as trials are more likely to be missing if they are not statistically significant. A case study of an IPD meta-analysis project with dramatic asymmetry is given in Figure 9.1.[19]

For each funnel plot, a test for asymmetry can quantify whether there is evidence of asymmetry beyond chance. This suffers from the pitfalls of any statistical hypothesis test; in particular, there is low power to detect genuine asymmetry when the number of trials is small (e.g. < 10), and high power to detect even minor (and non-important) asymmetry when the number of trials is very large. Nevertheless, a statistical test helps provide some quantification alongside visual, subjective judgement. Guidance provided by Sterne et al. for examining and interpreting funnel plot asymmetry suggests at least 10 trials are needed with a p-value < 0.10 used to indicate statistical evidence of asymmetry.[15] There are also methods to examine the potential impact of 'missing' trials on the summary meta-analysis result, such as the trim and fill method.[20] A simpler approach is to restrict the IPD meta-analysis to include just the larger trials, to gauge if the results are notably different to those from the analysis of all trials. The definition of a 'large trial' is subjective, but might be predefined in the trial protocol.

Potential publication bias is often ignored or not reported in IPD meta-analysis projects. Ahmed et al. surveyed a sample of 31 articles that each performed an IPD meta-analysis of randomised trials to establish whether a treatment was effective or not.[19] Only 10 of the 31 articles discussed (9 articles) or examined statistically (1 article) the potential for publication bias. Seven of those 10 articles inferred that the threat of publication bias was low. However, in the others asymmetrical funnel plots indicated small-study effects, thus raising the concern of potential publication bias.

De Luca et al.[21] performed an IPD meta-analysis of randomised trials to evaluate the benefits of early versus late use of Gp IIb-IIIa inhibitors in patients undergoing primary angioplasty for ST-segment elevation myocardial infarction. A primary angiographic endpoint was whether patients achieved a pre-procedural TIMI (thrombolysis in myocardial infarction) grade 3 flow distal embolisation. A systematic review identified 14 relevant trials; IPD were sought from all, and ultimately obtained for 11. Using the trial-specific results reported by De Luca et al., we performed a two-stage meta-analysis of the 11 IPD trials, assuming a random treatment effect, and using REML estimation and Hartung-Knapp-Sidik-Jonkman confidence interval derivation. This gave a summary odds ratio of 2.11 (95% CI: 1.46 to 3.05), with an approximate 95% prediction interval for the odds ratio in a single clinical setting from 1.00 to 4.44. Thus, there is strong evidence that early Gp IIb–IIIa inhibitors are associated with a significantly improved TIMI 3 flow.

However, all 11 trials were fully published and the contour-enhanced funnel plot (below) shows considerable asymmetry, with small trials systematically having larger effect sizes than larger trials (Peters' test for asymmetry: $p = 0.016$). This suggests potentially missing trials on the left-hand side of the plot, toward the bottom. Since such trials would predominantly be in the region of non-statistical significance (white background) close to an odds ratio of 1 (i.e. no difference between early and late use) or less than 1 (i.e. early use is not beneficial); this adds strength to the notion that publication bias mechanisms may be operating here, biasing the meta-analysis result in favour of early use. Indeed, when using a regression method to adjust for this asymmetry,[16,22] the adjusted summary odds ratio is 1.18 (95% CI: 0.79 to 1.76). The asymmetry remained even after incorporating treatment effect estimates from two of the other three trials not providing IPD.[19] This motivates further work to establish whether unpublished trials do indeed exist, and/or whether the causes of heterogeneity (e.g. study definitions of 'early') are driving the asymmetry in the funnel plot.

NB: The *p* in the plot denotes the *p*-value corresponding to a trial's treatment effect. The size of a trial's *p*-value is indicated by the shaded region within which the trial's circle lies.

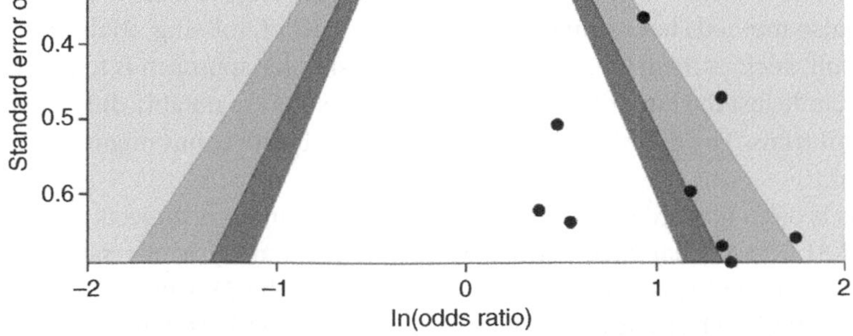

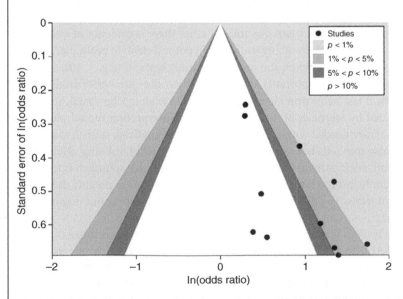

Figure 9.1 Examination of small-study effects in an IPD meta-analysis to evaluate the benefits of early versus late use of Gp IIb-IIIa inhibitors.[21] *Sources:* Richard Riley, adapting Figure 5 of Ahmed et al.,[19] with permission, © 2012 British Medical Journal Publishing Group (CC-BY-NC 2.0).

9.2.3 Small-study Effects May Arise Due to the Factors Causing Heterogeneity

Importantly, the factors that cause between-trial heterogeneity in treatment effect may also cause small-study effects and thus asymmetry in a funnel plot.[15,23] For example, larger effect estimates may be observed in the smaller trials if they were of lower quality (higher risk of bias), conducted in a more select group of participants (e.g. those at higher risk of poor outcomes), or used a different intended dose of treatment compared to larger trials. Thus, evidence of asymmetry is not proof of publication bias; rather it should trigger further work to examine why small trials are providing different results than larger trials. The following example illustrates this issue.

Martineau et al. conducted a systematic review and meta-analysis of IPD from randomised controlled trials on the efficacy of vitamin D supplementation to prevent acute respiratory tract infections.[24] Their meta-analysis was a substantial undertaking, included almost 11,000 participants across 25 trials. The authors conclude that their findings "support the introduction of public health measures such as food fortification to improve vitamin D status, particularly in settings where profound vitamin D deficiency is common", but they note that the corresponding funnel plot showed a "degree of asymmetry, raising the possibility that small trials showing adverse effects of vitamin D might not have been included in the meta-analysis".[24]

In a rapid response to the published paper, Holmes notes the dramatic difference between the results of the larger trials (defined by the total number of cases) and the smaller trials.[25] This is illustrated in Figure 9.2, which shows results from a two-stage random effects IPD meta-analysis using all trials, and also for each of three groups defined by the number of participants (<100, 100 to < 500, and 500 or more). Using all 25 trials, the summary odds ratio is 0.80 (95% CI: 0.67 to 0.95), suggesting that supplementation with vitamin D reduces the odds of acute respiratory tract infections. However, when using just the three largest trials (with > 500 participants), the summary odds ratio is 1.00 (95% CI: 0.79 to 1.26).

Thus, there is striking evidence of small-study effects, which raises concern that publication-related biases are acting. However, further inspection suggests that missing trials are unlikely in this IPD meta-analysis project because (i) collaborators were asked if they knew of any additional trials, (ii) searches were regularly updated and no language restrictions were imposed, (iii) searches were supplemented by searches of review articles and reference lists of trial publications, and (iv) the International Standard Randomised Controlled Trials Number (ISRCTN) registry was searched for unpublished and ongoing trials. Furthermore, investigators for all trials identified by the searches were contacted, and ultimately provided their IPD.

Therefore, rather than publication bias, the most plausible explanation is that small-study effects arise in this IPD meta-analysis due to the factors causing between-trial heterogeneity. That is, the observed differences in results for larger and smaller trials are likely to be due to intrinsic differences in the characteristics of the smaller and larger trials that lead to genuine differences in their treatment effects. For example, the authors note that "protective effects were seen in those receiving daily or weekly vitamin D without additional bolus doses but not in those receiving one or more bolus doses", and indeed the former set were more prevalent in the smaller trials.

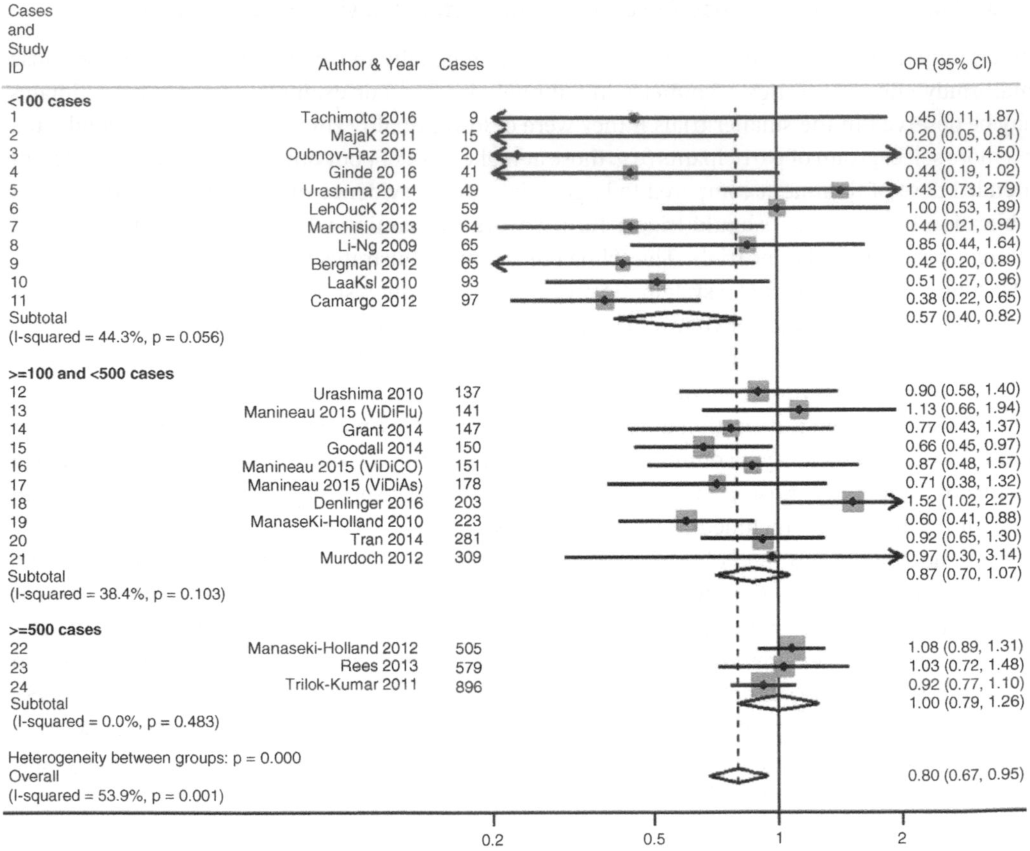

* Two-stage IPD meta-analysis model used, assuming a random treatment effect and estimated using the DerSimonian and Laird approach, with confidence intervals derived using the Hartung-Knapp Sidik-Jonkman approach.

Figure 9.2 Forest plot of the IPD meta-analysis* of Martineau et al.[24], with trials grouped by their size (defined by number of cases, i.e. those who developed acute respiratory tract infections) as demonstrated by Holmes.[25] *Sources:* Richard Riley, produced using data extracted from the article of Martineau et al.[24]

9.3 Biased Availability of the IPD from Trials

Availability bias can occur in an IPD meta-analysis project if IPD are unavailable for some trials and this unavailability is related to the trial results. As for publication bias, this leads to a set of trials from which the IPD available may not reflect the entire evidence base, and thus subsequent IPD meta-analysis results may be biased. However, the direction of any bias is hard to predict. If researchers of trials with non-significant or clinically unimportant results are more likely to have destroyed, lost or are unwilling to share their IPD, this will bias IPD meta-analyses toward a favourable treatment effect (unfavourable trials are missing). Conversely, if researchers of trials with favourable findings are unable or do not wish to provide their IPD, perhaps because they want to utilise it further (e.g. to examine subgroup effects or an extended follow-up), this may lead to IPD meta-analyses being biased toward less favourable findings.

When a high proportion of evidence is obtained, the impact of availability bias will usually be less of a concern. Encouragingly, empirical reviews show that IPD meta-analysis projects can obtain a large proportion of the eligible IPD.[19,26,27] For example, Riley et al. found that IPD from 90% or more of the total number of trials were obtained in 102 (58%) of 175 IPD meta-analysis projects examined.[26] Although this is encouraging, that still leaves many IPD meta-analysis projects that do not obtain IPD from a substantial proportion of eligible trials; for example, in the Riley et al. review, 51 (29%) of 175 articles obtained IPD for less than 80% of the eligible trials. Furthermore, the proportion of total participants (and not trials) is more important. For example, if only one trial does not provide their IPD, it may still represent a relatively large proportion of the total participants across all trials. Conversely, the lack of several very small trials may account for only a small fraction of the overall evidence.

In 2017, Nevitt et al. reviewed the data retrieval success for IPD meta-analysis projects published between 1987 and 2015[27], where the studies (of any design) in the IPD meta-analysis were identified by systematic methods. Only 324 (43%) of 760 IPD projects obtained IPD for 80% or more of the eligible IPD. There was no evidence that IPD retrieval success had improved over time. Common reasons for not obtaining IPD were that investigators could not be contacted, declined to share data, or failed to provide their IPD in time for the IPD meta-analysis; requested IPD had been lost or destroyed; or there were ethical or ownership restrictions on providing IPD.

Unavailability of IPD may be related to trial quality. As trials providing their IPD are open to more scrutiny, some trial investigators wishing to conceal errors or poor-quality data may withhold their IPD. An extreme example is that published trials with fabricated data are very unlikely to provide their IPD in case of being exposed. In such situations, an IPD meta-analysis of the subset of trials providing IPD may be more reliable that an analysis of all trials. Some IPD meta-analysis researchers may even prioritise obtaining IPD from the subset of better-quality trials. For example, in the Nevitt et al. review, 24 IPD meta-analysis projects reported that IPD were not requested for all trials,[27] mainly owing to the small size or low quality of those trials. Chapter 4 provides detailed discussion on the process of selecting and retrieving relevant IPD for meta-analysis.

9.3.1 Examining the Impact of Availability Bias

Tsujimoto et al. examined 31 IPD meta-analysis projects containing 728 randomised trials,[28] and found that 321 (44%) contributed IPD, whereas 407 (56%) did not. A trial was more likely to provide their IPD if it was recently published, had a large number of participants, had adequate allocation concealment, and was published in a journal with an impact factor ≥10. Encouragingly, on average across all the IPD meta-analysis projects, there was no systematic difference in the summary treatment effect (odds ratio) between trials contributing and not contributing IPD toward a primary binary outcome of interest (ratio of odds ratios: 1.01; 95% CI: 0.86 to 1.19). However, although similar on average across all projects, in a particular IPD meta-analysis project the differences between results from IPD and non-IPD trials could be substantial (95% prediction interval for ratio of odds ratios in a single IPD meta-analysis project: 0.60 to 1.42).[28]

Therefore, where possible, we recommend investigating the potential impact of unavailable IPD on the conclusions of an IPD meta-analysis. This requires suitable aggregate data (e.g. treatment effect estimates) to be obtained for non-IPD trials. For example, Vale et al. obtained aggregate data for three of their 10 missing trials,[29] and 'incorporating them into the meta-analysis did not materially change the results'. In the review of Nevitt et al.,[27] of the 571 IPD meta-analyses that failed to retrieve IPD from 100% of eligible studies, 201 (35%) supplemented IPD with aggregate data extracted from trial publications, enabling the inclusion of a median of 5 (range 1–541) extra studies representing a median of 683 (range 9–1,180,505) participants. In such situations, we suggest the meta-analysis of IPD should be the main analysis, whilst the meta-analysis combining IPD and aggregate data should be presented as a sensitivity analysis, to examine the robustness of findings.

Statistical approaches for combining IPD and aggregate data in a meta-analysis are described within each of Chapters 5 to 7,[26,30,31] with the simplest option to include the aggregate data in the second stage of the two-stage IPD meta-analysis framework. Incorporation of aggregate data may not always be possible, however. In particular, the required aggregate data (e.g. treatment-covariate interactions) may not be available from the publications of non-IPD trials, simply reinforcing why IPD were desired in the first place. In this case, it is worth asking trial investigators of non-IPD trials to derive and supply the required aggregate data directly, which they may sometimes be willing to do, even when not agreeing to supply their IPD.

Even when aggregate data are obtained for non-IPD trials, including the aggregate data alongside the IPD trials may introduce bias in the summary treatment effect (e.g. if non-IPD trials use inappropriate statistical analysis methods to produce their aggregate data) and could distort (often increase) between-trial heterogeneity (e.g. if non-IPD trials do not adjust for prognostic factors, but IPD trials do).

The characteristics and quality of IPD and non-IPD trials might also be compared. For example, McCormack et al. compared hernia trials providing IPD with those not providing IPD,[32] and conclude that 'other than the availability of unpublished data, there were no clear differences in trial characteristics between those with or without IPD.' Where characteristics do differ, researchers might identify a subset of IPD trials that can be matched to non-IPD trials (e.g. in terms of length of follow-up, statistical analysis methods, inclusion criteria, risk of bias etc) to enable a fairer comparison of whether effect estimates from IPD and non-IPD trials are systematically different. It is also worth remembering that the non-IPD trials cannot be scrutinised in the same way as the IPD trials; there may be differences between the IPD and non-IPD trials that are not apparent from the details available within publications. In particular, the quality of the non-IPD trials cannot be verified in the same way as for the IPD trials (one reason why the IPD analysis should be regarded as the main analysis).

9.3.2 Example: IPD Meta-Analysis Examining High-dose Chemotherapy for the Treatment of Non-Hodgkin Lymphoma

Greb et al. investigated whether high-dose chemotherapy with autologous stem cell transplantation as part of first-line treatment improved survival in adults with aggressive non-Hodgkin lymphoma.[33] Fifteen randomised trials comparing high-dose versus conventional chemotherapy were identified by a systematic review, and IPD were sought from all 15 trials. However, publication and availability biases were threats, as all trials were fully published and IPD were unavailable for five of them (33%). Greb et al. examined both these issues and we now summarise their work.[33]

A two-stage IPD meta-analysis of the 10 IPD trials (1,500 participants) assuming a common treatment effect gave a summary hazard ratio of 1.14 (95% CI: 0.98 to 1.34), favouring conventional chemotherapy and providing some evidence that high-dose chemotherapy decreased survival rates (top part of Figure 9.3). To investigate availability bias, Greb et al.[33] extracted hazard ratio estimates for four of the five non-IPD trials, containing a total of 944 participants. Then, these four results were included in the second stage of the IPD meta-analysis, such that there were now 14 trials containing 2,444 participants in the updated meta-analysis, with the four non-IPD trials contributing 39% of the total participants. Since the treatment effect estimates from non-IPD trials were more favourable toward high-dose chemotherapy than those from IPD trials (bottom part of Figure 9.3), the summary hazard ratio was closer to the null value of 1 after non-IPD trials were included (HR = 1.05; 95% CI: 0.92 to 1.19). Interestingly, there was less between-trial heterogeneity in the results

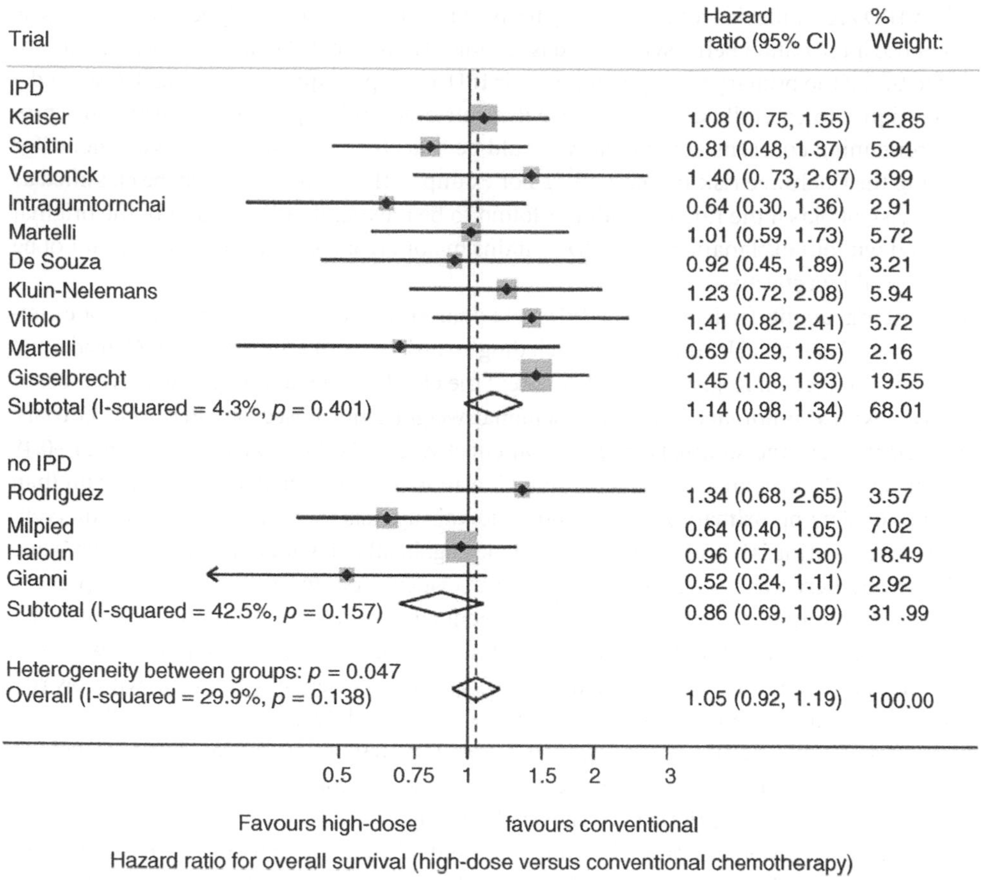

Figure 9.3 Example of combining IPD and non-IPD trials in an IPD meta-analysis of randomised trials examining high-dose chemotherapy for the treatment of non-Hodgkin lymphoma, as described by Greb et al.[33] and Ahmed et al.[19] *Sources:* Richard Riley, adapting Figure 2 of Ahmed et al.,[19] with permission, © 2012 British Medical Journal Publishing Group (CC-BY-NC 2.0).

of the IPD trials than the non-IPD trials, which may be due to the IPD approach enabling standardisation of participant inclusion criteria and statistical analysis methods across the IPD trials (whereas this is not possible for the non-IPD trials). Regardless, in all analyses there was no evidence that high-dose chemotherapy improved survival. There was also no evidence of small-study effects from a funnel plot.

9.4 Trial Quality (risk of bias)

> *"Public agencies are very keen on amassing statistics – they collect them, add them, raise them to the nth power, take the cube root and prepare wonderful diagrams. But what you must never forget is that every one of those figures comes in the first instance from the village watchman, who just puts down what he damn well pleases."*
>
> (attributed to Sir Josiah Stamp, 1880–1941)

Even when IPD are available from all existing trials, it is critical – as in any type of meta-analysis project – that the information being synthesised is reliable. Therefore, IPD meta-analysis results are susceptible to bias if the primary trials providing their IPD are of poor quality. Chapter 4 described a range of techniques to carefully check IPD once it is retrieved and, if possible, to rectify any problems. Any remaining concerns about quality should be reflected in a risk of bias assessment (for example, using the Cochrane risk-of-bias tool[34]). For example, IPD from a trial may be classified as being at high risk of bias if the randomisation is found to be flawed, if only a subset of the original IPD is provided without explanation, or if IPD contains major errors or inaccuracies that cannot be resolved with trial investigators.

The impact of trial quality (risk of bias) on IPD meta-analysis results should be checked. For example, a sensitivity analysis could be undertaken excluding any trials not at low risk of bias. Consider the IPD meta-analysis project of Rogisinzka et al. to assess the effects of diet and physical activity–based interventions,[35] with the primary outcome gestational weight gain. Based on IPD from 33 trials, including 9,320 women, the summary intervention effect was –0.70 kg (95% CI: –0.92 kg to –0.48 kg), indicating strongly that, on average, those receiving an intervention had lower weight gain than those that did not. An approximate 95% prediction interval suggests the range of potential intervention effects in a new setting is between –1.24 and –0.16 kg, again all in favour of the intervention being effective. However, there was strong visual and statistical evidence of funnel plot asymmetry (Egger's test: $p = 0.038$), with smaller trials having larger treatment effects (Figure 9.4(a)). Inclusion of aggregate data from an additional 27 trials did not resolve the issue, and indeed the asymmetry was even more pronounced (Egger's test: $p = 0.026$; Figure 9.4(b)). However, when only IPD trials with low risk of bias were included, the asymmetry in the funnel plot was removed (Egger's test: $p = 0.61$; Figure 9.4 (c)) and, reassuringly, the summary result of –0.67 (95% CI: –0.95 to –0.38) remained strongly in favour of the intervention (15 trials, 5,585 participants), with an approximate 95% prediction interval of –1.14 to –0.19 for the intervention effect in a single setting.

We note that availability of IPD may allow improved statistical analysis within each trial to (partially) mitigate against risk of bias concerns. For example, availability of IPD for a trial may reveal loss to follow-up and missing outcomes for some individuals; if the magnitude of this problem is different for treatment and control groups, this raises concerns of attrition bias, and thus perhaps a higher risk of bias classification for the trial than initially thought without IPD. However, having the IPD more easily allows the impact of missing outcomes to be investigated in such trials,[36] and sensitivity analyses performed to examine the impact of particular missing data assumptions. For example, the meta-analysis might adjust for prognostic factors in each trial so that a missing at random assumption is potentially plausible for the missing outcomes (Chapters 5 and 18 give further discussion on dealing with missing variables), and to reduce missing not at random concerns.[37]

9.5 Other Potential Biases Affecting IPD Meta-Analysis Results

We now consider three other biases that may impact IPD meta-analysis results.

9.5.1 Trial Selection Bias

Selection bias can occur if the IPD meta-analysis project deliberately seeks IPD only from a subset of all eligible trials, and this subset does not reflect the entire relevant evidence base for the target population of interest.[38] This is a particular concern when trials are not identified by a systematic review, but rather through contacts or colleagues in the field, and when the selection takes place

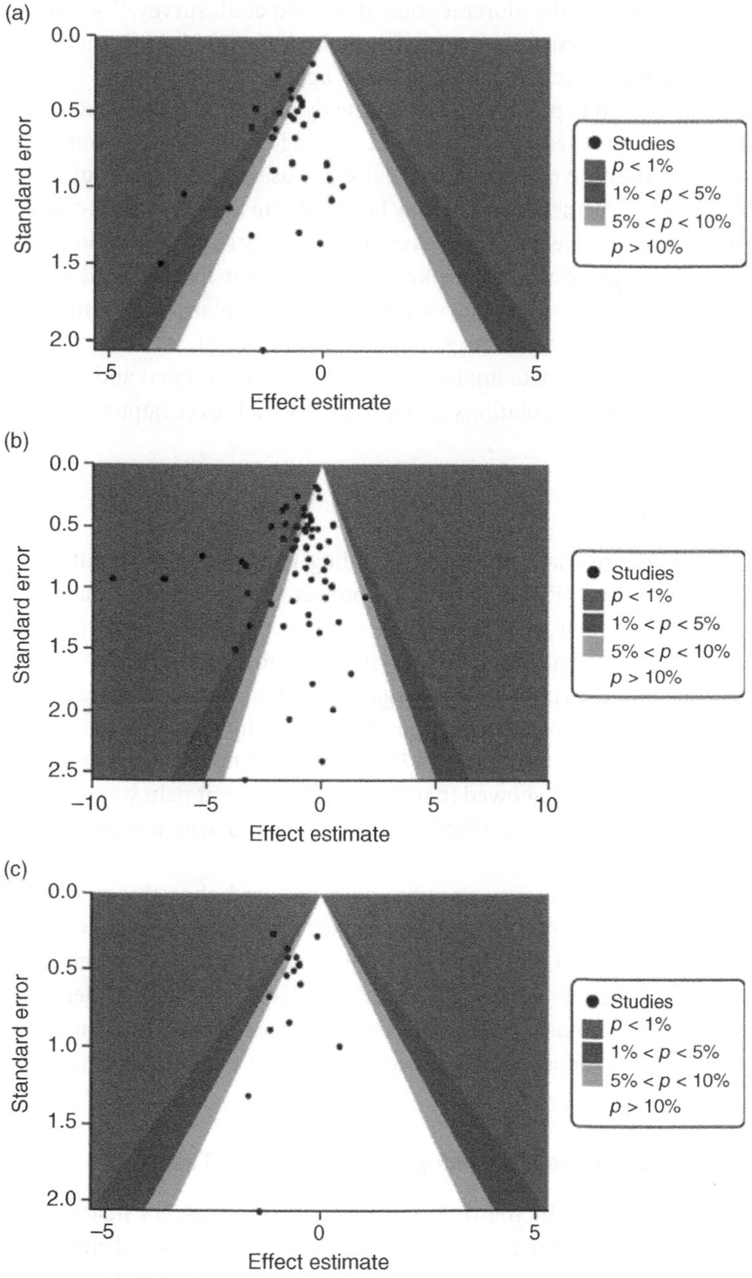

Figure 9.4 Contour-enhanced funnel plots for the IPD meta-analysis of Rogozinska et al.[35] that examined the effects of diet and physical activity-based interventions for the primary outcome gestational weight gain, for (a) all IPD trials, (b) all IPD trials and non-IPD trials providing aggregate data, and (c) only IPD trials at low risk of bias. *Source:* Figure taken from Figure 7 of Rogozinska et al.[35], with permission, © 2017 Queen's Printer and Controller of HMSO.

with knowledge of individual trial results. In the aforementioned Ahmed et al. survey,[19] selection bias was a concern in 9 of 31 IPD meta-analysis projects, as the method of trial identification was either not stated or was based on a more selective, non-systematic approach.

The direction of any selection bias is hard to predict, and can (directly or indirectly) be affected by the selectors' knowledge of the field, their research contacts and existing collaborations, and their informed opinion about the research question of interest. Crucially, the use of IPD from a subset of trials does not necessarily introduce bias. As mentioned, it may be legitimate to select (ideally based on pre-defined criteria) a subset of trials in a field on the basis of their quality (e.g. those at low risk of bias), but not because of their findings or any insider knowledge of what the IPD will show. Similarly, the subset of trials may be those recording key variables (e.g. particular participant-level variables or outcomes), or those that best reflect the target population of interest. Identifying such trials may not be apparent until after the IPD meta-analysis project has been initiated and contact with trial investigators made to clarify trial populations and available variables (Chapter 4).

9.5.2 Selective Outcome Availability

Selective outcome reporting occurs where trial outcomes (including particular time-points) are entirely excluded upon publication.[39] If an IPD meta-analysis project simply ignores trials that do not report the outcomes of interest, even though they are otherwise eligible, then relevant IPD may be missed. This is demonstrated by an IPD meta-analysis of laparoscopic versus open surgery for the repair of inguinal hernia. Based on published aggregate data from three trials, the risk of persistent pain was found to be significantly greater with laparoscopic repair (summary odds ratio = 2.03; 95% CI: 1.03 to 4.01).[40] Yet when IPD from a further 17 trials (that did not publish results for this outcome) were added, the combined results showed that the risk of persistent pain was actually *less* with laparoscopic repair (summary odds ratio = 0.54; 95% CI: 0.46 to 0.64), with a substantially narrower confidence interval.

If a trial does not provide IPD with all the outcomes or time-points desired, then this should be addressed with the original trial investigators (i.e. to confirm that such outcomes were never collected by the trial, or to ask for additional IPD that do provide the outcomes needed). Where outcomes remain missing in some trials, a multivariate IPD meta-analysis might be considered to borrow information across correlated outcomes.[41] This approach has been shown to reduce the impact of missing outcomes and outcome reporting bias,[42] and details are provided in Chapter 13.

9.5.3 Use of Inappropriate Methods by the IPD Meta-Analysis Research Team

IPD meta-analysis results may also be biased by the IPD researchers themselves, for instance by wrongly including or excluding relevant participants, or using inappropriate statistical methods. Parts 1 and 2 of this book outline good practice for designing and undertaking IPD meta-analysis projects, which should be considered at the onset, and specified in the project protocol including an analysis plan. Independent peer review of such protocols helps to flag sub-standard methods or areas for improvement. For example, common analysis mistakes include using one-stage models that analyse the IPD as if it all came from a single trial (Chapter 6) or amalgamate within-trial and across-trial relationships (Chapter 7).

9.6 Concluding Remarks

IPD meta-analysis projects cannot be assumed to be free from bias, even when best practice is followed throughout the project. Results may be affected by missing IPD due to publication and availability biases, and the inclusion of IPD from low-quality trials. Often the potential impact of such biases on IPD meta-analysis results can be examined, for example using funnel plots and sensitivity analyses, and such investigations should be clearly reported to ensure transparency and integrity (Chapter 10).[43] Later chapters also discuss how bias due to missing data can be reduced by multivariate (Chapter 13) and multiple imputation (Chapter 18) methods.

10

Reporting and Dissemination of IPD Meta-Analyses

Lesley A. Stewart, Richard D. Riley, and Jayne F. Tierney

Summary Points

- To maximise uptake, impact and usefulness, IPD meta-analysis projects must be carried out rigorously and reported well.
- Reporting and dissemination activity should be planned from the outset, with a broad range of potential stakeholders in mind, including patients and policy-makers.
- Owing to size and complexity, communicating the methods, results and implications of an IPD meta-analysis project can be challenging.
- Methods and results should be reported transparently and in sufficient detail to allow readers to judge the research quality, and consequently the credibility of findings.
- PRISMA-IPD, and its associated checklist and flow diagram, provides a framework to help authors describe essential elements of IPD meta-analysis design, conduct and findings in their journal article.
- Disseminating and mobilising the knowledge gained from IPD meta-analysis can benefit from additional activity over and above publishing in academic journals.
- Different types of outputs can be prepared and tailored for different audiences, including practitioners, guideline developers, policy-makers, patient advocacy and support groups, and members of the public.
- Effective use of social media, blogs, videos, press releases and lay summaries can enhance communication and reach a broader audience.

10.1 Introduction

The main purpose of evidence synthesis within healthcare is to generate reliable research-based evidence to inform decisions that ultimately improve the health and care of individuals. To achieve this, they must produce reliable results and be reported in a way that reaches and is understood by those who need to use the results. Previous chapters in this book explore the many advantages offered by IPD meta-analysis projects, and explain how to minimise potential biases and improve the robustness of findings. It is also essential that IPD meta-analysis projects are reported clearly and transparently, and in a way that can be understood by non-technical audiences. This is because good methods and conduct alone do not guarantee uptake and implementation of findings.[44]

Individual Participant Data Meta-Analysis: A Handbook for Healthcare Research, First Edition.
Edited by Richard D. Riley, Jayne F. Tierney, and Lesley A. Stewart.

In common with other types of research, using a range of outputs and approaches to dissemination will help to reach the different types of people who might be interested in IPD meta-analysis results. This may include the preparation of longer technical reports, more succinct journal articles, and shorter summaries tailored for different audiences including patients, policy-makers and other stakeholders. Social media can also be a useful dissemination tool, as can, where appropriate, engagement with the press. This chapter outlines how to report the methods and findings of IPD meta-analysis projects in technical reports and journal articles, and also briefly describes other methods of dissemination and knowledge mobilisation that may be adopted to increase their impact.

10.2 Reporting IPD Meta-Analysis Projects in Academic Reports

Parts 1 and 2 of this book describe how IPD meta-analysis projects provide a powerful way of assembling and conducting robust analyses of existing trial datasets. However, the flexibility and analytic advantages offered by IPD also allows data to be organised ('sliced and diced') in varying ways, and analyses done using different approaches, some of which are more appropriate than others. Therefore, it is particularly important that journal articles report IPD meta-analysis methods and findings transparently, paying attention to distinguishing between pre-specified and *post hoc* investigations, and documenting the reasons for making decisions and choices along the way.

One of the challenges in communicating the findings of IPD meta-analysis projects is that they can be large and complex, making them difficult to describe within a standard-length academic paper. They often require description of the approaches used to identify, obtain, check and harmonise relevant datasets and can involve non-standard statistical methods and large numbers of analyses. Reporting needs to be succinct and information presented in a way that helps readers navigate and understand the main findings and take-home messages, without becoming overwhelmed by unnecessary detail. Whilst transparency requires making results of all analyses available, careful thought is required about which results need detailed description and discussion within the article, and which may be described briefly with signposting to more detailed exposition in appendices or supplementary material.

The Preferred Reporting Items for Systematic Reviews and Meta-Analyses for Individual Participant Data (PRISMA-IPD) statement was developed as standalone guidance to aid those writing, peer reviewing or reading reports of IPD meta-analysis projects.[43] It was developed primarily for meta-analyses of IPD from randomised trials of treatments, but many items are also applicable to other types of IPD syntheses, including those addressing diagnosis and prognosis (Chapters 15 to 17). The PRISMA-IPD checklist (Tables 10.1 to 10.3) is largely self-explanatory and represents the minimum amount of information that should be reported in order to provide a full and transparent account of how the IPD meta-analysis project was conducted and what it found. It may be necessary to include additional material to deal with non-standard issues that occurred during the review process and to convey nuances of findings, or specialist applications such as multivariate or network meta-analysis (Chapters 13 and 14).[45] IPD syntheses of study designs other than randomised trials may require further or different information, particularly in relation to the meta-analysis methods and statistics of interest, and may draw on checklists such as STARD, REMARK and TRIPOD.[46–48] PRISMA-IPD has the same structure as the standard PRISMA checklist for conventional meta-analyses based on aggregate data,[49,50] but has additional items and modified wording to reflect the attributes of the IPD approach.

Like all reporting guidelines, PRISMA-IPD is intended as a tool to help ensure that important methods, results and implications used within an IPD meta-analysis project are covered in associated reports and journal articles; it is not mandatory and does not provide 'rules' or stipulate ordering of writing. However, it provides a good starting point to ensure that IPD meta-analysis projects are reported with sufficient detail to enable readers to judge their appropriateness and quality, and consequently the credibility of their findings.

The following section provides some further suggestions on how PRISMA-IPD might be implemented using the IMRAD format (Introduction, Methods, Results and Discussion), and assumes that the IPD meta-analysis project was carried out within a systematic review framework.

10.2.1 PRISMA-IPD Title and Abstract Sections (Table 10.1)

Title (PRISMA-IPD 1)

It is helpful to those reading the article if the title states explicitly that it reports a systematic review and IPD meta-analysis, as well as indicating the nature of the topic being addressed.

Structured abstract (PRISMA-IPD 2)

A structured abstract should include important details of methods and results. Journal format and word limits may make it difficult to include all the information outlined in the abstract section of the PRISMA-IPD checklist, but as much relevant information as possible should be captured. This is important because the abstract may be the only part of the paper that some readers access.

Table 10.1 Title and Introduction sections of the PRISMA-IPD Checklist as reported by Stewart et al.[43]

TITLE	1	Identify the report as a systematic review and meta-analysis of individual participant data.
ABSTRACT		
Structured summary	2	Provide a structured summary including as applicable: **Background**: state research question and main objectives, with information on participants, interventions, comparators and outcomes. **Methods**: report eligibility criteria; data sources including dates of last bibliographic search or elicitation, noting that IPD were sought; methods of assessing risk of bias. **Results**: provide number and type of studies and participants identified and number (%) obtained; summary effect estimates for main outcomes (benefits and harms) with confidence intervals and measures of statistical heterogeneity. Describe the direction and size of summary effects in terms meaningful to those who would put findings into practice. **Discussion:** state main strengths and limitations of the evidence, general interpretation of the results and any important implications. **Other:** report primary funding source, registration number and registry name for the systematic review and IPD meta-analysis.
INTRODUCTION		
Rationale	3	Describe the rationale for the review in the context of what is already known.
Objectives	4	Provide an explicit statement of the questions being addressed with reference, as applicable, to participants, interventions, comparisons, outcomes and study design (PICOS). Include any hypotheses that relate to particular types of participant-level subgroups.

Source: Items reproduced with permission from Table 1 of Stewart et al.,[43] © 2015 American Medical Association; also freely available at www.prisma-statement.org.

10.2.2 PRISMA-IPD Introduction Section (Table 10.1)

Background

An IPD meta-analysis article will usually start with a brief outline of the health area and topic under consideration, providing details about the condition, prevalence, outcomes and current prognosis, as appropriate. Current clinical practice may be described and, for therapeutic topics, information about the treatments under investigation provided. Where different types of participants may be expected to benefit differentially from treatment, the underlying reasons for this should be given and benefits of targeted approaches described, if appropriate.

Rationale (PRISMA-IPD 3)

The need for systematic review and meta-analysis should be explained in relation to the research question being addressed. This should include the specific rationale for adopting the IPD approach (Chapter 2); for example, the need for participant-level data to explore effectiveness in different types of participants, to address limitations revealed by a conventional systematic review of aggregate data (such as reporting bias), or the need to perform particular types of analysis that can only be done with participant-level data. As IPD meta-analysis projects remain a small (but important) minority of all systematic reviews,[51] if space permits it can be useful to include a brief explanation of the general benefits of using IPD.

Aims and objectives (PRISMA-IPD 4)

The aims and specific objectives being addressed should be set out clearly and provide information about participants, interventions, comparisons, outcomes and study design (PICOS), as applicable (Chapter 3). Importantly these should include any aims that relate to specific types of participant-level subgroups. Information about objectives may be presented as statements or posed as questions according to personal preference or the usual style of the journal or organisation to which it will be submitted.

10.2.3 PRISMA-IPD Methods Section (Table 10.2)

Protocols and registration (PRISMA-IPD 5)

As described in Chapter 4, the production of and adherence to a protocol and analysis plan is crucial for IPD meta-analysis projects. Deviation from the analyses planned in the protocol may be necessary, and might even improve on what was intended, but it is important that this is reported transparently. Providing the protocol registration number enables readers to access the registration record, for example, on the PROSPERO website (https://www.crd.york.ac.uk/PROSPERO/), to check how the completed IPD meta-analysis project aligns with the outcomes and analyses planned when the project was registered, and with any subsequent updates. If the full protocol has been published, this should also be cited. If not published in full, it may also be helpful to include a copy of the protocol as an appendix or supplementary material, or via a web link.

Eligibility criteria (PRISMA-IPD 6)

Criteria for inclusion or exclusion of trials and, if relevant, participants should be described in detail. For example, an IPD meta-analysis project concerned with treatments in paediatric populations might include data from trials that only recruited children and also data from the children enrolled in trials that recruited both adults and children. As well as being transparent, this information may help readers avoid confusion if the number of included participants differs markedly from the number reported in the original trial publication.

Table 10.2 Methods section of the PRISMA-IPD Checklist as reported by Stewart et al.[43]

METHODS		
Protocol and registration	5	Indicate if a protocol exists and where it can be accessed. If available, provide registration information, including registration number and registry name. Provide publication details, if applicable.
Eligibility criteria	6	Specify inclusion and exclusion criteria, including those relating to participants, interventions, comparisons, outcomes, study design and characteristics (e.g. years when conducted, required minimum follow-up). Note whether these were applied at the study or individual level, i.e. whether eligible participants were included (and ineligible participants excluded) from a study that included a wider population than specified by the review inclusion criteria. The rationale for criteria should be stated.
Identifying studies – information sources	7	Describe all methods of identifying published and unpublished studies, including, as applicable: which bibliographic databases were searched, with dates of coverage; details of any hand searching, including of conference proceedings; use of study registers and agency or company databases; contact with the original research team and experts in the field; open adverts and surveys. Give the date of last search or elicitation.
Identifying studies – search	8	Present the full electronic search strategy for at least one database, including any limits used, such that it could be repeated.
Study selection processes	9	State the process for determining which studies were eligible for inclusion.
Data collection processes	10	Describe how IPD were requested, collected and managed, including any processes for querying and confirming data with investigators. If IPD were not sought from any eligible study, the reason for this should be stated (for each such study).
		If applicable, describe how any studies for which IPD were not available were dealt with. This should include whether, how and what aggregate data were sought or extracted from study reports and publications (such as extracting data independently in duplicate) and any processes for obtaining and confirming these data with investigators.
Data items	11	Describe how the information and variables to be collected were chosen. List and define all study-level and participant-level data that were sought, including baseline and follow-up information. If applicable, describe methods of standardising or translating variables within the IPD datasets to ensure common scales or measurements across studies.
IPD integrity	A1	Describe what aspects of IPD were subject to data checking (such as sequence generation, data consistency and completeness, baseline imbalance) and how this was done.
Risk of bias assessment in individual studies	12	Describe methods used to assess risk of bias in the individual studies and whether this was applied separately for each outcome. If applicable, describe how findings of IPD checking were used to inform the assessment. Report if and how risk of bias assessment was used in any data synthesis.
Specification of outcomes and effect measures	13	State all treatment comparisons of interests. State all outcomes addressed and define them in detail. State whether they were pre-specified for the review and, if applicable, whether they were primary/main or secondary/additional outcomes. Give the principal

(Continued)

Table 10.2 (Continued)

		measures of effect (such as risk ratio, hazard ratio, difference in means) used for each outcome.
Synthesis methods	14	Describe the meta-analysis methods used to synthesise IPD. Specify any statistical methods and models used. Issues should include (but are not restricted to): • Use of a one-stage or two-stage approach. • How effect estimates were generated separately within each study and combined across studies (where applicable). • Specification of one-stage models (where applicable), including how clustering of patients within studies was accounted for. • Use of fixed or random effect models and any other model assumptions, such as proportional hazards. • How (summary) survival curves were generated (where applicable). • Methods for quantifying statistical heterogeneity (such as I^2 and τ^2). • How studies providing IPD and not providing IPD were analysed together (where applicable). • How missing data within the IPD were dealt with (where applicable).
Exploration of variation in effects	A2	If applicable, describe any methods used to explore variation in effects by study- or participant-level characteristics (such as estimation of interactions between effect and covariates). State all participant-level characteristics that were analysed as potential effect modifiers, and whether these were pre-specified.
Risk of bias across studies	15	Specify any assessment of risk of bias relating to the accumulated body of evidence, including any pertaining to not obtaining IPD for particular studies, outcomes or other variables.
Additional analyses	16	Describe methods of any additional analyses, including sensitivity analyses. State which of these were pre-specified.

Source: Items reproduced with permission from Table 1 of Stewart et al.,[43] © 2015 American Medical Association; also freely available at www.prisma-statement.org.

Identifying trials and trial selection processes (PRISMA-IPD 7, 8, 9)

Methods of identifying included trials should be described, including information about which bibliographic databases, trial registers and other sources of unpublished trials were searched and when this was done. An example search strategy for at least one database should be provided (generally as an appendix or in supplementary material). If trial investigators were asked to help identify eligible trials, this should be described, as should any additional means of identification such as open calls for evidence. The methods section should include a brief description of how screening was done and by whom. If trial investigators were asked to provide additional information to clarify eligibility this should be noted, as should the involvement of any advisory group members or trial investigators in making decisions about which trials were included.

Data collection (PRISMA-IPD 10, 11)

As discussed in Chapters 3 and 4, data collection is one area where IPD meta-analysis projects differs markedly from a conventional systematic review of aggregate data. Therefore, the methods section should include a description of how data were requested, obtained and managed. If IPD were not sought from any eligible trials, the reason for this should be given. How data were coded should also be described, for example stating whether a data dictionary/coding convention was developed (Chapter 4). Ideally, all trial-level and participant-level data that were sought should be listed. This may be done briefly in the text, and supported by a fuller list or table in an appendix or supplementary material.

For any trials not providing IPD, the methods of extracting their aggregate data (e.g. from trial reports and publications, or from trial investigators directly) should be described, including what key aggregate data items were sought and how extraction was done (e.g. independently in duplicate), along with any processes for confirming these data with investigators.

IPD integrity (PRISMA-IPD A1)

As described in Chapter 4, checking and verification of supplied data is a central aspect of IPD meta-analysis projects. The fact that an independent research team examined the provided IPD closely is an important aspect of credibility, but, in our experience, is typically not well reported. Brief information should be provided about the types of data checks that were carried out and how any identified issues were resolved. Any unresolved problems should be reported. This may naturally run on from the description of how data were collected and into risk of bias assessment, as these are interrelated. How checks were done (e.g. by running computer scripts that flag values above a certain threshold or by plotting the distribution of values for certain variables within and across trials) may also be described, if space permits.

Risk of bias assessment in individual trials (PRISMA-IPD 12)

The methods section should describe how potential for bias within included trials was assessed. This should include consideration of risk of bias assessments, data checking and the interplay between these. For example, there might be less concern about potential bias associated with sealed envelope allocation concealment if checking the IPD shows the treatment allocation to trial groups to be balanced over time and that there is no important imbalance in baseline participant characteristics across these allocation groups. Conversely, it may be necessary to highlight concerns that are only revealed by the IPD itself. If and how these assessments were used in the actual IPD meta-analysis should be explained; for example, if sensitivity analyses were done restricting the IPD meta-analysis to only those trials rated as low risk of bias, then this should be stated.

Specification of outcomes and effect measures (PRISMA-IPD 13)

IPD meta-analysis projects may offer flexibility in the choice of outcomes, outcome measurement (such as different rating scales for measuring depression) and subgroups examined. However, this also creates potential for 'data dredging' whereby the IPD project team could explore numerous subgroups, outcomes, and measurements, potentially even at multiple time-points, to find those that yield results most to their liking. This makes it particularly important to state all outcomes, outcome measurements and subgroups that were examined, and whether these were pre-specified, as well as clearly defining them and stating the effect measures used (e.g. risk ratio, standardised mean difference). Sometimes outcomes are examined at multiple time-points, and if so these time-points should also be described in full.

Meta-Analysis methods (PRISMA-IPD 14, A2, 16)

The meta-analysis methods used to synthesise the IPD and produce summary results are not always reported fully for IPD meta-analysis projects. This may be due to journal restrictions on length, or possibly because it is assumed that they are obvious, or that their details are not necessary. However, it is essential to give a clear description of the statistical methods used for IPD meta-analysis in the main text of the paper, potentially with more detailed statistical equations and explanations in an appendix or supplementary material. Details should include whether the IPD meta-analysis used a two-stage or one-stage approach (Chapters 5 and 6); the statistical models chosen (e.g. the regression models used) and how they were estimated (e.g. restricted maximum likelihood estimation); how clustering of participants within trials was accounted for (e.g. stratified intercept in a one-stage model); how between-trial heterogeneity was measured and incorporated in the analyses; and the methods used to measure and explore variation in effects by trial-level or participant-level characteristics, including how estimation of treatment-covariate interactions separated within-trial and across-trial relationships (Chapter 7). All participant-level characteristics that were analysed as potential effect modifiers should be listed, and whether these were pre-specified or not should be mentioned.

Risk of bias associated with the overall body of evidence (PRISMA-IPD 15)

Any assessment of risk of bias relating to the accumulated body of evidence should be described, including any pertaining to unavailable IPD for particular trials, outcomes or other variables. This may include sensitivity analyses comparing meta-analyses with and without aggregate data from trials for which IPD were not available (Chapter 9), or undertaking sensitivity analyses under different missing data assumptions.

IPD meta-analysis projects usually involve considerable efforts to try to identify and obtain data from unpublished trials, but any methods for considering publication bias should be reported, such as the production and inspection of funnel plots for small-study effects (Chapter 9). If assessment of the strength of evidence was made, for example by using GRADE,[52,53] then this should also be stated.

10.2.4 PRISMA-IPD Results Section (Table 10.3)

An important aspect of validity for an IPD meta-analysis project is the completeness and representativeness of the data obtained and analysed, which underpins the credibility of the IPD meta-analysis results and subsequent conclusions. The results section should, therefore, usually begin with a description of the trials and the IPD that were sought and which were available for analysis.

Trials identified and data obtained (PRISMA-IPD 18)

The PRISMA-IPD flowchart should be used to illustrate the numbers of potentially eligible trials returned by bibliographic searches, screened, and judged eligible for inclusion, and to present the numbers of trials and participants for which IPD were sought and obtained (Figure 10.1). For any eligible trials where IPD were not available, the numbers of trials and participants for which aggregate data were available should also be shown. Reasons why IPD were not available should be reported, as should any trials that were excluded from the project as a whole or for particular outcomes or analyses.

Trial characteristics (PRISMA-IPD 18)

Information on key trial and participant characteristics should be provided for each trial, including a description of treatments, numbers of participants, demographic data, any unavailable outcomes, funding source, and if applicable, the duration of follow-up, along with a main citation for each trial. It can be challenging to do this within the space constraints of a journal article, and even within a longer report. Expressing trial information in tabular and graphical format saves space and can make it easier for readers to see key features at a glance. One or more tables summarising main trial design features can capture relevant information about setting, treatment, main

Table 10.3 Results and discussion sections of the PRISMA-IPD Checklist as reported by Stewart et al.[43]

RESULTS		
Study selection and IPD obtained	17	Give numbers of studies screened, assessed for eligibility, and included in the systematic review with reasons for exclusions at each stage. Indicate the number of studies and participants for which IPD were sought and for which IPD were obtained. For those studies where IPD were not available, give the numbers of studies and participants for which aggregate data were available. Report reasons for non-availability of IPD. Include a flow diagram.
Study characteristics	18	For each study, present information on key study and participant characteristics (such as description of interventions, numbers of participants, demographic data, unavailability of outcomes, funding source, and if applicable duration of follow-up). Provide (main) citations for each study. Where applicable, also report similar study characteristics for any studies not providing IPD.
IPD integrity	A3	Report any important issues identified in checking IPD or state that there were none.
Risk of bias within studies	19	Present data on risk of bias assessments. If applicable, describe whether data checking led to the up-weighting or down-weighting of these assessments. Consider how any potential bias impacts on the robustness of meta-analysis conclusions.
Results of individual studies	20	For each comparison and for each main outcome (benefit or harm), for each individual study report the number of eligible participants for which data were obtained and show simple summary data for each intervention group (including, where applicable, the number of events), effect estimates and confidence intervals. These may be tabulated or included on a forest plot.
Results of syntheses	21	Present summary effects for each meta-analysis undertaken, including confidence intervals and measures of statistical heterogeneity. State whether the analysis was pre-specified, and report the numbers of studies and participants and, where applicable, the number of events on which it is based.
		When exploring variation in effects due to patient or study characteristics, present summary interaction estimates for each characteristic examined, including confidence intervals and measures of statistical heterogeneity. State whether the analysis was pre-specified. State whether any interaction is consistent across trials.
		Provide a description of the direction and size of effect in terms meaningful to those who would put findings into practice.
Risk of bias across studies	22	Present results of any assessment of risk of bias relating to the accumulated body of evidence, including any pertaining to the availability and representativeness of available studies, outcomes or other variables.
Additional analyses	23	Give results of any additional analyses (e.g. sensitivity analyses). If applicable, this should also include any analyses that incorporate aggregate data for studies that do not have IPD. If applicable, summarise the main meta-analysis results following the inclusion or exclusion of studies for which IPD were not available.

(Continued)

Table 10.3 (Continued)

DISCUSSION		
Summary of evidence	24	Summarise the main findings, including the strength of evidence for each main outcome.
Strengths and limitations	25	Discuss any important strengths and limitations of the evidence, including the benefits of access to IPD and any limitations arising from IPD that were not available.
Conclusions	26	Provide a general interpretation of the findings in the context of other evidence.
Implications	A4	Consider relevance to key groups (such as policy-makers, service providers and service users). Consider implications for future research.
FUNDING		
Funding	27	Describe sources of funding and other support (such as supply of IPD), and the role in the systematic review of those providing such support.

Source: Items reproduced with permission from Table 1 of Stewart et al.,[43] © 2015 American Medical Association; also freely available at www.prisma-statement.org.

eligibility criteria and the types of participant that each individual trial aimed to enrol. Similar information should also be provided for any eligible trials for which IPD were not available (possibly in an appendix). This should be done irrespective of whether aggregate data from these were able to be included in sensitivity analyses.

The distribution of participant characteristics for each included trial (calculated from the IPD) can be included in the trial design table, or in a separate table, and may include information such as the age distribution (mean, median, standard deviation, etc) of participants, the proportion of individuals according to disease stage, and the numbers of participants with key risk factors.

It is important to convey the extent and pattern of any missing data (Chapter 18). The extent of missing data should be described for each outcome reported in the IPD meta-analysis, but it may also be helpful to convey the overall pattern of data availability. For example, a grid or 'heat map' can be used for each trial to indicate whether each variable sought was available for all participants, for some participants, or for no participants, with grid boxes shaded with colours and shades to reflect completeness. An example plot using a grey colour scale is shown in Figure 10.2. A colour scale is preferable, where possible, for example with green boxes indicating that a high proportion of patients provided data, and red boxes indicating that most patients did not provide data.

IPD integrity and risk of bias within trials (PRISMA-IPD 18,19)

The results section should give information about the findings of the data checking and risk of bias assessment process. If any issues were identified, these should be stated honestly but diplomatically, and a description given of any action taken and subsequent impact on analyses. As readers may be familiar with the published results of trials included in the IPD meta-analysis project, or may check findings against the original papers, it is important to acknowledge whether there were important differences between published results and those derived from the IPD. It will usually be sufficient to deal with this in a general way noting that, for example, the numbers of events differ between the IPD meta-analysis and some original trial publications because of the way that outcomes were defined. In some instances, if there are substantial differences it may be necessary to describe this

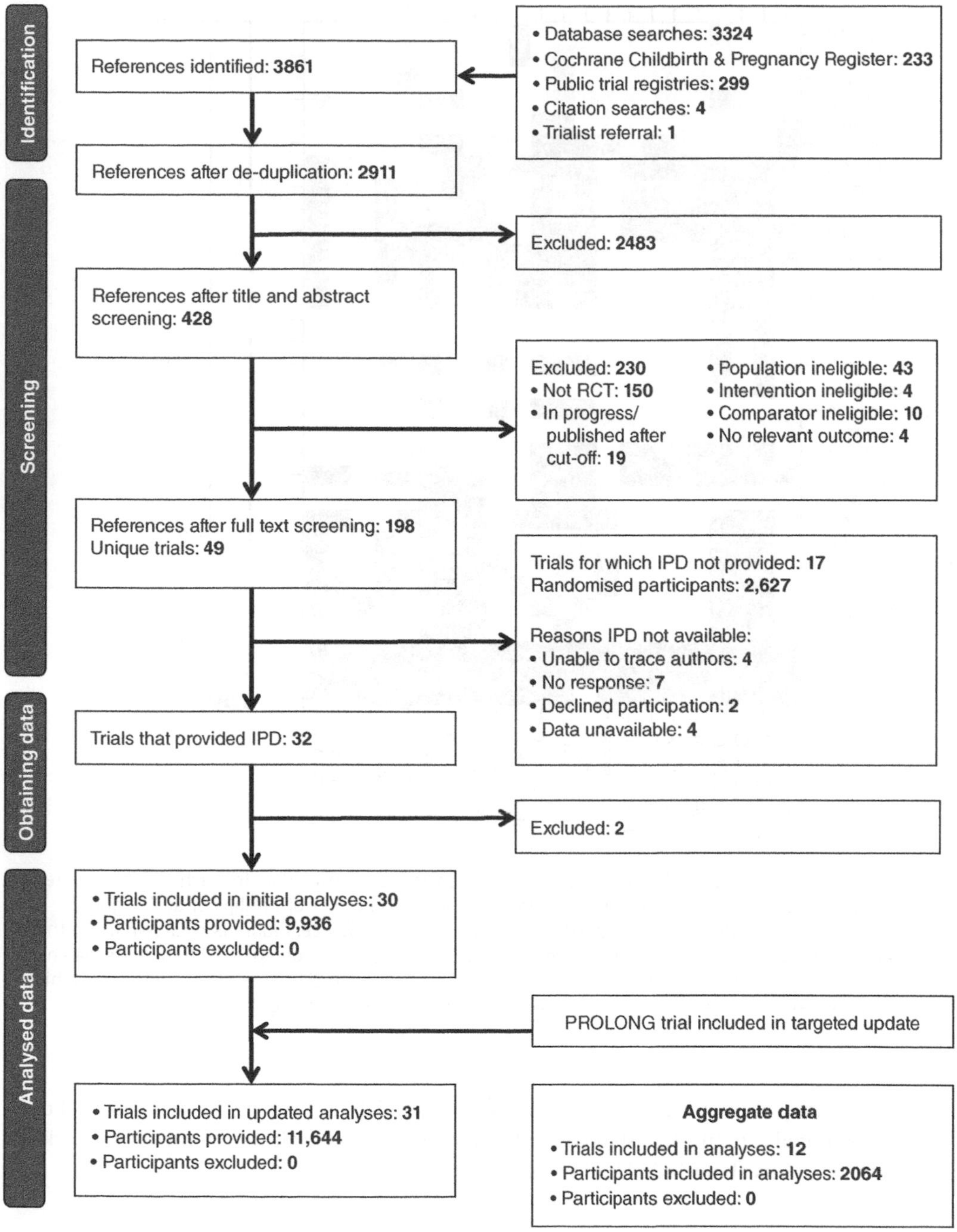

Figure 10.1 Example of the PRISMA-IPD flowchart applied to an IPD meta-analysis project.
Source: Lesley Stewart.

in more detail and specifically for each trial, either in the text or in the appendix, depending on how important the issues are.

Risk of bias assessments should be summarised for each trial (perhaps in the appendix), and a general statement made about the overall of risk of bias findings and any subsequent impact on

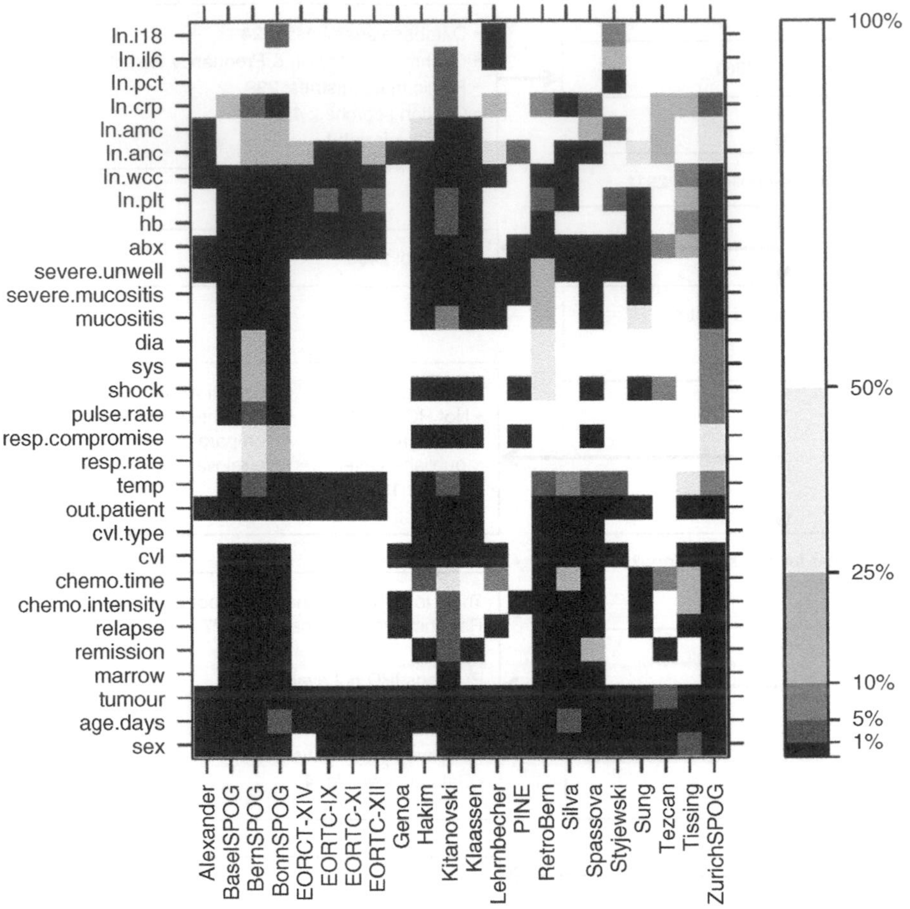

Figure 10.2 Example of a figure displaying the extent and pattern of missing data for each variable of interest (*y*-axis) in each of the studies (*x*-axis) within the IPD meta-analysis project of Phillips et al.[54] Lighter shading indicates a higher percentage of patients with missing data. *Source:* Figure is re-drawn using the original data, but is adapted from Figure 1 of Phillips et al.,[54] with permission, © 2016 Cancer Research UK (CC BY-NC-SA 4.0). Original figure uses colour (which is preferable), with shades of green indicating a high proportion of data available and red alerting to where there was much missing data.

analyses. There may be interrelations between risk of bias and data checking; these might be shown be adding additional columns to a standard risk of bias diagram to indicate whether data checking revealed any concerns about individual trials (Chapter 4).

Results of syntheses (PRISMA-IPD 20, 21, 23)

Results of all analyses should be reported, although not all need to be presented in detail within the main body of the paper. Some may be signposted and presented as appendix material available for readers who wish to explore them further. Care should be taken that this is done sensibly, and is not based on the direction or size of effects. Generally, all main outcomes should be described in the main body of the paper, but whether additional outcomes need to be included will be a matter of judgment. It is also important to note whether any planned analyses were not carried out and the reason for this.

Whether each outcome presented was pre-specified should be stated, alongside the numbers of trials and participants and, where applicable, the number of events on which it is based. Summary results and relevant statistics should be reported for each meta-analysis undertaken, including summary effect estimates and their confidence intervals, and measures of statistical heterogeneity. These may be tabulated or included on a forest plot (which also readily presents the numbers of included trials, participants and events). Results should be presented with a non-statistical audience in mind, so that as many people as possible can understand the findings. For example, coefficients from a one-stage logistic or Cox regression model relate to a log odds ratio or a log hazard ratio, respectively, which are not intuitively understood. Reporting these as odds ratios or hazard ratios makes them easier to understand, and it may be helpful to explain how to interpret each measure, at least for the first outcome presented. It may also be useful to present treatment effects for binary (or survival) outcomes as differences on the absolute risk scale (at a particular time-point), in addition to ratios such as risk ratios or hazard ratios. For example, a large risk ratio might at first sight appear dramatic, but may be of little clinical relevance if the underlying absolute risk, and absolute improvement, is small (a large percentage of a small number remains a small number). However, translation of treatment effects to the absolute scale is non-trivial, especially in the meta-analysis setting where they may be between-trial heterogeneity in the treatment effect, in addition to participant-level variability in baseline risk.[55–59] It is even more complex when there are genuine treatment-covariate interactions (Chapter 7). Using example baseline risks that are plausible for the populations considered may provide useful illustration, as might presenting a range of estimates that are representative of key patient groups.

Forest plots are recommended, as they enable readers to visually examine the overall meta-analysis estimates, any inconsistency in results across trials, and the precision and percentage weight of individual trials. They usually display two-stage IPD meta-analysis results, as the two-stage process naturally involves calculating trial-specific estimates, their percentage weights, and the summary meta-analysis result (Chapter 5). In contrast, a one-stage analysis avoids calculating trial-specific estimates and percentage trial weights can be calculated only after model estimation.[60] However, some software packages can force forest plots to display percentage trial weights and summary results from a one-stage meta-analysis (for example, using the option 'first' within the Stata package *metan*[61]), whilst still displaying trial-specific estimates.[60,62] A summary plot illustrating meta-analysis results for a number of outcomes (i.e. not showing individual trial results) can also be a useful way of presenting findings, particularly for IPD meta-analysis projects with many outcomes.

Any sensitivity and additional analyses should also be reported. These may be described very briefly if they indicate consistent patterns to the main analysis (along with a signpost to where the full results are presented in supplemental material), but require more detailed presentation and discussion if their findings are discrepant to the main analysis conclusions.

As described in earlier chapters, a major motivation for undertaking an IPD meta-analysis project is the ability to explore between-trial heterogeneity and participant-level variation in treatment response (Chapter 7). The latter is particularly important, as it allows analyses to assess whether there are any particular types (subgroups) of participants who benefit more or less from the treatment under investigation, and this is likely to be of real interest to decision-makers.[63,64] When reporting such analyses, it is vital to state whether or not there is any clear and convincing evidence of a difference in outcome by participant characteristics. As well as being of clinical relevance, any such variation may explain heterogeneity in results between trials.

Risk of bias across trials and other analyses (PRISMA-IPD 22)

Risk of bias in the body of evidence for which IPD are available should be described. As outlined in Chapter 9, this should include consideration of the impact that unavailable trials might have on the IPD meta-analysis results, including, where relevant, any differences in the characteristics or trial quality between available and unavailable trials. Where appropriate, sensitivity analyses that include extracted aggregate data for unavailable trials may provide an indication of the robustness of the IPD meta-analysis results to missing data. As described in Chapter 9, funnel plots may be used to examine whether there is evidence of small-study effects, and thus potential for unidentified trials due to publication-related biases. It may also be helpful to describe any concerns about reasons trial authors gave for not making their IPD available, and to note that trials not providing IPD could not be subject to the same independent scrutiny as those that did provide IPD. GRADE may provide a useful framework for considering the risk of bias for the whole body of evidence.[65]

10.2.5 PRISMA-IPD Discussion and Funding Sections (Table 10.3)

Discussion (PRISMA-IPD 24, 25, 26, A4)

The discussion should usually begin with a brief summary of the IPD obtained and main findings for the key outcomes. It is not necessary to repeat all the results or to restate them in detail. Results should be drawn together to form a coherent narrative examining the plausibility of findings and consistency (or not) of effect across outcomes and individuals, rather than reiterating a series of effect estimates. This narrative should reference benefits and harms as appropriate.

The discussion should also consider important strengths and limitations of the evidence, which again might usefully be considered in the GRADE framework.[52] This section will usually include a brief reminder of the benefits of the IPD approach and that data have been scrutinised and analysed by an independent team. How trial investigators were involved and how potential for academic bias was mitigated may be mentioned briefly. Any shortcomings of the data should be highlighted, along with the potential impact of data that were unavailable and any mitigation such as sensitivity analyses that incorporated aggregate data for missing trials or analyses that imputed missing data.

Results should also be considered with reference to any important existing evidence, for example existing good-quality reviews of aggregate data or existing, possibly smaller, IPD syntheses, noting similarity and dissimilarity of findings, including consideration of why results might differ (if they do). It may also be helpful to describe how findings align with current practice, for example recommendations in major national or international guidelines. The discussion is also the place to consider unexpected findings, to bring external evidence to bear and outline new ideas or hypotheses generated by findings, if appropriate.

Whether or not specific recommendations are made for practice will depend on the strength of evidence and also on the nature of funding and contract with commissioners. For example, some commissioners require that reports present the evidence, but do not make direct recommendations for practice. Clear recommendations regarding future research should be given where appropriate; vague statements such as the ubiquitous "further research is needed" are best avoided.

Funding (PRISMA-IPD 27)

The source of funding or other support for the review should be stated, along with the role of those providing funds or support.

10.3 Additional Means of Disseminating Findings

Whilst publishing an IPD meta-analysis project in an academic journal is important, it will not necessarily reach all intended audiences directly, and taking more active steps to engage with relevant audiences may improve uptake and implementation of research findings. Given their increased time and resource requirements, IPD meta-analysis projects are likely to be reserved for questions of significant public health importance, for questions that are intractable to conventional systematic review and meta-analysis, or in areas of controversy. Therefore, it is, perhaps, even more important than for conventional reviews that efforts are made to make sure that IPD meta-analysis findings are accessible to intended audiences. This may require using a variety of channels, media and approaches to reach different target audiences, and thinking creatively about how to present complex findings in ways that they are more readily understood. This is not straightforward, and it is important to think about developing a dissemination plan in the early stages of an IPD meta-analysis project (including through patient and public involvement and engagement), rather than it being something that is left until the end.

Next, we briefly consider three routes to brokering knowledge to key audiences of particular relevance to IPD meta-analysis projects: (i) the trial investigators involved in the project collaborative group, who may serve as a conduit to relevant clinical and research audiences; (ii) clinical guideline developers as a route to a broad clinical and policy-making audience; and (iii) support groups and charities as a means of reaching relevant patient and public audiences. We also consider also some types of materials that can be produced to help facilitate this engagement. There is a broad and more general literature on dissemination and knowledge translation and mobilisation that may be drawn on.[66–68]

10.3.1 Key Audiences

10.3.1.1 The IPD Collaborative Group

An added benefit of involving trial investigators in a collaborative IPD meta-analysis project is that they can provide a direct channel to relevant clinical and research communities, often on an international basis. Dissemination activity may start by holding a dedicated collaborators' meeting that brings trial investigators together to discuss projects results. As well as serving as an incentive to collaborate, such a meeting can be helpful in gaining a common understanding of findings, possibly highlighting a range of views and perspectives held by group members, which may also be reflective of the wider clinical community. Discussion of results and their implications can therefore provide important context and information that may be drawn on in the final report or publication. This can be followed by providing members of the group with dissemination materials that they may use to cascade information about the project findings within their own groups and communities. Materials can include, for example, a set of IPD meta-analysis project slides that they can use in their own presentations, copies of any evidence summaries or policy briefs produced, short statements, links or infograms that they may tweet or share on other social media.

10.3.1.2 Patient and Public Audiences

Working with patient support groups and charities, (groups that are often highly skilled in communication) provides a patient or public perspective that can help frame the project and findings, and provides a direct route to relevant patients and public audiences. As well as co-producing plain-language summaries and non-technical briefings, patient and public groups may provide an opportunity to produce material (blogs, videos, etc.) specifically for group newsletters, websites, and associated social media. Whilst IPD meta-analysis projects may benefit considerably from patient and public involvement and engagement, the nature of engagement differs from clinical trials, and therefore expectations need to be managed carefully. For example, an IPD meta-analysis project cannot obtain outcomes that matter to patients if they have not been recorded in the included trials, although the IPD meta-analysis publications may usefully highlight the lack of such outcomes in previous trials.

10.3.1.3 Guideline Developers

Although it might be expected that guideline developers would actively seek the results of IPD meta-analyses as best evidence to inform guidelines, this is not necessarily the case. A study comparing 33 IPD meta-analyses with 177 matched clinical guidelines (medical condition, treatments, populations, and dates of publication) found that only 37% of guidelines cited a matched IPD meta-analysis.[44] Recommendations based directly on a matched IPD meta-analysis were identified for only 18 guidelines, suggesting that IPD meta-analyses are being under-utilised in the development of clinical guidelines. Hence, an important target audience for IPD meta-analysis projects should be relevant clinical guidelines developers. As well as encouraging them to routinely seek good-quality up-to-date IPD meta-analyses to inform guidelines, those undertaking IPD meta-analyses could also reach out to relevant guideline developers to inform them of progress. Again, this is something that is best explored in the early stages of the project, as letting developers know in advance when an IPD meta-analysis project is likely to be completed may help them in planning their own timelines.

10.3.2 Communication Channels

10.3.2.1 Evidence Summaries and Policy Briefings

Short summaries or briefings may provide a useful way of reaching audiences who may not have the time to read, or skills to understand, academic journal publications. These can be presented in a visually appealing way, take a more conversational approach to describing the project (e.g. what problem did we address/what did we do/what did we find/what does it mean) and provide 'bottom line' messaging. If the summary comes from a reliable and trusted source this may be all the information that some decision-makers need to decide to pursue further and, for example, tasking someone within the organisation to read the associated full paper or report and explore implications within their own setting. Whilst briefings and bulletins are becoming increasingly used to broker information about health research, they have thus far not been widely used for IPD meta-analyses. We believe that they can provide a useful way to brief and catch the attention of those whom we would like to pay attention to our results.

10.3.2.2 Press Releases

Although not all research project findings are newsworthy, given the nature, scale and often high-profile topic areas of IPD meta-analysis projects, a press release will often be warranted. This is usually best done by working with an institutional or organisational press office to develop a clear and accurate statement that is engaging, but does not exaggerate, and which provides journalists with the basic background information and sources that they would need for a story. An example press release is given in Box 10.1. As most journals issue their own press releases it is important to

Box 10.1 Example of a press release issued for an IPD meta-analysis project[69]

York Researchers Question the Effectiveness and Safety of Bone Growth Product

The advantage of a controversial product used to promote bone growth has been questioned by research from the Centre for Reviews and Dissemination (CRD) at the University of York.

Recombinant human bone morphogenetic protein-2 (rhBMP-2) is an orthobiologic agent used to promote bone growth in spinal surgery. In 2011, after serious questions were raised about the product's safety and efficacy in the USA, Yale University brokered an unprecedented agreement with the manufacturer, Medtronic, to release all of its patient-level clinical research data for unrestricted independent scrutiny. Yale then appointed two teams, CRD and the Evidence-based Practice Center at Oregon Health & Science University, to separately assess and reanalyse the company's data.

Researchers at York conducted a systematic review of benefits and harms. They re-analysed individual participant data from all Medtronic-sponsored randomised controlled trials (RCTs) comparing rhBMP-2 with usual practice of ileac crest bone graft (ICBG), and from one other RCT. They also reviewed adverse event data from 35 published observational studies. Published in *Annals of Internal Medicine,* the research found that, compared to ICBG, rhBMP-2 increases the chance of joining the vertebrae, but that this does not translate to clinically meaningful reduction in pain or improvements in function or quality of life. The small benefits in these outcomes, which are seen from six months after operation, also come at the expense of more pain immediately after surgery and the possibility of an increased albeit small absolute risk of cancer.

CRD Director Professor Lesley Stewart, who led the York-based team, said, "This has been a ground-breaking project. As well as addressing an important clinical question, the project has set a new standard in transparency and release of trial data for independent scrutiny – a development that is in the public interest and an issue that is currently being examined by the UK Parliamentary Select Committee on clinical trials. It was also reassuring to find that working completely independently the two teams reached the same broad conclusions."

Professor Stewart added, "Clinicians should discuss these findings with their patients so that they can make informed choices about the type of surgery they would prefer."

Notes for Editors

1) Simmonds MC, Brown JA, Heirs MK, Higgins JT, Mannion RJ, Rodgers MA, Stewart LA. Safety and effectiveness of recombinant human bone morphogenetic protein-2 (BMP-2). *Annals of Internal Medicine* 2013;158(12):877–889).
2) *Annals of Internal Medicine* attribution is required for all coverage.
3) For an embargoed copy of a study, contact ...
4) This study used data obtained from the Yale University Open Data Access Project (http://medicine.yale.edu/core/projects/yodap/index.aspx) that included clinical trials of rhBMP-2 funded by Medtronic. Analysis, interpretation, and reporting of the data are the sole responsibility of the authors and do not necessarily represent the views of the Yale Project.
5) Further information can be obtained from ...

Source: Lesley Stewart.

liaise with them and to make sure that embargo timings (the time before which journalists cannot post stories) are aligned.

It is worth remembering that issuing a press release is the beginning rather than the end of a process, and that members of the team will need to be prepared to talk to journalists who decide to pick up the story. It can be helpful to share additional plain-language briefing materials and to think about what quotes are needed. As a journalist may wish to pursue several angles and perspectives, it is important to think about which members of the project team are willing, and best placed, to talk to the press. In particular, there may be an opportunity to draw on clinicians from different countries within the IPD meta-analysis collaboration, to disseminate the findings internationally. Clearly, those put forward for dissemination must have a shared understanding of the project and its findings.

10.3.2.3 Social Media

Twitter is becoming increasingly used to promote research findings, as it can quickly generate attention through retweets and comments. Tweeting and sharing links to journal articles can be a good way of encouraging people with an interest in the area to access and read an IPD meta-analysis paper. It can also be a way to provide plain-language summaries to a public audience. An interesting way of doing this may be to tweet an 'infogram' or pictorial representation of the project, which is an emerging means of communicating with non-technical audiences. Twitter can also direct those interested to visit project, departmental, institutional, organisational websites, blogs, videos and other media sources. Using other social media platforms such as Facebook to share content may also be valuable, but often these require people to seek out content, and may therefore be more effective as part of a larger endeavour that has already built an interested audience and following.

10.4 Concluding Remarks

IPD meta-analysis projects generally address important problems with the intent of improving health and well-being. To achieve this, they must be completed to high standards and their findings communicated in ways that reach and are understood by decision-makers, including patients, practitioners and policy-makers. Academic papers should be reported transparently and clearly, using as accessible language as possible. PRISMA-IPD, and associated checklist and flow diagram, provides a framework to help researchers ensure that the essential elements of an IPD meta-analysis project's design, conduct and findings are included in academic reports and journal articles. However, to maximise uptake and impact, dissemination should not stop at academic publication. Different types of outputs can be prepared and tailored for different audiences, and social media, blogs, videos, press releases and lay summaries can enhance communication and reach a broader audience.

11

A Tool for the Critical Appraisal of IPD Meta-Analysis Projects (CheckMAP)

Jayne F. Tierney, Lesley A. Stewart, Claire L. Vale, and Richard D. Riley

Summary Points

- Evidence suggests that not all published IPD meta-analysis projects are completed to the same standard.
- Collecting, checking and synthesising IPD is more complex than for conventional meta-analyses that use existing aggregate data, with a myriad of potential choices and issues to address, including those relating to data collection and integrity, bias assessment and statistical modelling.
- This complexity can make it challenging for researchers, clinicians, patients, policy-makers, funders and publishers to judge the quality of planned or completed IPD meta-analysis projects.
- CheckMAP is a tool for critically appraising a completed IPD meta-analysis project evaluating the effects of a treatment. It enables stakeholders to recognise a high-quality IPD meta-analysis project, to help ensure that the most robust findings are used to inform policy, practice and subsequent research.

11.1 Introduction

Part 1 of this book explains how the IPD approach can bring about substantial improvements to the quantity and quality of data included (for example, more trials, participants and outcomes) compared to conventional meta-analyses based on published aggregate data, as well as enabling standardisation of outcomes across trials and detailed data checking. IPD also allows greater scope and flexibility in the analyses (Part 2), including the ability to investigate whether a treatment is more or less effective for different types of participants (Chapter 7).[10,70,71,79] These advantages help provide more in-depth investigations, and potentially more detailed and robust meta-analysis results.[72–77]

However, not all IPD meta-analyses projects are done to the same standard,[11,19] and they too can suffer from bias in their design and conduct (Chapter 9). In particular, with greater analytical flexibility comes more opportunity for erroneous modelling decisions that can affect the reliability and robustness of the results. Added to that, the process of collecting, checking and meta-analysing IPD is more complex than for aggregate data. All these issues can make it difficult for researchers, clinicians, patients, policy-makers, funders and publishers to judge the quality of IPD meta-analysis

Individual Participant Data Meta-Analysis: A Handbook for Healthcare Research, First Edition.
Edited by Richard D. Riley, Jayne F. Tierney, and Lesley A. Stewart.

projects, which could in turn hinder their uptake and implementation, for example, in clinical guidelines,[44] clinical practice, and the design of new trials.[78] Our two previous chapters in Part 3 are aimed primarily at those conducting IPD meta-analysis projects, describing how to examine the impact of potential biases on their results (Chapter 9), and how to best report and disseminate findings (Chapter 10). In contrast, this chapter is written principally to guide those reading and using IPD meta-analysis proposals, protocols and particularly findings. It provides and describes the CheckMAP tool for Checking and appraising Meta-Analyses of Participant data that aim to evaluate the efficacy of treatments, and are based on randomised trials (Box 11.1).

11.2 The CheckMAP Tool

The CheckMAP tool provides a list of signalling questions to consider when checking and appraising an IPD meta-analysis project (Box 11.1), and answers of 'yes' to questions are indicative of higher quality. The following sections describe the different elements of the tool, and how it might be applied, and are illustrated using an IPD meta-analysis project that aimed to assess the effects of chemotherapy prior to local treatment on outcomes in operable non-small-cell lung cancer.[80]

A summary of the CheckMAP assessment provides a useful overview of the quality of a particular IPD meta-analysis project. The summary for the lung cancer example is shown in Table 11.1, and is based on information reported in the project's publication and, in some instances, the protocol. The answer to most of the CheckMAP signalling questions is 'yes', suggesting the project was of good quality, albeit with some caveats. In particular, it was done within the context of a systematic review, generally used appropriate methods, included a substantial proportion of eligible IPD, and, for the most part, the analyses were pre-specified and reported transparently. There is some lack of clarity regarding the checking of trial and data quality, but on balance, these are relatively minor issues. The absence of planned analyses of toxicity and quality of life analyses is perhaps a greater oversight, preventing a complete picture of the benefits and harms of pre-operative chemotherapy for non-small-cell lung cancer patients.

11.3 Was the IPD Meta-Analysis Project Done within a Systematic Review Framework?

A key component of appraising an IPD meta-analysis project evaluating treatment effects is determining whether it has been done as part of a systematic review.[10,70,71,79] If so, then the steps taken to minimise potential bias throughout the review process should be clear, for example in the identification and selection of trials, and in planned meta-analyses. When reading the report of an IPD meta-analysis project it may not be immediately clear whether the project was carried out within a systematic review framework, because the terminology of reviews and meta-analysis has evolved over time, and IPD meta-analyses are used in both systematic and non-systematic approaches to evidence synthesis (Chapter 2). In our lung cancer example, however, the publication title and introduction specifies that the IPD meta-analysis was in the context of a systematic review.[80]

Box 11.1 Checklist of signalling questions to consider when appraising an IPD meta-analysis project evaluating the effects of treatments (CheckMAP tool), adapted from Tierney et al.[79]

1) Was the IPD meta-analysis project done within a systematic review framework?
2) Were the methods of the IPD meta-analysis project pre-specified in a publicly available protocol?
3) Did the IPD meta-analysis project have a clear research question qualified by explicit eligibility criteria for trials and participants?
4) Did the IPD meta-analysis project use a systematic and comprehensive search to identify trials?
   - Were fully published trials sought?
   - Were trials published in the grey literature sought?
   - Were unpublished trials sought?
5) Was the approach to data collection consistent and thorough?
   - Were key baseline variables defined and sought?
   - Were key outcomes defined and sought?
6) Were IPD obtained for most of the eligible trials and their participants?
   - Were IPD obtained for a large proportion of eligible trials?
   - Were these trials likely to be representative of all high-quality trials?
   - Were IPD obtained for a large proportion of eligible participants?
   - Were the reasons for not obtaining IPD provided?
7) Was the quality of the IPD checked for each trial?
   - Were the data checked for missing, invalid, out-of-range or inconsistent items?
   - Were the data checked for discrepancies with the trial report?
   - Were any issues queried with trial investigators, and either resolved or addressed?
8) Was the risk of bias assessed for each trial and informed by checks of the associated IPD?
   - Was the randomisation process checked based on the IPD?
   - Were the IPD checked to ensure that all (or most) trial participants were included?
   - Were all important outcomes included in the IPD?
   - Were the outcomes measured/defined appropriately?
   - Was the quality of outcome data checked?
9) Were the methods of meta-analysis appropriate?
   - Were the analysis methods pre-specified in detail and the key estimands (target parameters) defined (e.g. average treatment effect; treatment-covariate interaction)?
   - Were the methods of summarising overall effects of treatments appropriate?
     - Did researchers account for clustering of participants within trials in their meta-analysis methods?
     - Was the choice of one- or two-stage meta-analysis framework appropriate, and was the choice specified in advance and/or were results for both approaches provided?
     - Was between-trial heterogeneity in treatment effects examined and accounted for?
     - Were other statistical intricacies accounted for (e.g. non-proportional hazards, clustering of trials with a cluster randomised design, etc)?
   - Were the methods of assessing whether effects of treatments varied by trial-level characteristics appropriate?

(Continued)

Box 11.1 (Continued)

- Were the methods of assessing whether effects of treatments vary by participant-level characteristics appropriate?
  - Did researchers estimate a treatment-covariate interaction separately for each trial and combine these across trials in a two-stage common-effect or random-effects meta-analysis? Or
  - Did researchers incorporate treatment-covariate interaction terms in a one-stage regression model, whilst also accounting for clustering of participants, and separating these participant-level interactions from any trial-level associations?
  - Were continuous covariates analysed on their continuous scale? Were potential non-linear relationships examined?
- Was the robustness of conclusions checked using relevant sensitivity or other analyses?
  - E.g. removing trials at high risk of bias, including aggregate data from trials that did not supply IPD, examining asymmetry on funnel plots

10) Did the IPD meta-analysis project's main report cover the items described in the Preferred Reporting Standards for Systematic Reviews and Meta-Analyses of IPD (The PRISMA-IPD Statement[43]), or explain why they were not relevant?

Source: Adapted from Tierney et al.[79] with permission.

In the absence of a clear statement, and to be convinced that a project reported as a systematic review is indeed one, the following hallmarks indicate whether this is likely:

- A publicly available protocol or other pre-specified plan
- A clear research question, qualified by unambiguous eligibility criteria relating to participants, settings, interventions, comparisons and outcomes
- An explicit, systematic and comprehensive search strategy, to ensure that all relevant trials are identified
- A thorough and consistent approach to data collection, including an explanation of which items were requested
- Assessment of risk of bias of included trials
- Meta-Analysis methods pre-planned in detail in a protocol or statistical analysis plan
- Two or more researchers independently checking classifications at each stage (e.g. trial inclusion, risk of bias), with any discrepancies resolved

11.4 Were the IPD Meta-Analysis Project Methods Pre-specified in a Publicly Available Protocol?

To limit bias, ensure transparency and allow scrutiny, all methods pertaining to the IPD meta-analysis project should have been set out in a protocol. Ideally, such a protocol would have been registered in the PROSPERO international prospective register of systematic reviews,[81] or the full protocol published in a journal or on a project website so that the planned methods could be accessed and evaluated more easily. Date 'stamping' of each version of the protocol provides important insurance against unscrupulous post-hoc posting of the protocol or protocol amendments, prior to publication. The report of the lung cancer IPD meta-analysis clearly states that all the

Table 11.1 Summary of completion of the CheckMAP tool for an IPD meta-analysis project of pre-operative chemotherapy for non-small-cell lung cancer.

CheckMAP signalling question	Answer and relevant supporting information for the non-small-cell lung cancer IPD meta-analysis project
1) Was the IPD meta-analysis done within a systematic review framework?	**Yes** Title and introduction states that it was part of a systematic review.
2) Were all of the methods pre-specified in a publicly available protocol?	**Yes** Protocol was available upon request (N.B. written before systematic review protocol registration or publication was commonplace).
3) Did it have a clear research question qualified by explicit eligibility criteria for trials and participants?	**Yes**
4) Did it use a systematic and comprehensive search to identify trials?	**Yes** Published and unpublished trials were sought from bibliographic databases, study registers and grey literature, and searches were updated regularly.
5) Was the approach to data collection consistent and thorough?	**Yes, mostly** IPD were sought for important baseline variables and outcomes, for all participants randomised, and updated follow-up was sought. Aggregate data on toxicity and quality of life were not analysed as planned
6) Were IPD obtained for most trials for most of the eligible trials and their participants?	**Yes** 15/19 trials, representing 92% of participants from all eligible trials
7) Was the quality of the IPD checked for each trial?	**Yes** IPD were checked for missing, invalid or inconsistent data, data validity and consistency, and these were resolved, and the final dataset verified with the trial contact.
8) Was the risk of bias assessed for each trial and informed by checks of the associated IPD?	**Yes** • Checked randomisation pattern and the balance of baseline characteristics by allocation group • Data on all but two participants from included trials were available and analysed on an intention-to-treat basis • All relevant outcomes were included except toxicity and quality of life • All outcomes were clearly defined, and some were constructed from the IPD to avoid bias in the comparison of groups. • Checked to see if follow-up was up-to-date and balanced by allocation group
9) Were the methods of meta-analysis appropriate?	**Yes** • Analyses were planned in considerable detail • Used a two-stage meta-analysis, assuming a common treatment effect, with a random-effects model to allow for between-study heterogeneity in treatment effect also applied as a sensitivity analysis

(Continued)

Table 11.1 (Continued)

CheckMAP signalling question	Answer and relevant supporting information for the non-small-cell lung cancer IPD meta-analysis project
	• Used a two-stage meta-analysis of within-trial interactions • Planned analyses of the effects of early stopping, plus exploratory analysis by trial and participant characteristics to investigate the main results
10) Did the project's report cover the items described in PRISMA-IPD,[43] or explain why they were not relevant?	**Yes, mostly** Project pre-dates PRISMA IPD. Most items were covered, but there was a lack of information or detail on eligibility screening, data management and risk of bias assessment

Source: Jayne Tierney.

methods had been pre-specified in a protocol,[80] and because this protocol was "available on request", users would be able to confirm which methods had been planned.

11.5 Did the IPD Meta-Analysis Project Have a Clear Research Question Qualified by Explicit Eligibility Criteria?

As for conventional systematic reviews, IPD meta-analysis projects require that explicit objectives and eligibility criteria are pre-specified to minimise bias in the selection of trials, participants and possibly outcomes for inclusion.[10,70,79] IPD meta-analysis projects must be viewed with caution if they have an unclear or unduly selective approach to including trials, or do not include known trials published in the grey literature (Chapter 9).[19] The objectives for the lung cancer project are clearly described in the main publication:[80] "Therefore, we did a systematic review and meta-analysis of individual participant data to provide more reliable and up-to-date evidence on the effect of pre-operative chemotherapy on survival and other key outcomes and whether this varies by patient subgroup." Also, the inclusion and exclusion criteria are summarised in the project publication,[7] with greater detail given in the protocol.

11.6 Did the IPD Meta-Analysis Project Have a Systematic and Comprehensive Search Strategy?

Clear objectives and eligibility criteria should have been backed up by a systematic and comprehensive search that seeks to identify all relevant trials.[82] In particular, given the substantial evidence that publication of research studies, including randomised trials, is influenced by the nature of study results,[83] ideally all relevant published and unpublished trials would have been sought to limit publication bias (Chapter 4). Of course, even with researchers' best efforts, all trials may not come to light, but the potential effects of missing trials can and should be explored (Chapter 9). Although not essential, a search strategy that extends to ongoing trials can be very useful for providing proper context. For example, if relevant ongoing trials are identified, the IPD meta-analysis results could change with their subsequent inclusion, and so the report might suggest a plan to update the meta-analysis at a later date, once IPD from those trials become available.

The lung cancer IPD meta-analysis protocol describes a comprehensive search for published and unpublished trials via bibliographic databases, conference proceedings, trial registers and reference lists of review article and trial publications, and these are summarised in the trial report. Whilst dates for all sources are not provided in the publication, it does say that searches were regularly updated until May 2013 (the manuscript was submitted in June 2013).[80]

11.7 Was the Approach to Data Collection Consistent and Thorough?

An IPD meta-analysis project should have adopted a thorough and consistent approach to IPD collection (Chapter 4). Hence, all key baseline and outcome variables of relevance to the objectives of the project should have been defined at the outset and sought from trial investigators.

For the lung cancer IPD meta-analysis project, a full list of the variables sought is listed in the protocol and summarised in the publication:[80] "For all eligible trials and all patients who were randomised, data were sought on the date of randomisation, treatment allocation, type of chemotherapy and number of cycles, age, sex, histology, performance status, date of surgery, extent of resection, clinical and pathological tumour stage, clinical and pathological response, recurrence, survival, cause of death, and date of last follow-up."

11.8 Were IPD Obtained from Most Eligible Trials and Their Participants?

Assuming that most trials are of good quality and considered to be at low risk of bias, IPD meta-analyses should include a large proportion of the eligible trials and participants to provide the greatest power (Chapter 12), and to limit the potential impact of unavailable trials (Chapter 9). If the available data can be shown to provide sufficient power to detect an effect reliably, and are suitably representative of the target population(s) and setting(s) of interest, then a lower proportion may be acceptable (Chapter 12). Either way, the proportion of trials and participants for which IPD are available, and reasons for unavailability of data, should have been reported (Chapter 10).[43]

If a substantial proportion of potentially eligible IPD is not obtained, data availability bias is a potential concern (Chapter 9). Sometimes this can be investigated by comparing or combining results based on IPD with those based on aggregate data, to check for compatibility.[26] However, this requires that suitable aggregate data are available for non-IPD trials, and this may not be possible. In certain situations, funnel plots may also help indicate the potential for missing trials, if they show funnel plot asymmetry (i.e. small study effects) (Chapter 9).[15]

The lung cancer IPD meta-analysis project's publication states that findings are based on IPD from 15 out of 19 eligible trials, representing 92% of participants randomised.[80] It also gives a clear account of the potential impact of the unavailable trials and participants on the results for the primary outcome of survival; in particular, the impact of an additional trial for which only aggregate data results could be obtained: "Although this meta-analysis included most patients known to have been randomised, four eligible trials (198 patients) could not be included. We could estimate an HR for survival for one trial of 90 patients, but not the remaining three trials ... When the single estimated HR was combined with the overall result for the meta-analysis, the effect on survival remained the same (HR 0.87, $p = 0.006$)."

Also, preceding the results for each outcome, the authors describe the amount of information included in the analysis and any limitations, for example, for mortality within 30 days of surgery: "Mortality within 30 days of surgery could be calculated for nine trials (1611 patients, 52 deaths) that supplied date of surgery. Four of these had no deaths within 30 days of surgery in either arm and an odds ratio was not estimable".

11.9 Was the Validity of the IPD Checked for Each Trial?

The IPD for each trial should have been checked for missing, invalid, out-of-range or inconsistent values, and for any discrepancies with those reported within the trial publication or other report (Chapter 4).[10,70] Any issues should be queried, and, where possible, resolved with the associated trial investigators, both improving data quality and ensuring that trials are represented accurately.

The lung cancer IPD meta-analysis publication states that:[80] "Standard methods were used to identify missing data and to assess data validity and consistency" and "any inconsistencies were resolved and the final dataset verified by the relevant trial contact." Whilst more detail would have been helpful, and the protocol did not help in this regard, the statement provides some reassurance that data had been checked for quality.

11.10 Was the Risk of Bias Assessed for Each Trial and Its Associated IPD?

Assessing the risk of bias of included trials is a key component of systematic reviews, and well-conducted IPD meta-analysis projects should be no exception.[34] Any issues with the included trials should be identified and acknowledged, and their impact on the reliability of subsequent IPD meta-analysis results should be examined (Chapter 9). This should include direct checking of the IPD (Chapter 4), and not just assessments based on trial publications and/or protocols. Collaborating trial investigators can then help to explain issues that arise, and may even help alleviate them by providing additional data or information (Chapter 4).[84]

Chapter 4 outlines the sort of risk of bias signalling questions that are needed in IPD meta-analysis projects, and in the following sections, the key issues to be summarised as part of the project report are explained briefly. Although neither the lung cancer IPD meta-analysis publication nor project protocol specifically mention using a risk of bias tool, quality checks of included trials were applied, as now described.

11.10.1 Was the Randomisation Process Checked Based on IPD?

It is vital that the IPD for each trial are checked to ensure that randomisation and allocation concealment were implemented appropriately, and therefore that each trial provides a fair comparison of treatments (Chapter 4).[85] For example, the IPD can be used to examine the pattern of allocation of participants to treatment groups over time, and to check whether participant characteristics are reasonably balanced by group (Chapter 4). IPD meta-analyses that have incorporated such checks will safeguard against the inclusion of trials that purport to be randomised, but turn out not to be, and the inclusion of non-randomised participants.

This was the approach taken in the lung cancer IPD meta-analysis project, as described in the publication: "Patterns of treatment allocation and the balance of baseline characteristics by treatment group were used to check randomisation integrity", and the risk of bias was judged to be low.[80]

11.10.2 Were the IPD Checked to Ensure That All (or Most) Randomised Participants Were Included?

IPD should have been checked to ensure that data on all or as many randomised participants as possible were collected and included in the meta-analysis, because even with adequate randomisation methods, fair comparison of treatment groups requires that all randomised participants are included, and then analysed using an intention-to-treat approach.[86–88] If participants have dropped out or been excluded from trial analyses in considerable numbers, and this is disproportionate by treatment group, this can cause attrition bias.[89] There may be good reasons why certain types of participants were excluded from an IPD meta-analysis, for example, if they represented a subset of participants from a trial that were not relevant to the meta-analysis objectives. However, to avoid bias, the intention to exclude particular subsets of participants should have been pre-specified as part of the meta-analysis eligibility criteria, and the exclusions applied consistently across trials and treatment groups.[90]

For the lung cancer IPD meta-analysis project, it is made clear in the publication that data were "sought for all patients randomised into each trial",[80] and indeed the researchers were able to obtain data for all participants who had been excluded from the original trial analyses (although not for two other participants): "... data were obtained for all 24 patients excluded from the investigators' original analyses, and reinstated in this meta-analysis." Also, the publication specifies that the analyses were conducted on an intention-to treat basis.[80]

11.10.3 Were All Important Outcomes Included in the IPD?

IPD meta-analysis projects should aim to include data on all relevant outcomes for all included trials, to provide a balanced view of benefits and harms, and pre-specify what these are. A major advantage is that the trial investigators may be able to supply IPD incorporating more outcomes than reported in their trial publications. This circumvents the potential for outcome reporting bias that can arise if the effect of a treatment varies by outcome, and only particular outcomes are reported, such as those showing benefit.[39] Even so, it is unlikely that all trials will have recorded all outcomes, in which case a multivariate IPD meta-analysis may also be useful, to synthesise all outcomes jointly and account for their correlation (Chapter 13).

The protocol for the lung cancer IPD meta-analysis project states that IPD would be sought for survival and progression outcomes, surgical resection rates and post-operative mortality, but not for toxicity or quality of life. Instead, the plan was to make use of "the available information on toxicity and quality of life reported in trial publications". However, the effects of pre-operative chemotherapy on toxicity are described only briefly in the discussion section of the project publication,[80] and quality of life is not included.

11.10.4 Were the Outcomes Measured/Defined Appropriately?

IPD meta-analysis projects should have included outcomes that have been measured, or at least defined, appropriately. Even if this was not done in the original trial, access to IPD allows the opportunity to rectify any inappropriate outcome measurement, by re-defining or constructing new ones and doing this consistently across trials (Chapter 4).[10,70,79] As well as facilitating subsequent pooling of data, this helps to provide the most reliable and readily interpretable results.

In the lung cancer IPD meta-analysis project all the outcomes are clearly defined, particularly in the appendix of the protocol, and in such a way that they could be standardised across trials. In addition, the cancer recurrence outcomes were re-defined based on a "landmark time of 6 months after the date of randomisation to allow for the difference in timing of surgery between the two treatment groups", in order to minimise bias in the comparison of the treatments.

11.10.5 Was the Quality of Outcome Data Checked?

The quality of trial outcome data should have been checked. For example, the timing of recording of continuous and binary outcomes should be similar for those in treatment and control groups, otherwise this may lead to bias in their comparison. For time-to-event outcomes, bias can occur if participants are followed up (monitored) more frequently or for a longer duration on one treatment group compared to another, as this may cause discrepant event rates between groups even when there are no genuine differences (Chapter 4).[79]

The publication of the lung cancer IPD meta-analysis project explains that "the follow-up of surviving patients was checked to ensure it was up to date and balanced by arm". In addition, up-to-date follow-up was requested in order that researchers could "report on longer-term outcomes", and whilst it was not clear how much extra follow-up was obtained for each of the included trials, the publication states that "the effects of early stopping" of some of the included trials "were minimised by the collection of updated follow-up".[80]

11.11 Were the Methods of Meta-Analysis Appropriate?

Unlike a conventional meta-analysis of existing aggregate data, an IPD meta-analysis project is not reliant on the analyses used in the original trials. Rather, the IPD can be utilised directly, and provides the opportunity for a whole range of statistical analysis methods, which generally are more complex than those used in aggregate data meta-analysis (Part 2), thereby making them more difficult to appraise by non-experts. To supplement Part 2, we now outline some key principles that should be considered when appraising the statistical methods used in an IPD meta-analysis project.

11.11.1 Were the Analyses Pre-specified in Detail and the Key Estimands Defined?

The objectives, broad analytical approach and corresponding statistical methods for an IPD meta-analysis project should have been pre-specified in a protocol and/or statistical analysis plan. This is because IPD offers the potential for substantially greater numbers of analyses, and there is a greater risk that data might be interrogated repeatedly until the desired results are obtained, with only those that are 'significant' being published subsequently. This is not to say that unplanned analyses are unjustified or invalid; rather they can play an important role in explaining or adding to per-protocol results. However, such exploratory analyses should have been justified and clearly labelled as such in any report of the results (Chapter 10).[43]

The main body of the protocol for the lung cancer IPD meta-analysis project gives an overview of the planned analytic approach, including: the primary and secondary outcomes; analyses of the overall effects of chemotherapy versus control, and by various trial-level and participant-level characteristics. In addition, an appendix provides greater detail, such as outcome definitions, the statistical models and how relative effects will be translated to absolute effects. The publication aligns closely to this pre-specified plan, and where it does not, usually a clear explanation is given. For example: "For the overall resection rate, ORs [odds ratios] could not be estimated for four trials because they had 100% resection rates in both arms. The remaining seven trials represented less than half of the total data and, with possible variation in the classification of extent of incomplete resection, this analysis was deemed unreliable." A number of analyses that were not pre-specified in the protocol are described in the publication, and are clearly flagged as exploratory, such as: "... exploratory analyses do suggest a synergistic effect of combining preoperative and postoperative chemotherapy on time to metastases".

11.11.2 Were the Methods of Summarising the Overall Effects of Treatments Appropriate?

A key component of an IPD meta-analysis is that it should have been stratified to account for clustering of participants within trials.[91] If, instead, IPD from all trials have been analysed as if coming from a single 'mega' trial, this could lead to biased comparisons of treatments and over-precise estimates of effect (Chapter 6). As described in Part 2, stratification can be achieved via a two-stage approach, or an appropriate one-stage model (e.g. linear, logistic, or Cox regression) that includes a separate intercept for each trial. One-stage and two-stage methods usually produce similar meta-analysis results, although differences can arise when trials have few events or participants, or when they use different estimation methods (Chapter 8).[92] It is important, therefore, that the choice (and specification) of one-stage or two-stage analysis is specified in advance (together with estimation methods), or that results for both approaches are reported.[93]

In the lung cancer IPD meta-analysis protocol, whilst not explicitly described as such, the detailed analysis appendix shows that a two-stage approach, assuming a common treatment effect, was planned for the primary analysis of all the outcomes, with a random-effects model used to examine the robustness of findings when between-trial heterogeneity in the treatment effect was allowed for. This is summarised in the project publication,[80] for example, for time-to-event outcomes: "... we used the log-rank expected number of events and variance to calculate hazard ratio (HR) estimates of effect for each individual trial, which were then combined across trials using a stratified-by-trial, two-stage, fixed [common]-effect model. The random-effects model was used to assess the robustness of the results."

11.11.3 Were the Methods of Assessing whether Effects of Treatments Varied by Trial-level Characteristics Appropriate?

Exploring whether the magnitude of a treatment effect is associated with *trial*-level characteristics, such as the duration of the treatment or dose of drugs, should have been investigated formally, for example using a meta-regression including trial-level covariates.[94] Meta-regression models in either the second stage of the two-stage approach, and as part of a one-stage model, are described in Chapters 5 and 6. A similar approach is when trials are grouped by trial-level characteristics, and their meta-analysis results compared using a formal test (for between-group heterogeneity).

The lung cancer meta-analysis pre-specified and reported on a number of such trial group analyses, for example:[80] "There is no clear evidence that the effect of chemotherapy on survival differed according to whether chemotherapy was given preoperatively or both preoperatively and postoperatively."

11.11.4 Were the Methods of Assessing whether Effects of Treatments Varied by Participant-level Characteristics Appropriate?

Establishing if particular types of participants gain importantly larger (or smaller) treatment effects than others should have been based on estimating and summarising within-trial treatment-covariate interactions, as this is the most reliable approach to inform clinical decision-making and policy. How to achieve this is detailed in Chapter 7 and elsewhere.[95] Many existing IPD meta-analyses have used inappropriate analyses, however.[96] In particular, one-stage analyses often include an interaction term, but without separating out within-trial and across-trial relationships, with the latter potentially introducing aggregation bias. [30,95,97] A related mistake is comparing a two-stage IPD meta-analysis of treatment effects in one participant group, say men, with a separate two-stage IPD meta-analysis of treatment effects in another, say women, using a test for interaction (sometimes called subgroup analyses).[95] This is a method that has, and continues to be been used by many groups worldwide,[96] even though it has now been shown to be inappropriate due to potential aggregation bias, and better methods are available (Chapter 7).[95–97]

The lung cancer project represents an early example of a two-stage IPD meta-analysis project estimating treatment-covariate interactions within trials, and pooling these across trials:[80] "Cox regressions including the relevant treatment by subgroup interaction term will be conducted within trials and the interaction coefficients (HRs) pooled across trials using a fixed [common]-effect model."

11.11.5 Was the Robustness of Conclusions Checked Using Relevant Sensitivity or Other Analyses?

Sensitivity or other analyses to test the robustness of the results are a frequent step for any systematic review and meta-analysis (e.g. to examine assumptions or to explain findings), and ideally, they would have been pre-specified in the protocol or analysis plan. However, given that the full nature of the results will not be known until the gamut of analyses have been conducted, it is perfectly reasonable for additional exploratory analyses to take place. As stated previously, it is important that such post-hoc analyses have been described as such in the IPD meta-analysis project's publication.

For example, in the lung cancer meta-analysis, the investigators wanted to check whether the difference in effect they observed between trials that did or did not stop before reaching their accrual target was being driven by small trials. Therefore, the researchers conducted an additional sensitivity analysis excluding these small trials, and the difference was no longer evident: "An exploratory analysis, excluding smaller trials (100 patients or fewer), was based on 80% of the data (77% of all deaths), and showed no clear difference in effect between trials stopping early and those reaching their target accrual."

11.11.6 Did the IPD Meta-Analysis Project's Report Cover the Items Described in PRISMA-IPD?

Ideally, IPD meta-analysis projects should have been reported according to PRISMA-IPD guidelines (Chapter 10),[43] or at least be described in sufficient detail so that users can thoroughly understand the methods used, and interpret the results appropriately.

Whilst the conduct and publication of the lung cancer IPD meta-analysis project precedes the publication of PRISMA-IPD, the paper does provide most of the items listed in the checklist. However, there is a lack of information or detail on the processes for eligibility screening, data management and risk of bias assessment, and the abstract does not include all the required elements.

11.12 Concluding Remarks

The CheckMAP tool (Box 11.1), and the associated guidance included in this chapter, should help stakeholders to critically check the quality and robustness of reported IPD meta-analysis projects. Specialist expertise may be required to navigate and appraise the more complicated items, in particular, those related to the statistical methods for IPD meta-analysis. Realistically, an IPD meta-analysis project is unlikely to be perfect in all respects, but if it is conducted in the context of a systematic review, includes a high proportion of good-quality data, and pre-specifies and uses appropriate analyses, it is more likely to provide reliable findings.

Our CheckMAP checklist and guidance on critical appraisal has focused on IPD meta-analyses projects that examine the efficacy of one particular treatment compared to a control. However, much is transferrable to other types of IPD meta-analysis, such as network meta-analysis of multiple treatments (Chapter 14) and those for diagnosis, prognosis and prediction (Part 5), although aspects relating to risk of bias and analytical approaches may need to be tailored accordingly.

Part III References

1 Simes RJ. Publication bias: the case for an international registry of clinical trials. *J Clin Oncol* 1986;4(10):1529–1541.

2 Sterne JA, Egger M, Smith GD. Systematic reviews in health care: investigating and dealing with publication and other biases in meta-analysis. *BMJ* 2001;323(7304):101–105.

3 Sutton AJ, Duval SJ, Tweedie RL, et al. Empirical assessment of effect of publication bias on meta-analyses. *BMJ* 2000;320(7249):1574–1577.

4 Rothstein HR, Sutton AJ, Borenstein ME. *Publication Bias in Meta-analysis*. Chichester, UK: Wiley 2005.

5 Turner EH, Matthews AM, Linardatos E, et al. Selective publication of antidepressant trials and its influence on apparent efficacy. *N Engl J Med* 2008;358(3):252–260.

6 Smith R. What is publication? *A continuum. BMJ* 1999;318:142.

7 Ioannidis JPA. Effect of the statistical significance of results on the time to completion and publication of randomized efficacy trials. *JAMA* 1998;279:281–286.

8 Clarke M, Stewart LA. Time lag bias in publishing clinical trials (letter). *JAMA* 1998;279:1952–1953.

9 Stewart L, Tierney J, Burdett S. Do systematic reviews based on individual patient data offer a means of circumventing biases associated with trial publications? In: Rothstein HR, Sutton AJ, Borenstein M, eds. *Publication Bias in Meta-Analysis: Prevention, Assessment and Adjustments*. Chichester, UK: Wiley 2006.

10 Stewart LA, Tierney JF. To IPD or not to IPD? Advantages and disadvantages of systematic reviews using individual patient data. *Eval Health Prof* 2002;25(1):76–97.

11 Riley RD, Lambert PC, Abo-Zaid G. Meta-analysis of individual participant data: rationale, conduct, and reporting. *BMJ* 2010;340:c221.

12 Riley RD. Commentary: like it and lump it? Meta-analysis using individual participant data. *Int J Epidemiol* 2010;39(5):1359–1361.

13 Burdett S, Stewart LA, Tierney JF. Publication bias and meta-analyses: a practical example. *Int J Technol Assess Health Care* 2003;19(1):129–134.

14 Egger M, Davey Smith G, Schneider M, et al. Bias in meta-analysis detected by a simple, graphical test. *BMJ* 1997;315(7109):629–634.

15 Sterne JAC, Sutton AJ, Ioannidis JPA, et al. Recommendations for examining and interpreting funnel plot asymmetry in meta-analyses of randomised controlled trials. *BMJ* 2011;342:d4002.

16 Moreno SG, Sutton AJ, Turner EH, et al. Novel methods to deal with publication biases: secondary analysis of antidepressant trials in the FDA trial registry database and related journal publications. *BMJ* 2009;339:b2981.

17 Peters JL, Sutton AJ, Jones DR, et al. Contour-enhanced meta-analysis funnel plots help distinguish publication bias from other causes of asymmetry. *J Clin Epidemiol* 2008;61:991–996.

Individual Participant Data Meta-Analysis: A Handbook for Healthcare Research, First Edition.
Edited by Richard D. Riley, Jayne F. Tierney, and Lesley A. Stewart.

18 Sterne JA, Gavaghan D, Egger M. Publication and related bias in meta-analysis: power of statistical tests and prevalence in the literature. *J Clin Epidemiol* 2000;53(11):1119–1129.

19 Ahmed I, Sutton AJ, Riley RD. Assessment of publication bias, selection bias and unavailable data in meta-analyses using individual participant data: a database survey. *BMJ* 2012;344:d7762.

20 Duval S, Tweedie R. Trim and fill: A simple funnel-plot-based method of testing and adjusting for publication bias in meta-analysis. *Biometrics* 2000;56(2):455–463.

21 DeLuca G, Gibson CM, Bellandi F, et al. Early glycoprotein IIb-IIIa inhibitors in primary angioplasty (EGYPT) cooperation: an individual patient data meta-analysis. *Heart* 2008;94 (12):1548–1558.

22 Moreno SG, Sutton AJ, Ades AE, et al. Assessment of regression-based methods to adjust for publication bias through a comprehensive simulation study. *BMC Med Res Methodol* 2009;9:2.

23 Terrin N, Schmid CH, Lau J, et al. Adjusting for publication bias in the presence of heterogeneity. *Stat Med* 2003;22(13):2113–2126.

24 Martineau AR, Jolliffe DA, Hooper RL, et al. Vitamin D supplementation to prevent acute respiratory tract infections: systematic review and meta-analysis of individual participant data. *BMJ* 2017;356:i6583.

25 Holmes MV. Rapid response to: Vitamin D supplementation to prevent acute respiratory tract infections: systematic review and meta-analysis of individual participant data. *BMJ* 2017;356:i6583.

26 Riley RD, Simmonds MC, Look MP. Evidence synthesis combining individual patient data and aggregate data: a systematic review identified current practice and possible methods. *J Clin Epidemiol* 2007;60(5):431–439.

27 Nevitt SJ, Marson AG, Davie B, et al. Exploring changes over time and characteristics associated with data retrieval across individual participant data meta-analyses: systematic review. *BMJ* 2017;357:j1390.

28 Tsujimoto Y, Fujii T, Onishi A, et al. No consistent evidence of data availability bias existed in recent individual participant data meta-analyses: a meta-epidemiological study. *J Clin Epidemiol* 2020;118:107–114.e5.

29 Vale C, Tierney JF, Stewart LA, et al. Reducing uncertainties about the effects of chemoradiotherapy for cervical cancer: a systematic review and meta-analysis of individual patient data from 18 randomized trials. *J Clin Oncol* 2008;26(35):5802–5812.

30 Riley RD, Lambert PC, Staessen JA, et al. Meta-analysis of continuous outcomes combining individual patient data and aggregate data. *Stat Med* 2008;27(11):1870–1893.

31 Sutton AJ, Kendrick D, Coupland CA. Meta-analysis of individual- and aggregate-level data. *Stat Med* 2008;27:651–669.

32 McCormack K, Scott N, Grant A. *Are trials with individual patient data available different from trials without individual patient data available? 9th Annual Cochrane Colloquium Abstracts*, Lyon, France, 2001.

33 Greb A, Bohlius J, Schiefer D, et al. High-dose chemotherapy with autologous stem cell transplantation in the first line treatment of aggressive non-Hodgkin lymphoma (NHL) in adults. *Cochrane Database of Systematic Reviews* 2008(1):CD004024.

34 Sterne JAC, Savovic J, Page MJ, et al. RoB 2: a revised tool for assessing risk of bias in randomised trials. *BMJ* 2019;366:l4898.

35 Rogozinska E, Marlin N, Jackson L, et al. Effects of antenatal diet and physical activity on maternal and fetal outcomes: individual patient data meta-analysis and health economic evaluation. *Health Technol Assess* 2017;21(41):1–158.

36 White IR, Higgins JP, Wood AM. Allowing for uncertainty due to missing data in meta-analysis – part 1: two-stage methods. *Stat Med* 2008;27(5):711–727.

37 Bell ML, Kenward MG, Fairclough DL, et al. Differential dropout and bias in randomised controlled trials: when it matters and when it may not. *BMJ* 2013;346:e8668.

38 Clarke MJ, Stewart LA. Obtaining data from randomised controlled trials: how much do we need for reliable and informative meta-analyses?. In: Chalmers I, Altman DG, eds. *Systematic Reviews*. London, UK: BMJ Publishing 1995:37–47.

39 Kirkham JJ, Dwan KM, Altman DG, et al. The impact of outcome reporting bias in randomised controlled trials on a cohort of systematic reviews. *BMJ* 2010;340:c365.

40 McCormack K, Grant A, Scott N. Value of updating a systematic review in surgery using individual patient data. *Br J Surg* 2004;91(4):495–499.

41 Riley RD, Price MJ, Jackson D, et al. Multivariate meta-analysis using individual participant data. *Res Synth Method* 2015;6:157–174.

42 Kirkham JJ, Riley RD, Williamson PR. A multivariate meta-analysis approach for reducing the impact of outcome reporting bias in systematic reviews. *Stat Med* 2012;31(20):2179–2195.

43 Stewart LA, Clarke M, Rovers M, et al. Preferred Reporting Items for Systematic Review and Meta-Analyses of individual participant data: the PRISMA-IPD Statement. *JAMA* 2015;313(16):1657–1665.

44 Vale CL, Rydzewska LH, Rovers MM, et al. Uptake of systematic reviews and meta-analyses based on individual participant data in clinical practice guidelines: descriptive study. *BMJ* 2015;350:h1088.

45 Hutton B, Salanti G, Caldwell DM, et al. The PRISMA extension statement for reporting of systematic reviews incorporating network meta-analyses of health care interventions: checklist and explanations. *Ann Intern Med* 2015;162(11):777–784.

46 Cohen JF, Korevaar DA, Altman DG, et al. STARD 2015 guidelines for reporting diagnostic accuracy studies: explanation and elaboration. *BMJ Open* 2016;6(11):e012799.

47 McShane LM, Altman DG, Sauerbrei W, et al. Reporting recommendations for tumor marker prognostic studies (REMARK). *J Natl Cancer Inst* 2005;97(16):1180–1184.

48 Collins GS, Reitsma JB, Altman DG, et al. Transparent reporting of a multivariable prediction model for individual prognosis or diagnosis (TRIPOD): the TRIPOD statement. *BMJ* 2015;350:g7594.

49 Moher D, Liberati A, Tetzlaff J, et al. Preferred reporting items for systematic reviews and meta-analyses: the PRISMA statement. *BMJ* 2009;339:b2535.

50 Liberati A, Altman DG, Tetzlaff J, et al. The PRISMA statement for reporting systematic reviews and meta-analyses of studies that evaluate healthcare interventions: explanation and elaboration. *BMJ* 2009;339:b2700.

51 Simmonds M, Stewart G, Stewart L. A decade of individual participant data meta-analyses: a review of current practice. *Contemp Clin Trials* 2015;45(Pt A):76–83.

52 Guyatt GH, Oxman AD, Vist GE, et al. GRADE: an emerging consensus on rating quality of evidence and strength of recommendations. *BMJ* 2008;336(7650):924–926.

53 Guyatt G, Oxman AD, Akl EA, et al. GRADE guidelines: 1. Introduction – GRADE evidence profiles and summary of findings tables. *J Clin Epidemiol* 2011;64(4):383–394.

54 Phillips RS, Sung L, Ammann RA, et al. Predicting microbiologically defined infection in febrile neutropenic episodes in children: global individual participant data multivariable meta-analysis. *Br J Cancer* 2016;114(12):e17.

55 Kent DM, van Klaveren D, Paulus JK, et al. The Predictive Approaches to Treatment effect Heterogeneity (PATH) statement: explanation and elaboration. *Ann Intern Med* 2020;172(1): W1–W25.

56 Kent DM, Paulus JK, van Klaveren D, et al. The Predictive Approaches to Treatment effect Heterogeneity (PATH) statement. *Ann Intern Med* 2019;172(1):35–45.

57 Kent DM, Nelson J, Dahabreh IJ, et al. Risk and treatment effect heterogeneity: re-analysis of individual participant data from 32 large clinical trials. *Int J Epidemiol* 2016;45(6):2075–2088.

58 Kent DM, Nelson J, Altman DG, et al. Treatment effect heterogeneity in clinical trials: an evaluation of 13 large clinical trials using individual patient data. *Value Health* 2014;17(7):A543–A544.

59 Kent DM, Steyerberg E, van Klaveren D. Personalized evidence based medicine: predictive approaches to heterogeneous treatment effects. *BMJ* 2018;363:k4245.

60 Riley RD, Ensor J, Jackson D, et al. Deriving percentage study weights in multi-parameter meta-analysis models: with application to meta-regression, network meta-analysis and one-stage individual participant data models. *Stat Methods Med Res* 2018;27(10):2885–2905.

61 Harris R, Bradburn M, Deeks J, et al. metan: fixed- and random-effects meta-analysis. *Stata Journal* 2008;8(1):3–28.

62 Burke DL, Ensor J, Snell KIE, et al. Guidance for deriving and presenting percentage study weights in meta-analysis of test accuracy studies. *Res Synth Methods* 2018;9(2):163–178.

63 Riley RD, van der Windt D, Croft P, et al., editors. *Prognosis Research in Healthcare: Concepts, Methods and Impact*. Oxford, UK: Oxford University Press, 2019.

64 Hingorani AD, Windt DA, Riley RD, et al. Prognosis research strategy (PROGRESS) 4: stratified medicine research. *BMJ* 2013;346:e5793.

65 Guyatt GH, Oxman AD, Vist G, et al. GRADE guidelines: 4. Rating the quality of evidence – study limitations (risk of bias). *J Clin Epidemiol* 2011;64(4):407–415.

66 Grimshaw JM, Eccles MP, Lavis JN, et al. Knowledge translation of research findings. *Implementation Science* 2012;7(1):50.

67 Straus S, Tetroe J, Graham ID. *Knowledge Translation in Health Care: Moving from Evidence to Practice*. West Sussex, UK: Wiley 2013.

68 https://www.nihr.ac.uk/documents/knowledge-mobilisation-research/22598

69 Simmonds MC, Brown JV, Heirs MK, et al. Safety and effectiveness of recombinant human bone morphogenetic protein-2 for spinal fusion: a meta-analysis of individual-participant data. *Ann Intern Med* 2013;158(12):877–889.

70 Stewart LA, Clarke MJ. Practical methodology of meta-analyses (overviews) using updated individual patient data. *Cochrane Working Group. Stat Med* 1995;14(19):2057–2079.

71 Tierney JF, Stewart LA, Clarke M. Individual participant data. In: Higgins JPT, Chandler TJ, Cumpston M, et al., eds. *Cochrane Handbook for Systematic Reviews of Interventions*. London, UK: Cochrane 2019.

72 Duchateau L, Pignon JP, Bijnens L, et al. Individual patient- versus literature-based meta-analysis of survival data: time to event and event rate at a particular time can make a difference, an example based on head and neck cancer. *Control Clin Trials* 2001;22(5):538–547.

73 Stewart LA, Parmar MK. Meta-analysis of the literature or of individual patient data: is there a difference? *Lancet* 1993;341:418–422.

74 Jeng GT, Scott JR, Burmeister LF. A comparison of meta-analytic results using literature vs individual patient data: paternal cell immunization for recurrent miscarriage. *JAMA* 1995;274(10):830–836.

75 EU Hernia Trialists Collaboration. Value of updating a systematic review in surgery using individual patient data. *Br J Surgery* 2004;91:495–499.

76 Tudur Smith C, Marcucci M, Nolan SJ, et al. Individual participant data meta-analyses compared with meta-analyses based on aggregate data. *Cochrane Database Syst Rev* 2016;9:MR000007.

77 Tierney JF, Fisher DJ, Burdett S, et al. Comparison of aggregate and individual participant data approaches to meta-analysis of randomised trials: an observational study. *PLoS Med* 2020;17(1): e1003019.

78 Tierney JF, Pignon J-P, Gueffyier F, et al. How individual participant data meta-analyses can influence trial design and conduct. *J Clin Epidemiol* 2015;68(11):1325–1335.

79 Tierney JF, Vale C, Riley R, et al. Individual participant data (IPD) meta-analyses of randomised controlled trials: guidance on their use. *PLoS Med* 2015;12(7):e1001855.

80 NSCLC Meta-analysis Collaborative Group. Preoperative chemotherapy for non-small cell lung cancer: a systematic review and meta-analysis of individual participant data. *Lancet* 2014;383:1561–1571.

81 Booth A, Clarke M, Ghersi D, et al. An international registry of systematic-review protocols. *Lancet* 2011;377(9760):108–109.

82 Lefebvre C, Glanville J, Briscoe S, et al. Chapter 4: Searching for and selecting studies. In: Higgins JPT, Thomas J, Chandler J, et al., eds. *Cochrane Handbook for Systematic Reviews of Interventions* version 60 (updated July 2019) (Available from www.training.cochrane.org/handbook): Cochrane, 2019.

83 Dickersin K. Publication bias: recognising the problem, understanding its origins and scope, and preventing harm. In: Rothstein H, Sutton A, Borenstein M, eds. *Publication Bias in Meta-Analysis: Prevention, Assessment and Adjustments*. Chichester, UK: Wiley 2005:261–286.

84 Stewart L, Tierney J, Burdett S. Do systematic reviews based on individual patient data offer a means of circumventing biases associated with trial publications? In: Rothstein H, Sutton A, Borenstein M, eds. *Publication Bias in Meta-Analysis: Prevention, Assessment and Adjustments*. Chichester, UK: Wiley 2005:261–286.

85 Higgins JPT, Altman DG, on behalf of the Cochrane Statistical Methods Group and the Cochrane Bias Methods Group. Assessing risk of bias in included studies. In: Higgins JPT, Green S, eds. *Cochrane Handbook for Systematic Reviews of Interventions*. Chichester, UK: Wiley 2008:187–241.

86 Altman DG. Randomisation. *BMJ* 1991;302:1481–1482.

87 Lachin JM. Statistical considerations in the intent-to-treat principle. *Contr Clin Trials* 2000;21:167–189.

88 Schulz KF, Grimes DA. Sample size slippages in randomised trials: exclusions and the lost and wayward. *Lancet* 2002;359:781–785.

89 Juni P, Altman DG, Egger M. Systematic reviews in health care: assessing the quality of controlled clinical trials. *BMJ* 2001;323(7303):42–46.

90 Tierney JF, Stewart LA. Investigating patient exclusion bias in meta-analysis. *Int J Epidemiol* 2005;34(1):79–87.

91 Abo-Zaid G, Guo B, Deeks JJ, et al. Individual participant data meta-analyses should not ignore clustering. *J Clin Epidemiol* 2013;66(8):865–873 e4.

92 Burke DL, Ensor J, Riley RD. Meta-analysis using individual participant data: one-stage and two-stage approaches, and why they may differ. *Stat Med* 2017;36(5):855–875.

93 Stewart GB, Altman DG, Askie LM, et al. Statistical analysis of individual participant data meta-analyses: a comparison of methods and recommendations for practice. *PLoS One* 2012;7(10):e46042.

94 Deeks JJ, Higgins JP, Altman DG. Analysing data and undertaking meta-analyses. In: Higgins JP, Green S, eds. *Cochrane Handbook for Systematic Reviews of Interventions*. Chichester, UK: Wiley 2008.

95 Riley RD, Debray TPA, Fisher D, et al. Individual participant data meta-analysis to examine interactions between treatment effect and participant-level covariates: statistical recommendations for conduct and planning. *Stat Med* 2020;39(15):2115–2137.

96 Fisher DJ, Carpenter JR, Morris TP, et al. Meta-analytical methods to identify who benefits most from treatments: daft, deluded, or deft approach? *BMJ* 2017;356:j573.

97 Fisher DJ, Copas AJ, Tierney JF, et al. A critical review of methods for the assessment of patient-level interactions in individual participant data meta-analysis of randomized trials, and guidance for practitioners. *J Clin Epidemiol* 2011;64(9):949–967.

Part IV

Special Topics in Statistics

12

Power Calculations for Planning an IPD Meta-Analysis

Richard D. Riley and Joie Ensor

Summary Points

- Before IPD collection, exploring the statistical power of a planned IPD meta-analysis can provide valuable insight about the value and viability of the project. It can indicate when the power is likely to be too low even if IPD were obtained from the majority of trials; conversely, it can provide reassurance that even with a conservative assumption about IPD availability, the resulting power is likely to be sufficient.
- The power of an IPD meta-analysis depends on the research aim (e.g. to examine a treatment-covariate interaction), the number of trials and the number of participants (and events) for which IPD can potentially be obtained, and many intricate aspects including the distribution of covariate values and magnitude of assumed effects.
- Closed-form solutions to calculate the power of an IPD meta-analysis for treatment-covariate interactions are available for continuous outcomes; these utilise likelihood-based solutions for the variance of the summary interaction estimate which depend only on sample sizes, residual variances, and variance of covariate values. Such information can be extracted from trial publications.
- Closed-form solutions for binary and time-to-event outcomes are difficult to derive reliably before IPD collection, due to participant-level response variances being conditional on their actual covariate values, which are unknown without IPD.
- A flexible alternative is to use simulation-based power calculations, where IPD meta-analysis datasets of a particular size (chosen to reflect the trials promising their IPD) are generated multiple (e.g. 10,000) times based on a particular data-generating model, and on each occasion an IPD meta-analysis is performed to estimate the effect of interest. The proportion of simulated datasets that give a p-value < 0.05 (or equivalently a confidence interval excluding the null) provides the estimated power.
- Power calculations also reveal which trials contribute most to the power, which can be useful if needed to prioritise IPD collection from a subset of trials (i.e. those that provide the most information) due to time and resource constraints. A trial's contribution does not just depend on sample size or number of events, but also other factors, in particular the variance of covariate values.
- In addition to calculating power, researchers may also want to check that their IPD meta-analysis will give precise enough estimates of the effect of interest, to ensure that confidence intervals will be sufficiently narrow to inform clinical decision making.
- IPD meta-analysis results might also inform the sample size required for a new primary study.

Individual Participant Data Meta-Analysis: A Handbook for Healthcare Research, First Edition.
Edited by Richard D. Riley, Jayne F. Tierney, and Lesley A. Stewart.

12.1 Introduction

12.1.1 Rationale for Power Calculations in an IPD Meta-Analysis

Part 1 of this book emphasises how IPD meta-analysis projects are time-consuming,[1,2] often taking upwards of two years to engage with trial investigators; obtain, clean, harmonise and meta-analyse the IPD; and publish and disseminate results. Therefore, *before* embarking on an IPD meta-analysis project, researchers and funders may want to be reassured that the time and resources required are worth the investment. This should include consideration of how many trials are likely to provide their IPD (Chapters 2 and 3) and, based on this, estimation of the potential power of the planned IPD meta-analysis.

In our experience, power calculations and sample size justifications are rarely considered in protocols or publications of IPD meta-analysis projects. It might be argued that obtaining IPD is almost always worth the investment, in order to best appraise, synthesise and summarise the existing evidence. However, if researchers knew before IPD collection that their planned IPD meta-analysis may have, say, only 30% power to detect a clinically important effect, then they might reconsider whether the project should be initiated. Conversely, if a planned IPD meta-analysis has a potential power of over 80%, then researchers and funders will be more reassured that the required resources are worth investment. Power calculations could also reveal which trials contribute most to the power, and so direct which trials are sought. This last point is contentious, as many will argue that IPD should *always* be sought from *all* trials. The counter-argument is that IPD meta-analysis projects are time-consuming, and sometimes limited resources are available or there is an urgent clinical need for evidence synthesis (e.g. in a pandemic); then, it may be justified to focus on obtaining IPD from the subset of trials that provide the most information to answer the research question reliably and in the shortest time frame.

12.1.2 Premise for This Chapter

In this chapter we explain how to estimate the power of a planned IPD meta-analysis, in advance of IPD collection. Our premise is that an IPD meta-analysis project is required to answer a particular research question, and that a set of existing randomised trials have been identified from which IPD will be sought. Further, we assume that basic aggregate data are available for each of these trials, such as the number of participants and events in each group, and the mean and standard deviation of continuous outcomes and covariates. We show how to use such aggregate data to estimate the power of the planned IPD meta-analysis. We mainly focus on projects that aim to examine treatment-covariate interactions (treatment effect modifiers), as this is often the main objective of an IPD meta-analysis of randomised trials (Chapter 7).

We begin by introducing a motivating example of an IPD meta-analysis of randomised trials of interventions to reduce unnecessary weight gain in pregnancy, for which treatment-covariate interactions were suspected. Then, Section 12.3 outlines power calculations for such IPD meta-analyses with a continuous outcome, based on either closed-form solutions or a simulation-based approach,[3–7] and applies these to the pregnancy example. Sections 12.4 and 12.5 consider how to ascertain the contribution of particular trials toward the power calculation, and how modelling assumptions about heterogeneity, residual variances, or linearity can impact power estimates. Extensions then follow to binary or time-to-event outcomes; calculating the expected precision (rather than power) of estimates from an IPD meta-analysis project; and deriving the sample size for a new trial, conditional on IPD meta-analysis results.

12.2 Motivating Example: Power of a Planned IPD Meta-Analysis of Trials of Interventions to Reduce Weight Gain in Pregnant Women

12.2.1 Background

Thangaratinam et al.[8] systematically reviewed the effects of weight management interventions during pregnancy on maternal and fetal outcomes. One of their main outcomes was maternal weight gain, and their meta-analysis of published aggregate data from 30 randomised trials suggests that, on average, weight gain is 0.97 kg lower (95% CI: 0.34 to 1.60) for lifestyle interventions compared with control. Their paper concludes that an "IPD meta-analysis is needed to provide robust evidence on the differential effect of intervention in various groups based on BMI, age, parity, socio-economic status and medical conditions in pregnancy", and so recommends synthesis of IPD to examine potential treatment-covariate interactions.

In 2012 the Weight Management in Pregnancy International IPD Collaboration (i-WIP) was established to carry out such an IPD meta-analysis project and subsequently a grant application was submitted for funding. At the time of developing the grant application, 14 trials (including 1183 women) had provisionally agreed to provide their IPD. A meta-analysis of the published treatment effect estimates from these 14 trials gives a summary mean difference of −0.84 kg (95% CI: −1.63 to −0.06), which is a similar result to the aforementioned aggregate data meta-analysis of 30 trials, suggesting that this subset of 14 trials promising their IPD is broadly representative of the original set of trials.

12.2.2 What Is the Power to Detect a Treatment-BMI Interaction?

A main objective of the i-WIP project was to examine a potential interaction between baseline BMI and intervention effect. The prior hypothesis was that those with high baseline BMI may benefit most from weight management interventions, and the grant application noted that "our IPD meta-analysis provides an efficient way to substantially increase the sample size, without the need for a new trial". However, no formal power calculation was performed. The remainder of this chapter will consider, retrospectively, how a power calculation could have helped the i-WIP collaborators and their prospective funders, by providing quantitative reassurance about the power of their project. In particular, we will describe power calculations that could have been implemented before IPD retrieval based on the published aggregate data for eligible trials.

12.3 Power of an IPD Meta-Analysis to Detect a Treatment-covariate Interaction for a Continuous Outcome

Consider an IPD meta-analysis of multiple randomised trials, each comparing the effect of a particular treatment relative to a control using a simple parallel group design. Let i denote trial ($i = 1$ to S), n_i denote the number of participants in the ith trial, j denote participant ($j = 1$ to n_i), and x_{ij} denote allocation to either the treatment ($x_{ij} = 1$) or control ($x_{ij} = 0$) group for the jth participant in the ith trial. Let z_{ij} be a participant-level covariate of interest (e.g. the sex of participant j in trial i), observed for all participants in each trial. Finally, let γ_W denote the assumed magnitude of a genuine treatment-covariate interaction, revealing how the treatment effect (as measured on a scale such as mean difference, log risk ratio, log odds ratio, or log hazard ratio) changes for a one-unit increase in the covariate value. W is used to emphasise that this relationship is based solely on within-trial information, as recommended in Chapter 7. In this section, we describe how to estimate the power of an IPD meta-analysis to detect such an interaction for a continuous outcome. Our website (www.ipdma.co.uk) provides examples of statistical code to implement the methods.

12.3.1 Closed-form Solutions

For an IPD meta-analysis of S randomised trials with a continuous outcome, closed-form solutions are obtainable for the power to detect a treatment-covariate interaction, γ_W.[3,9] Simmonds and Higgins provide the following analytic solution for the maximum likelihood estimate of a treatment-covariate interaction for a continuous outcome in a single randomised trial (i) with two parallel groups including a total of n_i participants:[3]

$$\hat{\gamma}_{Wi} = \frac{2}{\sum_{j=1}^{n_i} z_{ij}'^2}\left(\sum_{j\in T_i} y_{ij}z_{ij}' - \sum_{j\in C_i} y_{ij}z_{ij}'\right)$$

Here, T_i denotes the treatment group and C_i the control group in trial i, and z_{ij}' denotes that each z_{ij} is centered about the trial-specific mean value of z_{ij} (that is, $z_{ij}' = z_{ij} - \bar{z}_i$). Simmonds and Higgins used this to derive subsequent power calculations,[3] assuming residual variances are common to all trials. Riley et al. extended their work by allowing for different residual variances in each trial (σ_i^2) (though common for treatment and control groups in the same trial),[9] and derive the variance (var) of the interaction estimate in a particular trial i as:

$$\begin{aligned}\operatorname{var}(\hat{\gamma}_{Wi}) &= \operatorname{var}\left(\frac{2}{\sum_{j=1}^{n_i} z_{ij}'^2}\left(\sum_{j\in T_i} y_{ij}z_{ij}' - \sum_{j\in C_i} y_{ij}z_{ij}'\right)\right)\\ &= \frac{4}{\left(\sum_{j=1}^{n_i} z_{ij}'^2\right)^2}\left(\sum_{j\in T_i} z_{ij}'^2 \operatorname{var}(y_{ij}) + \sum_{j\in C_i} z_{ij}'^2 \operatorname{var}(y_{ij})\right) \\ &= \frac{4\sigma_i^2}{\left(\sum_{j=1}^{n_i} z_{ij}'^2\right)^2}\left(\sum_{j\in T_i} z_{ij}'^2 + \sum_{j\in C_i} z_{ij}'^2\right)\end{aligned} \tag{12.1}$$

Note that the solution does not depend on the actual value of $\hat{\gamma}_{Wi}$ itself. Assuming an equal number of participants in the treatment and control groups, and that the variance of the covariate ($\sigma_{z_i}^2$) in trial i is the same in each group (i.e. $\sigma^2_{z_{ij}\in T_i} = \sigma^2_{z_{ij}\in C_i} = \sigma^2_{z_i}$), then $\sum_{j=1}^{n_i} z_{ij}'^2 = n_i\sigma^2_{z_i}$ and equation (12.1) simplifies to:

$$\text{var}(\hat{\gamma}_{Wi}) = \frac{4\sigma_i^2}{\left(\sum_{j=1}^{n_i} z_{ij}'^2\right)^2}\left(\sum_{j=1}^{n_i} z_{ij}'^2\right) = \frac{4\sigma_i^2}{\sum_{j=1}^{n_i} z_{ij}'^2} = \frac{4\sigma_i^2}{n_i\sigma_{z_i}^2} \tag{12.2}$$

Using the solution for $\text{var}(\hat{\gamma}_{Wi})$ from either equation (12.1) or (12.2), Riley et al. derived a closed-form solution for the variance of the summary interaction estimate ($\hat{\gamma}_W$) from the second stage of a two-stage IPD meta-analysis.[9] Assuming a common interaction across trials (i.e. no between-trial heterogeneity), $\text{var}(\hat{\gamma})$ is simply the sum of the inverse of the variances from each trial:

$$\text{var}(\hat{\gamma}_W) = \left(\sum_{i=1}^{S} \frac{1}{\text{var}\left(\hat{\lambda}_{Wi}\right)}\right)^{-1} \tag{12.3}$$

The subsequent power to detect γ_W using the IPD meta-analysis is approximately:

$$\text{Power} = \text{Prob}\left(\frac{\hat{\gamma}_W}{\sqrt{\text{var}(\hat{\gamma}_W)}} > 1.96\right) + \text{Prob}\left(\frac{\hat{\gamma}_W}{\sqrt{\text{var}(\hat{\gamma}_W)}} < -1.96\right) \tag{12.4}$$

Thus, assuming a common interaction and that trials have equally sized groups, equations (12.2) to (12.4) lead to

$$\begin{aligned}\text{Power} &= \text{Prob}\left(\frac{\hat{\gamma}_W}{\sqrt{\text{var}(\hat{\gamma}_W)}} > 1.96\right) + \text{Prob}\left(\frac{\hat{\gamma}_W}{\sqrt{\text{var}(\hat{\gamma}_W)}} < -1.96\right)\\ &= \Phi\left(-1.96 + \hat{\gamma}_W\sqrt{\sum_{i=1}^{S}\frac{n_i\sigma_{z_i}^2}{4\sigma_i^2}}\right) + \Phi\left(-1.96 - \hat{\gamma}_W\sqrt{\sum_{i=1}^{S}\frac{n_i\sigma_{z_i}^2}{4\sigma_i^2}}\right)\end{aligned} \tag{12.5}$$

where $\Phi(x)$ is the probability of sampling a value $< x$ from the standard normal distribution. Allowing for different-sized groups in a trial (i.e. using equation (12.1) rather than (12.2)), the power calculation becomes:

$$\begin{aligned}\text{Power} = \Phi&\left(-1.96 + \hat{\gamma}_W\sqrt{\sum_{i=1}^{S}\left(\frac{\left(\sum_{j=1}^{n_i} z_{ij}'^2\right)^2}{4\sigma_i^2\left(\sum_{j\in T_i} z_{ij}'^2 + \sum_{j\in C_i} z_{ij}'^2\right)}\right)}\right)\\ + \Phi&\left(-1.96 - \hat{\gamma}_W\sqrt{\sum_{i=1}^{S}\left(\frac{\left(\sum_{j=1}^{n_i} z_{ij}'^2\right)^2}{4\sigma_i^2\left(\sum_{j\in T_i} z_{ij}'^2 + \sum_{j\in C_i} z_{ij}'^2\right)}\right)}\right)\end{aligned} \tag{12.6}$$

As before we could replace $\sum_{j=1}^{n_i} z_{ij}'^2$ with $n_i\sigma_{z_i}^2$, and similarly $\sum_{j\in T_i} z_{ij}'^2$ and $\sum_{j\in C_i} z_{ij}'^2$ could be replaced, respectively, with $n_{T_i}\sigma^2_{z_{ij}\in T_i}$ and $n_{C_i}\sigma^2_{z_{ij}\in C_i}$. Equation (12.6) is more difficult to implement than equation (12.5), and the latter should suffice when the number of participants and covariate distributions are reasonably similar in each group for all trials.

Equation (12.5) requires the user to specify $\hat{\gamma}_W$, which is unknown. We suggest replacing $\hat{\gamma}_W$ with a minimally important value for γ_W, as identified by discussion with clinical experts within the IPD meta-analysis project team. Other required values are S (the total trials either promising or assumed to provide their IPD) and, for each trial, n_i, σ_i^2, and $\sigma_{z_i}^2$ as obtained from published information (e.g. from the baseline characteristics table for a trial) or, if necessary, the original trial investigators. The residual variance (σ_i^2) might be unavailable, but a conservative approximation is to use the reported variance of outcome values (Section 12.5.3 discusses this further). Related power formulae are available for a one-stage IPD meta-analysis of continuous outcomes that amalgamates within-trial and across-trial interactions (available within the package *ipdmeta* in R)[3,5], but we do not recommend these as the interaction should be based solely on within-trial information (Chapter 7).

12.3.1.1 Application to the i-WIP Example

Recall that in the i-WIP example introduced in Section 12.2, a key objective was to examine a treatment-BMI interaction using 14 trials that promised their IPD. In advance of their IPD collection, equations (12.5) or (12.6) could have been used to estimate the power to detect a genuine treatment-BMI interaction, conditional on published aggregate data summarised in Table 12.1. To illustrate this, we applied equation (12.5) using the values for S, n_i, σ_i^2, and $\sigma_{z_i}^2$ given in

Table 12.1 Trial characteristics used in the power calculations of an IPD meta-analysis of 14 pregnancy trials aiming to estimate treatment-BMI interaction in regards to the effect on weight gain

Characteristic	Chosen values	Interpretation and justification
S	14	Number of trials in a previous aggregate data meta-analysis that had promised their IPD
n_i	Trials 1 to 14: 50, 931, 125, 85, 235, 327, 45, 12, 39, 142, 105, 84, 15, 124	Total sample size in each trial: taken from original trial publications.
σ_i^2	Trials 1 to 14: 43.25, 15.57, 119.26, 52.69, 16.98, 37.37, 33.89, 6.63, 12.93, 12.63, 15.22, 12.93, 13.78, 40.53	Residual variance: used average of the variance values for treatment and control groups as stated in original trial publications.
$\sigma_{z_i}^2$	Trial 1: 12.5, Trial 2: 25.51 Trial 3: 0.49, Trial 4: 14.77 Trial 7: 27.45, Trial 8: 12.25 Trial 10: 0.25, Trial 12: 13.45 Trial 13: 18.13, Other trials: 12.25	Variance of BMI values: taken from original trial publications (averaged across treatment groups if presented for each group separately), or if unavailable, based on average observed from other trials

Source: Table is adapted from Table 3 of Ensor et al.,[7] with permission, © 2018 Ensor et al. (CC-BY 4.0).

Table 12.1. A minimally important interaction size of −0.1 was used, as suggested by clinical experts, such that the reduction in weight is at least 1 kg larger for a 10-unit increase in BMI. Thus the power calculation is

$$\Phi\left(-1.96+\hat{\gamma}_W\sqrt{\sum_{i=1}^{S}\frac{n_i\sigma_{z_i}^2}{4\sigma_i^2}}\right)+\Phi\left(-1.96-\hat{\gamma}_W\sqrt{\sum_{i=1}^{S}\frac{n_i\sigma_{z_i}^2}{4\sigma_i^2}}\right)$$
$$=\Phi\left(-1.96-0.1\sqrt{542.02}\right)+\Phi\left(-1.96+0.1\sqrt{542.02}\right)$$
$$=\Phi(-4.288)+\Phi(0.368)$$
$$=0+0.644$$

revealing that – at the time of the funding application – the planned IPD meta-analysis had only a moderate power of 64.4% to detect a treatment-BMI interaction of −0.1. Even though there are many other benefits of undertaking an IPD meta-analysis project (Chapter 2), such low power signals that ideally additional IPD from other trials are still required, as their inclusion would improve power and increase the project's appeal to funders (Section 12.4.1).

12.3.2 Simulation-based Power Calculations for a Two-stage IPD Meta-Analysis

An alternative to using closed-form solutions is to adopt a simulation-based approach,[10–13] and this may offer more flexibility. Ensor et al. suggest simulation-based power calculations for IPD meta-analysis based on the two-stage framework described in Chapter 5.[7] The general set-up is that an IPD meta-analysis dataset of a given size is simulated and then a two-stage meta-analysis performed; that is, in the simulated IPD meta-analysis dataset, the IPD for each trial is estimated separately to obtain a treatment-covariate interaction estimate and then, in the second stage, these are combined using either a common-effect or random-effects meta-analysis model. This process is repeated m times (ideally thousands) and each time the resultant summary estimates, confidence intervals and p-values are stored. Based on a traditional frequentist paradigm, power can then be estimated by calculating the proportion of times the summary estimate was statistically significant (e.g. as defined by the associated 95% confidence interval excluding the null value, or equivalently an associated p-value < 0.05).

As in the closed-form approach, the simulation-based approach should ensure the numbers of trials and participants in each simulated trial are fixed to match those in the trials promising their IPD. This forms the basic IPD to be simulated, which is then appended with simulated covariate values for each participant in each trial (based on the distributions specified in trial publications). Finally, participant outcome values are simulated conditional on their covariate value and their treatment group allocation.[7] This requires the user to specify the information shown in Table 12.1, plus a data-generating model that includes assumed values for the prognostic effect of the covariate, the treatment effect at the average covariate value, and the treatment-covariate interaction. We refer to Ensor et al. for further details,[7] and our website (www.ipdma.co.uk) provides examples of statistical code. Papadimitropoulou et al. propose a related approach, which has the additional advantage of ensuring the basic IPD simulated for each trial always has an observed mean and standard deviation of the continuous outcome that matches exactly those reported in the trial publication for each treatment group (and thus the unadjusted treatment effect will also match that reported for each trial in every simulated dataset).[14] Covariate values then need to be appended to this basic IPD, conditional on the assumed magnitude of treatment-covariate interaction and any prognostic effect of the covariate.

The simulation-based approach allows uncertainty to be better reflected than the closed-form approach. For example, when we implemented closed-form equation (12.5) in Section 12.3.1, we replaced $\hat{\gamma}_W$ with the assumed true value of γ_W. This is not necessary when using the simulation-based approach, as the power is based on the proportion of datasets giving statistically significant results, which depends on the $\hat{\gamma}_W$ obtained from the actual IPD meta-analysis of each simulated dataset. Another advantage of the simulation-based approach is that for trials with missing information (such as the variance of the covariate of interest), the missing values can be randomly sampled from a distribution based on the observed values in other trials. For instance, in the i-WIP application the variance of BMI values was unknown in some trials (Table 12.1). When using the closed-form approach we simply replaced these with the average value from other trials (Table 12.1). However, in the simulation-based approach we could randomly draw the missing values from a uniform distribution reflecting the range of BMI variances observed in other trials.

12.3.2.1 Application to the i-WIP Example

Building on Ensor et al.,[7] we applied the simulation-based approach to the i-WIP example. Obtained power estimates are similar to those when using the closed-form approach. For example, when assuming the true treatment-BMI interaction is –0.1, the power is estimated to be 63.6% because 6,360 of 10,000 simulated IPD meta-analyses produced a statistically significant result. Recall that the corresponding closed-form estimate is very similar (64.4%), but was obtained in a few seconds, compared to about 30 minutes to run the simulation.

Further power estimates based on the simulation-based approach are shown in Figure 12.1, across a range of assumed treatment-BMI interactions of –0.01 (tiny) to –0.2 (large). Power increases as the

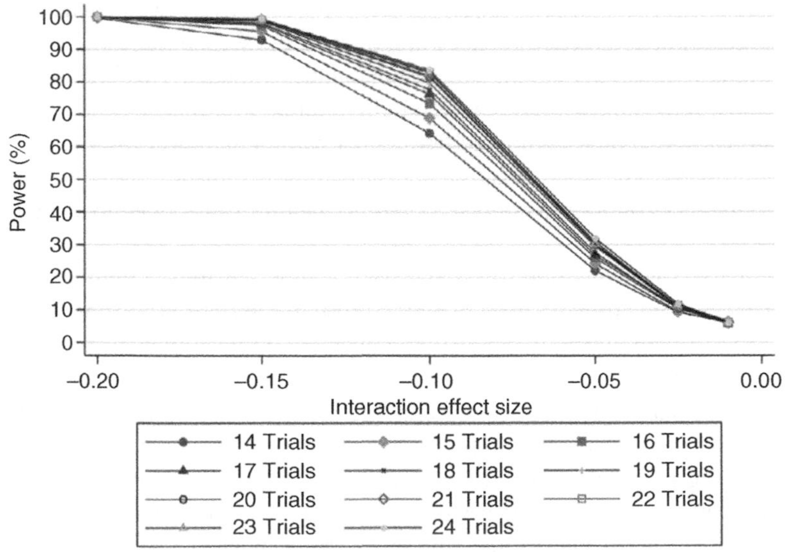

* Based on simulating an IPD meta-analysis with the same number of participants as in the trials promising their IPD, and accounting for reported distributions of BMI in each trial. For each of 10,000 simulated datasets, a two-stage IPD meta-analysis was undertaken, with the second stage using a common-effect meta-analysis of the interaction estimates.

Figure 12.1 Simulation-based power estimates (based on 10,000 replications) for the planned two-stage IPD meta-analysis of 14 to 24 trials for detecting a common treatment-BMI interaction (γ_W), across a range of assumed values for the interaction *Source:* Figure is adapted from Figure 1 of Ensor et al.,[7] with permission, © 2018 Ensor et al (CC-BY 4.0).

magnitude of the interaction estimate increases. Indeed, when the interaction is assumed to be –0.15 or larger, the power is over 90%. Therefore, the i-WIP meta-analysis of 14 trials was adequately powered to detect a genuinely large interaction, but not a minimally important one (–0.1).

12.3.3 Power Results Naively Assuming the IPD All Come from a Single Trial

It is not appropriate to approximate the power calculation for an IPD meta-analysis project by assuming the IPD comes from a single trial. This would ignore the clustering of participants and characteristics (e.g. variability of BMI) within trials, and so could lead to errors. For example, in the i-WIP application let us naively assume that the planned IPD meta-analysis of 14 trials is the same as a single trial with 2319 participants, with values for residual variance and BMI variance taken as the average values (weighted by sample size) across the 14 trials. Such an assumed trial has a power of 36.1%, which is very different from the 64% power obtained from either the simulation-based or closed-form approaches. The 'single trial' approach is naive, as there are large differences across trials in the residual variance and the BMI variance. In particular, it dilutes the contribution of the largest trial (Landon), which actually has a small residual variance and a large BMI variance, which are factors that improve power (Section 12.4.2).

12.4 The Contribution of Individual Trials Toward Power

In the i-WIP example the estimated power was about 64% when assuming γ_W was –0.1. When faced with such moderate power, IPD meta-analysis researchers might strive (even harder) to persuade additional trials to provide their IPD. A related issue is that sometimes the opportunity to obtain additional IPD arises *after* an IPD meta-analysis project has commenced and when deadlines (e.g. to funders) are on the horizon; then the decision to pursue this additional IPD (and perhaps apply for funding extensions) is more convincing when this additional IPD would substantially improve power. For such reasons, it is helpful to calculate the contribution of individual trials toward the power of an IPD meta-analysis.

12.4.1 Contribution According to Sample Size

Although 14 trials promised their IPD at the grant application stage, an additional 10 trials joined the i-WIP collaboration by the time funding was received, such that IPD from 24 trials were promised. Let us evaluate how these additional 10 trials improve the power, by adding each of the 10 new trials sequentially, from the largest to the smallest, and each time calculating the improvement in power. That is, we firstly add just the largest trial (contributing 399 additional participants) to form an IPD meta-analysis of 15 trials, and conclude with an IPD meta-analysis of 24 trials (with 1761 additional participants contributed by the additional 10 trials).

The simulation-based results are presented in Figure 12.1, which are very similar to those when rather using the closed-form approach of equation (12.5). Adding IPD from the largest trial improves power but it is still not sufficient. For example, assuming a true interaction of –0.1 the IPD meta-analysis of 15 trials has an estimated power of 69%, only a slight increase from the 64% based on the original set of 14 trials. Findings are more promising when *all* additional 10 trials are added. In particular, for a true interaction effect of –0.1, the IPD meta-analysis of 24 trials has an estimated power of 83%. This is above 80% for the first time, which is a threshold often used to indicate adequate power within a single randomised trial. Thus, with IPD from 24 trials there is large power to detect interaction effects of $\leq$ –0.1, which would have been reassuring for the i-WIP researchers to have known when their project commenced.

12.4.2 Contribution According to Covariate and Outcome Variability

Sample size is not the only criterion that will impact a trial's contribution toward power. For a treatment-covariate interaction, the standard deviation of covariate values (σ_{z_i}) is also important,[3] as evident by the variance of covariate values being included in the closed-form solution of equation (12.5). Other things being equal, those trials with larger variation in covariate values across participants will have the greater contribution. This makes sense as, hypothetically, if all participants in a trial had the same covariate value (e.g. all males), then it is not possible to examine how changes in that covariate value interact with treatment effect. Conversely, the more spread out the covariate values, the more information available to detect any interactions between the covariate and treatment effect.

The residual (i.e. unexplained) variability of outcome values (σ_i^2) also influences the contribution of each trial (equation (12.5)). Other things being equal, those trials with larger σ_i^2 values will have lesser contribution toward the total power of the IPD meta-analysis than those trials with smaller σ_i^2 values. Again this is intuitive, as larger unexplained outcome variability leads to larger variances of parameter estimates in a linear regression model.

12.5 The Impact of Model Assumptions on Power

Sections 12.3 and 12.4 make some important modelling assumptions; in particular, zero between-trial heterogeneity of the treatment-covariate interaction was assumed, and confidence intervals and p-values were derived using the standard normal-based approach rather than other options.[15] Our power calculations for the i-WIP project also assume a linear effect for the treatment-BMI interaction and that residual variances can be approximated by the variance of outcome values. In this section we examine the impact of these assumptions, focusing on the power of the i-WIP meta-analysis based on the full set of 24 trials.

12.5.1 Impact of Allowing for Heterogeneity in the Interaction

To allow for between-trial heterogeneity in a treatment-covariate interaction, we suggest extending the closed-form power calculation of equation (12.5) to:

$$\text{Power} = \mathrm{T}\left(-t_{S-1,0.975} + \gamma_W\sqrt{\sum_{i=1}^{S}\frac{1}{\frac{4\sigma_i^2}{n_i\sigma_{z_i}^2}+\tau_{\gamma_W}^2}}\right) + \mathrm{T}\left(-t_{S-1,0.975} - \gamma_W\sqrt{\sum_{i=1}^{S}\frac{1}{\frac{4\sigma_i^2}{n_i\sigma_{z_i}^2}+\tau_{\gamma_W}^2}}\right) \qquad (12.7)$$

where T(x) is the probability of sampling a value $< x$ from a t-distribution with a mean of zero and $S-1$ degrees of freedom, where S is the number of trials assumed to provide their IPD. Compared to equation (12.5), this power formula includes $\tau_{\gamma_W}^2$, which denotes the assumed between-trial variance of the interaction, and replaces 1.96 with $t_{S-1,0.975}$, the value of the 97.5 percentile value of the t-distribution with $S-1$ degrees of freedom, to help reflect extra uncertainty due to $\tau_{\gamma_W}^2$ being estimated in practice (akin to the use of the t-distribution in the Hartung-Knapp-Sidik-Jonkman (HKSJ) approach for deriving 95% confidence intervals after fitting a random-effects meta-analysis[15,16]). Applying equation (12.7) to the i-WIP example with 24 trials, and assuming γ_W is –0.1 and $\tau_{\gamma_W} = 0.01$, we obtain

$$T\left(-2.069 - 0.1\sqrt{863.16}\right) + T\left(-2.069 + 0.1\sqrt{863.16}\right) = T(-5.00) + T(0.87) = 0.80$$

and thus the estimated power is 80%, slightly lower than the 84% when assuming a common treatment-BMI interaction.

Equation (12.7) is only an approximation, and is likely to be an over-estimate as it assumes τ_{γ_W} is known when in practice it will be estimated. This is of most concern when there are only a small number of trials and the true τ_{γ_W} is close to zero, as then τ_{γ_W} is particularly poorly estimated (often with upward bias). This issue can be reflected by extending the simulation-based approach described in Section 12.3.2 to allow for heterogeneity in the interaction when generating the IPD, and by using a random-effects meta-analysis model to pool the interaction estimates from each trial. On application to the i-WIP example, such a simulation-based approach gives an estimated power of about 70% or less across a range of τ_{γ_W} values (Figure 12.2), which is somewhat lower than for the closed-form approach of equation (12.7).

A simulation-based approach also enables the HKSJ approach to be used for deriving confidence intervals after fitting a random-effects meta-analysis model in the second stage.[15] Figure 12.2 shows that when using the HKSJ approach to derive 95% confidence intervals the power was consistently lower (by about 3%) than when using a standard normal-based approach. This is expected, as standard 95% confidence intervals are typically too narrow and the HKSJ correction aims to address this, usually leading to wider confidence intervals and larger p-values (Chapter 5).

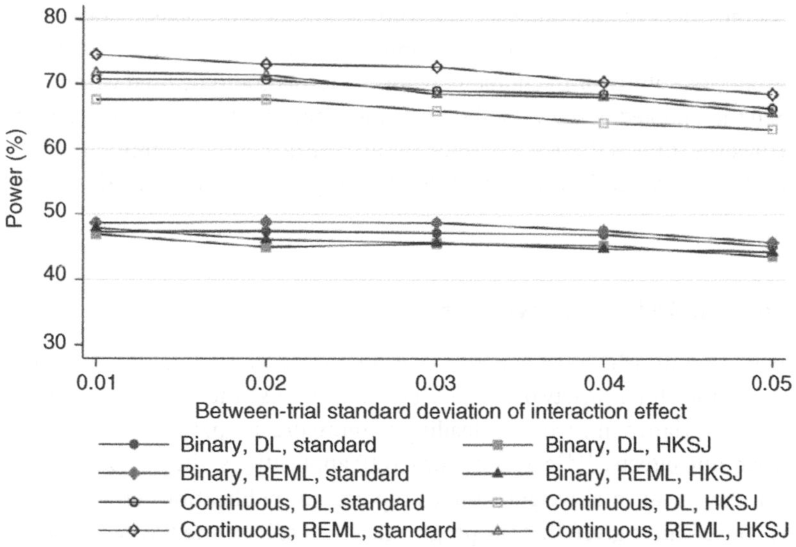

Figure 12.2 Simulation-based power estimates (based on 10,000 replications) for the planned two-stage IPD meta-analysis* of 24 trials for detecting a treatment-BMI interaction when the true interaction is −0.1, conditional on a range of values of the between-trial standard deviation (τ_{γ_W}) of the interaction effect, when either correctly analysing BMI as continuous or when wrongly analysing BMI as binary (≥ 30 versus < 30), and for different estimation techniques *Source:* Figure is adapted from Figure 2 of Ensor et al.,[7] with permission, © 2018 Ensor et al (CC-BY 4.0).

* DL = DerSimonian and Laird estimation used in second stage; REML = restricted maximum likelihood estimation used in second stage; Standard = p-values and CIs for interaction estimates in each meta-analysis derived using standard normal-based method; HKSJ = p-values and CIs for interaction estimates in each meta-analysis derived using approach of Hartung-Knapp-Sidik-Jonkman.

12.5.2 Impact of Wrongly Modelling BMI as a Binary Variable

In our i-WIP example, so far we chose to model BMI as a continuous variable with a linear association with outcome. In practice, many researchers dichotomise continuous variables but this will lose power to detect genuine linear (or non-linear) relationships.[17] To examine this we repeated our simulation-based approach, generating IPD with BMI on its continuous scale and assuming a common treatment-BMI interaction of –0.1, but then applying analyses that include BMI as a binary covariate, with a BMI ≥ 30 classed as 1 and a BMI < 30 classed as 0. This dichotomisation corresponds to a true interaction of about –0.65 kg between the treatment effect and binary BMI, such that the group of individuals with a BMI ≥ 30 have, on average, a 0.65 kg further reduction in weight gain by using the intervention rather than control, in comparison to those with a BMI < 30.

Assuming no heterogeneity in the interaction, and using all 24 trials, the estimated power to detect this interaction is 61%. This is an over 20% absolute reduction in power compared to when baseline BMI was analysed correctly as a continuous variable (84%), emphasising a huge loss of information by wrongly dichotomising BMI. Indeed, the estimated power of 61% is now similar to the power of 64% for the original IPD meta-analysis of just 14 trials when baseline BMI was analysed correctly as continuous using 1183 women. Therefore, in this particular example, the loss of power by dichotomising baseline BMI in the IPD meta-analysis of 24 trials is similar to throwing away the IPD from the additional 10 trials containing 1761 participants (about 60% of the total participants). Such cost of dichotomisation is well known in the single trial setting,[17–20] and the results here simply emphasise that it generalises to the IPD meta-analysis setting. Findings are similar when assuming between-trial heterogeneity in the interaction, with power estimates now less than 50% compared to about 65–70% when analysed correctly as continuous (Figure 12.2).

All these calculations assume linear relationships are the truth. The simulation-based power calculations could be modified to generate IPD assuming non-linear trends and interactions, if that is considered plausible. For example, splines or fractional polynomial terms could be used within the data-generating process, and then pooled in the second stage using a multivariate meta-analysis (as described in Chapter 7). However, unless there is evidence to the contrary, the assumption of linearity would appear a sensible and practical starting point for deriving power estimates *prior* to the IPD being collected.

12.5.3 Impact of Adjusting for Additional Covariates

Chapters 5 and 6 recommend that all IPD meta-analyses of randomised trials should adjust for a pre-defined set of prognostic factors, for a variety of reasons. For continuous outcomes, a key reason is that this reduces the residual variance in each trial, leading to more precise parameter estimates and larger power to detect genuine effects.[21–23] So far in our i-WIP applications, the size of residual variances (σ_i^2) was based on the variance of weight gain, as reported in publications (Table 12.1); however, this is potentially conservative given that the prognostic effect of baseline BMI will also be included in the IPD meta-analysis when estimating the treatment-BMI interaction. There are also other prognostic factors that could be included, such as age and parity.

To consider this, we repeated our simulation-based power calculations with residual variances reduced by between 10% and 90% in each trial. For brevity, we focus on a true interaction of –0.1, across a range of values on the between-trial standard deviation (τ_{γ_W}). The results in Figure 12.3 show that power improves as the residual variances decrease, and thus confirm why pre-specified adjustment for prognostic factors is recommended. However, the power consistently exceeds 80% across the entire range of τ_{γ_W} values only when the reduction in residual variances is at least 40%. Had this been known to the i-WIP researchers when planning their IPD project, it would have given even more credence for pre-specifying adjustment for key prognostic factors in their analyses.

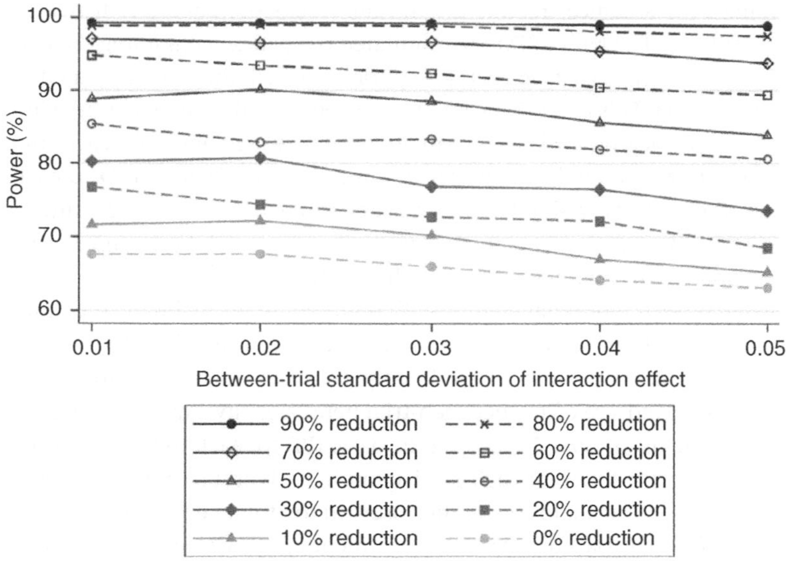

Figure 12.3 Simulation-based power estimates for the planned two-stage IPD meta-analysis of 24 trials allowing for a random interaction effect*. The true treatment-BMI interaction is −0.1, and results are shown for a range of scenarios conditional on values of the between-trial standard deviation (τ_{γ_W}) of the interaction effect, and an assumed % reduction in residual variances in each trial due to the inclusion of prognostic factors. *Source:* Richard Riley.

12.6 Extensions

12.6.1 Power Calculations for Binary and Time-to-event Outcomes

Closed-form solutions for non-continuous outcomes are problematic, because $\text{var}(\hat{\gamma}_W)$ will usually be correlated with $\hat{\gamma}_W$ itself, and similarly, $\text{var}(\hat{\gamma}_{Wi})$ will depend on the actual value of $\hat{\gamma}_{Wi}$. The reason is that for generalised linear models each participant-level variance is a function of the participant's predicted outcome values from the fitted model. In other words, rather than using a single σ_i^2 per trial as we have done for continuous outcomes, we need to specify a separate variance (σ_{ij}^2) for each participant in each trial, conditional on their covariate values. For example, for binary outcomes a participant's response variance is $p_{ij}(1 - p_{ij})$ and thus depends on their expected outcome probability (p_{ij}), which is conditional on the baseline risk in the trial and the effect of any covariates, including the interaction and treatment terms. This makes closed-form solutions problematic, and so Kovalchick and Cumberland suggest approximating these variances to enable a closed-form solution (based on matrix algebra implemented within the package *ipdmeta* in R).[5] Their approach requires strong assumptions, such as replacing each participant's $p_{ij}(1 - p_{ij})$ with $p_i(1 - p_i)$, where p_i is the overall outcome risk in the participant's corresponding group within trial *i*. Such approximations may not be reliable; for example, the error in the approximate closed-form power estimates of Kovalchick and Cumberland is often over 10%.[5] Their approach also assumes a one-stage model that amalgamates within-trial and across-trial information (which we do not recommend; see Chapter 7),[5] and so will over-estimate the actual power.

Hence, although their approach is a useful starting point, for non-continuous outcomes we prefer the simulation-based approach. For a binary outcome simulation, the required inputs include the number of participants and outcome events in each group in each trial, together with the distribution of covariate values, the assumed treatment-covariate interaction, and any between-trial heterogeneity in the interaction. The basic IPD to be simulated is a dataset containing the correct number of participants and outcome events in each group for each trial; this can be created as described in Chapter 6 (Section 6.4.1). This basic IPD should be forced to be the same in every simulation, to ensure the observed control group risk and the unadjusted treatment effect for each trial will always match those reported in trial publications. Then, appended to this basic IPD in each simulation should be a column containing simulated covariate values for each participant, as sampled conditional on their outcome value and treatment group allocation, and the assumed prognostic effect of the covariate and size of treatment-covariate interaction.

Simulating time-to-event outcomes is more challenging, with required inputs including the number of participants and events in each group, the distribution of survival times (magnitude and shape of baseline hazard function), maximum length of follow-up, censoring mechanism and level, the treatment-covariate interaction, and size of any between-trial heterogeneity. An excellent Stata module for simulating survival times is *survsim*.[24] Note that the basic IPD for each trial (i.e. number of participants, and event and censoring times for each participant in each group) might be reconstructed from the Kaplan-Meier curve,[25] again to ensure the observed treatment effect for each trial matches (in the simulated data for that trial) the observed treatment effect. Covariate values can then be simulated and appended to this basic IPD, conditional on the assumed interaction size and participant's outcome value and length of follow-up.

12.6.2 Simulation Using a One-stage IPD Meta-Analysis Approach

One-stage and two-stage approaches to IPD meta-analysis usually give similar results if their assumptions and estimation methods agree (Chapter 8).[26] When using a power-by-simulation approach, generally we prefer to incorporate a two-stage IPD meta-analysis, as it has many advantages. Firstly, it is relatively quick, and facilitated by the excellent package *ipdmetan* within Stata,[27] which undertakes both stages automatically. Secondly, it automatically avoids using across-trial information to inform treatment-covariate interactions, and thus interaction estimates are based solely on only within-trial information.

However, a two-stage approach is less appropriate when there are sparse outcome events or small sample sizes in most trials (Chapter 8).[26] In such situations, a one-stage IPD meta-analysis framework for simulation-based power calculations is appealing. Kontopantelis et al. have produced a package *ipdpower* in Stata,[6] which enables a simulation-based power estimates for one-stage IPD meta-analyses of continuous, binary or count outcomes. This follows a very similar approach to that described in Section 12.3.2, except with the two-stage IPD meta-analysis framework replaced by a one-stage IPD meta-analysis model. Note that the package currently amalgamates within-trial and across-trial information, and thus power estimates are likely to be too high.[28,29]

Simulations of one-stage models can be time-consuming, as the models can be hard to fit and may encounter convergence problems (e.g. when fitting one-stage models with both a random intercept and a random treatment effect). In R, simulation-based power calculations for one-stage IPD meta-analysis models might utilise the *SIMR* package,[30] which is designed to interoperate with the *lme4* package for generalised linear mixed models.[31] Other packages for simulation-based power calculations of mixed models are also emerging, including *powerlmm* and PASS.[32,33] However, many of these do not allow the user to specify the exact sample size (and outcome events) per trial, as is needed in the IPD meta-analysis setting to mirror situations where the researcher knows the basic characteristics of trials for which IPD are promised or desired.

12.6.3 Examining the Potential Precision of IPD Meta-Analysis Results

"If we ask researchers to present their results as confidence intervals rather than significance tests, I think we should also ask them to base sample size calculations on confidence intervals. It is inconsistent to say that we insist on the analysis using confidence intervals but that the sample size should be decided using significance tests."[34]

In addition to (or even instead of) calculating power, researchers may also want to check the potential precision of their planned IPD meta-analysis, in terms of whether confidence intervals will be sufficiently narrow to inform clinical decision-making. In the simulation-based approach, the average width of the 95% confidence interval could be recorded. When examining a treatment-covariate interaction for a continuous outcome, the closed-form variance solutions provided in Section 12.3.1 can be utilised. For example, assuming no between-trial heterogeneity in the treatment-covariate interaction, a 95% confidence interval for the interaction from an IPD meta-analysis can be calculated using $\hat{\gamma}_W \pm \left(1.96 \times \sqrt{\text{var}(\hat{\gamma}_W)}\right)$, where $\text{var}(\hat{\gamma}_W) = \sum_i \frac{4\sigma^2}{\sum_j z_{ij}^{\prime 2}}$ (equation (12.2)).

Returning to the i-WIP example of all 24 trials, for which the power to detect an interaction of at least –0.1 is 84% from the closed-form solution (Section 12.4.1), the anticipated confidence interval for an interaction $\hat{\gamma}_W$ of −0.1 from the IPD meta-analysis is

$$\hat{\gamma}_W \pm \left(1.96 \times \sqrt{\text{var}(\hat{\gamma}_W)}\right) = \hat{\gamma}_W \pm \left(1.96 \times \sqrt{\left(\sum_{i=1}^{S} \frac{1}{\frac{4\sigma_i^2}{n_i \sigma_{z_i}^2}}\right)^{-1}}\right)$$

$$= -0.1 \pm \left(1.96 \times \sqrt{0.00114}\right)$$

$$= -0.17 \text{ to} -0.03$$

Thus, under the assumptions made, the anticipated 95% confidence interval will be entirely below zero. However, the upper bound of –0.03 reflects a value that may not be clinically useful and so, if the true interaction is indeed –0.1, IPD from further trials may be needed to more precisely establish this value.

12.6.4 Estimating the Power of a New Trial Conditional on IPD Meta-Analysis Results

IPD meta-analysis projects may not resolve all questions, especially if their summary results are too imprecise to enable strong conclusions. Indeed, a key output of an IPD meta-analysis may be to inform whether a new primary study should be initiated and, if so, what its sample size should be. For example, Burke et al. considered the efficacy of bolus thrombolytic therapy versus standard infusion therapy for the in-hospital treatment of acute myocardial infarction,[35] and their article shows how to use an IPD meta-analysis of Phase II randomised trials to inform the sample size required for a new, subsequent Phase III trial. In brief, their approach uses a Bayesian framework and produces a predictive distribution for the treatment effect in a new Phase III trial (Figure 12.4), conditional on the Phase II IPD meta-analysis results, including the amount of between-trial heterogeneity. The sample size for the new trial is ascertained by repeatedly sampling from this predictive distribution (to obtain the true treatment effect) and then each time deriving a 95% credible interval for the treatment effect conditional on an assumed trial sample size and baseline risk. The Bayesian framework is crucial here, because it naturally accounts for uncertainty in parameter

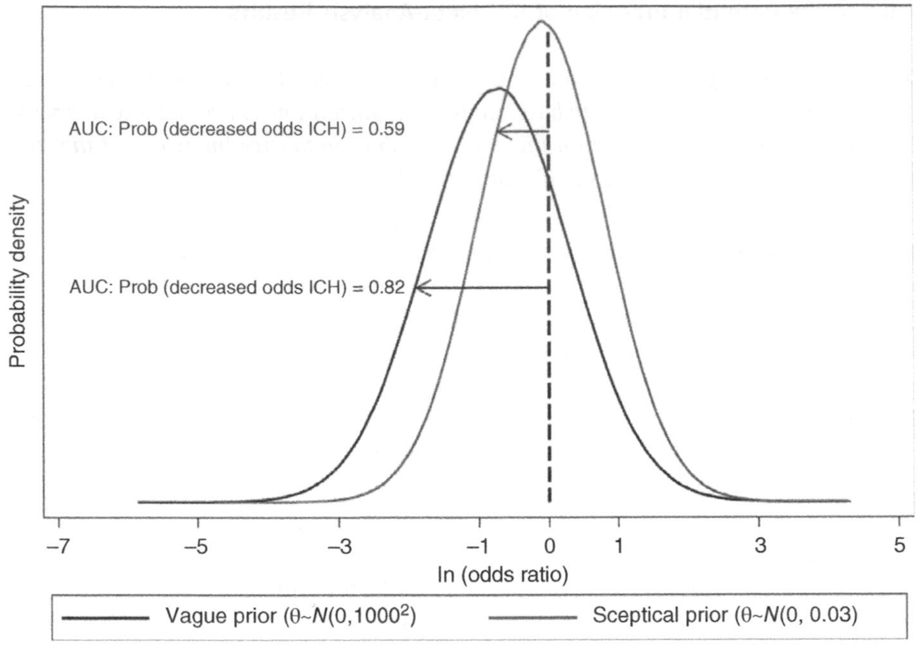

AUC = area under the curve to the left of dotted line, which gives the probability that bolus therapy will truly be effective in a new trial. ICH intracranial haemorrhage

Figure 12.4 Predictive distribution for the true treatment effect in a new Phase III trial, conditional on the results of an IPD meta-analysis of Phase II trials and assuming either a vague or sceptical prior distribution for the true treatment effect (θ) as measured by a log odds ratio. *Source:* Figure taken from Figure 7 of Burke et al.[35], with permission, © 2014 Burke et al., licensee BioMed Central Ltd. (CC-BY 4.0).

estimates from the IPD meta-analysis, including the uncertainty in the true treatment effect and the amount of between-trial heterogeneity. Furthermore, as Phase II trial results are particularly prone to optimism, it enables prior distributions to be incorporated that reflect sceptical clinical beliefs about the size of true treatment effect in the subsequent Phase III trial (Figure 12.4).

The minimum sample size required for a new trial is subjective, as it depends on many factors including costs and the potential risk-reward balance for the funders. However, ideally it should be large enough to give a high probability of identifying a clinically relevant treatment effect. In the Burke et al. example, a sample size of over 2000 per group only gives a 40% probability that the new trial will give a 95% credible interval for the treatment effect entirely in favour of bolus therapy for reducing the odds of intracranial hemorrhage.[35] This low probability is due to the large uncertainty in the results from the IPD meta-analysis of Phase II trials, partly due to the between-trial heterogeneity, and raises doubt about whether a new trial is likely to be worth the time and investment. Identifying causes of between-trial heterogeneity, and in particular settings where bolus therapy is likely to work best, would help tailor a subsequent trial and improve the probability of success.

Sometimes a new trial may be designed so that, after completion, its IPD can be added to an existing IPD meta-analysis. Then, the new trial's required sample size needs to be large enough to ensure sufficient power for the subsequent IPD meta-analysis, rather than the trial itself. For further details on that idea, we refer elsewhere.[36–39]

12.7 Concluding Remarks

Since IPD meta-analysis projects with high power are more likely to detect important effects of interest, they should (other things being equal) be a higher priority for funding. Careful assessments of power and sample size are, therefore, an important part of planning and commissioning IPD meta-analysis projects that aim to estimate a particular effect. A closed-form or simulated-based approach to power calculation can be used for this purpose, and applied in advance of IPD collection based on published aggregate data for trials whose IPD are desired. Results focused on treatment-covariate interactions in this chapter, but the principles (and especially the simulation-based framework) can be adapted to other types of IPD projects, such as those examining prognostic effects (Chapter 16) or differences in test accuracy between subgroups (Chapter 15). Funding applications for IPD meta-analysis projects might display a range of power calculations (or expected precision of estimates, Section 12.6.3) conditional on the assumed IPD acquired; for example, they might estimate power (or expected precision) when optimistically assuming IPD will be obtained from all trials, but also when cautiously assuming IPD will only be provided by trials that already provided verbal or written agreement.

13

Multivariate Meta-Analysis Using IPD

Richard D. Riley, Dan Jackson, and Ian R. White

Summary Points

- Often IPD meta-analysis projects are interested in a treatment's effect on each of multiple correlated outcomes (e.g. systolic and diastolic blood pressure); however, most perform a separate meta-analysis for each outcome, and ignore the correlation between them.
- Statistical models for multivariate IPD meta-analysis address this by analysing treatment effects for multiple outcomes simultaneously, whilst accounting for within-trial and between-trial correlation.
- In the first stage of a two-stage multivariate IPD meta-analysis, each trial is analysed separately to obtain a treatment effect estimate and its corresponding variance for each outcome, and the within-trial correlation between treatment effect estimates for each pair of outcomes.
- Within-trial correlation arises from participants in the same trial having correlated data for each of the multiple outcomes. It can be estimated by using joint models or, more generally, using bootstrapping.
- The second stage requires a multivariate meta-analysis model, which typically assumes multivariate normality, for both the treatment effect estimates within each trial and the true treatment effects across trials. When there is between-trial heterogeneity, the true treatment effects for the outcomes may also be correlated across trials, a phenomenon known as *between-trial correlation.*
- By accounting for correlation amongst outcomes, the multivariate meta-analysis can borrow strength across outcomes (i.e. gain information) to provide more precise summary results for each outcome; this is especially useful when some outcomes are not available in all trials.
- Accounting for correlation in a multivariate meta-analysis also enables more appropriate joint inferences across outcomes, such as the probability that a treatment is beneficial for *both* outcome 1 and outcome 2.
- Alternative one-stage IPD meta-analysis models are also possible to handle multiple outcomes, especially for multiple continuous outcomes or for a multinomial outcome.
- Multivariate IPD meta-analysis has many other applications; for example, for modelling multiple time-points (longitudinal data), examining surrogate outcomes, and joint synthesis of multiple model parameters, such as for dose-response relationships and non-linear trends.

Individual Participant Data Meta-Analysis: A Handbook for Healthcare Research, First Edition.
Edited by Richard D. Riley, Jayne F. Tierney, and Lesley A. Stewart.

13.1 Introduction

"Many clinical studies have more than one outcome variable; this is the norm rather than the exception. These variables are seldom independent and so each must carry some information about the others. If we can use this information, we should."[40]

Conventional methods for meta-analysis produce a single summary result, for example about a treatment effect or a treatment-covariate interaction for one particular outcome. In particular, the two-stage IPD meta-analysis methods described in Chapter 5 derive one effect estimate (and its variance) per trial in the first stage, which are then meta-analysed in the second stage. This process can be described as a *univariate* meta-analysis, with the word 'univariate' indicating that a single summary result is of interest. However, most IPD meta-analysis projects aim to produce multiple summary results, especially because multiple outcomes are of interest, such as a hypertensive participant's systolic blood pressure (SBP) and diastolic (DBP) blood pressure, a migraine sufferer's levels of pain and nausea, and a cancer participant's disease-free and overall survival times. A review of 75 systematic reviews published by the Cochrane Pregnancy and Childbirth Group found that the median number of forest plots per review was 52 (range 5 to 409),[41] mainly to address multiple outcomes for the mother and her baby. This potentially motivates a *multivariate* meta-analysis, to produce multiple summary results (one for each outcome) jointly from the same meta-analysis model.[42]

The key advantage of a multivariate meta-analysis is to account for correlation of the multiple outcomes.[43] At the participant level, multiple health outcomes are often correlated with each other, and this leads to correlation amongst multiple effect estimates from the same trial. Such correlation of a pair of effect estimates is known as *within-trial correlation* (or, more broadly, within-study correlation). For example, in a randomised trial of anti-hypertensive treatment, the estimated treatment effects for SBP and DBP are likely to have a positive within-trial correlation, caused by a positive correlation at the participant level between SBP and DBP. In other words, in each group the estimated mean change in SBP and mean change in DBP will be positively correlated, and this induces a correlation in the observed treatment effects on SBP and DBP. Similarly, within a cancer trial, the estimated treatment effects for disease-free survival and overall survival are likely to be positively correlated, because a treatment that prolongs participants' mean time to disease recurrence is also likely to prolong their mean time to death.

When there is between-trial heterogeneity, the true effect for each outcome may be correlated with the true effect for another outcome. This is known as *between-trial correlation* (or, more broadly, between-study correlation). For example, the true effect of anti-hypertensive treatment on SBP usually has a positive between-trial correlation with the true effect on DBP, caused by changes in trial and participant characteristics (such as dose and mean blood pressure at baseline) which modify the true treatment effects on SBP and DBP in the same direction. Similarly, the true prognostic effect of a biomarker on disease-free survival and overall survival may be positively correlated across studies, due to changes in the length of follow-up and diagnostic setting.

Many IPD meta-analysis projects ignore the correlation of multiple outcomes; that is, they conduct a standard univariate meta-analysis for each outcome separately, using the methods described in Part 2 of this book. A consequence is that trials that do not provide *direct evidence* about a particular outcome are excluded from the IPD meta-analysis of that outcome. This may be unwelcome, especially if their participants are otherwise representative of the population, clinical settings and condition of interest. Research studies require considerable costs and time, and involve precious participant involvement, and simply discarding them could be viewed as research waste if they still contain other outcomes that are correlated with (and thus contain indirect information about) the outcome of interest.[44–46] Statistical models for *multivariate IPD meta-analysis* address this by simultaneously analysing multiple outcomes, which allows more trials to contribute toward the meta-analysis for each outcome, which may improve efficiency and even decrease bias (e.g. due to selective outcome reporting[47]) in the summary results.

In particular, alongside any direct evidence, a multivariate meta-analysis allows the summary result for each outcome to depend on correlated results from other outcomes. The rationale is that by observing information from related outcomes we can learn something about the missing outcomes of interest, and thus gain some knowledge that is otherwise lost; a concept known statistically as *borrowing strength*.[48,49] Box 13.1 illustrates this for a motivating example in endometrial cancer,[50,51] where the borrowing of strength leads to important differences in the multivariate and univariate meta-analysis results. Post-estimation, joint inferences can also be made from the multivariate model to summarise overall effectiveness to inform decision-making and cost-effectiveness analyses. For example, we can quantify the probability that a particular treatment is beneficial for *both* SBP and DBP, or that the accuracy of a particular test is acceptable in terms

Box 13.1 Motivating example: Multivariate versus univariate meta-analysis of cohort studies examining the prognostic effect of progesterone receptor status for cancer-specific survival and progression-free survival in endometrial cancer.[50,51]

Background: Zhang et al. performed a meta-analysis to summarise the unadjusted prognostic effect of progesterone receptor status in endometrial cancer.[50] Four identified studies provided results for both cancer-specific survival (CSS) and progression-free survival (PFS), but other identified studies provided results for only CSS (2 studies) or only PFS (11 studies).

Methods: Prognostic results for CSS are missing in 11 studies (1412 participants) that provide results for PFS. Assuming there is between-study heterogeneity of the prognostic effect of progesterone receptor status, a conventional univariate meta-analysis for CSS simply discards these 11 studies, but they are retained in a multivariate meta-analysis of PFS and CSS, which accounts for their strong positive correlation to borrow strength across outcomes.

Results: There are important differences in summary results for the multivariate and univariate meta-analysis, as shown for CSS in the forest plot below. The univariate meta-analysis for CSS includes just the six studies with direct evidence and gives a summary hazard ratio (HR) of 0.61 (95%: 0.38 to 1.00), with the confidence interval just crossing the value of no effect. In contrast, the multivariate meta-analysis includes 17 studies and borrows strength from the correlated PFS result, especially in those 11 studies (containing 1412 participants) where CSS is not available; this leads to a summary HR for CSS of 0.48 (95% CI: 0.29 to 0.79), with a narrower confidence interval and stronger evidence that progesterone is prognostic for CSS than from univariate meta-analysis. The shift in the CSS summary HR from 0.61 to 0.48 occurs because the HRs for PFS and CSS are positively correlated, and the HRs for PFS in those studies without CSS results are lower than in those studies with CSS results.

(Continued)

Box 13.1 (Continued)

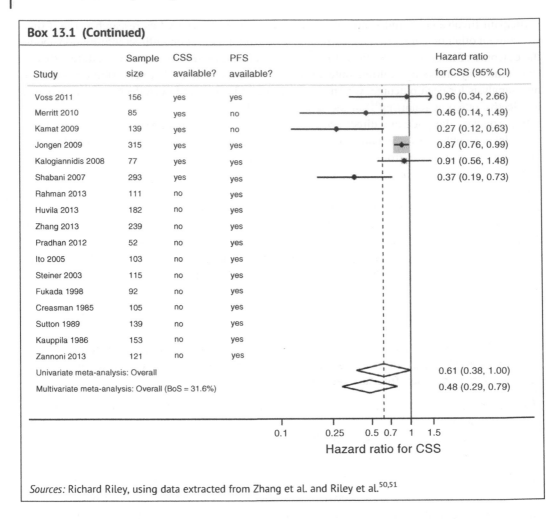

Study	Sample size	CSS available?	PFS available?	Hazard ratio for CSS (95% CI)
Voss 2011	156	yes	yes	0.96 (0.34, 2.66)
Merritt 2010	85	yes	no	0.46 (0.14, 1.49)
Kamat 2009	139	yes	no	0.27 (0.12, 0.63)
Jongen 2009	315	yes	yes	0.87 (0.76, 0.99)
Kalogiannidis 2008	77	yes	yes	0.91 (0.56, 1.48)
Shabani 2007	293	yes	yes	0.37 (0.19, 0.73)
Rahman 2013	111	no	yes	
Huvila 2013	182	no	yes	
Zhang 2013	239	no	yes	
Pradhan 2012	52	no	yes	
Ito 2005	103	no	yes	
Steiner 2003	115	no	yes	
Fukada 1998	92	no	yes	
Creasman 1985	105	no	yes	
Sutton 1989	139	no	yes	
Kauppila 1986	153	no	yes	
Zannoni 2013	121	no	yes	
Univariate meta-analysis: Overall				0.61 (0.38, 1.00)
Multivariate meta-analysis: Overall (BoS = 31.6%)				0.48 (0.29, 0.79)

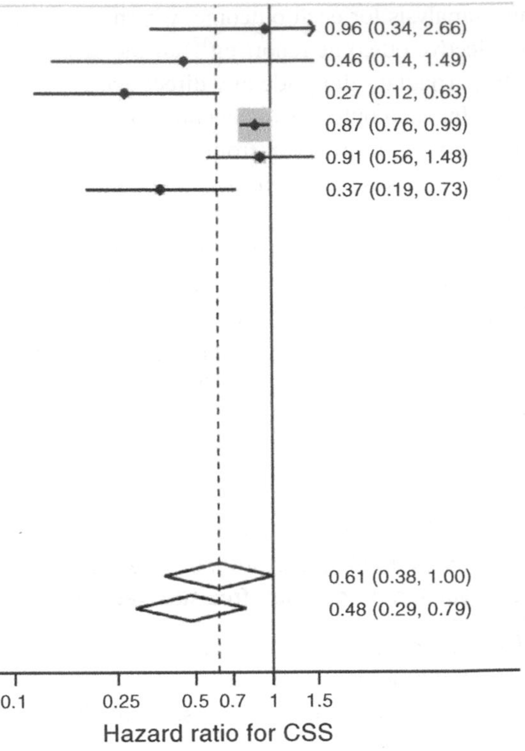

Sources: Richard Riley, using data extracted from Zhang et al. and Riley et al.[50,51]

of *both* sensitivity and specificity. This is more difficult, and potentially misleading, when assuming outcomes are independent and applying a univariate meta-analyses for each outcome separately.

In this chapter, we describe how to undertake a multivariate IPD meta-analysis of multiple correlated outcomes, and explain why it can lead to results that differ from those generated by analysing each outcome separately. The core theoretical material is covered in Section 13.2; more general readers may wish to focus on the applications, advantages and limitations described in Section 13.3 onwards.

13.2 General Two-stage Approach for Multivariate IPD Meta-Analysis

We begin by introducing the general two-stage approach to multivariate IPD meta-analysis of multiple outcomes.[52,53] To aid explanations, we extend our running example from Part 2 of this book of an IPD meta-analysis of 10 trials to examine the effects of anti-hypertensive treatment; here we focus on four outcomes: SBP and DBP at end of follow-up, and a diagnosis of cardiovascular disease (CVD) or stroke by end of follow-up.

13.2.1 First-stage Analyses

13.2.1.1 Obtaining Treatment Effect Estimates and Their Variances for Continuous Outcomes

We begin by considering IPD from S randomised trials with a parallel group design to compare treatment and control groups in regards to K continuous outcomes, such as SBP and DBP when $K = 2$. At baseline (i.e. before randomisation) the jth participant in the ith trial provides their initial (starting) values, which we denote by y_{0ijk}, where 0 indicates baseline and k denotes the outcome ($k = 1$ to K); for example, $k = 1$ for SBP and $k = 2$ for DBP. Also, each participant provides their final outcome values after treatment, which we denote by y_{ijk}. Let x_{ij} be 1 or 0 for participants in the treatment or control groups, respectively.

When such IPD are available, the first stage of a two-stage multivariate IPD meta-analysis estimates the treatment effects for each outcome in each trial, along with their corresponding variances. The following describes two possible options to do this, building on methods described in Chapter 5.

Option 1: Modelling outcomes separately within each trial

For each outcome and each trial separately, an analysis of covariance (ANCOVA) model could be applied,[54] where the outcome follow-up value is the response variable and the treatment effect is estimated adjusted for the baseline value:

$$\begin{aligned} y_{ijk} &= \phi_{ik} + \beta_{ik} y_{0ijk} + \theta_{ik} x_{ij} + e_{ijk} \\ e_{ijk} &\sim N\left(0, \sigma_{ik}^2\right) \end{aligned} \tag{13.1}$$

In this model, of key interest is θ_{ik}, the treatment effect for outcome k in trial i. The other parameters are essentially nuisance parameters: ϕ_{ik} is the model intercept for outcome k, β_{ik} denotes the mean change in y_{ijk} for a one-unit increase in y_{0ijk}, and σ_{ik}^2 is the residual variance of outcome k in trial i after accounting for treatment group and baseline values. The residual variance could also be made distinct for treatment and control groups, as discussed in Chapter 5.

Model (13.1) is a linear regression and so can be estimated in standard statistical software using, for example, restricted maximum likelihood (REML) estimation. After applying model (13.1) for each outcome and each trial separately, the treatment effect estimate, $\hat{\theta}_{ik}$, and its variance, s_{ik}^2, are obtained for each outcome in each trial. So, with two outcomes, $\hat{\theta}_{i1}$, $\hat{\theta}_{i2}$, s_{i1}^2, and s_{i2}^2 are obtained. If baseline values are unavailable for a trial, then fitting model (13.1) excluding the $\beta_{ik} y_{0ijk}$ term will still give unbiased estimates of θ_{ik}, though this is less efficient than adjusting for baseline.[54,55]

Option 2: Modelling outcomes jointly within each trial

An ANCOVA model could alternatively be applied to all of the continuous outcomes jointly. For example, with two outcomes ($k = 1$ or 2) we could write:

$$\begin{aligned} y_{ijk} &= \phi_{ik} + \beta_{ik} y_{0ijk} + \theta_{ik} x_{ij} + e_{ijk} \\ \begin{pmatrix} e_{ij1} \\ e_{ij2} \end{pmatrix} &\sim N\left(\begin{pmatrix} 0 \\ 0 \end{pmatrix}, \begin{pmatrix} \sigma_{i1}^2 & \sigma_{i(1,2)} \\ \sigma_{i(1,2)} & \sigma_{i2}^2 \end{pmatrix}\right) \end{aligned} \tag{13.2}$$

Now both outcomes are modelled jointly whilst accounting for the covariance of their residual errors ($\sigma_{i(1,2)}$); essentially each participant contributes two follow-up responses and two baseline values (one for each outcome) to a single joint model.[56] The approach is also known as 'seemingly unrelated regression' in some fields and software packages (e.g. *sureg* in Stata).[57] It is akin to a repeated measures model and the correlation in participant outcome responses is accounted for by the covariance term, $\sigma_{i(1,2)}$. The key results (i.e. $\hat{\theta}_{i1}$, $\hat{\theta}_{i2}$, s_{i1}^2, and s_{i2}^2) are now all obtained from this single analysis. For estimation purposes, it is helpful to re-write model (13.2) using dummy variables.[58]

In a trial where each participant provides all outcomes, model (13.2) will give approximately the same treatment effect estimates and variances as obtained from fitting model (13.1) to each outcome separately. However, model (13.2) can also include participants with one of the outcomes missing and, under a missing at random assumption, will use the participant-level correlation to borrow strength across outcomes at the participant-level. Thus, in a trial where some participants do not provide all outcomes, this will lead to more precise effect estimates than when analysing each outcome separately.

13.2.1.2 Obtaining Within-trial Correlations Directly or via Bootstrapping for Continuous Outcomes

In addition to the treatment effect estimates and their variances, the first stage of a two-stage multivariate IPD meta-analysis must also obtain the within-trial correlation (ρ_{Wi}, say) of each pair of treatment effect estimates from the same trial. For example, when using model (13.2) with two outcomes in a trial, a within-trial correlation ($\rho_{Wi(1,2)}$) between the two treatment effect estimates ($\hat{\theta}_{i1}$ and $\hat{\theta}_{i2}$) can naturally arise because the correlation of a participant's pair of outcome responses is accounted for through the covariance term, $\sigma_{i(1,2)}$. Larger correlation in outcomes at the participant level will usually lead to larger correlation in the treatment effect estimates for those outcomes. Without IPD, obtaining within-trial correlations is very difficult and presents a major stumbling block for implementing the multivariate approach (although novel solutions have been suggested, including formulae for deriving within-trial correlations from published aggregate data[59–63]).

With IPD, obtaining the within-trial correlations is relatively straightforward. After estimation of model (13.2), $\rho_{Wi(1,2)}$ can be obtained directly using $\rho_{Wi(1,2)} = cov(\hat{\theta}_{i1}, \hat{\theta}_{i2})/s_{i1}s_{i2}$, where s_{i1}^2 and s_{i2}^2 are the estimated variances of the treatment effect estimates ($\hat{\theta}_{i1}$ and $\hat{\theta}_{i2}$) and $\text{cov}(\hat{\theta}_{i1}, \hat{\theta}_{i2})$ is the estimated covariance of $\hat{\theta}_{i1}$ and $\hat{\theta}_{i2}$. These are routinely available in statistical software post-estimation of the equation, for example as derived from the inverse of Fisher's information matrix.

Model (13.1) does not account for participant-level correlation, as it analyses each outcome separately; therefore the within-trial correlations are not directly obtainable post-estimation. Rather, they can be estimated via non-parametric bootstrapping of the IPD in each trial separately. This approach randomly selects one participant with replacement, then randomly selects a second participant with replacement, and repeats until the same sample size is obtained as in the trial. This process is repeated *b* times, so that *b* bootstrap samples are obtained. Then, in each of the bootstrap samples, model (13.1) is fitted to outcome 1 (e.g. SBP) to obtain $\hat{\theta}_{i1}$ and then to outcome 2 (e.g. DBP) to obtain $\hat{\theta}_{i2}$, and so on. This produces *b* values of the multiple treatment effect estimates (e.g. *b* values of $\hat{\theta}_{i1}$ and $\hat{\theta}_{i2}$), and their observed correlation (e.g. Pearson's correlation) gives an estimate of their within-trial correlation (e.g. $\rho_{Wi(1,2)}$). When *b* is large (e.g. 10000), the $\rho_{Wi(1,2)}$ estimated from bootstrapping should be very similar to the $\rho_{Wi(1,2)}$ estimated directly from the joint modelling approach of model (13.2).

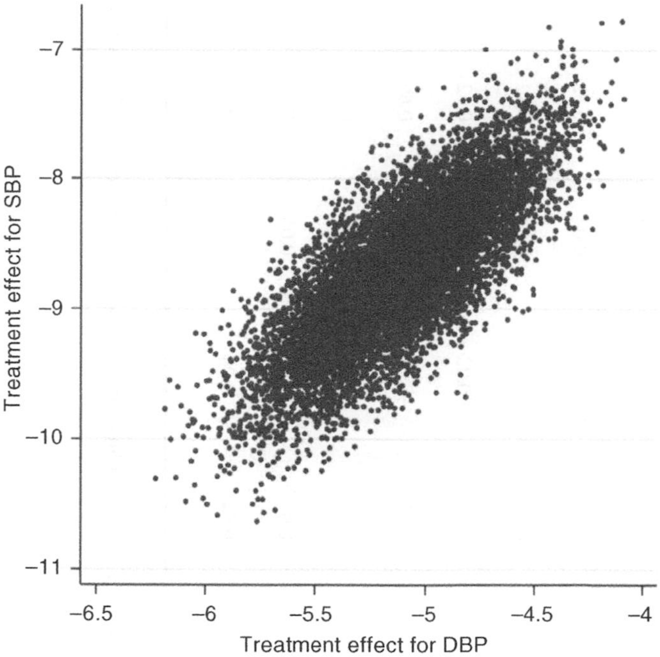

Figure 13.1 Scatterplot of 10,000 pairs of treatment effect estimates on systolic blood pressure (SBP) and diastolic blood pressure (DBP), obtained from 10,000 bootstrap samples of a single randomised trial examining the effect of anti-hypertensive treatment versus control. The observed correlation is +0.77, which provides an estimate of the within-trial correlation of the SBP and DBP treatment effect estimates in this trial. *Source:* Richard Riley.

Example: Application to a randomised trial of anti-hypertensive treatment

To illustrate the bootstrap approach, Figure 13.1 shows 10,000 pairs of treatment effect estimates obtained from 10,000 bootstrap samples of a single randomised trial examining the effect of anti-hypertensive treatment on SBP and DBP. In each bootstrap sample, ANCOVA model (13.1) was applied to estimate the adjusted mean difference (treatment minus control) in SBP at the end of follow-up, and then also applied to estimate the adjusted mean difference in DBP. Negative estimates indicate a greater reduction in blood pressure in the treatment group than in the control group. The figure shows a strong linear association between the estimates of treatment effect on SBP and DBP. Their observed Pearson's correlation is +0.77, and this provides an estimate of the within-trial correlation of the SBP effect estimate ($\hat{\theta}_{i1}$) and the DBP effect estimate ($\hat{\theta}_{i2}$) for this particular trial. When using the joint modelling approach of model (13.2), the estimate of within-trial correlation obtained post-estimation is also +0.77. Indeed, for all 10 trials the within-trial correlations from bootstrapping and joint modelling are almost identical (Table 13.1).

13.2.1.3 Extension to Binary, Time-to-event and Mixed Outcomes

Joint models are also possible for multiple binary outcomes or multiple survival outcomes.[65–68] However, they are sometimes less easy to fit and there may also be mixed outcomes, such as one continuous and one binary outcome, or one binary and one survival outcome. For example, in the IPD meta-analysis of anti-hypertensive treatment, the treatment effects on the time-to-event outcomes of stroke and cardiovascular disease (CVD) are of interest alongside the continuous

Table 13.1 Summary results for the 10 trials included in the meta-analysis of Wang et al.[64], as reported by Riley et al.[58]

	ANCOVA[2] treatment effect for outcomes 1 and 2		Cox regression treatment effect for outcomes 3 and 4		Within-trial correlations						
Trial name[1]	SBP Mean difference (var)	DBP Mean difference (var)	CVD log (HR) (var)	Stroke log (HR) (var)	SBP and DBP from model (13.2)	SBP and DBP from bootstrap	SBP and CVD from bootstrap	SBP and Stroke from bootstrap	DBP and CVD from bootstrap	DBP and Stroke from bootstrap	CVD and Stroke from bootstrap
ATMH	−6.66 (0.72)	−2.99 (0.27)	−0.09 (0.17)	−1.91 (1.17)	0.78	0.79	0.01	−0.01	−0.02	−0.02	0.16
HEP	−14.17 (4.73)	−7.87 (1.44)	0.06 (0.13)	−0.15 (0.17)	0.45	0.50	0.11	0.10	0.09	0.10	0.64
EWPHE	−12.88 (10.31)	−6.01 (1.77)	−0.17 (0.20)	0.75 (0.35)	0.59	0.59	−0.21	−0.05	−0.04	−0.04	0.10
HDFP	−8.71 (0.30)	−5.11 (0.10)	−0.24 (0.03)	−0.29 (0.07)	0.77	0.77	0.09	0.02	0.13	0.04	0.52
MRC-1	−8.70 (0.14)	−4.64 (0.05)	−0.18 (0.03)	−0.41 (0.11)	0.66	0.64	0.04	0.04	0.04	0.04	0.42
MRC-2	−10.60 (0.58)	−5.56 (0.18)	−0.23 (0.02)	−0.20 (0.03)	0.49	0.50	0.00	0.03	−0.02	0.00	0.62
SHEP	−11.36 (0.30)	−3.98 (0.075)	−0.32 (0.02)	−0.45 (0.02)	0.50	0.48	−0.01	−0.02	−0.03	−0.03	0.69
STOP	−17.93 (5.82)	−6.54 (1.31)	−1.87 (1.17)	0.32 (0.83)	0.61	0.59	−0.02	−0.07	−0.03	0.00	0.35
Sy-Chi	−6.55 (0.41)	−2.08 (0.11)	−0.33 (0.09)	−0.48 (0.04)	0.45	0.45	0.11	0.08	0.03	0.03	0.78
Sy-Eur	−10.26 (0.20)	−3.49 (0.04)	−0.26 (0.03)	−0.55 (0.03)	0.51	0.48	0.05	0.04	0.04	0.05	0.62

[1] Trial names are consistent with Wang et al.[64], where further details and trial publications can be found.
[2] Treatment effect is the mean difference (treatment group minus control group) in the participants' final blood pressure (follow-up minus baseline) after adjusting for baseline values, as derived by fitting model (13.1) in each trial separately;
SBP = systolic blood pressure; DBP = diastolic blood pressure; var = variance; CVD = cardiovascular disease
Source: From Table 1 of Riley et al.,[58] with permission, © 2014 Riley et al. (CC-BY 4.0).

outcomes of SBP and DBP. Joint models for mixed outcomes would typically require non-standard user-written likelihood functions. Therefore, a separate modelling approach for each outcome will often be the most convenient, with bootstrapping then used to derive within-trial correlations. That is, in the *b* bootstrap samples for each trial, different types of analyses (e.g. linear, logistic or Cox regressions) can be fitted to each outcome. For example, researchers might apply an ANCOVA model for SBP, an ANCOVA model for DBP, a Cox regression model for CVD, and a Cox regression model for stroke. These provide *b* sets of four treatment effect estimates, and the observed correlation between each pair of effect estimates provides an estimate of their within-trial correlation.[58] We applied this approach to each of the 10 randomised trials of anti-hypertensive treatment, and the within-trial correlation estimates are shown in Table 13.1.

Often researchers are interested in multiple binary outcomes, and these may also be related to one another, especially if they are nested or mutually exclusive. Nested outcomes occur when one outcome is a subset of the other, such as *unplanned caesarean section* and *any adverse maternal outcome* in pregnancy. Mutually exclusive outcomes occur when participants with one outcome cannot experience the other, for example *delivery by caesarean section* and *instrumental delivery other than caesarean section*. In each trial providing IPD, those nested or mutually exclusive binary outcomes can be identified, and the number of events obtained for each (although such information may also be available in trial publications, for example in contingency tables). Treatment effect estimates such as of log odds ratios or log risk ratios can then be estimated for each outcome in each trial, along with their within-trial variances. Then their within-trial correlations can be estimated via bootstrapping. Sometimes researchers will be interested in related binary outcomes that are neither nested nor mutually exclusive, such as *pain-free walking by one month* and *reduction in swelling by one month* after a knee operation.

One issue for bootstrapping is when the outcome event is rare, as then some bootstrap samples may contain zero outcome events in one or both groups and treatment effects may not be estimable. This will lead to some bootstrap samples being discarded, and may lead to bias in the subsequent estimate of within-trial correlation. In this situation, an alternative is to derive within-trial correlations after using seemingly unrelated estimation (e.g. via *suest* in Stata), which combines parameter estimates and their variance matrices from different regression models (i.e. one for each outcome) into a single parameter vector with variance matrix (including within-trial covariances) computed using a so-called sandwich or robust estimation method. Another option is to jointly fit different regression models after linking them via a copula function.[69]

13.2.2 Second-stage Analysis: Multivariate Meta-Analysis Model

Having completed the first-stage analyses, the treatment effect estimates ($\hat{\theta}_{ik}$) and their variances (s_{ik}^2) are available for each outcome in each trial, and their within-trial correlations (ρ_{Wi}) are also available. In the second stage, a multivariate meta-analysis model can now be fitted, which generalises the models for meta-analysis of a single outcome introduced in Chapter 5. These could assume that treatment effects are either random (referred to here as a multivariate random-effects meta-analysis) or common (a multivariate common-effect meta-analysis). We assume the random-effects model is more appropriate, to allow for potential between-trial heterogeneity in treatment effects.

13.2.2.1 Multivariate Model Structure

Let $\hat{\boldsymbol{\theta}}_i$ be a vector containing the available K effect estimates $(\hat{\theta}_{i1}, \hat{\theta}_{i2}, ..., \hat{\theta}_{iK})$ for the outcomes in the ith trial ($i = 1$ to S). The general specification of the multivariate meta-analysis model is:

$$\hat{\boldsymbol{\theta}}_i \big| \boldsymbol{\theta}_i \sim N(\boldsymbol{\theta}_i, \mathbf{S}_i)$$
$$\boldsymbol{\theta}_i \sim N(\boldsymbol{\theta}, \boldsymbol{\Sigma}) \tag{13.3}$$

Here N denotes a multivariate normal distribution, $\boldsymbol{\theta}_i$ contains the true underlying effects for the K outcomes for the ith trial, $\mathbf{S}_i$ is the within-trial variance-covariance matrix for the ith trial (assumed known) containing the K variances of the effect estimates (in the diagonal: $s_{i1}^2, s_{i2}^2, ..., s_{iK}^2$) and their covariances (in the off-diagonal; for example $\rho_{Wi(1,2)} s_{i1} s_{i2}$ is the within-trial covariance for outcomes 1 and 2), and $\boldsymbol{\theta}$ is a vector containing the K mean treatment effects (one for each outcome). The matrix $\boldsymbol{\Sigma}$ is the between-trial variance-covariance matrix, and in its unstructured form contains the K between-trial variances of the true treatment effects (in the diagonal: $\tau_1^2, \tau_2^2, ..., \tau_K^2$) and their between-trial covariances (in the off-diagonal; e.g. the between-trial covariance for outcomes 1 and 2 is $\rho_{B(1,2)} \tau_{i1} \tau_{i2}$, where $\rho_{B(1,2)}$ is their between-trial correlation). The number of rows in each vector and matrix is equal to the number of outcomes. The simplest form of model (13.3) is a bivariate meta-analysis of two correlated outcomes:

$$\begin{pmatrix} \hat{\theta}_{i1} \\ \hat{\theta}_{i2} \end{pmatrix} \sim N\left(\begin{pmatrix} \theta_{i1} \\ \theta_{i2} \end{pmatrix}, \begin{pmatrix} s_{i1}^2 & \rho_{Wi(1,2)} s_{i1} s_{i2} \\ \rho_{Wi(1,2)} s_{i1} s_{i2} & s_{i2}^2 \end{pmatrix} \right)$$
$$\begin{pmatrix} \theta_{i1} \\ \theta_{i2} \end{pmatrix} \sim N\left(\begin{pmatrix} \theta_{1} \\ \theta_{2} \end{pmatrix}, \begin{pmatrix} \tau_1^2 & \rho_{B(1,2)} \tau_1 \tau_2 \\ \rho_{B(1,2)} \tau_1 \tau_2 & \tau_2^2 \end{pmatrix} \right) \tag{13.4}$$

Sometimes it can be helpful to express the multivariate model in its marginal form, without the potential nuisance parameters of $\boldsymbol{\theta}_i$:

$$\hat{\boldsymbol{\theta}}_i \sim N(\boldsymbol{\theta}, \mathbf{S}_i + \boldsymbol{\Sigma}) \tag{13.5}$$

For example, the marginal bivariate model is:

$$\begin{pmatrix} \hat{\theta}_{i1} \\ \hat{\theta}_{i2} \end{pmatrix} \sim N\left(\begin{pmatrix} \theta_{1} \\ \theta_{2} \end{pmatrix}, \begin{pmatrix} s_{i1}^2 + \tau_1^2 & \rho_{Wi(1,2)} s_{i1} s_{i2} + \rho_{B(1,2)} \tau_1 \tau_2 \\ \rho_{Wi(1,2)} s_{i1} s_{i2} + \rho_{B(1,2)} \tau_1 \tau_2 & s_{i2}^2 + \tau_2^2 \end{pmatrix} \right) \tag{13.6}$$

The magnitude of correlation amongst outcomes drives any difference between multivariate and univariate results (Section 13.2.4). If the within-trial and between-trial correlations (i.e. the off-diagonal elements of $\mathbf{S}_i$ and $\boldsymbol{\Sigma}$) are all zero, the multivariate model simplifies to K separate univariate random-effects meta-analyses (one for each outcome).

13.2.2.2 Dealing with Missing Outcomes

Not all trials record the same outcomes. Hence, the treatment effect estimate for outcome k ($\hat{\theta}_{ik}$) may not be calculable for all trials in the IPD meta-analysis. Likelihood-based estimation of model (13.3) can handle such missing estimates under a missing at random assumption, which means that the probability of a particular pattern of missing data depends only on the data observed in that pattern (Chapter 18). This assumption implies that if, say, the treatment effect for outcome 1 is missing in a trial, the expected value of this missing treatment effect can be inferred conditional on the observed treatment effects for available outcomes in this trial and also other trials. A similar assumption is used when handling missing outcomes at the participant level using model (13.2).

The exact likelihood for the multivariate model can be written to accommodate missing data. For example, in a situation with two outcomes, the bivariate likelihood corresponding to model (13.3) is used for trials providing both outcomes; the likelihood corresponding to a univariate meta-analysis of outcome 1 is used for trials only providing outcome 1; and the likelihood corresponding to a univariate meta-analysis of outcome 2 is used for trials only providing outcome 2. The univariate likelihoods share some of the same parameters as the bivariate likelihood, and the product of all likelihoods forms the full likelihood, which is then used for parameter estimation. If a software package does not handle missing outcomes in this way, an alternative is to allocate missing effect estimates an arbitrary value (e.g. set $\hat{\theta}_{i1} = 0$ if outcome 1 is missing) with very large variances (e.g. set $s_{i1}^2 = 1000000$ if $\hat{\theta}_{i1}$ is missing) so that they have negligible weight in the meta-analysis, with any corresponding within-trial correlations set to 0. This approach is sometimes referred to as data augmentation.

13.2.2.3 Frequentist Estimation of the Multivariate Model

Estimation of the multivariate model can be achieved by a variety of options,[43] many of which extend estimation methods described in Chapter 5. Usually of most interest are $\hat{\boldsymbol{\theta}}$ and $\hat{\boldsymbol{\Sigma}}$. Given an estimate $\hat{\boldsymbol{\Sigma}}$, the maximum likelihood solution for the $\hat{\boldsymbol{\theta}}$, the vector of summary effect estimates, is

$$\hat{\boldsymbol{\theta}} = \left(\sum_{i=1}^{N} \hat{\mathbf{W}}_i\right)^{-1} \sum_{i=1}^{N} \hat{\mathbf{W}}_i \hat{\boldsymbol{\theta}}_i \tag{13.7}$$

where $\hat{\mathbf{W}}_i^{-1} = \mathbf{S}_i + \hat{\boldsymbol{\Sigma}}$. This is a multi-dimensional extension of the inverse-variance weighted solution for a single summary effect from a univariate model approach, with the weighting now determined by the matrix $\hat{\mathbf{W}}_i$.

A more difficult challenge is how to obtain $\hat{\boldsymbol{\Sigma}}$. Various frequentist options are available,[43] including approaches such as methods of moments (MM) that estimate $\boldsymbol{\Sigma}$ using a closed-form solution and then plug it into model (13.8),[70–72] and iterative approaches such as REML estimation.[42] REML requires the assumption of multivariate normality for the true treatment effects, $\boldsymbol{\theta}_i$, as made in model (13.3). The MM methods do not make any assumption about the between-trial distribution of true effects, and rather extend the DerSimonian and Laird approach for a single outcome (univariate setting).[73]

Assuming the $\hat{\mathbf{W}}_i$ are known in model (13.7), the variance-covariance matrix of $\hat{\boldsymbol{\theta}}$ is $\left(\sum_{i=1}^{N} \hat{\mathbf{W}}_i\right)^{-1}$, which contains (in the diagonal) the variances of the summary effect estimates and (in the off-diagonal) the covariance of each pair of summary effect estimates. Using the summary estimate and its corresponding variance, we can derive standard confidence intervals for the mean treatment effect (e.g. $\hat{\theta}_1 \pm 1.96\sqrt{\text{var}(\hat{\theta}_1)}$). However, as in the univariate setting, these ignore the uncertainty in the estimated between-trial variances and correlation. To better reflect the uncertainty, one approach is to invert the entire observed Fisher information matrix in order to obtain standard errors (rather than using the expected information matrix); this is implemented in the *mvmeta* package in Stata.[74] An alternative idea, which can be applied regardless of the estimation method used, is a multivariate extension of the univariate Hartung-Knapp-Sidik-Jonkman modification,[15,75] where the variance of each treatment effect is modified (usually inflated) post-estimation, and then 95% confidence intervals derived using the *t*-distribution rather than the normal distribution.

13.2.2.4 Bayesian Estimation of the Multivariate Model

A Bayesian estimation approach is also possible, which is especially important when probabilistic statements are desired, such as that the probability treatment is effective and clinically useful.[62,76,77] As Chapter 5 explains, the Bayesian approach uses computationally intensive methods such as Markov chain Monte Carlo (MCMC) to draw (after an initial burn-in period) thousands of samples from the joint posterior distribution of the unknown parameters, from which inferences (such as means, 95% probability intervals) can be made. It requires prior distributions to be specified for unknown parameters, such as $\mathbf{\Sigma}$ and $\boldsymbol{\theta}$. For example, without any prior beliefs, a vague normal prior distribution could be specified separately for each component of $\boldsymbol{\theta}$, with a mean of zero and a large variance of, say, 1,000,000. The prior distribution is harder to specify for $\mathbf{\Sigma}$, especially when there are three or more outcomes. The conjugate prior distribution for $\mathbf{\Sigma}$ is an inverse Wishart distribution, but this is known to be potentially informative and separation of the components of $\mathbf{\Sigma}$ is preferred to allow realistically vague prior distributions on each term.[77–79] $\mathbf{\Sigma}$ is first separated into variance and correlation matrices by $\mathbf{\Sigma} = \mathbf{V}^{1/2}\mathbf{R}\mathbf{V}^{1/2}$, where $\mathbf{V}^{1/2}$ is a diagonal matrix with between-trial standard deviations (τ_1, τ_2, etc) as elements and $\mathbf{R}$ is a $K \times K$ matrix of between-trial correlations (where k is the total number of outcomes). Then $\mathbf{R}$ is re-parameterised to enforce positive-definite constraints (i.e. correlations cannot be estimated <-1 or >1). Cholesky decomposition or spherical decomposition can achieve this, and we refer the reader to Wei and Higgins, who describe this in full.[77] A product-normal specification of $\mathbf{\Sigma}$ is also possible.[80]

In the bivariate setting, an example set of vague prior distributions for two binary outcomes is

$$\theta_1 \sim N(0, 1000000) \qquad \theta_2 \sim N(0, 1000000)$$
$$\tau_1 \sim N(0, 1)\mathrm{I}(0,) \qquad \tau_2 \sim N(0, 1)I(0,)$$
$$\rho_{B(1,2)} \sim \text{Uniform}(0, 1)$$

where the I(0,) notation denotes that the distribution is truncated at 0, so that non-negative values are avoided. The priors for τ_1 and τ_2 should be context specific, and realistically vague, such that they allow large but sensible values. A number of prior distributions might be examined, especially when the number of trials is small, as the choice of prior distributions may affect the posterior results.[81] As for the Wishart prior distribution, the use of an inverse gamma prior distribution for between-trial variances is best avoided, as it can be extremely influential.[79] Empirical prior distributions are more useful, such as those derived by Rhodes et al. and Turner et al.[82,83]

Burke et al. show that the use of a Uniform(−1,1) prior distribution for ρ_B is not necessarily vague.[79] Instead, researchers should identify a sensible prior distribution perhaps based on clinical, biological, or methodological rationale. For example, a Uniform(0,1) prior distribution corresponds to situations where only positive values are plausible, such as prognostic effects that are partially and fully adjusted, or treatment effects on two highly correlated outcomes like systolic and diastolic blood pressure. A Uniform(−1,0) prior distribution might be specified if only negative values are plausible, for example for sensitivity and specificity from multiple diagnostic test studies that use different thresholds (Chapter 15).

13.2.2.5 Joint Inferences and Predictions

In addition to borrowing strength, a major motivation for multivariate meta-analysis is to make *joint* inferences about the treatment effects across all the outcomes as a whole. This is most natural in a Bayesian MCMC framework. Within each posterior sample, K summary treatment effects are drawn, one for each outcome, and these can be used to make joint probabilistic statements. For example, the probability that the treatment is, on average, beneficial for *all* outcomes can be calculated by the proportion of samples where the drawn summary treatment effects for all outcomes suggest the treatment is beneficial. This can be mirrored after frequentist estimation by drawing samples from an assumed posterior distribution for $\boldsymbol{\theta}$, such as a multivariate normal distribution $\left(\text{i.e. } \boldsymbol{\theta} \sim N\left(\hat{\boldsymbol{\theta}}, \left(\sum_{i=1}^{N} \hat{\boldsymbol{W}}_i\right)^{-1}\right)\right)$ or perhaps a multivariate t-distribution to better reflect the uncertainty.[75]

Multivariate meta-analysis also allows (joint) predictive inferences for treatment effects in new settings for each outcome. Again this is most natural in a Bayesian MCMC approach. Let $\boldsymbol{\theta_{new}}$ be the vector of treatment effects in a new setting similar to those covered by the trials in the meta-analysis, and assume $\boldsymbol{\theta_{new}} \sim N(\boldsymbol{\theta}, \boldsymbol{\Sigma})$ (as in model (13.3)). Each posterior sample draws $\boldsymbol{\theta_{new}}$, and these can be used to make inferences whilst naturally accounting for the uncertainty in $\boldsymbol{\theta}$ and $\boldsymbol{\Sigma}$ (as these are also sampled from their posterior distributions). For example, a 95% probability interval for the first outcome's treatment effect in a new setting, θ_{1_new} (i.e. the first element of $\boldsymbol{\theta_{new}}$) can be calculated by ordering all the drawn samples for $\hat{\theta}_{1\_new}$ and taking those corresponding to the 2.5 and 97.5 percentiles. Joint predictive inferences can also made. For example, the probability that the treatment will be effective for all outcomes in a new setting is the proportion of samples where the drawn predicted effects (i.e. θ_{1_new}, θ_{2_new}, ..., θ_{K_new}) are all in favour of the treatment. Snell et al. suggest an approximate frequentist framework to achieve this, by drawing predicted treatment effects from a multivariate t-distribution.[84]

13.2.2.6 Alternative Specifications for the Between-trial Variance Matrix with Missing Outcomes

We generally prefer $\boldsymbol{\Sigma}$ to be unstructured where feasible, but simplifications are often necessary, especially where elements of $\boldsymbol{\Sigma}$ are not identifiable. In particular, allowing a distinct between-trial correlation per pair of outcomes is problematic when some pairs have no trials (or only a few trials) providing both outcomes. Frequentist estimates of between-trial correlations often converge at +1 or −1 when the number of trials is few, or the between-trial heterogeneity is small relative to the within-trial variability.[85] A practical simplification is to assume all between-trial correlations are the same, and perhaps even all between-trial variances are the same; however, this may be hard to justify, especially when the outcome scales differ. Sometimes there are estimation problems when the treatment effects for some outcomes have no observed heterogeneity. In this situation, it may help to force between-trial variances (and corresponding between-trial correlations) to zero for those apparently homogeneous outcomes. When all elements of the $\boldsymbol{\Sigma}$ matrix are set to zero, model (13.3) simplifies to a multivariate meta-analysis assuming common treatment effects.

13.2.2.7 Combining IPD and non-IPD Trials

Chapter 5 explains how aggregate data from trials not providing IPD could, at least in principle, be included in the second stage of the two-stage IPD meta-analysis approach. This remains true here, but a major issue is that the aggregate data for the non-IPD trials must include the within-trial correlation, but these are unlikely to be available.[60,85] Possible solutions include using a Bayesian framework for the second stage and including a prior distribution for the unknown within-trial correlations to bring in external information (potentially from those trials providing IPD) about the potential values.[62] An alternative is to fit approximate multivariate meta-analysis models that use the overall correlation (rather than decomposing into within-trial and between-trial correlations).[59,61,62,77,83]

13.2.3 Useful Measures to Accompany Multivariate Meta-Analysis Results

13.2.3.1 Heterogeneity Measures

As Chapter 5 explains, between-trial heterogeneity in treatment effects is best summarised directly by reporting the estimates of the between-trial standard deviations (τ_1, τ_2, ..., τ_K). In addition, approximate 95% prediction intervals for the true treatment effect in a new trial for each outcome are useful (Section 13.2.2.5). The between-trial correlations may themselves be of interest (Section 13.7.2).

Higgins and Thompson propose three univariate measures of the impact of heterogeneity, R^2, H^2 and I^2. Jackson and Riley show that the univariate R^2 statistic,[86] which is defined as the ratio of the variance (derived based on standard methods, i.e. not using an approach like HKSJ that modifies variances) for the estimated summary effect under the random-effects and common-effect models, most naturally generalises to the multivariate setting.[87] Let us denote the volumes of the confidence regions (using normal approximations for estimated effects but any fixed coverage probability) for all K estimated effects in $\hat{\boldsymbol{\theta}}$ that arise from the random-effects and common-effect model as V_R and V_C. In one dimension, V_R and V_C are the lengths of the confidence intervals from random-effects and common-effect models, respectively; in two dimensions they are areas; and in three dimensions they are volumes. In four or more dimensions, V_R and V_F are generalised notions of volumes. Jackson and Riley propose the following multivariate R statistic[87]:

$$R = \left(\frac{V_R}{V_C}\right)^{\frac{1}{K}}$$

This reverts to Higgins and Thompson's definition of R when $K = 1$. By taking the Kth root of V_R/V_C, this provides a single summary (across all K outcomes) of the amount of 'stretching' of confidence regions that follows from fitting the multivariate random-effects model, rather than the multivariate common-effect model. After estimation of a multivariate random-effects model and a multivariate common-effect model to a particular dataset, the R statistic can be conveniently calculated as

$$R = \left(\left|\mathrm{Var}_R\left(\hat{\boldsymbol{\theta}}\right)\mathrm{Var}_C\left(\hat{\boldsymbol{\theta}}\right)^{-1}\right|\right)^{\frac{1}{2K}} \tag{13.8}$$

where |.| denotes the determinant, and $\mathrm{Var}_R\left(\hat{\boldsymbol{\theta}}\right)$ and $\mathrm{Var}_C\left(\hat{\boldsymbol{\theta}}\right)$ are the estimated covariance matrices for $\hat{\boldsymbol{\theta}}$ from the multivariate random-effects and common-effect models, respectively. Following the relationships defined in Higgins and Thompson,[86] an overall I^2 for the multivariate meta-analysis can be calculated as:[87]

$$I_R^2 = \frac{R^2 - 1}{R^2}$$

This can be interpreted as a summary (across all K outcomes) of the proportion of the variance of the summary effect estimates that is due to heterogeneity between trials in a multivariate meta-analysis, rather than within-trial variability. This is subtly different from the conventional univariate I^2 statistic, which is broadly defined as the proportion of variability in the observed trial effect estimates that is due to heterogeneity, rather than within-trial variability. They are equivalent when all trials have the same $\mathbf{S}_i$, or there is no observed heterogeneity. I_R^2 is best reported as a percentage (i.e. $I_R^2 \times 100$), as is done for the conventional I^2. As mentioned, equation (13.8) assumes that conventional methods are used to derive variances of summary estimates. When using other approaches like HKSJ, the researcher might alternatively wish to scale up the R statistic based on the modified variances, or even the ratio of t-based and standard normal (z-based) quantiles.

An advantage of the R and I_R^2 statistics is that they can also be evaluated for subsets of the summary effects by using covariance matrices of reduced dimension in equation (13.8) and replacing K with this reduced dimension. Furthermore, R and I_R^2 statistics can be calculated for linear combinations of effects by using appropriate covariance matrices of the linear combinations in (13.8) and replacing K with the dimension of these covariance matrices. Alternative multivariate I^2measures have also been proposed that do reduce to the conventional interpretation,[74,87,88] but cannot be evaluated for subsets, or linear combinations of, the pooled effects. Many of the measures, including the R and I_R^2 statistics, are available within the *mvmeta* package in Stata.

13.2.3.2 Percentage Trial Weights

Riley et al. show how to derive percentage trial weights for one-stage and two-stage multi-parameter meta-analysis models, including multivariate meta-analysis.[89] The method uses a decomposition of Fisher's information matrix to split the total variance matrix of parameter estimates into trial-specific contributions, from which percentage weights are derived. This is equivalent to the approach of Jackson et al., who derived percentage trial weights for multivariate meta-analysis based on a decomposition of the score statistic.[49] It is implemented within the *mvmeta* package of Stata, and also leads to a measure of borrowing of strength (Section 13.2.3.3). Other suggestions for percentage trial weights based on data-point coefficients (Section 13.2.4.3) have been proposed,[60,90] but these are not invariant to transformations of the data.[49] An example displaying percentage trial weights is given in Section 13.3.3.

13.2.3.3 The Efficiency (E) and Borrowing of Strength (BoS) Statistics

Copas et al. suggest that, in comparison to a multivariate meta-analysis, a standard univariate meta-analysis of just the direct evidence is similar to throwing away $100 \times (1 - E)\%$ of the available studies.[91] For a particular outcome, the efficiency (E) is defined by

$$E = \frac{\text{Variance of summary result from multivariate analysis}}{\text{Variance of summary result from univariate analysis}}$$

where the variance relates to the original scale of the meta-analysis (so typically the log relative risk, log odds ratio, log hazard ratio, or mean difference). For example, if $E = 0.9$ then a univariate meta-analysis is similar to throwing away 10% of available trials and participants (and events). We recommend computing E whilst fixing the magnitude of between-trial heterogeneity to be the same in both multivariate and univariate meta-analyses;[91] we return to this issue in Section 13.2.4.2.

Let us define $n_{dir,\,k}$ as the number of available trials with direct evidence (i.e. those that would contribute toward a univariate meta-analysis) for outcome k. Then, the extra information gained for a particular summary meta-analysis result by using correlated evidence within a multivariate meta-analysis can also be considered similar to having found direct evidence from a further

$$n_{dir,k} \times \frac{(1-E)}{E} \text{ trials}$$

of a similar size to the $n_{dir,\,k}$ trials. For example, if nine trials provide direct evidence about an outcome for a standard univariate meta-analysis and $E = 0.9$, then the advantage of using a multivariate meta-analysis is like finding direct evidence for that outcome from a further $9 \times \frac{(1-0.9)}{0.9} = 1$ trial. We thus gain the considerable time, effort and money invested in about one trial.

Jackson et al. also propose the borrowing of strength (*BoS*) statistic,[49] which can be calculated for each summary result within a multivariate meta-analysis by

$$BoS = 100 \times (1 - E)\%$$

BoS provides the percentage reduction in the variance of a particular summary result that is due to (borrowed from) data from other correlated outcomes. As for *E*, it assumes that the between-trial variance estimates are the same in both multivariate and univariate models. To calculate *E* or *BoS*, we recommend using the between-trial variance values estimated from the multivariate analysis.[49]

An equivalent way of interpreting *BoS* for a particular outcome *k* is the percentage weight toward the summary result for outcome *k* that is given to the data for the correlated outcomes ($\neq k$) in the multivariate meta-analysis.[49] For example, in bivariate meta-analysis of two outcomes, a *BoS* of 0% for outcome 1 indicates that the summary result for outcome 1 is based only on data for outcome 1, whereas a *BoS* of 100% indicates that it is based entirely on the correlated data from outcome 2.

In the progesterone example (Box 13.1), the univariate meta-analysis for cancer-specific survival (CSS) includes just the six studies with direct evidence and gives a summary hazard ratio (HR) of 0.61 (95%: 0.38 to 1.00; $I^2 = 70\%$). The multivariate meta-analysis includes an additional 11 studies by borrowing strength from progression-free survival results, and gives a summary HR for CSS of 0.48 (95% CI: 0.29 to 0.79). Here, *BoS* is 33% for CSS, indicating that using the correlated PFS results reduces the variance of the summary log hazard ratio for CSS by 33%. This corresponds to an *E* of 0.67, and the information gained from the multivariate meta-analysis can be considered similar to having found CSS results for an additional $6 \times \dfrac{(1-0.67)}{0.67} \approx 3$ studies.

13.2.4 Understanding the Impact of Correlation and Borrowing of Strength

13.2.4.1 Anticipating the Value of BoS When Assuming Common Treatment Effects

Assume that there is no between-trial heterogeneity, such that the true treatment effect for an outcome is common to all trials. For this situation, Riley et al.[92] show that a multivariate meta-analysis assuming common treatment effects will always produce summary treatment effect estimates with precision equal to or larger than those from separate univariate meta-analyses. The precision will be equal when within-trial correlations are all zero. Copas et al.[91] show that, even when within-trial correlations are non-zero, the precision of multivariate and univariate summary results will be equal if data are complete and the $\mathbf{S}_i$ are exactly the same or proportional to one another across trials. In other situations, the precision of summary treatment effects will be larger (and confidence intervals narrower) following a multivariate meta-analysis, and thus we should anticipate $BoS > 0\%$ in most applications.

Sometimes it may be useful to gauge, in advance of data analysis, the extent of efficiency that could be gained by a multivariate meta-analysis compared to separate univariate meta-analyses. For a multivariate meta-analysis assuming common treatment effects, an approximate rule of thumb is that *BoS* for a particular outcome is bounded by the percentage of trials with missing data for that outcome. For example, consider a bivariate common-effect meta-analysis of two outcomes, with outcome 2 available in all *S* trials, but outcome 1 missing in *m* trials. In terms of *BoS* for outcome 1, the maximum gain in information that a bivariate meta-analysis could achieve (compared to a univariate meta-analysis) is to completely recover the lost information for outcome 1. If trials missing outcome 1 are similar (e.g. in terms of size, events, etc) to other trials that do present outcome 1 (such that trial weights would have been similar had outcome 1 been available in all trials), then the $\max(BoS) \approx 100 \times \left(\frac{m}{S}\right)\%$. We emphasise this is only an approximation, as the weights might not be similar in trials with and without missing outcomes (e.g. if there is a systematic difference in their size or number of events), and other aspects are important.[91] Nevertheless, this rule of thumb for max(*BoS*) may help flag when a multivariate meta-analysis could add value;[93] in particular, if max(*BoS*) is large then researchers may be more motivated to invest their time and resources to collect IPD so that within-trial correlations can be derived.

13.2.4.2 BoS When Assuming Random Treatment Effects

Now consider that there is between-trial heterogeneity in treatment effects for each outcome. In this situation, simulation studies show that a multivariate meta-analysis allowing random treatment effects (i.e. model (13.3)) will also improve precision of summary estimates, *on average*.[85] However, in a particular application, the precision of summary effect estimates may actually decrease in a multivariate random-effects meta-analysis if it estimates larger between-trial variances than univariate meta-analysis. This can occur where the observed heterogeneity of effects in the univariate meta-analysis is artificially narrow, either by chance or because a biased set of the evidence is available due to outcome reporting bias. By borrowing strength from more completely reported outcomes, a multivariate meta-analysis can reduce this bias but, as a consequence, will correctly give larger between-trial variance estimates.[47] For this reason, we recommend that calculation of the *BoS* statistic forces between-trial variances to be the same in univariate and multivariate meta-analysis, as otherwise *BoS* could be negative even though borrowing of strength occurs.[49]

13.2.4.3 How the Borrowing of Strength Impacts upon the Summary Meta-Analysis Estimates

The extra information used in a multivariate IPD meta-analysis may lead to different summary effect estimates compared to univariate meta-analysis.[94] To illustrate this for a bivariate IPD meta-analysis of two outcomes, consider that two trials are available with outcome 2 available in both, but outcome 1 available only in trial two (so $\hat{\theta}_{11}$ is missing). Also let us assume, for simplicity, the between-trial covariance matrix is known. In this situation the analytic solution for the summary treatment effect estimate for outcome 1 from bivariate random-effects model (13.6) is:[60]

$$\hat{\theta}_1 = \hat{\theta}_{21} - \frac{\left(s_{21}s_{22}\rho_{W2(1,2)} + \tau_1\tau_2\rho_{B(1,2)}\right)}{2\tau_2^2 + s_{12}^2 + s_{22}^2}\left(\hat{\theta}_{22} - \hat{\theta}_{12}\right)$$

In other words, the pooled estimate for outcome 1 equals the observed estimate for outcome 1 in trial 2, minus an adjustment due to borrowing of strength from outcome 2. The adjustment depends on the within-trial correlation in trial 2 and the between-trial correlation: if both are zero, then $\hat{\theta}_1 = \hat{\theta}_{21}$, and there is no borrowing of strength from outcome 2.

The adjustment also depends on the value of $\left(\hat{\theta}_{22} - \hat{\theta}_{12}\right)$, the difference in observed estimates for outcome 2 between the trial with outcome 1 observed and the trial with outcome 1 unobserved. This is sensible; when $\hat{\theta}_{22}$ is very different from $\hat{\theta}_{12}$, and given high within- and between-trial correlations, the unknown $\hat{\theta}_{11}$ is likely to be very different from the known $\hat{\theta}_{21}$, thus shifting $\hat{\theta}_1$ away from $\hat{\theta}_{21}$. For example let $\hat{\theta}_{12} = -1$, $\hat{\theta}_{21} = 1$ and $\hat{\theta}_{22} = 1$. Further, let $s_{21} = s_{22} = s_{12} = \tau_1 = \tau_2 = 1$, and $\rho_{W2(1,2)} = \rho_{B(1,2)} = 0.5$ such that there is moderate correlation. In this situation a univariate meta-analysis gives $\hat{\theta}_1 = 1$, but a bivariate meta-analysis gives:

$$\hat{\theta}_1 = 1 - \frac{(0.5 + 0.5)}{4}(1 - (-1)) = 0.5$$

Hence, the correlation allows outcome 1 to borrow strength from outcome 2, and this moves the summary result to 0.5, away from the univariate solution of 1. If the within-trial and between-trial correlations are, rather, set to 1 (i.e. perfect correlation), then the bivariate meta-analysis gives a summary result for $\hat{\theta}_1$ of 0. Thus with larger correlation, the larger the potential shift in summary results from univariate and multivariate meta-analyses.

13.2.4.4 How the Correlation Impacts upon Joint Inferences across Outcomes

As well as deriving summary inferences for each outcome, researchers are often interested in joint inferences across the outcomes. For example, they might want a hypothesis test about whether the treatment is effective for at least one outcome, or wish to estimate a function of the pooled estimates, such as the difference in summary treatment effect on SBP and DBP (i.e. effect on pulse pressure). In order to obtain valid inference, the correlation (or covariance) of summary outcome results must be accounted for. For instance, the variance of $\hat{\theta}_1 - \hat{\theta}_2$ is derived by $\text{var}(\hat{\theta}_1) + \text{var}(\hat{\theta}_2) - 2\text{cov}(\hat{\theta}_1, \hat{\theta}_2)$, where $\text{cov}(\hat{\theta}_1, \hat{\theta}_2)$ is the covariance of $\hat{\theta}_1$ and $\hat{\theta}_2$. If separate univariate analyses are performed, then (unless one of the approaches suggested by Chen and colleagues is adopted,[95,96] which do not provide borrowing of strength) such covariances are either not taken into account or are implicitly assumed to be zero. A major area where functions of pooled estimates are of interest is network meta-analysis (Chapter 14).

13.2.5 Software

Our website (www.ipdma.co.uk) provides examples of statistical code for various case studies used in this chapter. For the first stage of a two-stage multivariate IPD meta-analysis, standard regression methods (e.g. linear, logistic and Cox) can be applied to the IPD in each trial separately to obtain effect estimates and their variances for each trial. More problematic is obtaining within-trial correlations, which generally requires user-written code to perform bootstrapping, or to fit joint ('seemingly unrelated') regression models for the outcomes (such as model (13.2)). The Stata package *mvmeta_make* automates the derivation of effect estimates, their within-trial variances and correlations for each trial, ready for the second stage.[74,97] However, this package only applies to the special situation where the 'outcomes' are multiple parameter estimates from the same regression model (e.g. intercepts and slopes in model (13.1); treatment effects on multiple outcomes in model (13.2); the effect of different categories of a particular covariate; or non-linear dose-response relationships). After the multiple effect estimates are obtained, a bubble plot is useful to summarise the effects for pairs of outcomes and to depict within-trial correlations (Section 13.3.1). This can be produced using the *bubble* option (currently undocumented) in the *mvmeta* package in Stata.

For the second stage, the multivariate meta-analysis model (13.3) can be fitted in standard statistical software packages such as SAS, R, Stata and WinBugs. In SAS, PROC MIXED allows users enormous flexibility in their multivariate model specification, especially for the between-trial covariance matrix, $\boldsymbol{\Sigma}$. An introduction to the basic use of PROC MIXED for multivariate meta-analysis is given by Van Houwelingen et al.[42] The *parms* statement is crucial for specifying (and holding fixed) the within-trial variances and correlations. A potential disadvantage of the PROC MIXED is that it only allows ML or REML estimation. As it is a general package for mixed models, it also does not provide the latest developments such as I_R^2, *BoS* and percentage trial weights.

In contrast, the *mvmeta* packages in Stata and R are regularly updated and tailored to the multivariate meta-analysis field,[74,97,98] and thus have a wider range of estimation and output options, including MM in addition to REML estimation. The Stata package also implements the alternative multivariate model of Riley et al.[59], which is useful in situations where within-trial correlations are not available (i.e. in non-IPD settings). The *mvmeta* package in Stata can also be used to perform network meta-analysis in a frequentist setting, via the package *network*.[99] Nevertheless, non-standard multivariate models may require maximisation of user-written likelihoods. Bayesian multivariate meta-analysis models can be fitted using MCMC simulation, for example using WinBugs, with careful specification of prior distributions as discussed in Section 13.2.2.4.[58,77]

13.3 Application to an IPD Meta-Analysis of Anti-hypertensive Trials

We applied the two-stage multivariate IPD meta-analysis approach to the 10 trials of anti-hypertensive treatment. Firstly, we performed a bivariate meta-analysis of SBP and DBP, then a bivariate meta-analysis of CVD and stroke, and finally a multivariate meta-analysis of all four outcomes. The results obtained using REML estimation are summarised in Table 13.2.

13.3.1 Bivariate Meta-Analysis of SBP and DBP

13.3.1.1 First-stage Results

We applied the ANCOVA model (13.2) to each of the hypertension trials separately, to estimate the treatment effect on SBP and DBP after adjusting for baseline values. The treatment effect estimates and their variances for SBP and DBP are shown in Table 13.1 together with their within-trial correlations, which are all positive and quite high (ranging from +0.45 to +0.79), a consequence of the high correlation between SBP and DBP values at the participant level. The within-trial correlations are shown visually through the angle of the confidence ellipse for the effects in each trial (Figure 13.2).

13.3.1.2 Second-stage Results

We combined the trial estimates obtained from the first stage using bivariate random-effects meta-analysis model (13.4). The frequentist results after REML estimation are shown in Table 13.2. There is a large positive between-trial correlation estimate of +0.78, indicating that trials with a higher than average true treatment effect on SBP also have a higher than average true treatment effect on DBP.

The REML summary treatment effect estimates suggest that, on average, anti-hypertensive treatment reduces both SBP ($\hat{\theta}_1 = -10.21$, 95% CI: –12.11 to –8.30) and DBP ($\hat{\theta}_2 = -4.59$, 95% CI: –5.61 to –3.57) by more than control. A Bayesian approach obtains similar estimates and gives a posterior probability of almost 1 that $\theta_1 < 0$, and a probability of almost 1 that $\theta_2 < 0$, providing very strong evidence that on average anti-hypertensive treatment is effective at reducing each outcome.

As there are no missing outcomes across trials, summary results for both SBP and DBP are very similar to those from univariate meta-analysis.[58] This is reflected by small *BoS* values of 0.6% and 0.1%, indicating that the summary results for each outcome have gained barely anything from the other outcome. However, unlike separate univariate analyses, the multivariate approach enables *joint* inferences. For example, the Bayesian approach estimates a probability of 0.12 that anti-hypertensive treatment will reduce *both* SBP and DBP by at least 5 mmHg on average, which illustrates the use of a more stringent minimum reduction for clinical acceptability. Researchers might also be interested in the average treatment effect on pulse pressure (SBP – DBP), which was $\hat{\theta}_1 - \hat{\theta}_2 = -5.61$ (95% CI: –6.94 to –4.29) from the REML analysis. Wrongly applying two separate univariate analyses (and thus ignoring the correlation amongst outcomes) gave a more conservative confidence interval of –7.73 to –3.42 for the effect on pulse pressure.

Table 13.2 Bivariate and multivariate results for the IPD meta-analysis of 10 trials of anti-hypertensive treatment, as obtained from REML estimation, building on those originally shown by Riley et al.[58]

Model	Outcome	Effect type	Summary treatment effect (95% CI^)	Borrowing of strength, *BoS*	Impact of between-trial heterogeneity (I_R^2)	Between-trial standard deviation*	Between-trial correlation
Bivariate	SBP	Mean difference	−10.21 (−12.11 to −8.30)	0.6%	96.0%	2.71	SBP, DBP: +0.78
	DBP	Mean difference	−4.59 (−5.61 to −3.57)	0.1%	95.8%	1.48	
Bivariate	CVD	HR	0.78 (0.69 to 0.89)	1.4%	0%	<0.000001	CVD, Stroke: 1.00**
	Stroke	HR	0.68 (0.60 to 0.78)	11.1%	0%	<0.000001	
Multivariate	SBP	Mean difference	−10.22 (−12.14 to −8.30)	0.9%	96.0%	2.73	SBP, DBP: +0.79 SBP, CVD: −0.31 SBP, Stroke: −0.53 DBP, CVD: −0.83 DBP, Stroke: −0.94 CVD, Stroke: +0.97
	DBP	Mean difference	−4.63 (−5.67 to −3.60)	0.5%	95.9%	1.51	
	CVD	HR	0.79 (0.69 to 0.91)	4.2%	9.3%	0.05	
	Stroke	HR	0.73 (0.61 to 0.87)	20.8%	43.6%	0.14	

^ Inflated to account for uncertainty in the estimation of between-trial variances and correlation, using the method of White.[74]

* Measured on the log HR scale for stroke and CVD.

** Estimation at edge of boundary space is a consequence of between-trial variance estimates close to zero.

Source: Table adapted from Table 2 of Riley et al.[58], with permission,

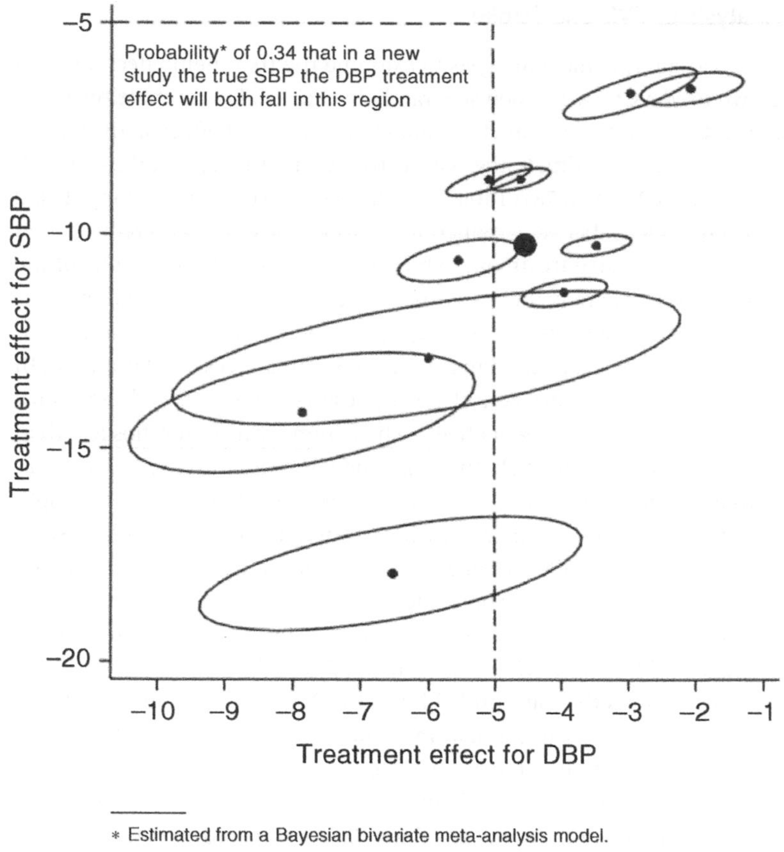

Figure 13.2 Relationship between the observed treatment effect estimates on pressure (SBP) and diastolic blood pressure (DBP), with 50% confidence ellipses around each trial's pair of estimates. The small solid points indicate a pair of estimates from one trial, and the ellipse around each point gives a 50% confidence ellipse. Thus smaller ellipses indicate more precise estimates (i.e. bigger trials). The angle of the ellipse indicates the within-trial correlation. The largest solid point (i.e. the one without an ellipse around it) denotes the pair of summary estimates from the meta-analysis. 50% (rather than 95%) confidence ellipses are given for cosmetic reasons, as otherwise the regions are large and overlap considerably. *Source:* Figure adapted from Figure 1 of Riley et al.[58], with permission, © 2014 Riley et al. (CC-BY 4.0).

13.3.1.3 Predictive Inferences

There is considerable heterogeneity in the treatment effects across trials ($\hat{\tau}_1 = 2.71$, $\hat{\tau}_2 = 1.48$ from REML estimation). The impact of between-trial heterogeneity on the summary result is large for both SBP ($I_R^2 = 96\%$) and DBP ($I_R^2 = 96\%$). Given the heterogeneity, clinicians might not be interested in the average treatment effect across trials, but rather the predicted true treatment effects (θ_{1_new} and θ_{2_new}) in a new trial population. Interest then lies in the bivariate distribution of θ_{1_new} and θ_{2_new} for a new trial; that is, the joint distribution of true treatment effects across new trials for the two outcomes. The Bayesian approach gives a 95% prediction (probability) interval of −14.11 to −5.82 for the true treatment effect for SBP, and −7.28 to −1.75 for the treatment effect for DBP. There is a probability of 0.99 that anti-hypertensive treatment will reduce *both* SBP and DBP more than control in a new population. Further, taking a more stringent level for clinical acceptability, there is a probability of 0.34 that the treatment will reduce both SBP and DBP by at least 5 mmHg more than placebo in a new population. This is the probability that the two predicted effects will fall in the area defined by the dashed lines shown in Figure 13.2.

13.3.2 Bivariate Meta-Analysis of CVD and Stroke

Next, we applied a two-stage bivariate IPD meta-analysis to examine the treatment effect on CVD and stroke. In the first stage, we used a Cox regression separately in each trial to estimate the treatment effect on the hazard rate of CVD, and then again to estimate the treatment effect on the hazard rate of stroke. Bootstrapping was used to estimate the within-trial correlations, and these are all positive and often high (ranging from 0.10 to 0.78) (Table 13.1). This suggests an underlying strong positive association at the participant level between reduction in stroke incidence and reduction in CVD incidence from using anti-hypertensive treatment, which is expected, as stroke is one of the main reasons for a diagnosis of CVD (others include angina, heart attack, and heart failure).

REML estimation of bivariate meta-analysis model (13.4) gives a between-trial correlation of +1; however, this is poorly estimated and has very little impact on the summary results, because both between-trial variances are estimated to be almost zero. Thus the results are similar to those from a bivariate meta-analysis assuming common treatment effects. The summary hazard ratios less than 1 indicate that the treatment is effective at reducing both stroke and CVD risk (Table 13.2). In comparison to univariate meta-analyses, the large within-trial correlations allow borrowing of strength across outcomes. Due to the complete outcome data, borrowing of strength is small. It is largest for stroke ($BoS = 11.1\%$), perhaps due to the smaller number of events for stroke in some trials (and thus more potential to gain from the correlated CVD outcome), which leads to a slight reduction in the standard error of the summary log hazard ratio for stroke from 0.074 in the univariate analysis to 0.070 in the bivariate analysis, and thus a narrower confidence interval.

Joint inferences are important, such as the joint probability of a clinically accepted benefit on both outcomes. For example, following Bayesian estimation of model (13.4), the estimated probability that anti-hypertensive treatment will reduce the hazard rate of stroke *and* CVD by at least 20% in a new trial is 0.52. Wrongly ignoring the correlation between outcomes gives a lower estimated probability of 0.47. Although this difference may appear minor (0.52 compared to 0.47), in situations where different treatment options are being compared (e.g. when multiple treatments exist for the same disease, or when resource limits the number of treatments that can be purchased by a particular healthcare body), such discrepancies in the estimated probability of success may impact upon the priority ranking of each treatment (Section 14.6.4 gives an example).

13.3.3 Multivariate Meta-Analysis of SBP, DBP, CVD and Stroke

So far we have considered bivariate meta-analyses of the same outcome type. But treatment effects may also be correlated for mixed outcomes, such as continuous and survival outcomes, and joint inferences of interest across them. Therefore, a more complete analysis is a multivariate meta-analysis of all four outcomes (SBP, DBP, stroke and CVD), undertaken by fitting model (13.3) using REML estimation. The results in Table 13.2 strongly indicate that anti-hypertensive treatment is effective for all four outcomes on average, with the summary effect for SBP and DBP < 0 and the summary hazard ratio for stroke and CVD < 1. Compared to the bivariate meta-analyses, there are larger *BoS* values for CVD (4.2%) and stroke (20.8%) after additionally accounting for the correlation with SBP and DBP outcomes.

Figure 13.3 shows a forest plot comparing the univariate and multivariate meta-analysis results for stroke, and it includes the percentage trial weights. Due to the borrowing of strength, there is a shift in the summary treatment effect on stroke from univariate (0.68) to multivariate (0.73), and a change in the percentage trial weights; for example, the SHEP trial has 34.2% weight in the univariate analysis and 24.9% weight in the bivariate meta-analysis. There was also a wider confidence interval for the summary treatment effect on stroke in the multivariate meta-analysis, which is

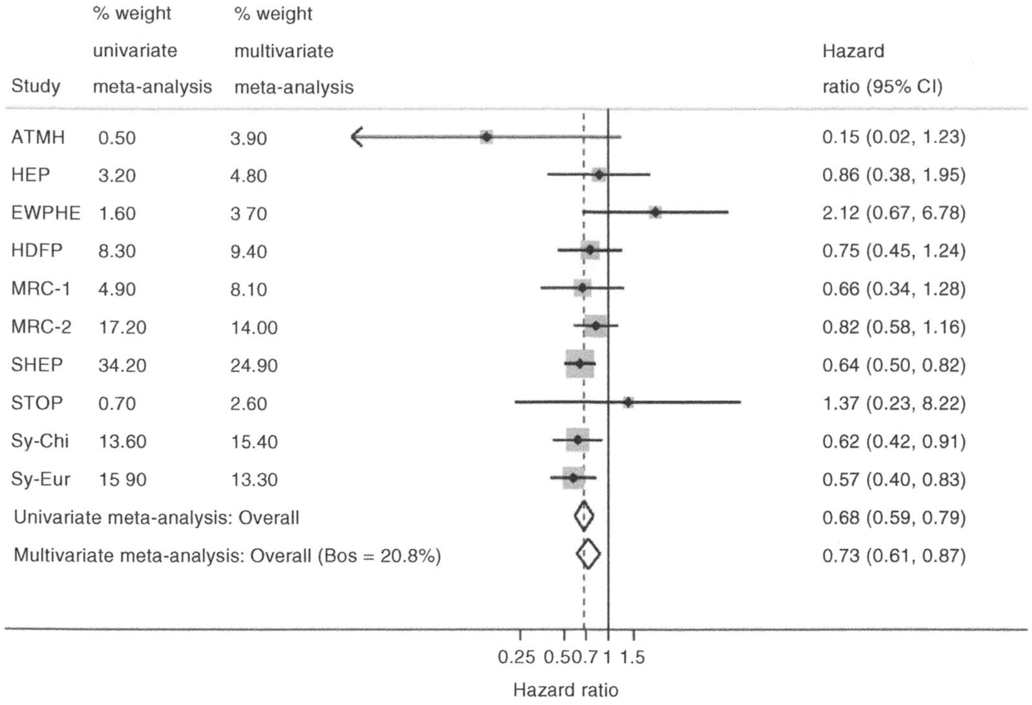

Figure 13.3 Forest plot comparing the summary treatment effect results and percentage trial weights for the stroke outcome from univariate and multivariate random-effects meta-analyses of 10 randomised trials of anti-hypertensive treatment. *Source:* Richard Riley.

due to a larger estimate of between-trial heterogeneity ($\hat{\tau}_4 = 0.14$) compared to univariate meta-analysis ($\hat{\tau}_4 = 0$) (Section 13.2.4.2).

A Bayesian multivariate IPD meta-analysis estimates that, if applied to a new trial population, there is a probability of 0.82 that anti-hypertensive treatment will reduce SBP by at least 5 mmHg *and* reduce the hazard of stroke by at least 20%. This is illustrated by the probability of the effects falling in the dashed area marked in Figure 13.4. Blood pressure outcomes are often viewed as a surrogate for clinical outcomes; that is, treatment effects on blood pressure predict treatment effects on clinical outcomes. Surrogacy would require positive between-trial correlations between blood pressure and clinical outcomes. However, Table 13.2 shows negative correlations. Rather than reflecting a genuine negative relationship (i.e. increase the treatment effect on blood pressure but decrease its effect on survival), this finding may be due to chance, or a consequence of inconsistent definitions of exactly when last follow-up values of SBP and DBP were recorded in each trial, and how they are linked to survival events (e.g. last blood pressure recorded close to death in those who died). A proper evaluation of surrogacy would require clearer understanding of the pathway between SBP and DBP measurements and subsequent survival outcomes, which was not available in the hypertension IPD meta-analysis dataset used here. Surrogate outcomes are considered further in Section 13.7.2.

13.4 Extension to Multivariate Meta-regression

The second stage of the two-stage multivariate IPD meta-analysis can be extended to a multivariate meta-regression by including trial-level covariates.[100] For example, with two outcomes, model (13.4) can be extended to a bivariate meta-regression including a covariate for year of trial publication, z_i, as follows:

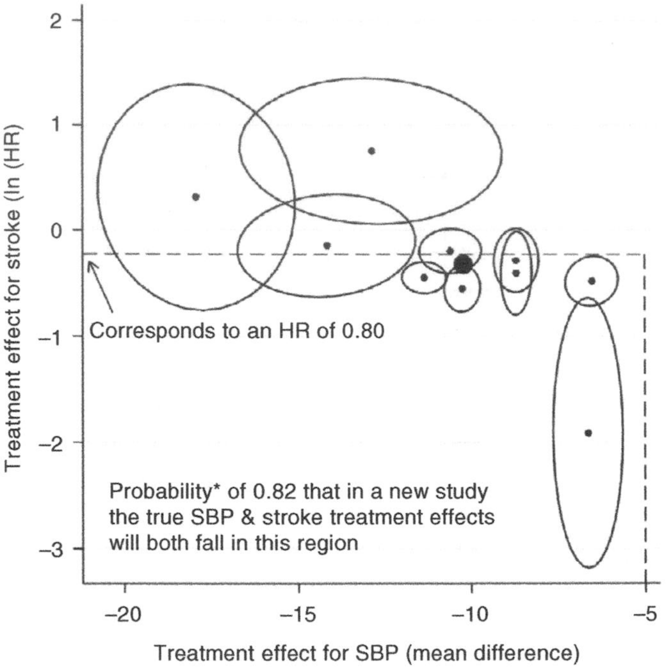

* Estimated from a Bayesian four-outcome multivariate meta-analysis model.

Figure 13.4 Relationship between the observed treatment effect estimates on systolic blood pressure (SBP) and stroke, with 50% confidence ellipses and a joint predictive inference.

The smaller points indicate a pair of estimates from one trial, and the ellipse around each point gives a 50% confidence ellipse. Thus smaller ellipses indicate more precise estimates (i.e. bigger trials). The angle of the ellipse indicates the within-trial correlation. 50% (rather than 95%) confidence ellipses are given for cosmetic reasons, as otherwise the regions are large and overlap considerably. The larger point (without an ellipse) denotes the pair of summary estimates from the meta-analysis. *Source:* Figure adapted from Figure 2 of Riley et al.[58], with permission, © 2014 Riley et al. (CC-BY 4.0).

$$\begin{pmatrix} \hat{\theta}_{i1} \\ \hat{\theta}_{i2} \end{pmatrix} \sim N\left(\begin{pmatrix} \theta_{i1} \\ \theta_{i2} \end{pmatrix}, \begin{pmatrix} s_{i1}^2 & \rho_{Wi(1,2)} s_{i1} s_{i2} \\ \rho_{Wi(1,2)} s_{i1} s_{i2} & s_{i2}^2 \end{pmatrix} \right)$$
$$\begin{pmatrix} \theta_{i1} \\ \theta_{i2} \end{pmatrix} \sim N\left(\begin{pmatrix} \alpha_1 + \lambda_1 z_i \\ \alpha_2 + \lambda_2 z_i \end{pmatrix}, \begin{pmatrix} \tau_1^2 & \rho_{B(1,2)} \tau_1 \tau_2 \\ \rho_{B(1,2)} \tau_1 \tau_2 & \tau_2^2 \end{pmatrix} \right) \tag{13.9}$$

After fitting model (13.9), of key interest are the estimates of λ_1 and λ_2, which reveal whether a one-unit increase in z_i is associated with a change (across trials) in the true treatment effect for outcomes 1 and 2, respectively. As emphasised for meta-regression of a single outcome in Chapters 5 and 7, across-trial relationships are especially prone to aggregation bias, confounding, and low power, and so should be used with caution. An example of a multivariate meta-regression to examine trial-level covariates is given in Section 13.6.2.1, and more extensively elsewhere.[42,56,100]

13.5 Potential Limitations of Multivariate Meta-Analysis

The previous sections showcase the value of multivariate meta-analysis, but the approach is not without potential challenges, as now described.

13.5.1 The Benefits of a Multivariate Meta-Analysis for Each Outcome Are Often Small

> "... *multivariate and univariate models generally give similar point estimates, although the multivariate models tend to give more precise estimates. It is unclear, however, how often this added precision will qualitatively change conclusions of systematic reviews.*"[101]

This argument is based on empirical evidence,[93,101,102] and might be levelled at our IPD meta-analysis of the 10 anti-hypertensive trials (Table 13.2), as the borrowing of strength is small for most outcomes, and so conclusions are similar in both univariate and multivariate analyses. Figure 13.5 shows that in the empirical review by Trikalinos et al.,[101,103] the *BoS* value is often small (<20%) and the summary estimates and confidence intervals are generally similar for multivariate and univariate analyses.[93]

As mentioned in Section 13.2.4, the potential importance of a multivariate IPD meta-analysis is greatest when *BoS* and $1 - E$ are large. This is evident in Figure 13.5, with observed differences between multivariate and univariate summary results increasing as the magnitude of *BoS* increases; in some examples (e.g. review ID 10 and 38 in Figure 13.5) the conclusions are importantly affected, either based on size of summary effect and/or confidence intervals overlapping the null value.

In general, *BoS* and $1 - E$ will be largest in situations where the outcomes are highly correlated and some trials have missing outcomes (Section 13.2.4.1). Yet, even with complete outcomes in all trials, there may be broader reasons why a multivariate analysis is important. In particular, if joint (summary or predictive) inferences are of interest across correlated outcomes, then these are best derived using multivariate framework (regardless of the amount of missing data and potential *BoS*), in order to account for correlations between outcomes and thus avoid erroneous confidence intervals and *p*-values (Section 13.2.4.4)[92].

13.5.2 Model Specification and Estimation Is Non-trivial

Even when *BoS* is anticipated to be large, challenges may remain.[43] Multivariate meta-analysis models are often complex, and achieving convergence (i.e. reliable parameter estimates) may require simplification (e.g. common between-trial variance terms for each outcome; multivariate normality assumption), which may be open to debate.[43,104,105] Convergence and estimation problems increase as the number of outcomes (and hence unknown parameters) increase, and so applications of multivariate meta-analysis beyond two or three outcomes are rare.

13.5.3 Benefits Arise under Assumptions

> "*But borrowing strength builds weakness. It builds weakness in the borrower because it reinforces dependence on external factors to get things done.*"[106]

As mentioned in Section 13.2.2.2, the benefits of multivariate meta-analysis depend on missing outcomes being missing at random.[107] We are assuming that the relationships that we *do* observe in some trials are transferable to other trials where they are unobserved. Further, assuming multivariate normal distributions within and between trials implies that the observed linear association (correlation) of effects for pairs of outcomes (both within trials and between trials) is transferable to other trials where only one of the outcomes is available. This relationship is especially important to justify surrogate outcomes,[108] where it is often subject to criticism and debate.[109] Some

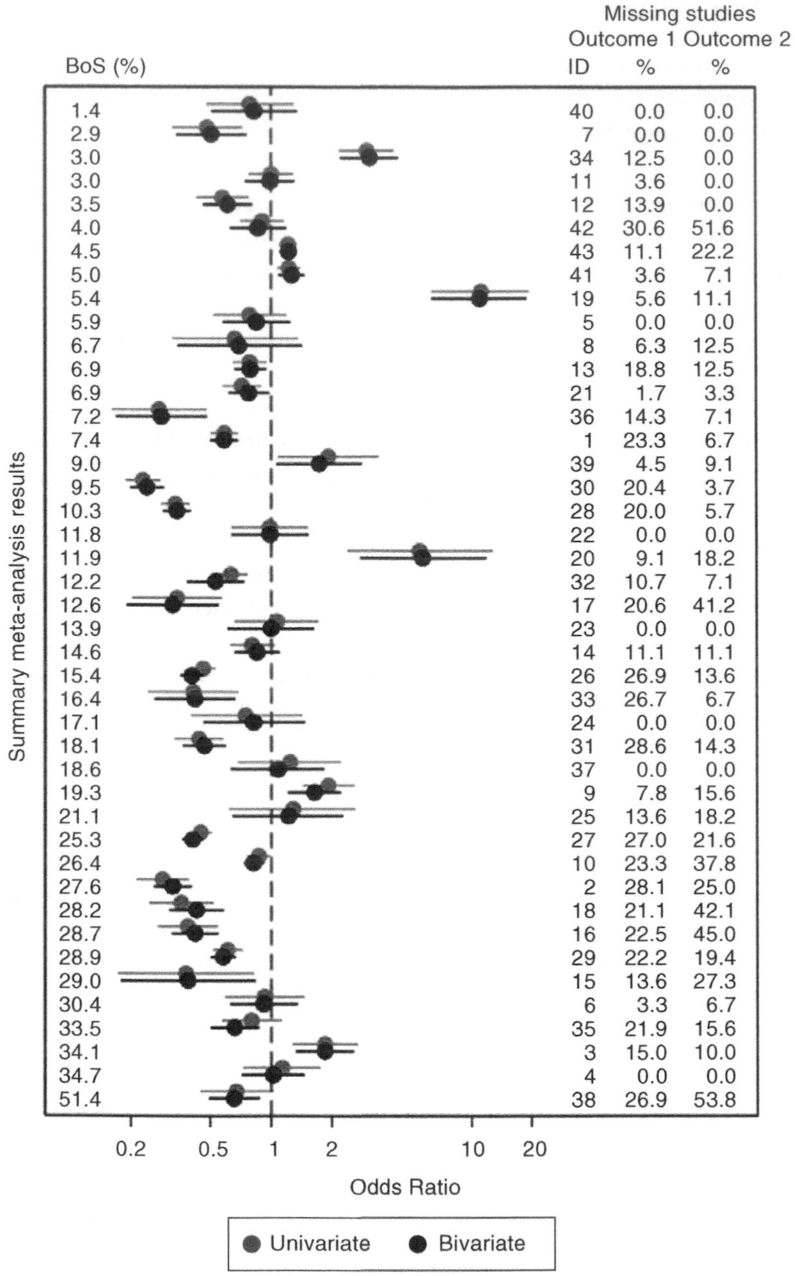

Figure 13.5 Comparison of summary meta-analysis results for outcome 1 in the empirical review by Trikalinos et al.,[101] with corresponding *BoS* and missing outcome information. *Source:* Richard Riley, produced using results provided by Hattle et al.[93]

researchers prefer to allow different (non-linear) associations between trials, for example via copula methods,[69,104,110] which is outside the scope of this book.

Missing *not* at random may be more appropriate when results are missing due to selective outcome reporting[111] or selective choice of analyses.[112] However, IPD meta-analysis projects should seek to retrieve all outcomes of interest from those trials providing their IPD; hence, outcome availability bias should not be a concern in an IPD meta-analysis project. The exception is when there are trials providing their IPD that decide to withhold some recorded outcomes; if they do, this raises concerns about the overall integrity of those trials and whether they should be included in the IPD meta-analysis at all. If including such trials, a multivariate IPD meta-analysis approach may help reduce selective outcome availability biases in this situation,[47] and thus be preferable to separate univariate meta-analyses. However, to remove the bias completely, the exact mechanism for causing the missing outcomes should be modelled.[113]

13.6 One-stage Multivariate IPD Meta-Analysis Applications

So far we have focused on a two-stage approach to multivariate meta-analysis, but multiple outcomes might also be handled via a one-stage approach. As explained in Chapter 8, one-stage and two-stage models will usually give very similar results; however, differences may arise, and one-stage methods are especially useful when participants or outcome events are sparse. Therefore, in this section we consider one-stage IPD meta-analysis models, through a series of applications.

13.6.1 Summary Treatment Effects

One-stage multivariate IPD meta-analysis models come with all the potential advantages and disadvantages outlined for a one-stage meta-analysis of a single outcome (as detailed in Chapters 6 and 8). Additionally for multiple outcomes, a key advantage of a one-stage approach is that it avoids having to derive within-trial correlations; a key disadvantage is that the number of parameters to estimate will quickly become large and potentially unwieldy.

Consider a one-stage IPD meta-analysis of two continuous outcomes, such as SBP and DBP, that extends the ANCOVA approach for analysing a single trial given in model (13.2). Essentially the one-stage model jointly estimates model (13.2) and the second part of model (13.4):

$$
\begin{aligned}
&y_{ijk} = \phi_{ik} + \beta_{ik} y_{0ijk} + \theta_{ik} x_{ij} + e_{ijk} \\
&e_{ijk} \sim N\left(0, \sigma_{ik}^2\right) \qquad cov\left(e_{ij1}, e_{ij2}\right) = \sigma_{i(1,2)} \\
&\begin{pmatrix} \theta_{i1} \\ \theta_{i2} \end{pmatrix} \sim N\left(\begin{pmatrix} \theta_1 \\ \theta_2 \end{pmatrix}, \begin{pmatrix} \tau_1^2 & \rho_{B(1,2)}\tau_1\tau_2 \\ \rho_{B(1,2)}\tau_1\tau_2 & \tau_2^2 \end{pmatrix} \right)
\end{aligned}
\tag{13.10}
$$

13.6.1.1 Applied Example

Using REML estimation to fit one-stage model (13.10) to the IPD from the 10 anti-hypertensive trials, with SBP and DBP as the outcomes, and deriving confidence intervals using the Kenward-Roger approach (as recommended in Chapter 6), the summary results are almost identical to those for the two-stage multivariate IPD meta-analysis approach (Table 13.3). This echoes the main message of Chapter 8: when the assumptions and estimation methods are the same, and the data are not sparse, then one-stage and two-stage IPD meta-analysis results will be very similar.

13.6.2 Multiple Treatment-covariate Interactions

Perhaps the main motivation for a one-stage multivariate IPD model is to analyse both multiple participant-level and trial-level covariates, to reduce within-trial and between-trial variability respectively, and to examine treatment-covariate interactions for all the outcomes simultaneously.

Table 13.3 Results from two-stage and one-stage bivariate meta-analysis of SBP and DBP for the hypertension data as obtained from REML estimation.

Model	Outcome	Effect type	Summary treatment effect (95% CI^)	Between-trial standard deviation*	Between-trial correlation
Two-stage (model (13.1) then model (13.3))	SBP	Mean difference	−10.21 (−12.11 to −8.30)	2.71	SBP, DBP: +0.78
	DBP	Mean difference	−4.59 (−5.61 to −3.57)	1.48	
One-stage (model (13.10))	SBP	Mean difference	−10.23 (−12.09 to −8.36)	2.75	SBP, DBP: +0.78
	DBP	Mean difference	−4.60 (−5.59 to −3.60)	1.48	

* 95% CIs calculated using the Kenward-Roger method in the one-stage analysis, and using the method of White in a two-stage analysis[74] to account for uncertainty in between-trial variance estimates.
Source: Richard Riley.

Riley et al. suggest a framework for this,[56] which allows all the correlation amongst outcomes and parameters to be accounted for in the modelling. As emphasised in Chapter 7, it is important to avoid aggregation bias in one-stage models, including treatment-covariate interaction terms. One way to achieve this is to include participant-level covariates centered about their means, and include an additional term for their mean values. For example, with one participant-level covariate (z_{ij}), such as age, and one trial-level covariate ($\bar{z}_i$) that represents the mean of z_{ij}, such as mean age, the one-stage bivariate meta-analysis of model (13.10) can be extended to:

$$\begin{gathered} y_{ijk} = \phi_{ik} + \beta_{ik} y_{0ijk} + \theta_{ik} x_{ij} + \mu_{ik} z_{ij} + \gamma_{Wk} x_{ij} \left(z_{ij} - \bar{z}_i \right) + e_{ijk} \\ e_{ijk} \sim N\left(0, \sigma_{ik}^2\right) \quad cov\left(e_{ij1}, e_{ij2}\right) = \sigma_{i(1,2)} \\ \begin{pmatrix} \theta_{i1} \\ \theta_{i2} \end{pmatrix} \sim N\left(\begin{pmatrix} \alpha_1 + \gamma_{A1}\bar{z}_i \\ \alpha_2 + \gamma_{A2}\bar{z}_i \end{pmatrix}, \begin{pmatrix} \tau_1^2 & \rho_{B(1,2)}\tau_1\tau_2 \\ \rho_{B(1,2)}\tau_1\tau_2 & \tau_2^2 \end{pmatrix} \right) \end{gathered} \tag{13.11}$$

Here, we stratify nuisance parameters by trial; that is, we have separate trial intercepts per outcome (ϕ_{ik}), and separate adjustment effects for the baseline outcome value (β_{ik}) and the baseline age (μ_{ik}). Of key interest are λ_{W1} and λ_{W2}, together with γ_{A1} and γ_{A2}. The γ_{W1} and γ_{W2} denote interactions between the treatment effect and the participant-level covariate for outcomes 1 and 2, respectively. These are assumed common for simplicity, although this could be relaxed by adding additional random effects. The W notation emphasises that the interactions are based only on within-trial information. In contrast, the A notation emphasises an association based only on across-trial information, with γ_{A1} and γ_{A2} representing the across-trial association of the trial treatment effects and the mean covariate value ($\bar{z}_i$), for outcomes 1 and 2 respectively. Riley et al. show how to combine IPD trials with non-IPD trials in this one-stage framework.[56] An alternative two-stage approach is also possible; the multiple treatment-covariate interactions are estimated in each trial separately (first stage), and then these estimates are combined in a multivariate model that accounts for their correlation (second stage).

Table 13.4 Results from one-stage bivariate IPD meta-analysis of 10 randomised trials of anti-hypertensive treatment to examine within-trial interactions and across-trial associations for age and the effect of treatment on SBP and DBP

Parameter from model (13.11)	Outcome	Interpretation of parameter	Summary estimate (95% CI)
Within-trial interaction, γ_{W1}	SBP	The change in treatment effect on SBP within trials for a one-unit increase in age	−0.049 (−0.114 to 0.015)
Within-trial interaction, γ_{W2}	DBP	The change in treatment effect on DBP within trials for a one-unit increase in age	0.001 (−0.034 to 0.036)
Across-trial association, γ_{A1}	SBP	The change in a trial's overall treatment effect on SBP for a one-unit increase in mean age	−0.138 (−0.249 to −0.027)
Across-trial association, γ_{A2}	DBP	The change in a trial's overall treatment effect on DBP for a one-unit increase in mean age	−0.028 (−0.106 to 0.051)

Source: Richard Riley.

13.6.2.1 Applied Example

Using the IPD meta-analysis of anti-hypertensive trials, let us apply model (13.11) to examine whether there are interactions between age and the treatment effects on SBP and DBP. The results are shown in Table 13.4. There is no strong evidence of a treatment-age interaction within trials, for either SBP or DBP. Thus, after adjusting for baseline blood pressure, anti-hypertensive treatment appears to have the same benefit on SBP and DBP regardless of an individual's age. In contrast, the mean age is strongly associated with a larger overall treatment effect for SBP (although not DBP); those trials with a higher mean age have a larger (more negative) treatment effect for SBP, and thus mean age explains some of the between-trial variability in treatment effects for SBP. This across-trial association is most likely due to other trial-level factors that change across trials, and it does not arise from an underlying participant-level relationship between age and treatment effect.

13.6.3 Multinomial Outcomes

A two-stage multivariate meta-analysis is problematic when outcome events are sparse, as it is for univariate meta-analysis (Chapter 8), as trial-specific estimates may require the use of continuity corrections and may not be normally distributed. In contrast, a one-stage approach allows the IPD to be modelled more exactly.[114] For example, for nested or mutually exclusive outcomes, Trikalinos et al.[101] show how multinomial distributions can be used to model the number of outcome events within trials whilst incorporating random effects to allow for any between-trial heterogeneity in the true log odds ratios and their between-trial correlation.

When outcomes are missing in some trials, the categories that define the multinomial model are not all available in all trials. In such trials, the within-trial likelihood becomes a reduced multinomial (or binomial) likelihood, but can still be written in terms of the full set of probabilities (for the full set of categories), such as p_{ij1}, p_{ij12} and p_{ij3} for three categories.[115] For example, the probability of being in either category 1 or 2 could be written as $p_{ij1} + p_{ij2}$ in trials that do not provide the numbers in categories 1 and 2 separately. This is a non-standard model, and requires a user-written likelihood, as most software packages would otherwise remove the trials with missing categories, which would lose precision.

In our experience, convergence problems can arise with one-stage multinomial models, especially when the proportion of missing outcome data is large and frequentist estimation is used. The problem is that category probabilities must sum to one within trials, and also across trials (on average); this constraint can lead to estimation difficulties, especially when the true probabilities vary considerably across trials. In this situation, a Bayesian approach with informative prior distributions may be useful.[101,103,115] Alternatively, a multiple imputation approach could be used. Here, in each trial separately, the missing categories are imputed for each participant, conditional on the observed categories (and potentially other participant-level information in the IPD). Then, the one-stage multinomial IPD meta-analysis is applied. This process is repeated a certain number of times, and then Rubin's rules used to combined results across the set of imputations, to obtain the summary results. Multiple imputation within an IPD meta-analysis is considered further in Chapter 18.

13.7 Special Applications of Multivariate Meta-Analysis

Potential applications of multivariate IPD meta-analysis are broad. In this section, we highlight some further applications that warrant special mention.

13.7.1 Longitudinal Data and Multiple Time-points

A natural extension of multivariate IPD meta-analysis models is to longitudinal data (or repeated measures data), where summary results at two or more follow-up time-points are of interest. Randomised trials often report results for multiple time-points, but usually the set of time-points only partly overlaps across trials. Therefore, a multivariate IPD meta-analysis is warranted to borrow strength across time-points, and improve efficiency compared to a univariate meta-analysis at each time-point separately. An IPD meta-analysis that wrongly assumes time-points are independent can result in less precise summary results, and may even produce biased estimates at particular time-points if the subset of IPD trials that provide those time-points is a biased subset of all trials that recorded those time-points.[116–118]

The article by Jones et al. describes how to undertake a two-stage multivariate IPD meta-analysis of randomised trials with a longitudinal continuous outcome.[119] The approach to use depends on whether time is modelled as a discrete or continuous factor. When time is taken as discrete, the approach is analogous to a two-stage multivariate IPD meta-analysis of multiple outcomes; essentially the discrete time-points (e.g. 1 month, 3 months, 6 months, and 12 months) are considered to be 'outcomes'. In the first step a repeated measures linear regression model is fitted to the IPD in each trial separately, treating time as a discrete factor and estimating a separate treatment effect at each time-point, whilst accounting for the correlation amongst multiple responses over time from the same participant (and potentially allowing a separate residual variance at each time-point). This produces a vector of treatment effect estimates in each trial ($\hat{\boldsymbol{\theta}}_i$) spanning the time-points of interest, and the corresponding estimated within-trial covariance matrix, $\mathbf{S}_i$. Jones et al. also provide an equation for deriving within-trial correlations between treatment effect estimates at a pair of time-points within a randomised trial of a continuous outcome.[119] The equation depends on the residual variances and correlation in participant responses at the two time-points, as well as the number of participants contributing to each time-point and the number contributing to both. Occasionally, such information may be available without IPD, for example from trial reports or authors.

The second step fits a multivariate meta-analysis model, to estimate the vector of mean treatment effects ($\boldsymbol{\theta}$), as specified in Section 13.2.2. Ideally an unstructured between-trial covariance matrix is assumed. However, when estimates for some time-points are sparse, it may be necessary for simplifying assumptions such as a common between-trial variance at all time-points or an autoregressive correlation structure, such that between-correlations are largest between pairs of neighbouring time-points and gradually reduce as time-points become further apart.

A difficulty with modelling time as a discrete factor is that trials give different follow-up times, and therefore 'similar' time-points may need to be grouped to facilitate meta-analysis. For example, 24 weeks in trial 2, 28 weeks in trial 4, and 30 weeks in trial 5 might all be classed as '6 months' in order to synthesise results across trials. To avoid this, an alternative is to model responses over time as a continuous trend. Here, in the first stage, a repeated measures regression model is fitted to the IPD in each trial separately, usually assuming a linear trend in mean responses over time but with a separate intercept and slope for control and treatment groups. Correlation amongst multiple responses from the same participant is again accounted for. This leads to a vector $\hat{\boldsymbol{\theta}}_i$ containing two estimates per trial: the estimated differences in intercepts and slopes of the mean regression lines for the treatment and control groups, and the corresponding (here, two-by-two) within-trial covariance matrix ($\mathbf{S}_i$). The second stage is then a bivariate meta-analysis model, assuming either common or random effects for the intercept and slope differences. This leads to an estimated summary mean difference in intercepts ($\hat{\alpha}_D$ say), and an estimated summary mean difference in slopes ($\hat{\beta}_D$ say), which can then be used to obtain the treatment effect at any time-point of interest (including those not actually reported by any of the original trials). For example, assuming that the time scale was modelled in months, the treatment effect at six months would be $\hat{\alpha}_D + \left(6 \times \hat{\beta}_D\right)$. Extension to non-linear trends is possible,[120] for example using splines or fractional polynomials in each treatment group, which is then similar to a multivariate meta-analysis of a dose-response relationship (Section 13.7.3 and Chapter 16).

A limitation with a meta-analysis of trend parameters is that trials with a single time-point will be excluded, as they do not allow a trend to be estimated. To address this, Jones et al.[119] propose a further approach, essentially a hybrid between the aforementioned approaches for time as discrete and continuous factors. In the first stage, time is taken as a factor and a repeated measures model fitted to the IPD in each trial separately, to give the vector of treatment effect estimates ($\hat{\boldsymbol{\theta}}_i$) and within-trial covariance matrix ($\mathbf{S}_i$) in each trial. Then, in the second approach, a summary (linear or non-linear) trend is fitted through the data points ($\hat{\boldsymbol{\theta}}_i$), weighting by the $\mathbf{S}_i$ and potentially allowing for between-trial heterogeneity (and correlation) in the trend parameters (e.g. intercept and slope) across trials. The estimated summary trend can then be used to estimate a summary treatment effect at any time-point of interest.

13.7.1.1 Applied Example

Jones et al. show that accounting for the correlation amongst time-points is important,[119] as the estimate and standard error of the multivariate meta-analysis summary result at each time-point can differ dramatically from those from separate univariate analyses. They considered an IPD meta-analysis of five trials investigating the effects of selegiline (10 mg/day) versus placebo for the treatment of Alzheimer's disease,[19] with respect to the Mini-Mental State Examination (MMSE) score, a measure of cognitive function ranging 0 and 30, with higher values being regarded as good. When time was treated as a discrete factor, the available time-points were grouped to create common time-points across trials. That is: month 1 = weeks 4 and 5; month 2 = weeks 8 and 9; month 4 = week 17; month 6 = weeks 24, 25 and 30; month 9 = week 35 and 43; month 12 = weeks 56 and 65. Not all time-points were available in all trials.

A two-stage multivariate common effect meta-analysis, with time as a factor, provides no strong evidence of differences between selegiline and placebo at any of the time-points (Table 13.5). When the time-points were wrongly assumed uncorrelated and a series of separate univariate meta-analyses conducted at each time-point, the summary estimates and standard errors are very different. For example, assuming zero correlation the summary difference (between selegiline and placebo groups) at 9 months is 0.69 with standard error of 0.63, compared to the multivariate summary estimate of 0.34 with standard error of 0.52. Notably, the standard error is consistently smaller when accounting for correlation, due to the borrowing of strength.

When considering time as continuous, one trial was removed as it provided only one time-point. The subsequent summary results give no evidence that the difference between selegiline and placebo follows a linear trend over time or that selegiline is better than placebo (Table 13.5). Ignoring correlation between intercept and slope estimates gives underestimated standard errors of the summary treatment effect estimates. Very similar conclusions are also found when using the hybrid approach (time modelled as a discrete factor in first stage, then a linear trend modelled in the second stage).

13.7.1.2 Extensions

An alternative one-stage IPD meta-analysis approach is also feasible, where the longitudinal participant-level responses from all trials are analysed in a single model, accounting for the correlation of multiple responses from the same participant and the clustering of participants within trials (via stratified intercepts). Again, time could be considered as either a factor or continuous.[119] In the Jones et al. MMSE example, one-stage results are almost identical to the two-stage results shown in Table 13.1 when using REML estimation.

The same principles of one-stage or two-stage, or treating time as a factor or continuous, also apply to meta-analysing repeated binary outcome data. Trikalinos and Olkin consider multivariate meta-analysis of treatment effect estimates for binary outcomes as measured by four common metrics (log odds ratio, log risk ratio, risk difference, and arcsine difference at multiple time-points).[121] For a two-stage approach, they provide formulae for estimating within-trial variances and within-trial correlations between effect estimates at pairs of time-points, which depend on the total numbers of participants and the proportion with the outcome of interest in each group at each time-point. Such information may be available even without IPD.

Further novel extensions for meta-analysis of longitudinal data include network meta-analysis applications,[120,122] and joint modelling of longitudinal and survival outcomes.[123–125] IPD also allows the transition between outcomes to be modelled directly (for example, the rate to recurrence, and then the subsequent rate to death), which would facilitate multi-state modelling.[126] Similarly, multivariate meta-analysis can summarise survival proportions over time.[127–129]

13.7.2 Surrogate Outcomes

Sometimes the magnitude of correlation between a pair of outcomes is of key interest, for example in the evaluation of surrogate outcomes where a treatment's effect on one outcome (such as disease-free survival) is used as a surrogate (proxy) for the treatment's effect on another outcome that is of more interest clinically (such as overall survival), but would take longer to evaluate. The use of

Table 13.5 Summary results following REML estimation of a two-stage multivariate IPD meta-analysis with time either as a discrete or continuous factor, as reported by Jones et al.[119] A common treatment effect is assumed for each time-point.

	Time as a discrete factor (five trials)^		**Time as a continuous factor (four trials)^^**
	Multivariate meta-analysis (accounts for within-trial correlation of effect estimates across time-points)	**Separate univariate meta-analyses (ignores within-trial correlation of effect estimates across time-points)**	**Multivariate meta-analysis (accounts for correlation of within-trial intercept and slope estimates)**
Parameter	**Estimate (s.e.)**	**Estimate (s.e.)**	**Estimate (s.e.)**
Intercept	N/A	N/A	0.37 (0.52)
Slope	N/A	N/A	–0.005 (0.036)
Summary treatment effect* at 1 month	0.30 (0.47)	0.43 (0.54)	0.37 (0.51)
Summary treatment effect* at 2 months	–0.47 (0.59)	–0.84 (0.97)	0.36 (0.51)
Summary treatment effect* at 4 months	0.33 (0.47)	0.75 (0.57)	0.35 (0.51)
Summary treatment effect* at 6 months	0.19 (0.48)	0.31 (0.50)	0.34 (0.52)
Summary treatment effect* at 9 months	0.34 (0.52)	0.69 (0.63)	0.32 (0.55)
Summary treatment effect* at 12 months	–0.03 (0.55)	0.29 (0.66)	0.31 (0.60)

* Difference in mean MMSE score for selegiline versus placebo.

^ Time as a discrete factor: treatment effect was estimated at distinct time-points in each trial and these were then jointly meta-analysed to produce summary results for each time-point directly.

^^ Time as continuous factor: a linear trend of the treatment effect over time was estimated in each trial and then meta-analysed to produce a pooled linear trend, which is then used to derive summary treatment effects at each time-point.

Source: Richard Riley, using data extracted from Jones et al.[119]

multivariate meta-analysis to evaluate potential surrogate outcomes (or so-called surrogate markers) has been well-discussed,[68,130–134] including how it can be used to predict the effect of a treatment on the clinical outcome(s) of interest, based on the observed effect of the treatment on the surrogate outcome(s) of interest.

Buyse and Molenberghs emphasise the importance of considering both participant-level and trial-level correlations in the evaluation of a candidate surrogate,[130] and also suggest that a surrogate is only 'valid' if both trial-level and participant-level correlations are high.[133] IPD enables Prentice's criteria for validation of surrogate endpoints to be checked at the participant level.[135–137] If the participant-level correlation is high then this adds credence to the outcomes being causally linked to each other, whilst a high between-trial correlation indicates that a large proportion of the variation in treatment effect for the clinical outcome(s) of interest is captured by the variation in treatment effect for the surrogate outcome(s). If participant-level correlation is low, then there is unlikely to be a surrogate relationship even if the trial-level association is high. Further, trial-level correlations are prone to aggregation bias and confounding, and thus it is important to check whether correlations are consistent at the participant level and trial level.

Participant-level outcome relationships can be derived in the first stage of a two-stage multivariate IPD meta-analysis, and are rarely available without IPD. For a pair of continuous outcomes, in each trial we can calculate the correlation of the observed outcome values (y_{ij1} and y_{ij2}); the correlation of the pair of residuals (e.g. $\hat{\sigma}_{i(1,2)}/\hat{\sigma}_{i1}\hat{\sigma}_{i2}$ from model (13.2)); and the within-trial correlation of the pair of treatment effect estimates ($\rho_{Wi(1,2)}$). For non-continuous outcomes, the focus is on the within-trial correlation of the pair of treatment effect estimates (which is produced as a consequence of participant-level associations of outcomes), which can be obtained using bootstrapping post-estimation (as outlined in Section 13.2.1.2) or after incorporating a copula function to link otherwise separate regression models for each outcome during estimation (e.g. to link two hazard functions[138]).

In the second step of a multivariate IPD meta-analysis, the between-trial correlation of the true treatment effects for the main and surrogate outcome is estimated (e.g. $\rho_{B(1,2)}$ in model (13.4)). This is then used (alongside the summary results and their uncertainty) to predict the treatment effect for the main outcome in new trials where only the surrogate is available.[139] A Bayesian framework is often recommended,[140] to make predictions whilst accounting for parameter uncertainty,[141] although measurement error models might be used to address this in a frequentist setting.[138] To test performance of a surrogate outcome, cross-validation can be employed to compare predicted (i.e. from the surrogate) and observed treatment effects in new trials.[131,138,139] In each cycle of cross-validation, a trial is either entirely removed,[131] or its main clinical outcome considered missing;[139] then the meta-analysis model is fitted to the remaining data, and used to predict the treatment effect for the main clinical outcome in the omitted trial, which can be compared to the actual observed effect. This is repeated across all permutations of the trial omitted for validation. Ideally predicted treatment effects will closely agree with observed treatment effects. A package called *surrosurv* is available for R, which implements many of the aforementioned approaches,[138] whilst producing important summary measures and graphs.

Traditionally a bivariate framework is used to evaluate one surrogate outcome in regards to one main clinical outcome. Bujkiewicz et al. considered extension to trivariate and high-order multivariate models,[139] to allow a single framework for evaluating the joint use of two or more surrogate endpoints to predict the clinical outcome. By using multiple surrogate outcomes, there is a potential for more precise predictive inferences about the treatment effect for the main outcome of interest.

13.7.3 Development of Multi-parameter Models for Dose Response and Prediction

Section 13.7.1 describes the synthesis of intercepts and slopes from randomised trials with longitudinal outcomes. Another area where the whole regression equation (including the intercept or, for survival models, the baseline hazard) is important is for clinical prediction models,[142] where the fitted equation (e.g. whole logistic regression model) is needed to predict outcome risk for individuals based on their covariate values. Given IPD from multiple studies, the same model could be fitted in each study and the estimated regression coefficients combined in a multivariate meta-analysis, to produce an overall model. Chapter 17 provides detailed explanation of the use of IPD meta-analysis methods for developing and validating clinical prediction models.

Another important application is for examining dose-response relationships,[88,98,143] for example between the amount of alcohol intake and risk of cancer.[144,145] Interest is in how increasing the dose or value of a factor increases (or decreases) the risk of a poor outcome. In the first stage a suitable linear or non-linear dose-response model can be fitted in each study; in the second stage, a multivariate meta-analysis is used to synthesise intercepts and slopes (for linearity), and additionally other terms (such as spline terms, quadratic terms, etc) that allow for non-linearity, whilst accounting for the correlations amongst each pair of parameters.[88,146] This produces a summary relationship across studies, and misleading inferences are possible if correlation is ignored. For example, Orsini et al. found strong evidence for a linear trend between alcohol intake and lung cancer risk when using the multivariate approach ($p = 0.03$),[145] but not when wrongly ignoring correlation ($p = 0.58$). IPD meta-analysis for risk and prognostic factor research is described in Chapter 16, including the synthesis of non-linear associations.

13.7.4 Test Accuracy

In diagnostic or screening test research, multivariate meta-analysis methods are being used to deal with correlation between sensitivity and specificity. Typically such methods have allowed one pair of sensitivity and specificity estimates per study.[147] However, extended multivariate meta-analysis models can accommodate multiple pairs of results per study, which arise when test accuracy estimates are available at multiple thresholds,[148,149] as is the case when IPD are available. Monotonic relationships can be enforced within and between studies, such that sensitivity decreases and specificity increases as the threshold increases, and this enables a summary ROC curve to be produced. Further discussion is given in Chapter 15.

13.7.5 Treatment-covariate Interactions

Multivariate IPD meta-analysis can also enhance examinations of treatment-covariate interactions, as follows.

13.7.5.1 Non-linear Trends

A two-stage multivariate IPD meta-analysis also allows the synthesis of multiple parameter estimates defining a non-linear treatment-covariate interaction, for example as defined by a restricted cubic spline function or a fractional polynomial function. Further details are given in Chapter 7.

13.7.5.2 Multiple Treatment-covariate Interactions

Section 13.6.2 proposes a multivariate model for examining two treatment-covariate interactions, one for each of two outcomes. However, often multiple treatment-covariate interactions are of interest for the *same* outcome, and these may be correlated with each other due to the covariates themselves being correlated, such as age, BMI, blood pressure, and biomarker measurements. Accounting for this correlation in a multivariate meta-analysis may be useful, especially when the IPD for some trials does not include all the covariates of interest. For example, when considering interactions with treatment for each of two biomarkers, some trials may only measure biomarker A and not biomarker B. In this situation, the second stage of a two-stage multivariate IPD meta-analysis synthesises the pair of interactions jointly, and allows the interaction with treatment effect for biomarker B to borrow strength from the interaction with treatment effect observed for biomarker A. In this way, the impact of missing data for biomarker B is reduced. An example accounting for correlation of biomarkers Ch1p and MYCN in neuroblastoma patients is given by Riley et al.[60] Related discussion is given in Chapter 18 on missing data.

13.8 Concluding Remarks

Enabling multivariate meta-analysis is a major advantage of having IPD. Longitudinal data and multiple outcomes are common within IPD from multiple randomised trials, and this chapter shows how the multivariate approach allows them to be modelled more effectively by accounting for their correlation. Extended applications include synthesis of multiple model parameters, synthesis of correlated prognostic effects, and summaries of non-linear associations. Various other potential uses are possible, and we refer readers to further topics.[42,150–152] Examples in later chapters include novel applications to diagnosis, prognosis and prediction (Chapters 15 to 17) and missing data (Chapter 18). Network meta-analysis can also be expressed in a multivariate framework, as described in the next chapter.

14

Network Meta-Analysis Using IPD

Richard D. Riley, David M. Phillippo, and Sofia Dias

Summary Points

- There are often multiple treatments available for the same clinical condition; evidence synthesis of existing randomised trials can inform decisions about which treatments are best.
- Existing randomised trials rarely directly compare all the available treatments; rather, each directly compares a subset of treatments of interest.
- A network meta-analysis simultaneously synthesises such trials, allowing the direct evidence about available treatment comparisons to be combined with indirect evidence propagated through the network. This produces summary treatment effect estimates, and provides a coherent framework for all the treatments to be compared and ranked.
- Rankings can be very sensitive to the uncertainty in summary results and do not reveal clinical value. In particular, focusing on the probability of being ranked first is potentially misleading: a treatment ranked first may also have a high probability of being ranked last, and its benefit over other treatments may be of little clinical relevance.
- A network meta-analysis combines direct and indirect evidence by assuming consistency between these two sources of evidence.
- The consistency assumption should be evaluated in each network where possible. There is usually low power to detect inconsistency, which mainly arises when trial-level or participant-level effect modifiers are systematically different in the subsets of trials providing direct and indirect evidence.
- IPD has the same potential advantages for network meta-analysis as it does for pairwise meta-analysis, including standardising participant inclusion criteria, outcome definitions and length of follow-up in each trial; allowing analyses that adjust for prognostic factors and treatment effect modifiers; and conducting analyses within subgroups of individuals.
- The main *additional* advantages of IPD for network meta-analysis pertain to inconsistency and its detection or reduction. In particular, IPD enables researchers to examine and plot covariate distributions to improve detection, and allows statistical models to include adjustment for covariates that cause inconsistency (e.g. effect modifiers, and prognostic factors when modelling non-collapsible measures such as odds ratios).
- Even if IPD are available from just one or a few trials in the network, it may be possible to adjust for effect modifiers by fitting a multi-level network meta-regression model, and to produce estimates of population-adjusted average treatment effects.

Individual Participant Data Meta-Analysis: A Handbook for Healthcare Research, First Edition.
Edited by Richard D. Riley, Jayne F. Tierney, and Lesley A. Stewart.

14.1 Introduction

Healthcare organisations and decision makers, such as the National Institute for Health and Care Excellence (NICE) in the United Kingdom, require evidence synthesis of existing studies to inform their policies. In particular, decisions about the best available treatments can be informed by meta-analysis of data from multiple randomised trials. However, individual trials rarely provide direct evidence about *all* the available treatments, and rather each trial compares a different subset of treatments. For example, in a meta-analysis of 28 trials to compare eight thrombolytic treatments after acute myocardial infarction, it is unrealistic to expect every trial to compare all eight treatments;[153] in fact a different set of treatments was examined in each trial, and the maximum number of trials per treatment was only eight.[153] This creates problems for meta-analysis. For example, if a separate meta-analysis is performed for each treatment contrast (e.g. treatment A versus treatment B), then the available trials for each meta-analysis will differ. Furthermore, for each meta-analysis, any trials that do not provide *direct evidence* about the treatment comparison of interest will be excluded. This is unwelcome, especially if their participants are otherwise representative of the population, clinical settings and condition of interest. Research studies require considerable costs and time, and involve precious patient involvement, and simply discarding them could be viewed as research waste.[44–46] Statistical models for *network meta-analysis* address this by meta-analysing all relevant trials in a single framework to summarise and compare the multiple treatments simultaneously.[51] For each treatment contrast, this also allows direct evidence to be combined with indirect evidence from other sets of treatment contrasts available in the network, which may lead to a considerable gain in precision of summary results and inferences (also known as 'borrowing of strength', as described in Chapter 12).[48]

In this chapter, we explain the key concepts, methods, and assumptions of network meta-analysis. This is a large field, and readers who require a more complete overview are referred to the book by Dias et al.[154] and other technical documents.[155–161] Here, we provide a practical overview in the context of having IPD from all or a subset of randomised trials to be included in a network meta-analysis. We begin by explaining the key assumptions, statistical models and summary measures for network meta-analysis (Sections 14.2 to 14.5), and then detail why the availability of IPD can improve the application and robustness of network meta-analysis compared to the conventional use of published aggregate data (Sections 14.6 to 14.8). We focus on statistical analysis issues, as other tasks such as identifying relevant trials, examining risk of bias, and obtaining, cleaning and harmonising IPD are the same as those described in Part 1 of this book.

14.2 Rationale and Assumptions for Network Meta-Analysis

A meta-analysis that evaluates a particular treatment comparison (e.g. treatment A versus B) using only direct evidence is known as a 'pair-wise meta-analysis'. When the set of treatments compared differs across trials, this approach may greatly reduce the number of trials per meta-analysis, and makes it hard to formally compare more than two treatments. A network meta-analysis addresses this by synthesising all trials in the same analysis whilst utilising both the *direct* and *indirect evidence*.[74,99,162]

Consider a simple network meta-analysis of three treatments (A, B and C) evaluated in previous randomised trials. Assume that the relative treatment effect (i.e. the treatment contrast) of A versus B is of key interest, and that some trials compare A and B directly. However, there are also other trials of A versus C, and of B versus C, which provide no direct evidence of the benefit of A versus B, as they did not examine both A and B. Indirect evidence of A versus B can still be obtained from these trials under the so-called "consistency" assumption which states that, on average across all trials regardless of the treatments compared, the

$$\text{Treatment contrast of A versus B} = (\text{treatment contrast of A versus C}) - (\text{treatment contrast of B versus C})$$

where 'treatment contrast' is a measure that compares the relative effect of two treatments, such as a log relative risk, log odds ratio, log hazard ratio or mean difference. This relationship will always hold *exactly* within any randomised trial where A, B and C are all examined. However, it is plausible that it will also hold (on average) across those trials that only compare a reduced set of treatments, if their clinical and methodological characteristics (such as quality, length of follow-up, case-mix) are similar in each subset (here, A versus B, A versus C, and B versus C trials). In this situation, the benefit of A versus B can be inferred from the indirect evidence from comparing trials of just A versus C with trials of just B versus C, in addition to the direct evidence coming from trials of A versus B (Figure 14.1).

Another way of expressing this is that a network meta-analysis assumes any missing treatment comparisons are *missing at random*.[107] That is, the relationships between treatments that we *do* observe in some trials are assumed transferable to other trials where they are unobserved. This is also known as *transitivity*;[163,164] it implies that the *relative* effects of three or more treatments observed directly in some trials would be the same in other trials where they are unobserved, such that the treatment effects are 'exchangeable'.[165] Based on this, the consistency assumption then holds. When the direct and indirect evidence disagree, this is known as inconsistency (incoherence).

Note that a network meta-analysis comparing three or more treatments makes no additional assumptions to a conventional pairwise meta-analysis comparing two treatments. In both cases, we require that relative treatment effects are exchangeable across trials. Furthermore, comparing three or more treatments using results from separate pairwise meta-analyses is not guaranteed to give consistent estimates (i.e. inconsistency may occur), and does not utilise any indirect evidence

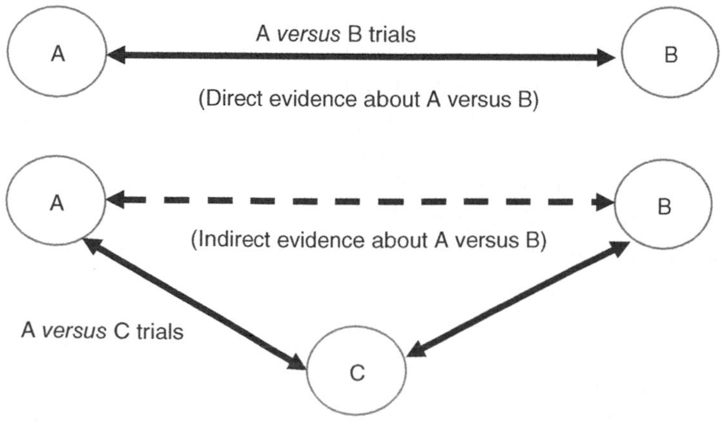

Figure 14.1 Visual representation of direct and indirect evidence toward the comparison of A versus B. *Source:* Richard Riley.

on each treatment comparison. In contrast, a network meta-analysis is a comprehensive framework that utilises all the available (direct and indirect) evidence to provide coherent summary results that inform clinical decision making about the efficacy of each of multiple treatments.

14.3 Network Meta-Analysis Models Assuming Consistency

In this section we outline the general statistical framework for conducting a network IPD meta-analysis model assuming consistency. This framework uses either two-stage or one-stage approaches that build on those described in Part 2 of this book. Initially we assume that IPD are available from all randomised trials of interest, although the models described are also applicable if relevant aggregate data (such as treatment effect estimates or two-by-two tables) can be obtained directly for each trial (e.g. from publications). The additional advantages of having IPD for network meta-analysis are the focus of Section 14.6, and how to incorporate aggregate data from any trials not providing IPD is considered in Section 14.7.

14.3.1 A Two-stage Approach

In the first stage of a two-stage network IPD meta-analysis, the IPD are analysed separately for each trial to calculate treatment effect estimates and their corresponding within-trial variances and correlations. That is, for each pair of treatments available in a particular trial, the IPD are used to estimate the treatment effect estimate (a measure such as a log risk ratio, log odds ratio, log hazard ratio or mean difference that provides a relative contrast of the two treatments) and its variance, plus the correlation for each pair of treatment effect estimates in that trial (Chapter 13 provides more details on within-trial correlation and why IPD are often required to estimate it). Generally, this requires a linear, logistic or Cox regression model to be fitted to the IPD in each trial separately, similar to (or extensions of) those introduced for the first stage of the two-stage IPD meta-analyses described in Chapter 5. As IPD are available, the regression model might adjust for a pre-defined set of key prognostic factors at the participant level (e.g. stage of disease at baseline when modelling treatments to improve survival after cancer diagnosis, or baseline blood pressure when modelling treatments to reduce blood pressure at one year after hypertension diagnosis); the benefit of this is considered further in Section 14.6.2.

In the second stage, a multivariate meta-regression model is used to synthesise all the effect estimates jointly, whilst accounting for their within-trial and between-trial correlations, akin to the models introduced in Chapter 13 (e.g. Sections 13.2.2 and 13.4). A common reference group is needed for the whole network, and a design matrix used to express all available treatment comparison estimates (contrasts) in relation to this reference group. The reference group does not need to be present in every trial. The meta-regression model requires the use of indicator variables (i.e. –1/0/1 values), which specify each available treatment effect estimate relative to the chosen reference group, and enable both direct and indirect evidence to contribute toward each summary treatment effect. For example, with treatment A as the reference group in the network, the log odds ratio estimate for C versus B can be expressed (using indicator variables) in terms of the log odds ratio estimate for C versus A and the log odds ratio for B versus A; more specifically, as $\log OR_{(C,B)} = \log OR_{(C,A)} - \log OR_{(B,A)}$, we require indicator variable codings of CA = 1 and BA = –1 for any treatment effect estimates comparing C and B when A is the chosen reference treatment in the network. The choice of reference treatment is arbitrary, and makes no difference to the meta-analysis results.

Under the consistency assumption, the multivariate meta-regression model used in the second stage can be written as[99,166]

$$\hat{\boldsymbol{\theta}}_i \sim N(\mathbf{X}_i\boldsymbol{\theta}, \mathbf{S}_i + \boldsymbol{\Sigma}) \tag{14.1}$$

where $\hat{\boldsymbol{\theta}}_i$ is a vector of treatment effect estimates from trial i, which has a corresponding within-trial variance matrix $\mathbf{S}_i$ containing the (assumed known) within-trial variances and correlations of the treatment effect estimates; $\boldsymbol{\theta}$ is a column vector containing the basic parameters, which are the average treatment effects (for each treatment compared to the chosen reference treatment in the network); $\mathbf{X}_i$ is a design matrix linking the treatment effect estimates in trial i to the basic parameters; and $\boldsymbol{\Sigma}$ contains the variances and covariance of the random effects. Typically $\boldsymbol{\Sigma}$ is simplified to contains diagonal entries of τ^2, such that the between-trial variance is assumed to be the same regardless of the treatment comparison; similarly, the off-diagonal entries are typically set to $0.5\tau^2$, which again ensures there is a common between-trial variance of τ^2 for all treatment contrasts in the network. These decisions are mainly for pragmatic reasons, as they considerably reduce the number of variance parameters to be estimated (and thus improve convergence) and aid interpretation across the network.

Estimation of model (14.1) could be via a frequentist or Bayesian approach (Sections 13.2.2.3 and 13.2.2.4). The package *network* in Stata implements the two-stage approach, including restricted maximum likelihood (REML) estimation of model (14.1), and allows comprehensive summaries and plots.[99,166] Note that if there are only two treatments (i.e. one treatment contrast) per trial, then model (14.1) reduces to a standard meta-regression, and within-trial correlations are not an issue. When there are trials with three or more groups (often called 'multi-arm trials'),[166,167] then to fit the multivariate meta-regression of model (14.1) the user needs to provide effect estimates that are expressed relative to the chosen reference group in the network. For example, if treatments A, B and C are available for a particular trial, and A is the reference in the network, then the user only needs to provide estimates of B versus A and C versus A (and their corresponding within-trial variances and correlations) for that trial; essentially this information already contains the C versus B result and so the treatment effect estimate for C versus B is not directly required. If the network's reference treatment is missing in a trial (e.g. B and C are available, but not A), then this can be accommodated in a frequentist framework using data augmentation, where some information about A is added to that trial but with huge uncertainty, so that it has barely any weight in the meta-analysis. Data augmentation is part of the *network* module in Stata, and for further details we refer elsewhere.[99,166] Data augmentation is not required in a Bayesian framework.[154,156]

14.3.2 A One-stage Approach

The two-stage approach assumes treatment effects follow a multivariate normal distribution both within and between trials. This is an approximation, and a more exact approach is to model the IPD directly in a one-stage (sometimes called 'arm-based') model. For example, given a binary outcome and assuming participant-level covariates are not of interest, the IPD can be used to model the number of participants and outcome events for each available treatment group (arm) directly using a binomial distribution via a hierarchical logistic regression framework with random effects to allow for between-trial heterogeneity in the magnitude of treatment effects,[168,169] as follows:

$$\begin{aligned} r_{ik} &\sim \text{Binomial}(n_{ik}, p_{ik}) \\ \text{logit}(p_{ik}) &= \alpha_i + \mathbf{X}_i\boldsymbol{\beta}_i \\ \boldsymbol{\beta}_i &\sim N(\boldsymbol{\theta}, \boldsymbol{\Sigma}) \end{aligned} \tag{14.2}$$

Here, p_{ik} is the probability of death for participants in treatment group k of trial i; n_{ik} and r_{ik} are the number of participants and events, respectively, in trial i for treatment group k; the α_i are separate trial intercept terms (to account for within-trial clustering) which relate to the chosen reference group in each trial; $\boldsymbol{\beta}_i$ is a vector containing the trial-specific true treatment effects (in relation to the reference group); and $\mathbf{X}_i$, $\boldsymbol{\theta}$ and $\boldsymbol{\Sigma}$ are as defined previously for the two-stage approach. Similarly, a hierarchical linear or Poisson regression with random effects could be used to directly model continuous outcomes and rates, respectively, in each group in each trial. When interest is in including participant-level covariates, then a participant-level model must be specified, for example, using a Bernoulli rather than binomial distribution for a binary outcome. This is considered further in Section 14.6.3.

When fitting one-stage network meta-analysis models such as model (14.2), it is important to maintain the clustering of participants within trials,[167] as otherwise within-trial randomisation may be compromised and misleading summary results obtained (Chapter 6).[170–174] This can be done by stratifying the intercept by trial (i.e. specifying a separate intercept per trial), with each intercept relating to the chosen reference group for that trial, as illustrated in model (14.2). In terms of software to fit one-stage network meta-analysis models in a frequentist framework, REML estimation is recommended for continuous outcomes and, as long as most trials are not small in terms of the number of participants or outcome events, pseudo-REML estimation can be used for other outcomes.[175–177] Conventional (unrestricted) ML estimation of one-stage models may suffer from considerable downward bias of between-trial variances and thus lead to artificially narrow confidence intervals for the summary treatment effects. More generally, Bayesian estimation may be preferable using, for example, WinBUGS (code available at www.nicedsu.org.uk) or in dedicated packages such as *gemtc* or *multinma* in R.[178–180] Further discussion of estimation methods for one-stage IPD meta-analysis models is given in Chapter 6.

14.3.3 Summary Results after a Network Meta-Analysis

After estimation of either a one-stage or two-stage network IPD meta-analysis, a summary result is obtained for each treatment relative to the chosen reference treatment. Subsequently, other comparisons (treatment contrasts) can then be derived using the consistency relationship. In other words, each comparison (summary treatment effect) can be obtained by calculating contrasts of the estimated parameters from the fitted meta-analysis model. For example, if C is the reference treatment in a network meta-analysis of a binary outcome, then the summary log odds ratio (logOR) for A versus B is obtained by the difference in the summary logOR estimate for A versus C and the summary logOR estimate for B versus C. The choice of the reference group is immaterial as summary results will be the same regardless. Derivation of standard errors of summary treatment effects should account for the correlation amongst parameter estimates. It is important to calculate 95% confidence (or credible) intervals for the summary treatment effects, to reveal the uncertainty of the results. Other relevant statistics include the estimated between-trial variance(s), percentage trial contributions, and the borrowing of strength (*BoS*).[49,99,181–184] The *BoS* statistic was introduced in Section 13.2.3.3 for multivariate meta-analysis of multiple outcomes. In our experience, *BoS* is usually greater in a network meta-analysis; that is, more information is usually gained about multiple treatments via the consistency assumption than is gained about multiple outcomes via correlation.

14.3.4 Example: Comparison of Eight Thrombolytic Treatments after Acute Myocardial Infarction

In the previously mentioned thrombolytics meta-analysis,[153] the aim was to estimate the relative efficacy of eight competing treatments in reducing the odds of mortality by 30–35 days; these

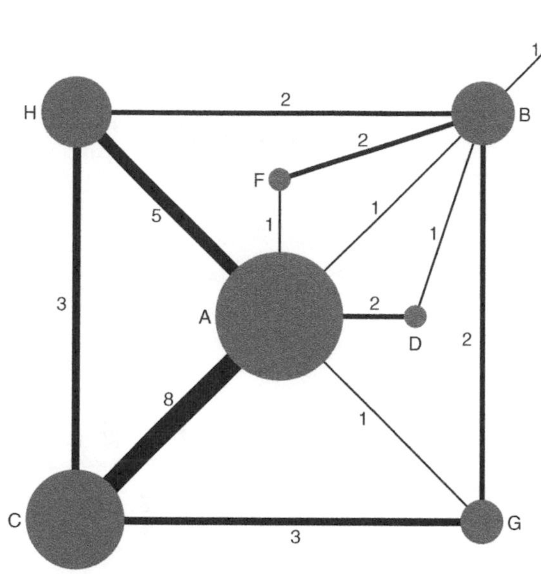

A = streptokinase; B = accelerated altepase; C = alteplase; D = streptokinase + alteplase; E = tenecteplase; F = reteplase; G = urokinase; H = anti-streptilase

Figure 14.2 Network map of the direct comparisons available in the 28 trials examining the effect of eight thrombolytics (labelled A to H) on 30- to 35-day mortality in patients with acute myocardial infarction. Numbers shown on the connecting lines give the number of trials making that direct comparison. As two trials have three treatment arms, the sum of the numbers above the lines is greater than the total number of trials. *Source:* Figure adapted from Figure 5 of Riley et al.,[51] with permission, © 2017 British Medical Journal Publishing Group (CC-BY 4.0).

treatments are labelled as A to H for brevity (Figure 14.2 gives full names). A version of this dataset containing seven treatments was introduced by Caldwell et al.,[185] but our investigations follow the updated analysis of Riley et al.[51] The IPD are summarised by the group-level data in Table 14.1. In this section, we do not consider adjustment for participant-level covariates, and so Table 14.1 is essentially the IPD.

With eight treatments, there are 28 pair-wise comparisons of potential interest; however, only 13 of these were available in at least one trial. This is shown by the network diagram in Figure 14.2, where each node is a particular treatment, and a line connects two nodes when at least one trial directly compares the two respective treatments. The width of the line joining two nodes is proportional to the number of trials that directly compare the two respective treatments (the number is also shown next to the line). For example, a direct comparison of C versus A is available in eight trials, whilst a direct comparison of F versus A is only available in one trial. Where no line directly joins two nodes (e.g. C and D), this indicates there was no trial that directly compared the two respective treatments. We applied two-stage and one-stage network IPD meta-analysis models to this dataset, using a frequentist estimation framework.

14.3.4.1 Two-stage Approach

We applied a two-stage network IPD meta-analysis to this dataset. In the first stage, log odds ratios (treatment effect estimates) and their corresponding within-trial variances and correlations were

Table 14.1 Trials in the thrombolytic network meta-analysis summarised in terms of r (number of events) and n (total participants) for eight treatment groups (A–H)

Trial	Treatments evaluated (design)	rA	nA	rB	nB	rC	nC	rD	nD	rE	nE	rF	nF	rG	nG	rH	nH
1	A B D	1472	20173	652	10344			723	10328								
2	A C H	1455	13780			1418	13746									1448	13773
3	A C	9	130			6	123										
4	A C	5	63			2	59										
5	A C	3	65			3	64										
6	A C	887	10396			929	10372										
7	A C	7	85			4	86										
8	A C	12	147			7	143										
9	A C	10	135			5	135										
10	A D	4	107					6	109								
11	A F	285	2992									270	2994				
12	A G	10	203											7	198		
13	A H	3	58													2	52
14	A H	3	86													6	89
15	A H	3	58													2	58
16	A H	13	182													11	188
17	B E			522	8488					523	8461						
18	B F			356	4921							757	10138				
19	B F			13	155							7	169				

20	B G	2	26			7	54		
21	B G	12	268			16	350		
22	B H	5	210					17	211
23	B H	3	138					13	147
24	C G			8	132	4	66		
25	C G			10	164	6	166		
26	C G			6	124	5	121		
27	C H			13	164			10	161
28	C H			7	93			5	90

Source: Table adapted from information published by Riley et al.,[89] with permission, © 2017 Riley et al. (CC-BY 3.0).

derived; then, in the second stage a multivariate random effects meta-regression model (14.1) was fitted using REML estimation, with treatment A chosen as the reference treatment. This produced the summary odds ratios for treatments B to H versus A, and subsequently all other contrasts (e.g. B versus C) could be derived from the parameter estimates using the consistency relationship.[99,166] This allowed all 28 trials to be incorporated and all eight treatments to be compared simultaneously, utilising direct evidence and also indirect evidence propagated through the network via the consistency assumption.

The summary results are displayed in Figure 14.3 and Table 14.2. The indirect evidence has an important impact on some treatment comparisons. For example, the summary treatment effect of H versus B in the network meta-analysis of all 28 trials (OR 1.19, 95% CI: 1.06 to 1.35) is substantially different from a standard pair-wise meta-analysis of two trials (summary OR 3.87; 95% CI: 1.74 to 8.58). *BoS* is often large (Figure 14.3). For example, the comparison of H versus B has a *BoS* of 97.8%, as there are only two trials with direct evidence. This is similar to having found direct evidence for H versus B from an additional $2 \times \frac{(1-0.022)}{0.022} \approx 89$ trials of similar size to those existing two trials (Section 13.2.3.3). *BoS* is 0% for E versus B, as there was no indirect evidence toward this comparison. For comparisons not shown in Figure 14.3, such as C versus B, *BoS* was 100% because there was no direct evidence.

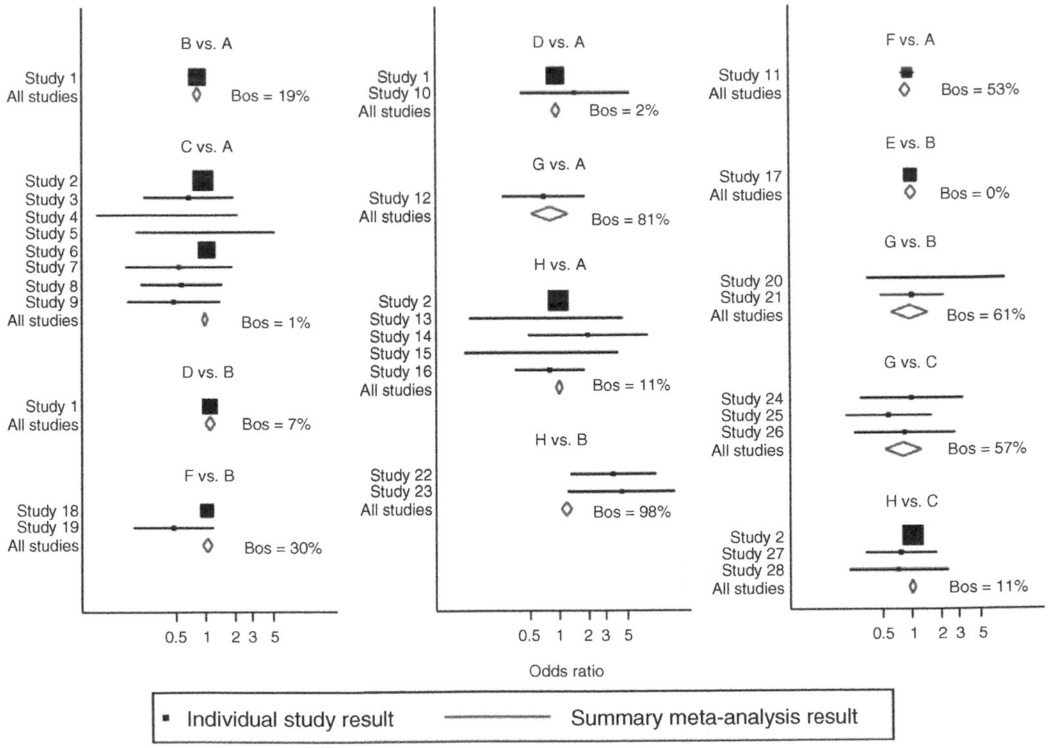

Figure 14.3 Extended forest plot showing the thrombolytics network meta-analysis results for all comparisons where direct evidence was available in at least one trial. *Source:* Figure adapted from Figure 6 of Riley et al.,[51] with permission, © 2017 British Medical Journal Publishing Group (CC-BY 4.0).

Table 14.2 Summary results from the thrombolytics network meta-analysis comparing treatments B to H versus reference treatment A

Comparison	Summary odds ratio	95% CI
B vs. A	0.85	0.78 to 0.93
C vs. A	1.00	0.94 to 1.07
D vs. A	0.96	0.87 to 1.05
E vs. A	0.86	0.73 to 1.00
F vs. A	0.89	0.79 to 1.01
G vs A	0.82	0.53 to 1.27
H vs A	1.01	0.94 to 1.10

14.3.4.2 One-stage Approach

We also fitted the following one-stage network meta-analysis model to the group-level data shown in Table 14.1:

$$
\begin{aligned}
&r_{ik} \sim \text{Binomial}(n_{ik}, p_{ik}) \\
&\text{logit}(p_{ik}) = \alpha_i + \beta_{1i}BA_{ik} + \beta_{2i}CA_{ik} + \beta_{3i}DA_{ik} + \beta_{4i}EA_{ik} + \beta_{5i}FA_{ik} + \beta_{6i}GA_{ik} + \beta_{7i}HA_{ik} \\
&\begin{pmatrix} \beta_{1i} \\ \vdots \\ \beta_{7i} \end{pmatrix} \sim N(\boldsymbol{\beta}, \mathbf{G})
\end{aligned}
\tag{14.3}
$$

Here, α_i denotes a separate intercept term per trial and each one corresponds to the chosen reference group for that trial; the BA_{ij} to HA_{ij} terms are either 1, 0, or −1 depending on the treatment groups compared in trial i; $\boldsymbol{\beta}$ is a seven-by-one column vector containing the basic parameters, which are the seven summary treatment effects (for B compared to A, up to H compared to A); and $\mathbf{G}$ is a seven-by-seven matrix with diagonal entries of τ^2 and off-diagonal entries of $0.5\tau^2$.

When using ML estimation the estimate of τ^2 is zero, which may often occur due to downward bias in ML estimation,[176] as previously mentioned. When using REML estimation of the pseudo-likelihood,[175–177] the estimate of τ^2 is 0.0002, and very similar to the REML estimate from the two-stage approach. Indeed, the summary treatment effect estimates are almost identical for both one-stage and two-stage models. Thus the two-stage multivariate normal approximation to the one-stage binomial approach performs well in this example, which is not surprising because many trials have large numbers of participants and outcome events.

14.4 Ranking Treatments

Following a network meta-analysis it is helpful to rank treatments according to their effectiveness. This process usually, though not always,[186] requires using simulation or resampling methods.[99,166,187] These use thousands of samples from the estimated distribution of summary treatment effects, to identify the percentage of samples (i.e. the probability) that each treatment has the most (or least) beneficial effect. Figure 14.4(a) shows the probability that each thrombolytic treatment was ranked most effective out of all treatments, and similarly second, third, and so on

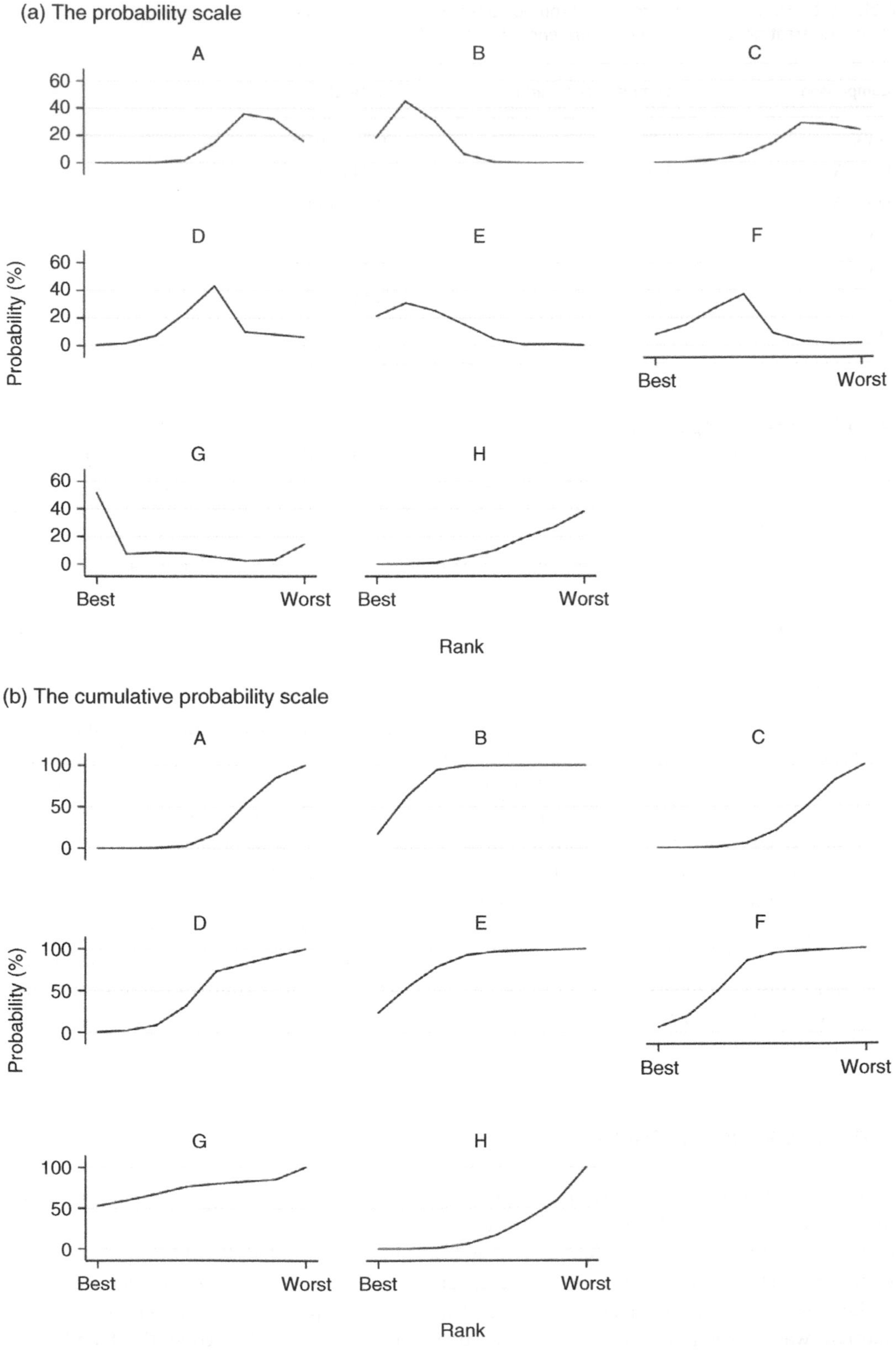

Figure 14.4 Plots of the ranking probability for each treatment considered in the thrombolytics network meta-analysis. *Source:* Figure adapted from Figure 7 of Riley et al.,[51] with permission, © 2017 British Medical Journal Publishing Group (CC-BY 4.0).

down to the least effective. Treatment G has the highest probability (51.7%) of being the most effective at reducing the odds of mortality by 30–35 days, followed by treatment E (21.5%) and B (18.3%).

Focusing on the probability of being ranked first is potentially misleading: a treatment ranked first may also have a high probability of being ranked last,[188] and its benefit over other treatments may be of little clinical value. In our example, treatment G has the highest probability of being most effective, but the summary effect for G is very similar to that for B and E, and the difference in their summary effects is unlikely to be clinically important. Furthermore, treatment G is also fourth most likely to be the least effective (14.4%), reflecting a large summary treatment effect with a wide confidence interval. In contrast, treatments B, E and F have very low probability (close to 0%) of being least effective. Thus, a treatment may have the highest probability of being ranked first, when actually there is no strong evidence (beyond chance) that it is better than other available treatments. To illustrate this, Riley et al. added to the thrombolytics network a hypothetical new drug, called *Brexitocin*, for which no direct or indirect evidence exists.[51] Given the lack of evidence, Brexitocin essentially has a 50% chance of being the most effective treatment but also a 50% chance of being the least effective.

To help address this, the mean rank and the surface under the cumulative ranking curve (SUCRA) are useful.[181,183] The mean rank gives the average ranking place for each treatment. The SUCRA is the area under a line plot of the cumulative probability over ranks (from most effective to least effective) (Figure 14.4(b)), and is just the mean rank scaled to be between 0 and 1. A similar measure is the P-score.[186] For the thrombolytic network (now excluding Brexitocin), treatments B and E have the best mean ranks (2.3 and 2.6, respectively), followed by treatment G (3.0). Thus, although treatment G had the highest probability of being ranked first, based on the mean rank it is now in third place.

The SUCRA or the mean rank still only provide a single value and do not quantify the uncertainty in the ranking; two similar SUCRA values or two similar mean ranks may have very different levels of uncertainty in the rankings. Therefore, alongside the mean rank it is helpful to also provide quantiles (e.g. 25%, 50%, and 75%) of the ranks sampled for each treatment. In the thrombolytics example, for both treatments B and E their 25%, 50%, and 75% quantile values of rankings are 2, 2, and 3, respectively. In contrast, for treatment G the uncertainty in the rankings is larger, reflected by 25%, 50%, and 75% quantile values of rankings of 1, 1, and 4, respectively.

14.5 How Do We Examine Inconsistency between Direct and Indirect Evidence?

Treatment effect modifiers relate to methodological or clinical characteristics of the trials that influence the magnitude of treatment effects (on a given scale), and may include follow-up length, outcome definitions, trial quality (risk of bias), and participant-level characteristics.[189–192] When such effect modifiers are systematically different in trials making the same comparison(s), this manifests itself as between-trial heterogeneity in treatment effects. When such effect modifiers are systematically different in the subsets of trials providing direct and indirect evidence about a particular comparison, this causes inconsistency (i.e. disagreement between the direct and indirect evidence for that comparison). For example, if follow-up length is an effect modifier, and follow-up is generally longer in trials that provide direct evidence about a comparison compared to trials that provide indirect evidence about the same comparison, this causes inconsistency.

Similarly, for measures of treatment effect such as odds ratios or hazard ratios which are non-collapsible across different groups that vary in baseline risk, if distributions of prognostic factors are systematically different in the subsets of trials providing direct and indirect evidence, this may lead to inconsistency in the direct and indirect evidence for a particular treatment comparison due to changes in the baseline risk (Section 14.6.2).[192]

Thus, before undertaking a network meta-analysis it is important to select only those trials relevant for the population of clinical interest, and to then identify any systematic differences in variables that might affect measures of relative treatment effect; such variables are either effect modifiers or, specifically when analysing on non-collapsible scales, prognostic factors that modify baseline risk. For example, when planning the thrombolytics network meta-analysis, researchers might ask: are identified trials of A versus C and A versus H systematically different from trials of C versus H in terms of the distributions of potential effect modifiers or (because the effect of interest is the odds ratio which is non-collapsible) prognostic factors?[193] If so, inconsistency is likely and the decision to pool the data in a network meta-analysis is questionable and best avoided.

It may be difficult to gauge the potential for inconsistency in advance of a meta-analysis, although the availability of IPD and careful inspection of participant characteristics can help (Section 14.6.1). Regardless, following any network meta-analysis, inconsistency should be examined statistically, though unfortunately this is often not done.[194] The consistency assumption can be examined for each treatment comparison where there is direct and indirect evidence (seen as a closed loop within the network plot):[158,195,196] here the 'separating indirect from direct evidence'[195] approach (sometimes called 'node-splitting' or 'side-splitting') involves estimating relative treatment effects using only direct or indirect evidence, and comparing the results. The consistency assumption can also be examined across the whole network using 'design-by-treatment interaction' models,[166,197] or 'unrelated mean effects' models,[158,198] which allow an overall significance test for inconsistency. If evidence of inconsistency is found, explanations should be sought: for example, whether inconsistency arises from particular trials with a different design, at a higher risk of bias or with particular participant characteristics.[163] The network models could then be extended to include suitable explanatory covariates or reduced to exclude certain trials.[193]

If inconsistency remains unexplained then making coherent inferences is difficult. Some authors suggest modelling inconsistency terms as random effects with mean zero, thus allowing overall summary estimates allowing for unexplained inconsistency; however, sensible interpretation of such summary results is challenging.[199–201]

Usually there is low power to detect genuine inconsistency.[202] In our experience, most network meta-analyses with strong evidence of inconsistency have broad inclusion criteria leading to the inclusion of a heterogeneous set of trials covering a wide range of populations and settings. Therefore, when planning a network meta-analysis, the best way for researchers to increase their assurance in the approach (and that the consistency assumption is likely to be valid) is to use strict trial inclusion criteria, including only sufficiently homogenous trials that best represent the target population of interest.[154]

In the thrombolytics example, the 'separating indirect from direct evidence' approach found evidence for inconsistency for H versus B, visible in Figure 14.3 as the discrepancy between "Study 22", "Study 23" and "All studies" under the subheading "H vs. B". If the H versus B trials differed in design from the other trials then it might be reasonable to exclude them from the network, or consider adjustment for effect modifiers to remove the inconsistency. However, when we applied the 'design-by-treatment interaction' model there was no evidence of overall inconsistency, and the only statistically significant inconsistency parameter ($p = 0.024$) relates to the indirect evidence toward the H versus B treatment comparison, and so this may be a chance finding.

14.6 Benefits of IPD for Network Meta-Analysis

The thrombolytics network meta-analysis example used throughout this chapter synthesised binomial data for each treatment group within each trial. In the absence of covariates, binomial data is akin, statistically speaking, to having the IPD itself. Nevertheless, if IPD are truly available for each trial then additional participant-level information will be available, bringing important advantages for the network meta-analysis compared to using published aggregate data.[192] Most advantages are the same as for IPD meta-analysis of a single treatment effect in Parts 1 and 2 of this book.[53] For example, IPD enables more consistent inclusion criteria, exclusion criteria, outcome definitions (e.g. time-points) and statistical methods across trials; more up-to-date follow-up information; further insight toward risk of bias classifications; better handling of missing participant data, longitudinal outcomes, and time-to-event outcomes; adjustment for prognostic factors; and checking of modelling assumptions (e.g. non-proportional hazards). However, a specific advantage of IPD for network meta-analysis is to reduce inconsistency, and to tailor results to specific subgroups when there are participant-level effect modifiers. This is possible when the IPD allows relevant participant-level covariates (representing prognostic factors and/or treatment effect modifiers) to be included in the statistical modelling. This is especially important if particular covariates act as effect modifiers *and* their observed distribution differs across comparisons, as otherwise this may cause inconsistency in the network (Section 14.5).

14.6.1 Benefit 1: Examining and Plotting Distributions of Covariates across Trials Providing Different Comparisons

As discussed in Section 14.5, for each treatment comparison a fundamental assumption for network meta-analysis is that the distributions of any variables that affect relative treatment effects in trials that provide direct evidence are similar to their distributions in trials that provide indirect evidence; otherwise, the consistency assumption is unreliable. Without IPD, distributions of participant-level characteristics need to be extracted from the trial publications (or obtained from the trial investigators), such as the mean and standard deviation for a continuous covariate, or the proportion of participants in each category for a categorical covariate. Such information may not always be provided for all covariates that were recorded. In contrast, when IPD are available for each trial, researchers can plot and derive covariate distributions themselves, and may have access to a broader set of recorded covariates than summarised in the original trial publication. This allows better comparison of how covariate distributions differ across trials with different treatment comparisons. Donegan et al. illustrated various graphical approaches for this purpose,[203] whilst Batson et al. suggest a novel 3-D plot system.[204]

14.6.2 Benefit 2: Adjusting for Prognostic Factors to Improve Consistency and Reduce Heterogeneity

Part 2 of this book recommends that IPD meta-analyses of randomised trials adjust for a pre-defined set of prognostic factors; key reasons including producing conditional (rather than marginal) treatment effects and potentially improving efficiency and between-trial homogeneity of treatment effects (e.g. see Section 5.2.4).[21] This recommendation also applies to the network IPD meta-analysis setting, especially as it may also alleviate inconsistency between direct and indirect evidence. Even in situations where there are no effect modifiers, inconsistency can arise if differences exist in the distribution of prognostic factors between trials with different comparisons,[192] when measuring treatment effects on non-collapsible scales, such as the odds ratio or the hazard ratio, that are affected by differences in baseline risk. If there are differences in the distribution of key prognostic factors across trials and they are not adjusted for in the model, this will artificially increase the heterogeneity in the observed odds or hazard ratios across trials. Similarly, if the distributions of prognostic factors differ across trials with different comparisons, then without adjustment this may induce inconsistency in direct and indirect evidence for the odds or hazard ratios.

For example, consider that the underlying probability (p_{ij}) of having an adverse outcome depends on whether treatment B or A is used and, in particular, whether a participant smokes, as defined by the equation

$$\text{logit}\left(p_{ij}\right) = -0.5 + (4 \times \text{smoker}) - (0.5 \times \text{B})$$

where B = 1 if in treatment group B and B = 0 if treatment group A, and smoker = 1 if a participant currently smokes and 0 otherwise. Hence, after adjusting for the strong prognostic effect of smoking (corresponding to an odds ratio of exp(2) = 7.4), the true treatment effect for B versus A is an odds ratio of exp(−0.5) = 0.61. Note that there are no treatment effect modifiers (i.e. no treatment-smoker interaction). Now consider that two randomised trials of B versus A were conducted: trial 1 used a population where 20% of participants smoked, and trial 2 had a population where 80% of participants smoked. Regardless of the proportion of smokers, the equation tells us that both trials have a true odds ratio of 0.61 for the treatment effect adjusted for the prognostic effect of smoking. However, without adjustment for smoking, the unadjusted treatment effect estimates will be considerably different in the two trials. Simulating large data for such trials shows that the unadjusted odds ratio for B versus A is about 0.69 for trial 1 and 0.77 for trial 2. Hence, there is genuine between-trial heterogeneity in the *unadjusted* odds ratio for trials 1 and 2; however, such heterogeneity is removed when considering the treatment effect adjusted for the prognostic effect of smoking, as is more possible when IPD are available. Similarly, unadjusted odds ratios will differ for subsets of trials that provide direct and indirect evidence if the distribution of smokers is different in each subset. This will lead to inconsistency. However, with IPD this can be alleviated by estimating odds ratios adjusted for smoking.

14.6.3 Benefit 3: Including Treatment-covariate Interactions

Chapter 7 describes one-stage and two-stage IPD meta-analysis models for estimating treatment-covariate interactions (i.e. participant-level effect modifiers) in the context of a single treatment effect, and emphasises how using IPD increases statistical power and (when done appropriately) avoids aggregation bias compared to a meta-regression of aggregate data. Treatment-covariate interactions may also be included in IPD network meta-analysis models in a similar way as shown in Chapter 7; in particular, one-stage models must separate out within-trial and across-trial information to disentangle treatment-covariate interactions at the participant level from aggregated relationships at the trial level.[28,205] However, in a network meta-analysis setting there are multiple treatment effects, and so require further considerations of whether the treatment-covariate interactions for each treatment effect are related to each other.

Consider the example of Donegan et al.,[191] who used IPD to examine three artemisinin-based combination therapies for uncomplicated malaria: amodiaquine-artesunate (AQ+AS), dihydroartemisinin-piperaquine (DHAPQ), and artemether-lumefantrine (AL). The binary outcome of interest was treatment success at 28 days. IPD were available from a single multicentre randomised trial (the 4ABC trial[206]), where 11 sites were separately randomised to two or three of the treatments; the trial analysis therefore included a network meta-analysis of IPD from the 11 sites, which for simplicity can be considered as 11 'trials' here. Age was pre-specified as a potential treatment effect modifier, since in areas with endemic malaria older patients are more likely to achieve success on treatment because they have greater immunity. The following one-stage network IPD meta-analysis model was fitted, which extends that of model (14.2) by modelling at the participant-level (rather than group-level) and by including age (z_{ikj}) and mean age ($\bar{z}_i$) as covariates:

$$
\begin{aligned}
&y_{ikj} \sim \text{Bernoulli}\left(p_{ikj}\right)\\
&\text{logit}\left(p_{ikj}\right) = \alpha_i + \beta_{2,it_{i1}t_{ik}} + \beta_{1,i}z_{ikj} + \gamma_{Wt_{i1}t_{ik}}\left(z_{ikj} - \bar{z}_i\right) + \gamma_{At_{i1}t_{ik}}\bar{z}_i \quad \text{for all } k \geq 1\\
&\beta_{2,it_{i1}t_{ik}} \sim \text{N}\left(\theta_{t_{ik}} - \theta_{t_{i1}}, \tau^2\right) \quad \text{for all } k > 1\\
&\gamma_{Wt_{i1}t_{ik}} = \gamma_{Wt_{ik}} - \gamma_{Wt_{i1}}, \;\; \gamma_{At_{i1}t_{ik}} = \gamma_{At_{ik}} - \gamma_{At_{i1}}\\
&\gamma_{Wt_{i1}t_{i1}} = \gamma_{At_{i1}t_{i1}} = 0, \;\; \gamma_{W1} = \gamma_{A1} = 0,\\
&\beta_{2,it_{i1}t_{i1}} = 0, \;\; \theta_1 = 0
\end{aligned}
\tag{14.4}
$$

Here, individuals j in arm k of trial i receive treatment t_{ik}. The model parameters are interpreted in the same manner as those one-stage models described in Chapter 7 that separate within-trial and across-trial information. The α_i is a trial-specific intercept, the $\beta_{1,i}$ are trial-specific prognostic effects of age, the $\beta_{2,iab}$ are trial-specific relative treatment effects (log odds ratios) of any two treatments b versus a, and θ_t is the average relative effect (log odds ratio) of treatment t compared to the overall reference treatment 1. The within-trial treatment-age interaction γ_{Wab} and the across-trial association γ_{Aab} modify the b versus a relative treatment effect, according to the values of the age covariate z_{ikj} and mean trial value $\bar{z}_i$, respectively. As specified, there is assumed to be no heterogeneity in the within-trial interactions $\gamma_{Wt_{ik}}$; if this assumption is questionable, the model could be extended to include random effects on these parameters. Similar models are possible for other outcome types, by replacing the Bernoulli within-trial likelihood distribution and logit link function in model (14.4) with other choices appropriate for the outcome data being analysed (Chapter 6). It can also be extended to multiple outcomes.[205]

Importantly, model (14.4) invokes the consistency assumption for each within-trial interaction $\gamma_{Wt_{i1}t_{ik}}$, and similarly for the across-trial associations $\gamma_{At_{i1}t_{ik}}$. That is, as for the consistency assumption for the average relative treatment effects $\theta_{t_{i1}t_{ik}}$, direct and indirect evidence is assumed consistent for each of these terms, and this should (data permitting) be checked. Donegan et al. discuss this issue in the context of aggregate data network meta-regression,[207] and present graphical approaches to checking consistency of both treatment effects and interactions simultaneously.

When fitting model (14.4) different assumptions may be made regarding the γ_{Wt} for each treatment, and also the γ_{At} for each treatment. The least restrictive assumption is that all these terms are entirely independent and unrelated; in a Bayesian analysis, each γ_{Wt} and γ_{At} would then be given independent prior distributions. The most restrictive assumption is that the terms are common across all treatments:

$$\gamma_{Wt} = \gamma_W, \;\; \gamma_{At} = \gamma_A \quad \text{for all } t$$

A compromise is to assume terms are exchangeable across trials, such that they are similar and drawn from a common distribution such as

$$\gamma_{Wt} \sim \text{N}\left(m_W, \sigma_W^2\right), \;\; \gamma_{At} \sim \text{N}\left(m_A, \sigma_A^2\right)$$

where m_W and m_A are the means, and σ_W and σ_A are the between-trial standard deviations for the within-trial interactions and across-trial associations, respectively.

Donegan et al. applied model (14.4) in a Bayesian framework, making each of these assumptions, to the malaria data,[191] along with a standard model including no covariates (model (14.2)). Unfortunately, as the mean age value was very similar in all sites, estimating the across-trial associations was problematic and model (14.4) did not converge. Therefore, to aid model convergence, the authors made a further assumption that the within-trial interaction and across-trial association are identical for each treatment effect (i.e. there is no aggregation bias). The summary treatment effect estimates obtained are shown in Table 14.3. Regardless of whether common, independent or exchangeable interaction terms are assumed, there is quite strong evidence of an interaction between treatment effects and age, with larger effects at higher ages for both AQ + AS versus DHAPQ and AL versus DHAPQ. For example, assuming common interaction terms for all treatment effects, the estimated treatment-age interaction is −0.24 (95% −0.47 to −0.01). Hence, the

Table 14.3 Results reported by Donegan et al.[191] after estimation of network IPD meta-analysis model (14.4)* applied to the three treatments for malaria using IPD from 11 sites

		Assumptions about within-trial interactions and across-trial associations for the multiple treatment effects			
		Not included (equivalent to model (14.2))	Independent for all treatment effects	Exchangeable across treatment effects	Common to all treatment effects
Number of model parameters		14	27	27	26
Log odds ratio (95% CI)	AQ + AS versus DHAPQ	−0.98 (−1.79, −0.21)	At mean age: −1.01 (−1.88, −0.16)	At mean age: −1.01 (−1.90, −0.17)	At mean age: −1.01 (−1.89, −0.17)
			At zero age: −0.46 (−1.50, 0.59)	At zero age: −0.45 (−1.49, 0.57)	At zero age: −0.42 (−1.41, 0.57)
	AL versus DHAPQ	−1.08 (−1.77, −0.31)	At mean age: −1.12 (−1.90, −0.29)	At mean age: −1.12 (−1.90, −0.30)	At mean age: −1.12 (−1.88, −0.30)
			At zero age: −0.50 (−1.44, 0.52)	At zero age: −0.51 (−1.45, 0.50)	At zero age: −0.52 (−1.43, 0.45)
Mean of random effects distribution (95% CI)		–	–	−0.23 (−1.40, 0.95)	–
Variance of random effects distribution		–	–	0.09	–
Between-site variance		0.69	0.82	0.82	0.82

* To aid model convergence, the authors made a further assumption that the within-trial interaction and across-trial association are identical for each treatment effect.

** Calculated at the mean age in the models including interaction terms.

Source: Table created using information extracted from Supplementary Table 2 of Donegan et al.,[191] with permission, © 2012 Wiley.

benefit of the treatments vary according to age. At the mean age, there is evidence of a benefit of AQ + AS versus DHAPQ and AL versus DHAPQ (Table 14.3). However, at young ages, there is no clear evidence of a difference between the three treatments, with credible intervals for the treatment effects considerably overlapping the null value (Table 14.3).

14.6.4 Benefit 4: Multiple Outcomes

So far we have considered the comparison of multiple treatments for a single outcome. However, there is growing interest in accommodating multiple outcomes within the network meta-analysis framework, in order to help identify the best treatment across multiple clinically relevant outcomes.[208–212] This is achieved by extending the multivariate framework outlined in Chapter 13 for multiple outcomes of a single treatment comparison. IPD helps implement such models, in particular by enabling within-trial correlations between pairs of outcomes to be derived as described in Section 13.2.1.2. For example, Efthimiou et al.[209] performed a network meta-analysis of 68 trials comparing 13 active antimanic drugs and placebo for acute mania. Two main outcomes of interest were *efficacy* (defined as the proportion of participants with at least a 50% reduction in manic symptoms from baseline to week 3) and *acceptability* (defined as the proportion of participants with treatment discontinuation before 3 weeks). These are negatively correlated (as participants often discontinue treatment due to lack of efficacy), so the authors extend a network meta-analysis framework to jointly analyse these outcomes and account for this negative correlation. This is especially important as 19 of the 68 trials provided data on only one of the two outcomes. Compared to considering each outcome separately, this approach produces narrower confidence intervals for summary treatment effects and has an impact on the relative ranking of some of the treatments. In particular, carbamazepine ranks as the most effective treatment in terms of response when considering outcomes separately, but falls to fourth place when accounting for their correlation (Figure 14.5). As mentioned in Section 14.4, uncertainty in rankings should also be considered, but is omitted here for brevity. Hong et al. consider how to incorporate treatment-covariate interactions in a multiple outcomes network IPD meta-analysis framework.[205]

14.7 Combining IPD and Aggregate Data in Network Meta-Analysis

As mentioned throughout this book, IPD may not always be available from every eligible trial. For example, in health technology submissions to reimbursement agencies such as NICE, a submitting company has IPD available on its own trials, but typically only has published aggregate data from its competitors' trials. This has led to much interest in network meta-analysis methods that combine available IPD with aggregate data (e.g. treatment effect estimates, two-by-two tables, etc) from those trials not providing their IPD. If IPD and non-IPD trials are similar in terms of the distribution of any effect modifiers, then combining IPD and aggregate data is straightforward. In particular, the second stage of the two-stage approach allows treatment effect estimates derived directly for IPD trials to be combined with treatment effect estimates extracted (e.g. from trial publications) for non-IPD trials (Section 14.3.1). Alternatively, for binary outcomes, two-by-two tables obtained for non-IPD trials can be combined with two-by-two tables derived for IPD trials in the one-stage framework outlined in Section 14.3.2. Of course, this assumes suitable aggregate data are available for the non-IPD trials, and does not allow the many other advantages of having IPD to manifest in the non-IPD trials (e.g. adjusting for prognostic factors, examining non-proportional hazards, etc).

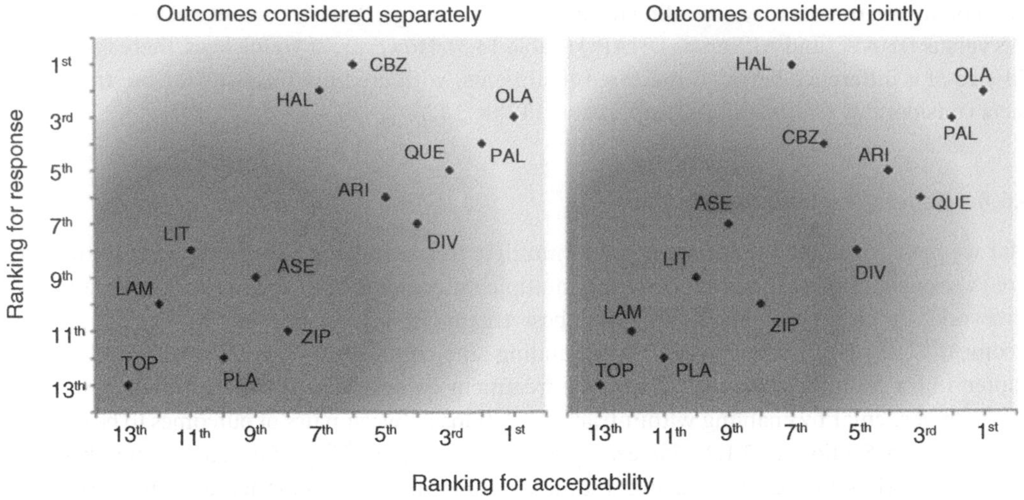

ARI = aripiprazole, ARI = aripiprazole, ASE = asenapine, CBZ = carbamazepine, VAL = divalproex, HAL = haloperidol, LAM = lamotrigine, LIT = lithium, OLZ = olanzapine, PBO = placebo, QTP = quetiapine, PAL = paliperidone, TOP = topiramate, ZIP = ziprasidone

Figure 14.5 Ranking of antimanic drugs for response and acceptability, based on either (a) a network meta-analysis of each outcome separately or (b) a network meta-analysis of both outcomes jointly, accounting for their negative correlation. Treatments located in the darker areas of the plots have the worst rankings, and those in the lighter areas have the best rankings. Figure adapted from Riley et al.[51] *Source:* Figure adapted from information published in the supplementary material of Riley et al.,[51] with permission, © 2017 British Medical Journal Publishing Group (CC-BY 4.0).

The required approach is more complex when adjustment for differences in effect modifiers between trials is needed. A special case of this scenario is that of a *population-adjusted indirect comparison*, where IPD are available on one trial comparing treatments A and B, and aggregate data are available on another trial comparing treatments A and C, and the researcher wants to perform an indirect comparison between these two trials to compare B and C.[213,214] An indirect comparison is a special case of network meta-analysis (as explained in Sections 14.2 and 14.5), where two treatments (here B and C) are compared indirectly via trials against a common comparator (A). A population-adjusted indirect comparison adjusts for differences in the distribution of effect modifiers between the AB and AC trials; without such adjustment, there would be bias in an indirect comparison of B and C obtained from a standard network meta-analysis of these two trials. Two proposed methods for population-adjusted indirect comparisons are matching-adjusted indirect comparison (MAIC),[215–217] and simulated treatment comparison (STC).[217,218]

MAIC is a weighting method, where IPD are used to derive weights for the individuals in the AB trial to match their covariate distributions with participants of the AC trial. The weights are then used to estimate the treatment effect of B versus A in the population of the AC trial (e.g. using a weighted regression), which is then compared with the observed treatment effect of C versus A in the AC trial to obtain a population-adjusted indirect comparison. STC is a regression method, where a regression model is fitted to the IPD in the AB trial, and used to predict average outcomes on treatments A and B in the AC trial population, from which the predicted treatment effect of

B versus A can be estimated. Again, this predicted treatment effect of B versus A in the AC trial population is compared with the observed treatment effect of C versus A in the AC trial to obtain a population-adjusted indirect comparison.

Both MAIC and STC produce estimates which are valid for the population of the AC trial, which may not represent the target population for a treatment decision. If (and only if) the effect modifiers of treatments B and C are the same and interact with each treatment in the same way (the "shared effect modifier assumption"), may the population-adjusted estimate of B versus C be valid in any target population since the effect modifiers are cancelled out.[213,214] Otherwise, companies may find themselves in the awkward situation of arguing that their competitor's trial is more representative than their own, for the purposes of deciding on the best treatment. This problem has already arisen in analyses from competing companies: Novartis and AbbVie presented MAIC analyses of the same two trials comparing secukinumab and adalimumab to placebo as treatments for ankylosing spondylitis.[219,220] Each company had IPD on their own trial, but not on their competitor's trial. The results from each company's MAIC appear to be in conflict, with one company claiming significant differences in efficacy in favour of secukinumab, and the other claiming comparable efficacy but improvements in cost effectiveness for adalimumab. However, since MAIC (and STC) attempt to produce estimates in the population of the trial providing aggregate data, the two MAIC analyses are aiming to provide estimates in two different target populations – the population of the competitor's trial in each case.

MAIC and STC also do not easily generalise to larger networks of treatments and trials. Some researchers have proposed combining IPD and aggregate data in (network) meta-regression models that allow mean values of participant-level covariates to be included (see Chapter 7).[56,169,191,221,222] However, this is unlikely to be adequate to adjust for participant-level effect modifiers, as the relationship between participant-level covariates and aggregate-level outcomes often depends on the entire covariate distribution and not just the mean covariate values.

14.7.1 Multilevel Network Meta-regression

Multilevel network meta-regression (ML-NMR) aims to address the limitations of MAIC, STC, and meta-regression approaches that incorporate mean covariate values.[180,223] It generalises (beyond binary covariates) an approach proposed by Jansen,[224] and is based on an approach proposed in the ecological inference literature.[225,226]

ML-NMR can be seen as a natural extension of IPD network meta-regression (Section 14.6.3) for incorporating aggregate data. In brief, the approach simultaneously fits a participant-level model (to the IPD trials) and an aggregate-level model (to the aggregate data trials). The approach recognises that aggregate data arise from averaging over a population of individuals (trial participants), and so the included aggregate-level model arises from averaging (i.e. integrating) the included participant-level model over the population in each aggregate data trial. Notably, ML-NMR reduces to a one-stage network IPD meta-regression when every trial has IPD (Section 14.3.2), and reduces to a network meta-analysis of aggregate data when no adjustment is to be performed (i.e. the second stage of the two-stage approach in Section 14.3.1). ML-NMR models can be fitted using the R package *multinma*.[180]

The participant-level and aggregate-level models must specify appropriate likelihood distributions, where the choice of participant-level likelihood depends on the outcome type (e.g. continuous, binary, count, etc) and will determine the corresponding aggregate-level likelihood (e.g. the mean of independent normal outcomes is normally distributed, the sum of independent Bernoulli outcomes is approximately binomially distributed, and the sum of independent Poisson outcomes is Poisson distributed, etc). For example, for a binary outcome assuming common treatment effects, the ML-NMR framework can be written as:

Participant-level model:	$y_{ikj} \sim \text{Bernoulli}(p_{ikj})$
	$g\left(p_{ikj}\right) = \eta_{ik}\left(z_{ikj}\right) = \alpha_i + z_{ikj}^T\left(\beta_1 + \gamma_{t_{ik}}\right) + \theta_{t_{ik}}$
Aggregate-level model:	$y_{ik\cdot} \sim \text{Binomial}(p_{ik\cdot})$
	$p_{ik\cdot} = \int_{\mathcal{Z}} g^{-1}(\eta_{ik}(z))\, f_{ik}(z)\, dz$

Here, p_{ikj} is the conditional mean outcome for participant j in arm k of trial i, assigned to treatment t_{ik}, with covariate vector z_{ikj} (i.e. the vector that contains the individual's values of all included prognostic and/or effect-modifying variables). Also, $p_{ik\cdot}$ is the marginal mean outcome in arm k of trial i, and $f_{ik}(z)$ is the distribution of z among those in arm k of trial i. Further, $g(\cdot)$ is a suitable link function (e.g. logit), and $\mathcal{Z}$ denotes the support of z. The coefficients α_i are trial-specific baseline terms, β_1 contains coefficients for prognostic factors. Note that, contrary to the recommendation in Chapter 6 to stratify prognostic factor effects by trial, the prognostic effects within β_1 are not trial-specific, as they would not be estimable in aggregate data trials, and so are assumed common out of necessity.

The remaining parameters refer to treatment effects ($\theta_{t_{ik}}$) and effect modifiers ($\gamma_{t_{ik}}$); as these are specific to treatments, rather than arms or trials, we can drop the i and k subscripts when discussing these parameters (e.g. $\gamma_{t_{ik}} = \gamma_t$). The vector γ_t contains coefficients for effect modifiers specific to each treatment t (each assumed common across trials, though this could be extended to allow heterogeneity via random effects). The effect of treatment t (at the participant level), θ_t, is defined with respect to the reference treatment 1 and we set $\theta_1 = 0$ and $\gamma_1 = \mathbf{0}$. Some coefficients of β_1 or γ_t may be set to zero, if it is known that a particular covariate is not prognostic or effect modifying, respectively. Numerical integration may be used to evaluate the aggregate-level model.[180,223] The joint covariate distributions $f_{ik}(\cdot)$ in each of the aggregate data trials are inferred from the obtained aggregate data (e.g. means and standard deviations for continuous covariates, proportions for binary covariates, etc), along with assumed forms for the marginal distributions (e.g. normal, gamma, Bernoulli) and information on the correlation structure typically taken from the available IPD.

In population adjustment scenarios, the focus is on estimating population-adjusted average treatment effects (rather than on estimating interactions, which is the focus of Chapter 7); therefore the key assumption is that there are no unobserved effect modifiers, in order that unbiased estimates of population-adjusted average treatment effects may be produced. Based on the model parameters, the treatment effect of any two treatments b versus a in population P is given by $d_{ab(P)} = \bar{z}_{(P)}^T(\gamma_b - \gamma_a) + \theta_b - \theta_a$, where $\bar{z}_{(P)}$ is the vector of mean covariate values in population P. Population average estimates of other quantities may be produced by integration over the respective covariate distribution.[180,223]

As described in Section 14.6.3, different assumptions can be made regarding the effect modifier (treatment-covariate interaction) coefficients γ_t. These can be independent for each treatment, but this requires IPD or sufficient amounts of aggregate data on each treatment. Alternatively, the interactions may be set to be equal across a class $\mathcal{T}$ of treatments, $\gamma_a = \gamma_b$ for all a, b in $\mathcal{T}$, which shares the data requirements within each treatment class. As a middle ground between independent and equal, the interactions may be assumed to be similar (exchangeable) within a class, following a distribution with common mean and variance such as $\gamma_t \sim N(\boldsymbol{m}, I\sigma^2)$. Unobserved effect modifiers should be checked for by examining residual heterogeneity and inconsistency in the network, and if data allow, by splitting participant-level interactions into within-trial and across-trial relationships as discussed in Chapter 7.

14.7.2 Example: Treatments to Reduce Plaque Psoriasis

Phillippo et al. present an analysis of a network of five treatment regimens (plus placebo) for moderate to severe plaque psoriasis, shown in Figure 14.6.[180,223] IPD were available from the UNCOVER-1, UNCOVER-2, and UNCOVER-3 trials (comparing ixekizumab Q2W and Q4W with etanercept in all trials, and also placebo in UNCOVER-1 and UNCOVER-2), and aggregate data were obtained for the FIXTURE trial (comparing secukinumab 150 mg and 300 mg, etanercept and placebo).[227–229]

The binary outcome of interest was success/failure to achieve a 75% reduction in symptoms on the psoriasis area and severity index (PASI 75). Although modelling the PASI 75 as a continuous outcome is preferable, this binary outcome was reported by trials not providing IPD and so was used to allow all trials to be included. There were five potential participant-level effect modifiers to adjust for: duration of psoriasis, body surface area, previous systemic treatment, psoriatic arthritis, and weight (Table 14.4). A previous MAIC analysis had compared ixekizumab Q2W and secukinumab 300mg via etanercept but the approach ignored all information from the common placebo arms, and required exclusion of an entire IPD trial which did not include an etanercept arm. To address this, the previously defined ML-NMR model was fitted to the data using a probit link function. In order to ensure model parameters were identifiable, interaction coefficients were shared between

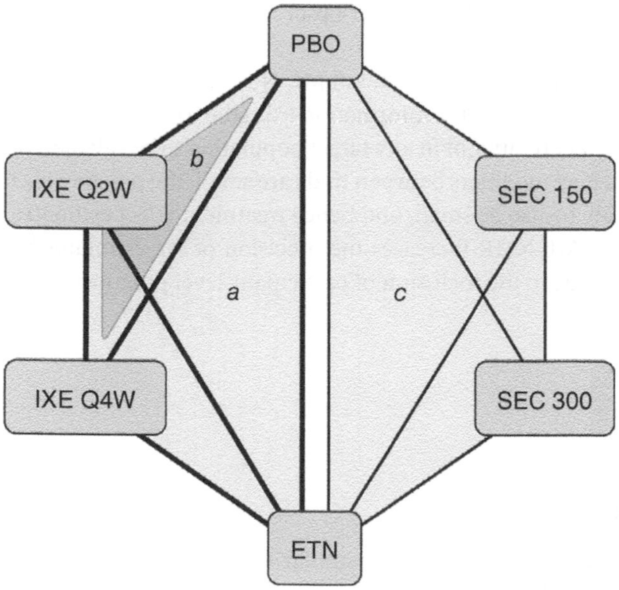

PBO = placebo, IXE = ixekizumab, SEC = secukinumab, ETN = etanercept. IXE and SEC were each investigated with two different dosing regimens.

Figure 14.6 The UNCOVER[228,229] and FIXTURE[227] trials form a network of six treatments, as summarised by Phillippo.[180] Shading indicates comparisons made in: (a) UNCOVER-2 and UNCOVER-3; (b) UNCOVER-1; (c) FIXTURE. The thick and thin lines represent availability of IPD and aggregate data on a comparison, respectively. *Source:* David Phillippo, reproduced from Phillippo,[180] with permission.

Table 14.4 Baseline covariate summaries from the UNCOVER and FIXTURE trials. Reported sample size for UNCOVER-2 and UNCOVER-3 are after removing two individuals from each trial with missing weight values. Statistics are mean (SD) unless otherwise specified. Modified from Phillippo.[180]

	UNCOVER-1 (*N* = 1296)	UNCOVER-2 (*N* = 1219)	UNCOVER-3 (*N* = 1339)	FIXTURE (*N* = 1306)
Body surface area, per cent	27.7 (17.3)	26.0 (16.5)	28.3 (17.1)	34.4 (18.9)
Duration of psoriasis, years	19.6 (11.9)	18.7 (12.5)	18.2 (12.2)	16.5 (12.0)
Previous systemic treatment (%)	71.3	64.2	57.1	64.0
Psoriatic arthritis (%)	26.3	23.6	20.5	14.7
Weight, kg	92.2 (23.8)	91.6 (22.2)	91.2 (23.5)	83.3 (20.8)

Source: David Phillippo, adapted from Phillippo,[180] with permission.

ixekizumab and secukinumab treatments (which are all interleukin-17A blockers). This model was fitted in a Bayesian framework using Stan.[230]

The resulting treatment effect estimates (expressed as standardised mean differences in PASI score due to the probit link function) in each trial population are shown in Figure 14.7. There are differences in the estimated average treatment effects in each population; for example, etanercept appears slightly more effective relative to placebo in the FIXTURE trial population than in the UNCOVER trial populations. However, the differences are small, as the distributions of effect modifiers are quite similar across populations. Moreover, a conventional random-effects network meta-analysis (i.e. using model (14.1)) gives little evidence of heterogeneity, meaning that there is likely to be little difference between trials in any effect modifiers (either observed or unobserved, at the participant or trial level).

The point estimates are similar between MAIC and ML-NMR, but ML-NMR has reduced uncertainty compared to MAIC due to incorporating all available information from the trials. In addition, ML-NMR enables relative effects between every treatment in any target population to be calculated. Since the differences in the distribution of effect modifiers between trials are small, the possible bias in the random effects NMA estimate is likely to also be small, and hence treatment effect estimates are quite similar for all methods. However, ML-NMR increases the precision of the estimates by explaining variation at the participant level due to the inclusion of participant-level prognostic factors and effect modifiers.

14.8 Further Topics

14.8.1 Accounting for Dose and Class

Standard network meta-analysis models make no allowance for similarities between treatments. When the treatments can be grouped into multiple classes, network meta-analysis models may be extended to allow treatments in the same class to have more similar effects than treatments in different classes.[231] Similarly, when some treatments represent different doses of the same drug, network meta-analysis models may be extended to incorporate sensible dose-response relationships.[232,233] Availability of IPD, and communication with the IPD providers (trial investigators), may help reveal more information about drugs than would otherwise be understood from

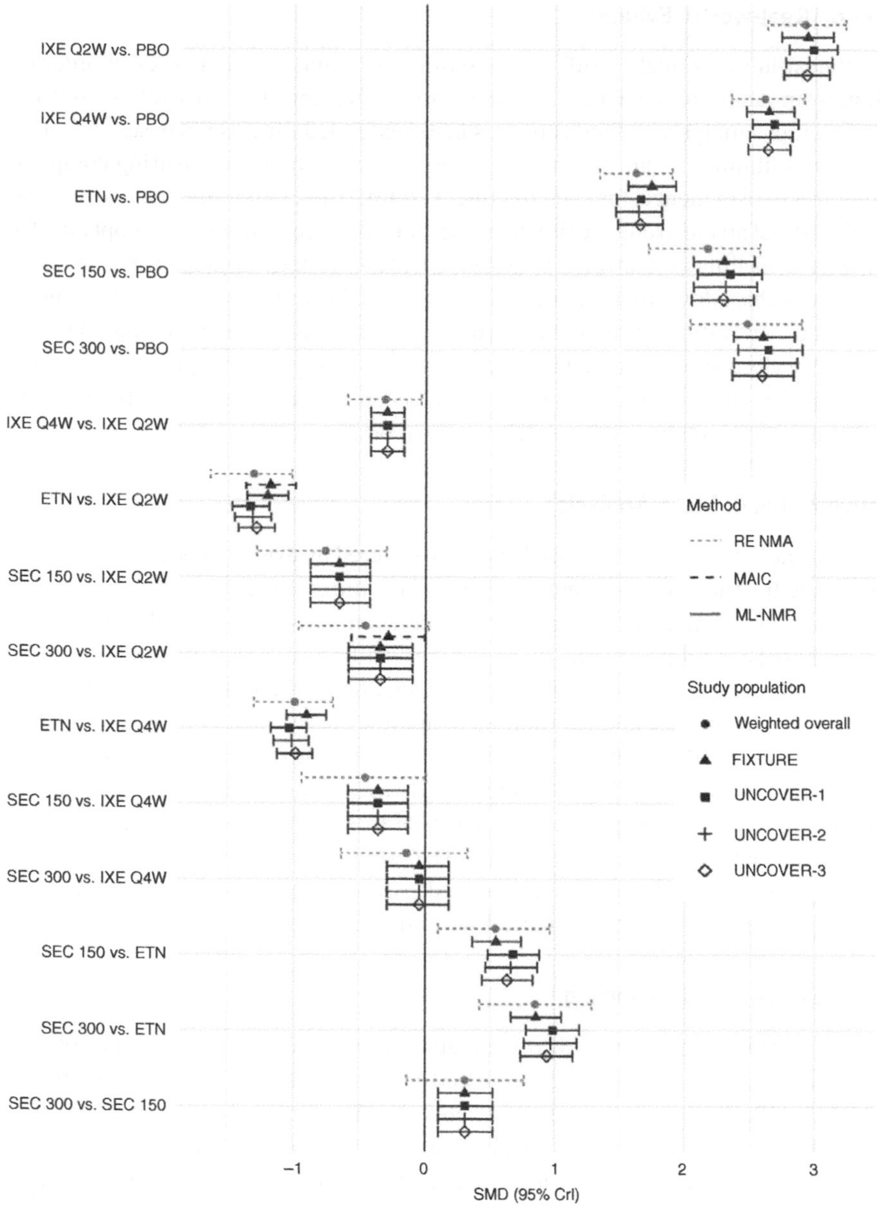

Figure 14.7 Average treatment effect estimates at the population level, for each pair of treatments in each trial population, for each of ML-NMR, a conventional random effects network meta-analysis (RE NMA, model (14.1)), and MAIC, as shown by Phillippo.[180] The interval for MAIC is a 95% confidence interval, as MAIC is a frequentist method. *Source:* David Phillippo, reproduced from Phillippo,[180] with permission.

reading a trial publication, which may help inform such extended network meta-analysis models. For example, the specific doses and timings of treatments may be more detailed within IPD, and it may even reveal that doses and other features (e.g. timing, adherence) differ across participants in the same trial.

14.8.2 Inclusion of 'Real-world' Evidence

There is growing interest in using 'real-world' evidence from non-randomised studies in order to corroborate findings from randomised trials, and to increase the evidence being used toward decision-making. Network meta-analysis methods are thus being extended for this purpose,[234,235] and an overview is given by Efthimiou et al.,[236] who emphasise the importance of ensuring compatibility of the different pieces of evidence, for each treatment comparison. Often the 'real-world' evidence comes from the IPD of an electronic health database, and so the researcher can adopt an IPD network meta-analysis modelling framework; in particular the two-stage approach may be best suited, as in the first stage this allows treatment effect estimates to be derived using different modelling techniques for each study depending on their type (e.g. propensity score modelling might be used to analyse IPD from electronic health databases, whilst simpler regression approaches can be used to analyse IPD from randomised trials), and then in the second stage these effect estimates can be combined using a network meta-analysis model such as model).

14.8.3 Cumulative Network Meta-Analysis

Créquit et al. show that the amount of randomized evidence covered by existing systematic reviews of competing second-line treatments for advanced non-small cell lung cancer was always substantially incomplete,[237] with 40% or more of treatments, treatment comparisons, and trials missing. To address this, they proposed a new paradigm "by switching: (1) from a series of standard meta-analyses focused on specific treatments (many treatments being not considered) to a single network meta-analysis covering all treatments; and (2) from meta-analyses performed at a given time and frequently out-of-date to a cumulative network meta-analysis systematically updated as soon as the results of a new trial become available." The latter is referred to as a "live cumulative network meta-analysis", and the various steps, advantages and challenges of this approach warrant further consideration in the context of obtaining and synthesising IPD. A similar concept is the framework for adaptive meta-analysis (FAME)[238], which requires knowledge of ongoing trials and suggests timing meta-analysis updates to coincide with new publications and availability of IPD.

14.8.4 Quality Assessment and Reporting

We encourage quality assessment of network IPD meta-analyses according to the guidance of Salanti et al,[239] and clear reporting of results using the PRISMA-NMA guidelines,[240] which should be used alongside PRISMA-IPD.[241] When the results of a network IPD meta-analysis inform decision-making, it is important to consider both the quality of evidence (or risk of bias) and the influence of evidence on the decision. Salanti et al. present an extension to the GRADE framework that combines quality ratings across the network in a coherent manner according to the relative weights,[239] implemented in the online tool CINeMA.[242] Threshold analysis is a form of sensitivity analysis that determines how much the evidence could change before a new decision is reached, described by a set of thresholds.[243,244] Combined with a quality or risk of bias assessment, these thresholds aid judgements of whether a decision may be robust or sensitive to plausible biases in the evidence.

14.9 Concluding Remarks

By using IPD, rather than published aggregate data, novel opportunities arise to improve the robustness and relevance of network meta-analysis results for clinical practice. Alongside various examples and emerging topics, this chapter has described the core principles and methods of a network IPD meta-analysis. Doing a network IPD meta-analysis project requires specific expertise, especially in terms of the statistical analysis. We anticipate future methodological research to improve and extend network IPD meta-analysis models even further. Of particular interest are methods for combining IPD and aggregate data, which is a common issue for network meta-analyses led by pharmaceutical companies and decision-makers. Lastly, we encourage readers to monitor ongoing developments and software. For those interested, www.ipdma.co.uk will provide signposts to new developments.

Part IV References

1 Hróbjartsson A. Why did it take 19 months to retrieve clinical trial data from a non-profit organisation? *BMJ* 2013;347:f6927.

2 Altman DG, Trivella M, Pezzella F, et al. Systematic review of multiple studies of prognosis: the feasibility of obtaining individual patient data. In: Auget J-L, Balakrishnan N, Mesbah M, et al., eds. *Advances in Statistical Methods for the Health Sciences*. Boston: Birkhäuser 2006:3–18.

3 Simmonds MC, Higgins JP. Covariate heterogeneity in meta-analysis: criteria for deciding between meta-regression and individual patient data. *Stat Med* 2007;26(15):2982–2999.

4 Kovalchik SA. Aggregate-data estimation of an individual patient data linear random effects meta-analysis with a patient covariate-treatment interaction term. *Biostatistics* 2013;14(2):273–283.

5 Kovalchik SA, Cumberland WG. Using aggregate data to estimate the standard error of a treatment-covariate interaction in an individual patient data meta-analysis. *Biom J* 2012;54(3):370–384.

6 Kontopantelis E, Springate DA, Parisi R, et al. Simulation-based power calculations for mixed effects modeling: ipdpower in Stata. *J Stat Softw* 2016;74(12):25.

7 Ensor J, Burke DL, Snell KIE, et al. Simulation-based power calculations for planning a two-stage individual participant data meta-analysis. *BMC Med Res Methodol* 2018;18(1):41.

8 Thangaratinam S, Rogozinska E, Jolly K, et al. Effects of interventions in pregnancy on maternal weight and obstetric outcomes: meta-analysis of randomised evidence. *BMJ* 2012;344:e2088.

9 Riley RD, Debray TPA, Fisher D, et al. Individual participant data meta-analysis to examine interactions between treatment effect and participant-level covariates: statistical recommendations for conduct and planning. *Stat Med* 2020;39(15):2115–2137.

10 Arnold BF, Hogan DR, Colford JM, Jr., et al. Simulation methods to estimate design power: an overview for applied research. *BMC Med Res Methodol* 2011;11:94.

11 Landau S, Stahl D. Sample size and power calculations for medical studies by simulation when closed form expressions are not available. *Stat Methods Med Res* 2013 22(3):324–345.

12 Feiveson AH. Power by simulation. *Stata J* 2002;2(2):107–124.

13 Browne WJ, Lahi MG, Parker RMA. A guide to sample size calculation for random effects models via simulation and the MLPowSim software package. MLPowSim Manual. University of Bristol 2009.

14 Papadimitropoulou K, Stijnen T, Dekkers OM, et al. One-stage random effects meta-analysis using linear mixed models for aggregate continuous outcome data. *Res Synth Methods* 2019;10(3):360–375.

15 Hartung J, Knapp G. A refined method for the meta-analysis of controlled clinical trials with binary outcome. *Stat Med* 2001;20(24):3875–3889.

16 Sidik K, Jonkman JN. A simple confidence interval for meta-analysis. *Stat Med* 2002;21 (21):3153–3159.

Individual Participant Data Meta-Analysis: A Handbook for Healthcare Research, First Edition.
Edited by Richard D. Riley, Jayne F. Tierney, and Lesley A. Stewart.

17 Royston P, Altman DG, Sauerbrei W. Dichotomizing continuous predictors in multiple regression: a bad idea. *Stat Med* 2006;25(1):127–141.

18 Altman DG, Royston P. Statistics notes: the cost of dichotomising continuous variables. *BMJ* 2006;332:1080.

19 Cohen J. The cost of dichotomization. *Appl Psychol Meas* 1983;7:249–253.

20 Cox DR. Note on grouping. *J Am Stat Assoc* 1957;52(280):543–547.

21 Senn S. Testing for basline balance in clinical trials. *Stat Med* 1994;13:1715–1726.

22 Teerenstra S, Eldridge S, Graff M, et al. A simple sample size formula for analysis of covariance in cluster randomized trials. *Stat Med* 2012;31(20):2169–2178.

23 Borm GF, Fransen J, Lemmens WA. A simple sample size formula for analysis of covariance in randomized clinical trials. *J Clin Epidemiol* 2007;60(12):1234–1238.

24 Crowther MJ, Lambert PC. Simulating biologically plausible complex survival data. *Stat Med* 2013;32(23):4118–4134.

25 Wei Y, Royston P. Reconstructing time-to-event data from published Kaplan-Meier curves. *Stata J* 2017;17(4):786–802.

26 Burke DL, Ensor J, Riley RD. Meta-analysis using individual participant data: one-stage and two-stage approaches, and why they may differ. *Stat Med* 2017;36(5):855–875.

27 Fisher DJ. Two-stage individual participant data meta-analysis and generalized forest plots. *Stata J* 2015;15(2):369–496.

28 Hua H, Burke DL, Crowther MJ, et al. One-stage individual participant data meta-analysis models: estimation of treatment-covariate interactions must avoid ecological bias by separating out within-trial and across-trial information. *Stat Med* 2017;36(5):772–789.

29 Fisher DJ, Copas AJ, Tierney JF, et al. A critical review of methods for the assessment of patient-level interactions in individual participant data meta-analysis of randomized trials, and guidance for practitioners. *J Clin Epidemiol* 2011;64(9):949–967.

30 Green P, MacLeod CJ. SIMR: an R package for power analysis of generalized linear mixed models by simulation. *Methods Ecol Evoln* 2016;7(4):493–498.

31 Bates D, Mächler M, Bolker B, et al. Fitting linear mixed-effects models using lme4. *J Stat Softw* 2015;67(1):1–48.

32 powerlmm: Power analysis for longitudinal multilevel models (available at https://github.com/rpsychologist/powerlmm) [program], 2018.

33 PASS 2019 Power analysis and sample size software (ncss.com/software/pass) [program]. Kaysville, Utah, 2019.

34 Bland JM. The tyranny of power: is there a better way to calculate sample size? *BMJ* 2009;339:b3985.

35 Burke DL, Billingham LJ, Girling AJ, et al. Meta-analysis of randomized phase II trials to inform subsequent phase III decisions. *Trials* 2014;15:346.

36 Sutton AJ, Cooper NJ, Jones DR, et al. Evidence-based sample size calculations based upon updated meta-analysis. *Stat Med* 2007;26(12):2479–2500.

37 Higgins JP, Whitehead A, Simmonds M. Sequential methods for random-effects meta-analysis. *Stat Med* 2011;30(9):903–921.

38 Jackson D, Turner R. Power analysis for random-effects meta-analysis. *Res Synth Methods* 2017;8 (3):290–302.

39 Jones HE, Ades AE, Sutton AJ, et al. Use of a random effects meta-analysis in the design and analysis of a new clinical trial. *Stat Med* 2018;37(30):4665–4679.

40 Bland JM. Comments on 'Multivariate meta-analysis: Potential and promise' by Jackson et al. *Stat Med* 2011;30:2502–2503.

41 Riley RD, Gates SG, Neilson J, et al. Statistical methods can be improved within Cochrane Pregnancy and Childbirth Reviews. *J Clin Epidemiol* 2011;64(6):608–618.

42 Van Houwelingen HC, Arends LR, Stijnen T. Advanced methods in meta-analysis: multivariate approach and meta-regression. *Stat Med* 2002;21(4):589–624.

43 Jackson D, Riley RD, White IR. Multivariate meta-analysis: potential and promise. *Stat Med* 2011;30:2481–2498.

44 Macleod MR, Michie S, Roberts I, et al. Biomedical research: increasing value, reducing waste. *Lancet* 2014;383(9912):101–104.

45 Glasziou P, Altman DG, Bossuyt P, et al. Reducing waste from incomplete or unusable reports of biomedical research. *Lancet* 2014;383(9913):267–276.

46 Chan AW, Song F, Vickers A, et al. Increasing value and reducing waste: addressing inaccessible research. *Lancet* 2014;383(9913):257–266.

47 Kirkham JJ, Riley RD, Williamson PR. A multivariate meta-analysis approach for reducing the impact of outcome reporting bias in systematic reviews. *Stat Med* 2012;31(20):2179–2195.

48 Higgins JP, Whitehead A. Borrowing strength from external trials in a meta-analysis. *Stat Med* 1996;15(24):2733–2749.

49 Jackson D, White IR, Price M, et al. Borrowing of strength and study weights in multivariate and network meta-analysis. *Stat Methods Med Res* 2017;26(6):2853–2868.

50 Zhang Y, Zhao D, Gong C, et al. Prognostic role of hormone receptors in endometrial cancer: a systematic review and meta-analysis. *World Jf Surg Oncol* 2015;13:208.

51 Riley RD, Jackson D, Salanti G, et al. Multivariate and network meta-analysis of multiple outcomes and multiple treatments: rationale, concepts, and examples. *BMJ* 2017;358:j3932.

52 Simmonds MC, Higgins JPT, Stewart LA, et al. Meta-analysis of individual patient data from randomized trials: a review of methods used in practice. *Clin Trials* 2005;2:209–217.

53 Riley RD, Lambert PC, Abo-Zaid G. Meta-analysis of individual participant data: rationale, conduct, and reporting. *BMJ* 2010;340:c221.

54 Riley RD, Kauser I, Bland M, et al. Meta-analysis of randomised trials with a continuous outcome according to baseline imbalance and availability of individual participant data. *Stat Med* 2013;32 (16):2747–2766.

55 Vickers AJ, Altman DG. Statistics notes: analysing controlled trials with baseline and follow up measurements. *BMJ* 2001;323(7321):1123–1124.

56 Riley RD, Lambert PC, Staessen JA, et al. Meta-analysis of continuous outcomes combining individual patient data and aggregate data. *Stat Med* 2008;27(11):1870–1893.

57 Zellner A. An efficient method for estimating seemingly unrelated regressions and tests of aggregation bias. *J Am Stat Assoc* 1962;57:500–509.

58 Riley RD, Price MJ, Jackson D, et al. Multivariate meta-analysis using individual participant data. *Res Synth Method* 2015;6 157–174.

59 Riley RD, Thompson JR, Abrams KR. An alternative model for bivariate random-effects meta-analysis when the within-study correlations are unknown. *Biostatistics* 2008;9(1):172–186.

60 Riley RD. Multivariate meta-analysis: the effect of ignoring within-study correlation. *J Royal Stat Soc A Stat Soc* 2009;172(4):701–951.

61 Wei Y, Higgins JP. Estimating within-study covariances in multivariate meta-analysis with multiple outcomes. *Stat Med* 2013;32(7):1191–1205.

62 Bujkiewicz S, Thompson JR, Sutton AJ, et al. Multivariate meta-analysis of mixed outcomes: a Bayesian approach. *Stat Med* 2013;32(22):3926–3943.

63 Trikalinos TA, Olkin I. A method for the meta-analysis of mutually exclusive binary outcomes. *Stat Med* 2008;27(21):4279–4300.

64 Wang JG, Staessen JA, Franklin SS, et al. Systolic and diastolic blood pressure lowering as determinants of cardiovascular outcome. *Hypertension* 2005;45(5):907–913.

65 Wassell JT, Moeschberger ML. A bivariate survival model with modified gamma frailty for assessing the impact of interventions. *Stat Med* 1993;12(3-4):241–248.

66 Hougaard P. *Analysis of Multivariate Survival Data*. New York: Springer-Verlag 2000.

67 Burzykowski T, Molenberghs G, Buyse M, et al. Validation of surrogate end points in multiple randomized clinical trials with failure time end points. *J Royal Stat Soc Series C Appl Stat* 2001;50:405–422.

68 Michiels S, Le Maitre A, Buyse M, et al. Surrogate endpoints for overall survival in locally advanced head and neck cancer: meta-analyses of individual patient data. *Lancet Oncol* 2009;10(4):341–350.

69 Nikoloulopoulos AK. A vine copula mixed effect model for trivariate meta-analysis of diagnostic test accuracy studies accounting for disease prevalence. *Stat Methods Med Res* 2017;26(5):2270–2286.

70 Jackson D, White IR, Thompson SG. Extending DerSimonian and Laird's methodology to perform multivariate random effects meta-analyses. *Stat Med* 2010;29:1282–1297.

71 Jackson D, White IR, Riley RD. A matrix-based method of moments for fitting the multivariate random effects model for meta-analysis and meta-regression. *Biom J* 2013;55(2):231–245.

72 Chen H, Manning AK, Dupuis J. A method of moments estimator for random effect multivariate meta-analysis. *Biometrics* 2012;68(4):1278–1284.

73 DerSimonian R, Laird N. Meta-analysis in clinical trials. *Control Clin Trials* 1986;7:177–188.

74 White IR. Multivariate random-effects meta-regression: updates to mvmeta. *Stata J* 2011;11:255–270.

75 Jackson D, Riley RD. A refined method for multivariate meta-analysis and meta-regression. *Stat Med* 2014;33(33):541–554.

76 Nam IS, Mengersen K, Garthwaite P. Multivariate meta-analysis. *Stat Med* 2003;22(14):2309–333.

77 Wei Y, Higgins JP. Bayesian multivariate meta-analysis with multiple outcomes. *Stat Med* 2013;32 (17):2911–2934.

78 Barnard J, McCulloch R, Meng XL. Modeling covariance matrices in terms of standard deviations and correlations, *with application to shrinkage. Statistica Sinica* 2000;10(4):1281–1331.

79 Burke DL, Bujkiewicz S, Riley RD. Bayesian bivariate meta-analysis of correlated effects: impact of the prior distributions on the between-study correlation, borrowing of strength, and joint inferences. *Stat Methods Med Res* 2018;27(2):428–450.

80 Spiegelhalter DJ, Thomas A, Best NG. *WinBUGS version 1.3 User Manual*. Cambridge: MRC Biostatistics Unit 2000.

81 Lambert PC, Sutton AJ, Burton PR, et al. How vague is vague? A simulation study of the impact of the use of vague prior distributions in MCMC. *Stat Med* 2005;24:2401–2428.

82 Rhodes KM, Turner RM, Higgins JP. Predictive distributions were developed for the extent of heterogeneity in meta-analyses of continuous outcome data. *J Clin Epidemiol* 2015;68(1):52–60.

83 Turner RM, Davey J, Clarke MJ, et al. Predicting the extent of heterogeneity in meta-analysis, using empirical data from the Cochrane Database of Systematic Reviews. *Int J Epidemiol* 2012;41 (3):818–827.

84 Snell KI, Hua H, Debray TP, et al. Multivariate meta-analysis of individual participant data helped externally validate the performance and implementation of a prediction model. *J Clin Epidemiol* 2016;69:40–50.

85 Riley RD, Abrams KR, Sutton AJ, et al. Bivariate random-effects meta-analysis and the estimation of between-study correlation. *BMC Med Res Methodol* 2007;7(1):3.

86 Higgins JP, Thompson SG. Quantifying heterogeneity in a meta-analysis. *Stat Med* 2002;21 (11):1539–1558.

87 Jackson D, White IR, Riley RD. Quantifying the impact of between-study heterogeneity in multivariate meta-analyses. *Stat Med* 2012;31(29):3805–3820.

88 Gasparrini A, Armstrong B, Kenward MG. Multivariate meta-analysis for non-linear and other multi-parameter associations. *Stat Med* 2012;31:3821–3839.

89 Riley RD, Ensor J, Jackson D, et al. Deriving percentage study weights in multi-parameter meta-analysis models: with application to meta-regression, network meta-analysis and one-stage individual participant data models. *Stat Methods Med Res* 2018;27(10):2885–2905.

90 Konig J, Krahn U, Binder H. Visualizing the flow of evidence in network meta-analysis and characterizing mixed treatment comparisons. *Stat Med* 2013;32(30):5414–5429.

91 Copas JB, Jackson D, White IR, et al. The role of secondary outcomes in multivariate meta-analysis. *J Royal Stat Soc Series C Appl Stat* 2018;67(5):1177–1205.

92 Riley RD, Abrams KR, Lambert PC, et al. An evaluation of bivariate random-effects meta-analysis for the joint synthesis of two correlated outcomes. *Stat Med* 2007;26(1):78–97.

93 Hattle M. Development and application of multivariate meta-analysis in medical research: borrowing of strength across multiple correlated outcomes (PhD thesis). Keele University 2020.

94 Riley RD. Evidence Synthesis of Prognostic Marker Studies (PhD thesis). University of Leicester 2005.

95 Chen Y, Hong C, Riley RD. An alternative pseudolikelihood method for multivariate random-effects meta-analysis. *Stat Med* 2015;34(3):361–380.

96 Chen Y, Cai Y, Hong C, et al. Inference for correlated effect sizes using multiple univariate meta-analyses. *Stat Med* 2016;35(9):1405–1422.

97 White IR. Multivariate meta-analysis. *Stata J* 2009;9:40–56.

98 Gasparrini A, Armstrong B. Multivariate meta-analysis: A method to summarize non-linear associations. *Stat Med* 2011;30:2504–2506.

99 White IR. Network meta-analysis. *Stata J* 2015;15:951–985.

100 Berkey CS, Hoaglin DC, Antczak-Bouckoms A, et al. Meta-analysis of multiple outcomes by regression with random effects. *Stat Med* 1998;17(22):2537–2550.

101 Trikalinos TA, Hoaglin DC, Schmid CH. An empirical comparison of univariate and multivariate meta-analyses for categorical outcomes. *Stat Med* 2014;33(9):1441–1459.

102 Price MJ, Blake HA, Kenyon S, et al. Empirical comparison of univariate and multivariate meta-analyses in Cochrane Pregnancy and Childbirth reviews with multiple binary outcomes. *Res Synth Methods* 2019;10(3):440–451.

103 Trikalinos TA, Hoaglin DC, Schmid CH. Empirical and simulation-based comparison of univariate and multivariate meta-analysis for binary outcomes. Methods Research Report. Agency for Healthcare Research and Quality 2013:Publication No. 13-EHC066-EF.

104 Nikoloulopoulos AK. A mixed effect model for bivariate meta-analysis of diagnostic test accuracy studies using a copula representation of the random effects distribution. *Stat Med* 2015;34 (29):3842–3865.

105 Senn S, Gavini F, Magrez D, et al. Issues in performing a network meta-analysis. *Stat Methods Med Res* 2013;22(2):169–189.

106 Covey SR. *The 7 Habits of Highly Effective People Personal Workbook.* Simon & Schuster UK 2008.

107 Seaman S, Galati J, Jackson D, et al. What is meant by "missing at random"? *StatSci* 2013;28 (2):257–268.

108 Nixon RM, Duffy SW, Fender GR. Imputation of a true endpoint from a surrogate: application to a cluster randomized controlled trial with partial information on the true endpoint. *BMC Med Res Methodol* 2003;3(1):17.

109 D'Agostino RB. Debate: the slippery slope of surrogate outcomes. *Trials* 2000;1(2):76.

110 Kuss O, Hoyer A, Solms A. Meta-analysis for diagnostic accuracy studies: a new statistical model using beta-binomial distributions and bivariate copulas. *Stat Med* 2014;33(1):17–30.

111 Kirkham JJ, Dwan KM, Altman DG, et al. The impact of outcome reporting bias in randomised controlled trials on a cohort of systematic reviews. *BMJ* 2010;340:c365.

112 Dwan K, Altman DG, Clarke M, et al. Evidence for the selective reporting of analyses and discrepancies in clinical trials: a systematic review of cohort studies of clinical trials. *PLoS Med* 2014;11(6):e1001666.

113 Copas J. What works? Selectivity models and meta-analysis. *J Royal Stat Soc Series A* 1999;162:95–109.

114 Stijnen T, Hamza TH, Özdemir P. Random effects meta-analysis of event outcome in the framework of the generalized linear mixed model with applications in sparse data. *Stat Med* 2010;29:3046–3067.

115 Schmid CH, Trikalinos TA, Olkin I. Bayesian network meta-analysis for unordered categorical outcomes with incomplete data. *Res Synth Methods* 2014;5(2):162–185.

116 Liang K-Y, Zeger SL. Longitudinal data analysis using generalized linear models. *Biometrika* 1986;73 (1):13–22.

117 Peters JL, Mengersen KL. Meta-analysis of repeated measures study designs. *J Eval Clin Pract* 2008;14(5):941–950.

118 Ishak KJ, Platt RW, Joseph L, et al. Meta-analysis of longitudinal studies. *Clin Trials* 2007;4 (5):525–539.

119 Jones AP, Riley RD, Williamson PR, et al. Meta-analysis of individual patient data versus aggregate data from longitudinal clinical trials. *Clin Trials* 2009;6(1):16–27.

120 Jansen JP, Vieira MC, Cope S. Network meta-analysis of longitudinal data using fractional polynomials. *Stat Med* 2015;34(15):2294–2311.

121 Trikalinos TA, Olkin I. Meta-analysis of effect sizes reported at multiple time points: A multivariate approach. *Clin Trials* 2012;9(5):610–620.

122 Dakin HA, Welton NJ, Ades AE, et al. Mixed treatment comparison of repeated measurements of a continuous endpoint: an example using topical treatments for primary open-angle glaucoma and ocular hypertension. *Stat Med* 2011;30(20):2511–2535.

123 Sudell M, Tudur Smith C, Gueyffier F, et al. Investigation of 2-stage meta-analysis methods for joint longitudinal and time-to-event data through simulation and real data application. *Stat Med* 2018;37 (8):1227–1244.

124 Sudell M, Kolamunnage-Dona R, Tudur-Smith C. Joint models for longitudinal and time-to-event data: a review of reporting quality with a view to meta-analysis. *BMC Med Res Methodol* 2016;16(1):168.

125 Sudell M, Kolamunnage-Dona R, Gueyffier F, et al. Investigation of one-stage meta-analysis methods for joint longitudinal and time-to-event data through simulation and real data application. *Stat Med* 2019;38(2):247–268.

126 Crowther MJ, Lambert PC. Parametric multistate survival models: flexible modelling allowing transition-specific distributions with application to estimating clinically useful measures of effect differences. *Stat Med* 2017;36(29):4719–4742.

127 Dear KB. Iterative generalized least squares for meta-analysis of survival data at multiple times. *Biometrics* 1994;50(4):989–1002.

128 Jackson D, Rollins K, Coughlin P. A multivariate model for the meta-analysis of study level survival data at multiple times. *Res Synth Meth* 2014;5(3):264–272.

129 Arends LR, Hunink MG, Stijnen T. Meta-analysis of summary survival curve data. *Stat Med* 2008;27 (22):4381–4396.

130 Buyse M, Molenberghs G. Criteria for the validation of surrogate endpoints in randomized experiments. *Biometrics* 1998;54(3):1014–1029.

131 Daniels MJ, Hughes MD. Meta-analysis for the evaluation of potential surrogate markers. *Stat Med* 1997;16(17):1965–1982.

132 Gail MH, Pfeiffer R, Van Houwelingen HC, et al. On meta-analytic assessment of surrogate outcomes. *Biostatistics* 2000;1(3):231–246.

133 Buyse M, Molenberghs G, Burzykowski T, et al. The validation of surrogate endpoints in meta-analyses of randomized experiments. *Biostatistics* 2000;1(1):49–67.

134 Buyse M. Use of meta-analysis for the validation of surrogate endpoints and biomarkers in cancer trials. *Cancer J* 2009;15(5):421–425.

135 Prentice RL. Surrogate and mediating endpoints: current status and future directions. *J Natl Cancer Inst* 2009;101(4):216–217.

136 Prentice RL. Surrogate endpoints in clinical trials: definition and operational criteria. *Stat Med* 1989;8(4):431–440.

137 De Gruttola VG, Clax P, DeMets DL, et al. Considerations in the evaluation of surrogate endpoints in clinical trials. Summary of a National Institutes of Health workshop. *Control Clin Trials* 2001;22 (5):485–502.

138 Rotolo F, Paoletti X, Michiels S. surrosurv: an R package for the evaluation of failure time surrogate endpoints in individual patient data meta-analyses of randomized clinical trials. *Comput Methods Programs Biomed* 2018;155:189–198.

139 Bujkiewicz S, Thompson JR, Riley RD, et al. Bayesian meta-analytical methods to incorporate multiple surrogate endpoints in drug development process. *Stat Med* 2016;35(7):1063–1089.

140 Renfro LA, Shi Q, Sargent DJ, et al. Bayesian adjusted R^2 for the meta-analytic evaluation of surrogate time-to-event endpoints in clinical trials. *Stat Med* 2012;31(8):743–761.

141 Bujkiewicz S, Thompson JR, Spata E, et al. Uncertainty in the Bayesian meta-analysis of normally distributed surrogate endpoints. *Stat Methods Med Res* 2017;26(5):2287–2318.

142 Steyerberg EW, Moons KG, van der Windt DA, et al. Prognosis Research Strategy (PROGRESS) 3: prognostic model research. *PLoS Med* 2013;10(2):e1001381.

143 Sauerbrei W, Royston P. A new strategy for meta-analysis of continuous covariates in observational studies. *Stat Med* 2011;30(28):3341–3360.

144 Greenland S, Longnecker MP. Methods for trend estimation from summarized dose-response data, with applications to meta-analysis. *Am J Epidemiol* 1992;135(11):1301–1309.

145 Orsini N, Li R, Wolk A, et al. Meta-analysis for linear and nonlinear dose-response relations: examples, an evaluation of approximations, *and software. Am J Epidemiol* 2012;175(1):66–73.

146 White IR, Kaptoge S, Royston P, et al. Meta-analysis of non-linear exposure-outcome relationships using individual participant data: a comparison of two methods. *Stat Med* 2019;38(3):326–338.

147 Harbord RM, Deeks JJ, Egger M, et al. A unification of models for meta-analysis of diagnostic accuracy studies. *Biostatistics* 2007;8(2):239–251.

148 Hamza TH, Arends LR, van Houwelingen HC, et al. Multivariate random effects meta-analysis of diagnostic tests with multiple thresholds. *BMC Med Res Methodol* 2009;9:73.

149 Riley RD, Takwoingi Y, Trikalinos T, et al. Meta-analysis of test accuracy studies with multiple and missing thresholds: a multivariate-normal model. *J Biomet Biostat* 2014;5:3.

150 Sharp SJ, Thompson SG, Altman DG. The relation between treatment benefit and underlying risk in meta-analysis. *BMJ* 1996;313(7059):735–738.

151 Thompson SG, Smith TC, Sharp SJ. Investigating underlying risk as a source of heterogeneity in meta-analysis. *Stat Med* 1997;16(23):2741–2758.

152 Van Houwelingen HC, Zwinderman KH, Stijnen T. A bivariate approach to meta-analysis. *Stat Med* 1993;12(24):2273–2284.

153 Lu G, Ades AE. Assessing evidence inconsistency in mixed treatment comparisons. *J Am Stat Assoc* 2006;101(474):447–459.

154 Dias S, Ades AE, Welton NJ, et al. *Network Meta-Analysis for Decision Making*. Chichester, UK: Wiley 2018.

155 Dias S, Welton NJ, Sutton AJ, et al. Evidence synthesis for decision making 1: introduction. *Med Decis Making* 2013;33(5):597–606.

156 Dias S, Sutton AJ, Ades AE, et al. Evidence synthesis for decision making 2: a generalized linear modeling framework for pairwise and network meta-analysis of randomized controlled trials. *Med Decis Making* 2013;33(5):607–617.

157 Dias S, Sutton AJ, Welton NJ, et al. Evidence synthesis for decision making 3: heterogeneity – subgroups, meta-regression, bias, and bias-adjustment. *Med Decis Making* 2013;33(5):618–640.

158 Dias S, Welton NJ, Sutton AJ, et al. Evidence synthesis for decision making 4: inconsistency in networks of evidence based on randomized controlled trials. *Med Decis Making* 2013;33(5):641–656.

159 Dias S, Welton NJ, Sutton AJ, et al. Evidence synthesis for decision making 5: the baseline natural history model. *Med Decis Making* 2013;33(5):657–670.

160 Dias S, Sutton AJ, Welton NJ, et al. Evidence synthesis for decision making 6: embedding evidence synthesis in probabilistic cost-effectiveness analysis. *Med Decis Making* 2013;33(5):671–678.

161 Ades AE, Caldwell DM, Reken S, et al. Evidence synthesis for decision making 7: a reviewer's checklist. *Med Decis Making* 2013;33(5):679–691.

162 Salanti G. Indirect and mixed-treatment comparison, network, or multiple-treatments meta-analysis: many names, many benefits, many concerns for the next generation evidence synthesis tool. *Res Synth Methods* 2012;3(2):80–97.

163 Cipriani A, Higgins JP, Geddes JR, et al. Conceptual and technical challenges in network meta-analysis. *Ann Intern Med* 2013;159(2):130–137.

164 Jansen JP, Trikalinos T, Cappelleri JC, et al. Indirect treatment comparison/network meta-analysis study questionnaire to assess relevance and credibility to inform health care decision making: an ISPOR-AMCP-NPC Good Practice Task Force report. *Value Health* 2014;17(2):157–173.

165 Lu G, Ades A. Modeling between-trial variance structure in mixed treatment comparisons. *Biostatistics* 2009;10(4):792–805.

166 White IR, Barrett JK, Jackson D, et al. Consistency and inconsistency in network meta-analysis: model estimation using multivariate meta-regression. *Res Synth Method* 2012;3:111–125.

167 Salanti G, Higgins JP, Ades AE, et al. Evaluation of networks of randomized trials. *Stat Methods Med Res* 2008;17(3):279–301.

168 Riley RD, Higgins JP, Deeks JJ. Interpretation of random effects meta-analyses. *BMJ* 2011;342:d549.

169 Saramago P, Sutton AJ, Cooper NJ, et al. Mixed treatment comparisons using aggregate and individual participant level data. *Stat Med* 2012;31(28):3516–3536.

170 Dias S, Ades AE. Absolute or relative effects? Arm-based synthesis of trial data. *Res Synth Methods* 2016;7(1):23–28.

171 Bafeta A, Trinquart L, Seror R, et al. Reporting of results from network meta-analyses: methodological systematic review. *BMJ* 2014;348:g1741.

172 Mills EJ, Thorlund K, Ioannidis JP. Demystifying trial networks and network meta-analysis. *BMJ* 2013;346:f2914.

173 Glenny AM, Altman DG, Song F, et al. Indirect comparisons of competing interventions. *Health Technol Assess* 2005;9(26):1–134, iii–iv.

174 White IR, Turner RM, Karahalios A, et al. A comparison of arm-based and contrast-based models for network meta-analysis. *Stat Med* 2019;38(27):5197–5213.

175 Piepho HP, Madden LV, Roger J, et al. Estimating the variance for heterogeneity in arm-based network meta-analysis. *Pharm Stat* 2018;17(3):264–277.

176 Riley RD, Legha A, Jackson D, et al. One-stage individual participant data meta-analysis models for continuous and binary outcomes: comparison of treatment coding options and estimation methods. *Stat Med* 2020;39(11).

177 Wolfinger R, O'Connell M. Generalized linear mixed models: a pseudo-likelihood approach. *J Stat Comput Simul* 1993;48:233–243.

178 Lunn DJ, Thomas A, Best N, et al. WinBUGS – a Bayesian modelling framework: concepts, structure, and extensibility. *Stat Comput* 2000;10:325–337.

179 van Valkenhoef G, Lu G, de Brock B, et al. Automating network meta-analysis. *Res Synth Methods* 2012;3(4):285–299.

180 Phillippo DM. Calibration of treatment effects in network meta-analysis using individual patient data. PhD thesis, University of Bristol, 2019.

181 Chaimani A, Higgins JP, Mavridis D, et al. Graphical tools for network meta-analysis in STATA. *PLoS One* 2013;8(10):e76654.

182 Chaimani A, Salanti G. Visualizing assumptions and results in network meta-analysis: the network graphs package. *Stata J* 2015;15:905–950.

183 Salanti G, Ades AE, Ioannidis JP. Graphical methods and numerical summaries for presenting results from multiple-treatment meta-analysis: an overview and tutorial. *J Clin Epidemiol* 2011;64 (2):163–171.

184 Papakonstantinou T, Nikolakopoulou A, Rücker G, et al. Estimating the contribution of studies in network meta-analysis: paths, *flows and streams. F1000Res* 2018;7:610–610.

185 Caldwell DM, Ades AE, Higgins JP. Simultaneous comparison of multiple treatments: combining direct and indirect evidence. *BMJ* 2005;331(7521):897–900.

186 Rucker G, Schwarzer G. Ranking treatments in frequentist network meta-analysis works without resampling methods. *BMC Med Res Methodol* 2015;15:58.

187 Lu G, Ades AE. Combination of direct and indirect evidence in mixed treatment comparisons. *Stat Med* 2004;23(20):3105–3124.

188 Trinquart L, Attiche N, Bafeta A, et al. Uncertainty in treatment rankings: reanalysis of network meta-analyses of randomized trials. *Ann Intern Med* 2016;164(10):666–673.

189 Song F, Xiong T, Parekh-Bhurke S, et al. Inconsistency between direct and indirect comparisons of competing interventions: meta-epidemiological study. *BMJ* 2011;343:d4909.

190 Jansen JP, Naci H. Is network meta-analysis as valid as standard pairwise meta-analysis? It all depends on the distribution of effect modifiers. *BMC Med* 2013;11:159.

191 Donegan S, Williamson P, D'Alessandro U, et al. Combining individual patient data and aggregate data in mixed treatment comparison meta-analysis: individual patient data may be beneficial if only for a subset of trials. *Stat Med* 2013;32(6):914–930.

192 Debray TP, Schuit E, Efthimiou O, et al. An overview of methods for network meta-analysis using individual participant data: when do benefits arise? *Stat Methods Med Res* 2018;27(5):1351–1364.

193 Salanti G, Marinho V, Higgins JP. A case study of multiple-treatments meta-analysis demonstrates that covariates should be considered. *J Clin Epidemiol* 2009;62(8):857–864.

194 Nikolakopoulou A, Chaimani A, Veroniki AA, et al. Characteristics of networks of interventions: a description of a database of 186 published networks. *PLoS One* 2014;9(1):e86754.

195 Dias S, Welton NJ, Caldwell DM, et al. Checking consistency in mixed treatment comparison meta-analysis. *Stat Med* 2010;29(7–8):932–944.

196 Veroniki AA, Vasiliadis HS, Higgins JP, et al. Evaluation of inconsistency in networks of interventions. *Int J Epidemiol* 2013;42(1):332–345.

197 Higgins JPT, Jackson D, Barrett JK, et al. Consistency and inconsistency in network meta-analysis: concepts and models for multi-arm studies. *Res Synth Methods* 2012;3:98–110.

198 Dias S, Welton NJ, Sutton AJ, et al. NICE DSU Technical Support Document 4: Inconsistency in networks of evidence based on randomised controlled trials. Available from http://www.nicedsu.org.uk 2011.

199 Law M, Jackson D, Turner R, et al. Two new methods to fit models for network meta-analysis with random inconsistency effects. *BMC Med Res Methodol* 2016;16:87.

200 Jackson D, Law M, Barrett JK, et al. Extending DerSimonian and Laird's methodology to perform network meta-analyses with random inconsistency effects. *Stat Med* 2016;35(6):819–839.

201 Jackson D, Barrett JK, Rice S, et al. A design-by-treatment interaction model for network meta-analysis with random inconsistency effects. *Stat Med* 2014;33(21):3639–3654.

202 Veroniki AA, Mavridis D, Higgins JP, et al. Characteristics of a loop of evidence that affect detection and estimation of inconsistency: a simulation study. *BMC Med ResMethodol* 2014;14(1):106.

203 Donegan S, Dias S, Tudur-Smith C, et al. Graphs of study contributions and covariate distributions for network meta-regression. *Res Synth Methods* 2018;9(2):243–260.

204 Batson S, Score R, Sutton AJ. Three-dimensional evidence network plot system: covariate imbalances and effects in network meta-analysis explored using a new software tool. *J Clin Epidemiol* 2017;86:182–195.

205 Hong H, Fu H, Price KL, et al. Incorporation of individual-patient data in network meta-analysis for multiple continuous endpoints, with application to diabetes treatment. *Stat Med* 2015;34(20):2794–2819.

206 Four Artemisinin-Based Combinations Study Group. A head-to-head comparison of four artemisinin-based combinations for treating uncomplicated malaria in African children: a randomized trial. *PLoS Med* 2011;8(11):e1001119.

207 Donegan S, Dias S, Welton NJ. Assessing the consistency assumptions underlying network meta-regression using aggregate data. *Res Synth Methods* 2019;10(2):207–224.

208 Efthimiou O, Mavridis D, Cipriani A, et al. An approach for modelling multiple correlated outcomes in a network of interventions using odds ratios. *Stat Med* 2014;33(13):2275–2287.

209 Efthimiou O, Mavridis D, Riley RD, et al. Joint synthesis of multiple correlated outcomes in networks of interventions. *Biostatistics* 2015;16(1):84–97.

210 Hong H, Carlin BP, Chu H, et al. *A Bayesian missing data framework for multiple continuous outcome mixed treatment comparisons. Methods Research Report (Prepared by the Minnesota Evidence-based Practice Center under Contract No 290-2007-10064-I) AHRQ Publication No 13-EHC004-EF.* Rockville, MD: Agency for Healthcare Research and Quality; January 2013.

211 Hong H, Chu H, Zhang J, et al. A Bayesian missing data framework for generalized multiple outcome mixed treatment comparisons. *Res Synth Methods* 2016;7(1):6–22.

212 Jackson D, Bujkiewicz S, Law M, et al. A matrix-based method of moments for fitting multivariate network meta-analysis models with multiple outcomes and random inconsistency effects. *Biometrics* 2018;74(2):548–556.

213 Phillippo DM, Ades AE, Dias S, et al. Methods for population-adjusted indirect comparisons in health technology appraisal. *Med Decis Making* 2018;38(2):200–211.

214 Phillippo DM, Ades AE, Dias S, et al. NICE DSU Technical Support Document 18: Methods for population-adjusted indirect comparisons in submission to NICE. National Institute for Health and Care Excellence (available from www.nicedsu.org.uk) 2016.

215 Signorovitch JE, Sikirica V, Erder MH, et al. Matching-adjusted indirect comparisons: a new tool for timely comparative effectiveness research. *Value in Health* 2012;15(6):940–947.

216 Signorovitch J, Wu E, Yu A, et al. Comparative effectiveness without head-to-head trials: a method for matching-adjusted indirect comparisons applied to psoriasis treatment with adalimumab or etanercept. *PharmacoEconomics* 2010;28:935–945.

217 Ishak KJ, Proskorovsky I, Benedict A. Simulation and matching-based approaches for indirect comparison of treatments. *Pharmacoeconomics* 2015;33(6):537–549.

218 Caro JJ, Ishak KJ. No head-to-head trial? Simulate the missing arms. *Pharmacoeconomics* 2010;28(10):957–967.

219 Betts KA, Mittal M, Song J, et al. OP0115 Relative efficacy of adalimumab versus secukinumab in active ankylosing spondylitis: a matching-adjusted indirect comparison. *Ann Rheum Dis* 2016;75(Suppl 2):98–99.

220 Maksymowych W, Strand V, Baeten D, et al. OP0114 Secukinumab for The Treatment of Ankylosing Spondylitis: Comparative Effectiveness Results versus Adalimumab Using A Matching-Adjusted Indirect Comparison. *Ann Rheum Dis* 2016;75(Suppl 2):98.

221 Sutton AJ, Kendrick D, Coupland CA. Meta-analysis of individual- and aggregate-level data. *Stat Med* 2008;27:651–669.

222 Riley RD, Steyerberg EW. Meta-analysis of a binary outcome using individual participant data and aggregate data. *Res Synth Methods* 2010;1:2–9.

223 Phillippo DM, Dias S, Ades AE, et al. Multilevel network meta-regression for population-adjusted treatment comparisons. *J Royal Stat Soc Series A Stat Soc* 2020;183(3):1189–1210.

224 Jansen JP. Network meta-analysis of individual and aggregate level data. *Res Synth Methods* 2012;3(2):177–190.

225 Jackson C, Best N, Richardson S. Hierarchical related regression for combining aggregate and individual data in studies of socio-economic disease risk factors. *J Royal Stat Soc Series A* 2008;171:159–178.

226 Jackson C, Best N, Richardson S. Improving ecological inference using individual-level data. *Stat Med* 2006;25(12):2136–2159.

227 Langley RG, Elewski BE, Lebwohl M, et al. Secukinumab in plaque psoriasis – results of two phase 3 trials. *N Engl J Med* 2014;371(4):326–338.

228 Griffiths CE, Reich K, Lebwohl M, et al. Comparison of ixekizumab with etanercept or placebo in moderate-to-severe psoriasis (UNCOVER-2 and UNCOVER-3): results from two phase 3 randomised trials. *Lancet* 2015;386(9993):541–551.

229 Gordon KB, Blauvelt A, Papp KA, et al. Phase 3 trials of ixekizumab in moderate-to-severe plaque psoriasis. *N Engl J Med* 2016;375(4):345–356.

230 Carpenter B, Gelman A, Hoffman MD, et al. Stan: A probabilistic programming language. *J Stat Softw* 2017;76(1):1–32.

231 Owen RK, Tincello DG, Abrams KR. Network meta-analysis: development of a three-level hierarchical modeling approach incorporating dose-related constraints. *Value Health* 2015;18 (1):116–126.

232 Del Giovane C, Vacchi L, Mavridis D, et al. Network meta-analysis models to account for variability in treatment definitions: application to dose effects. *Stat Med* 2013;32(1):25–39.

233 Mawdsley D, Bennetts M, Dias S, et al. Model-based network meta-analysis: a framework for evidence synthesis of clinical trial data. *CPT Pharmacometrics Syst Pharmacol* 2016;5(8):393–401.

234 Jenkins D, Czachorowski M, Bujkiewicz S, et al. Evaluation of methods for the inclusion of real world evidence in network meta-analysis – a case study in multiple sclerosis. *Value Health* 2014;17(7):A576.

235 Thom HH, Capkun G, Cerulli A, et al. Network meta-analysis combining individual patient and aggregate data from a mixture of study designs with an application to pulmonary arterial hypertension. *BMC Med Res Methodol* 2015;15:34.

236 Efthimiou O, Mavridis D, Debray TP, et al. Combining randomized and non-randomized evidence in network meta-analysis. *Stat Med* 2017;36(8):1210–1226.

237 Crequit P, Trinquart L, Yavchitz A, et al. Wasted research when systematic reviews fail to provide a complete and up-to-date evidence synthesis: the example of lung cancer. *BMC Med* 2016;14:8.

238 Vale CL, Burdett S, Rydzewska LH, et al. Addition of docetaxel or bisphosphonates to standard of care in men with localised or metastatic, hormone-sensitive prostate cancer: a systematic review and meta-analyses of aggregate data. *Lancet Oncol* 2016;17(2):243–256.

239 Salanti G, Del Giovane C, Chaimani A, et al. Evaluating the quality of evidence from a network meta-analysis. *PLoS One* 2014;9(7):e99682.

240 Hutton B, Salanti G, Caldwell DM, et al. The PRISMA extension statement for reporting of systematic reviews incorporating network meta-analyses of health care interventions: checklist and explanations. *Ann Intern Med* 2015;162(11):777–784.

241 Stewart LA, Clarke M, Rovers M, et al. Preferred reporting items for systematic review and meta-analyses of individual participant data: the PRISMA-IPD Statement. *JAMA* 2015;313(16):1657–1665.

242 Nikolakopoulou A, Higgins JPT, Papakonstantinou T, et al. CINeMA: An approach for assessing confidence in the results of a network meta-analysis. *PLOS Medicine* 2020;17(4):e1003082.

243 Phillippo DM, Dias S, Ades AE, et al. Sensitivity of treatment recommendations to bias in network meta-analysis. *J Royal Stat Soc Series A Stat Soc*2018;181(3):843–867.

244 Phillippo DM, Dias S, Welton NJ, et al. Threshold analysis as an alternative to GRADE for assessing confidence in guideline recommendations based on network meta-analyses. *Ann Int Med* 2019;170 (8):538–546.

Part V

Diagnosis, Prognosis and Prediction

15

IPD Meta-Analysis for Test Accuracy Research

Richard D. Riley, Brooke Levis, and Yemisi Takwoingi

Summary Points

- Test accuracy studies aim to evaluate the performance of a particular medical test, usually for screening or diagnostic purposes.
- Meta-Analysis summarises the accuracy of one or more tests across multiple studies, in terms of sensitivity and specificity, and positive and negative predictive values.
- The use of IPD, rather than aggregate data, has important potential to improve test accuracy meta-analyses. For example, it allows the standardisation of participant inclusion criteria, reference standards, and thresholds to define positive and negative test results; it also enables the examination of how participant-level characteristics are associated with test accuracy.
- Eights steps are proposed to guide those conducting an IPD meta-analysis of test accuracy. These include defining the research question, searching and classifying relevant studies, examining risk of bias, requesting and cleaning IPD, performing meta-analysis, and interpreting results.
- The QUADAS-2 tool can be used to examine each study's risk of bias and applicability for the IPD meta-analysis research question.
- A one-stage IPD meta-analysis model can be used to summarise sensitivity and specificity (or predictive values), with a Bernoulli distribution to model test results within studies, and a bivariate normal distribution to model between-study heterogeneity of the true logit sensitivity and logit specificity, and their between-study correlation.
- The approach can be extended to include participant-level and study-level covariates, to identify factors associated with changes in test accuracy. To avoid aggregation bias, participant-level covariates should be centered by their mean value and an additional term for the mean value should be included.
- For tests which give results as ordered categories or continuous measurements, a separate meta-analysis can be performed at each threshold of interest. More sophisticated analyses that model multiple thresholds simultaneously may sometimes be warranted, especially when some studies do not provide their IPD but report results for a subset of thresholds.
- The clinical utility of a test can be summarised by fitting a trivariate meta-analysis of sensitivity, specificity and prevalence, and subsequently deriving a decision curve that summarises a test's net benefit across a range of plausible risk thresholds that define clinical action.
- The bivariate model can also be extended to compare the accuracy of multiple tests; however, caution is needed if including studies with only a subset of the tests of interest, as this introduces indirect (across-study) comparisons which may be subject to study-level confounding.

Individual Participant Data Meta-Analysis: A Handbook for Healthcare Research, First Edition.
Edited by Richard D. Riley, Jayne F. Tierney, and Lesley A. Stewart.

15.1 Introduction

Test accuracy studies aim to evaluate the performance of medical tests, such as those being considered for screening or diagnostic purposes. A screening test is used to identify those who warrant further clinical investigations, whilst a diagnostic test is used to diagnose the presence of a target condition (e.g. disease). Such tests include biomarkers, imaging and endoscopic investigations, physiologic measurements (e.g. blood pressure and temperature) and questionnaires, or may reflect a clinician's judgment after a physical examination. Well-known examples include ultrasound and serum biomarkers for Down's syndrome screening, and X-ray for diagnosing bone fractures.

Test accuracy describes the ability of a test to correctly classify individuals with and without the target condition as test-positive or test-negative, respectively. Primary studies of test accuracy typically report two-by-two tables of the results of the index test cross classified against those of the reference standard (Table 15.1). The *index test* is the test of interest whilst the *reference standard* is considered the best available way of verifying whether or not the target condition is present. The reference standard may be a single test or a combination of several tests (e.g. often based on scans or invasive investigatory procedures) with clinical information. The most commonly reported test accuracy measures of sensitivity, specificity, and predictive values are defined in Table 15.2.

Test results may not always be binary but rather an ordered set of categories (e.g. the Breast Imaging Reporting and Data System (BI-RADS) score for reporting mammograms) or continuous measurements (e.g. ear temperature for diagnosing fever). With an ordered or continuous test, a threshold value (also known as a cut-point or cut-off) is usually used to dichotomise the test results into positive or negative. For example, an ear temperature $\geq 38.0\,°\text{C}$ might be used to define a positive test for diagnosing fever in children. If a test measurement increases with the presence of the target condition (e.g. temperature measurement for fever), then decreasing the threshold will increase sensitivity and decrease specificity, whilst increasing the threshold will decrease sensitivity and increase specificity. This trade-off between sensitivity and specificity as the threshold changes can be illustrated using a receiver operating characteristic (ROC) plot of sensitivity against specificity. Examples will be given later in the chapter.

15.1.1 Meta-Analysis of Test Accuracy Studies

Most primary studies of test accuracy aim to assess the accuracy of a single index test. When multiple primary studies evaluate the accuracy of the same test, meta-analysis methods can synthesise the study results to help establish if and how the test can be used in practice.[1–4] Most test accuracy meta-analyses use aggregate data (i.e. the two-by-two tables shown in Table 15.1) from published

Table 15.1 Cross classification of index test results and reference standard results (two-by-two table) in a single study i

	Reference standard positive	**Reference standard negative**	**Total**
Index test positive	r_{11i} (number of true positives)	r_{01i} (number of false positives)	$r_{11i} + r_{01i}$ (number test positive)
Index test negative	r_{10i} (number of false negatives)	r_{00i} (number of true negatives)	$r_{10i} + r_{00i}$ (number test negative)
Total	n_{1i} (number with condition)	n_{0i} (number without condition)	$n_{1i} + n_{0i}$ (number of participants)

Source: Richard Riley.

Table 15.2 Typical statistical measures of test accuracy in a single study i

Measure	Formula	Definition
Sensitivity$_i$	$r_{11i}/(r_{11i} + r_{10i})$	Probability of testing positive for those truly with the condition
Specificity$_i$	$r_{00i}/(r_{01i} + r_{00i})$	Probability of testing negative for those truly without the condition
Positive predictive value* (PPV$_i$)	$r_{11i}/(r_{11i} + r_{01i})$	Probability of having the condition for those who test positive
Negative predictive value* (NPV$_i$)	$r_{00i}/(r_{10i} + r_{00i})$	Probability of not having the condition for those who test negative

* Formula shown for PPV and NPV assumes the study has a consecutive or random sample of participants from the population of interest; otherwise, Bayes' theorem needs to be used to estimate PPV and NPV conditional on the observed sensitivity and specificity, and an estimated prevalence of the target condition from external evidence.
Source: Richard Riley.

studies, and focus on producing pooled estimates that summarise *average* test performance across the multiple studies,[2–6] usually in terms of either the test's sensitivity and specificity when the threshold is the same in each study, or a summary ROC curve when the primary studies assess test accuracy at different thresholds.[7]

Test accuracy studies often exhibit between-study heterogeneity in test accuracy, which refers to genuine differences in the accuracy of a test from study to study caused by study differences in, for example, clinical setting (such as primary, secondary and community care), participant selection (such as symptom severity and previous testing), choice of healthcare practitioners implementing/reading the test, reference standard, test methodology (e.g. choice of measurement methods for index test and reference standard), participant characteristics (e.g. the distribution of age), and unknown factors. Meta-Analysis must, therefore, allow for heterogeneity by using models with random effects that allow test accuracy to vary across studies.[2,4,7] In particular, a bivariate random-effects meta-analysis of sensitivity and specificity is often used,[2] which is identical, in situations without covariates, to using a hierarchical summary receiver operating characteristic (HSROC) model.[3,8,9] The aim of the bivariate model is to estimate a summary point (i.e. summary sensitivity and summary specificity), whilst the aim of the HSROC model is to estimate a summary ROC curve. Regardless, in the presence of heterogeneity, both approaches produce summary meta-analysis results that may be difficult to interpret or translate into clinical practice.

15.1.2 The Need for IPD

The use of IPD, rather than aggregate data, has great potential to improve test accuracy meta-analyses. The key advantages are outlined in Box 15.1, and many are the same as those described for IPD meta-analyses of randomised trials in Chapter 2. In particular, IPD helps reduce between-study heterogeneity and enables the inclusion of participants that more strictly adhere to the eligibility criteria for the meta-analysis research question. For example, IPD allows the selection of subsets of study participants that represent the target population (such as participants over/under a certain age, those with/without a particular co-morbidity), the timing of index test assessment (such as first trimester of pregnancy, rather than the second or third), and the target

Box 15.1 Potential advantages of examining test accuracy using IPD meta-analysis rather than a conventional meta-analysis of published aggregate data.[18–22]

- Encourages greater collaboration across researchers, and increases the opportunity to identify and incorporate relevant studies (or datasets), including those unpublished, thereby increasing total sample size (and number of cases).
- Allows communication with original study investigators to clarify aspects such as the underlying design, recruitment strategy, definition of the target condition and criteria for test positivity.
- Allows more consistent participant inclusion and exclusion criteria across studies, and if appropriate, participants who were originally excluded (e.g. those with inconclusive test result) can be reinstated into the analysis.
- Enables results presented in the original study publications to be verified, and may allow a more enhanced assessment of each study's risk of bias and eligibility for the IPD meta-analysis research question.
- Uses more up-to-date information than in original study publication, such as longer follow-up information which may provide clarification on true condition status for each participant.
- Improves the identification of participants contributing IPD to each of multiple studies.
- Improves standardisation of the definitions of tests and target condition (reference standards) across studies.
- Allows the calculation of results (e.g. test accuracy at particular thresholds and proportion of inconclusive test results) previously not reported in sufficient detail; it may thus reduce the problem of selective within-study reporting.
- Allows the calculation of results for unpublished studies providing IPD; it may thus reduce the potential for publication bias (small-study effects).
- Ability to standardise the strategy of statistical analysis across datasets and potentially improve upon the methods used in original publications, to reduce statistical heterogeneity; notably, choice of thresholds and use of multiple imputation to deal with missing data (e.g. in covariate information).
- (Improved) ability to examine causes of heterogeneity in test accuracy across participants and across datasets; in particular, to compare test accuracy across subgroups, and to summarise within-study associations between test accuracy and participant-level covariates.
- Facilitates comparison of tests and the assessment of diagnostic strategies involving a sequence (combination) of tests in contrast to the assessment of individual tests in isolation.
- Ability to develop and validate (across multiple settings) diagnostic prediction models containing multiple tests and other information (e.g. risk factors, participant characteristics).
- Ability to discuss the implications of findings with the wide network of study investigators involved.

Source: Richard Riley.

condition definition (such as major depression, rather than a broader definition of depression) of interest to the IPD meta-analysis project. For example, in an IPD meta-analysis of magnetic resonance imaging (MRI) and mammography for breast cancer screening in BRCA mutation carriers, only women with BRCA1/2 mutations who had both MRI and mammography results from the same screening round were selected for analysis from the six studies included (this example is revisited in Section 15.6.2).[10] Similarly, IPD may improve consistency in reference standard definition and length of follow-up, such as in cancer test accuracy studies, where you may need an element of follow-up to confidently rule out the condition in those not sent for confirmatory testing.

IPD also allows test accuracy results to be obtained directly from study investigators, and thus may enable more results to be obtained for some studies than originally presented in study publications. A major advantage for tests measured on a continuous or ordinal scale is that IPD can provide the original (non-dichotomised) value of the test measurement (e.g. blood pressure value), which allows the meta-analyst to evaluate the test's accuracy at the same threshold value in each study and to assess performance across multiple thresholds. In contrast, published aggregate data for a study may only relate to one or a few thresholds, and the number and set of reported thresholds will usually differ across studies; such information is problematic to handle using conventional meta-analytic methods (i.e. the aforementioned bivariate or HSROC approaches).[11–14]

Furthermore, Levis et al. show that selective threshold reporting in primary studies can bias estimates of test accuracy obtained from a conventional aggregate data meta-analysis.[15] This is illustrated in Figure 15.1 by their summary ROC curves based on IPD from 13 studies, showing the test accuracy of the Patient Health Questionnaire-9 (PHQ-9) when used as a screening test for major

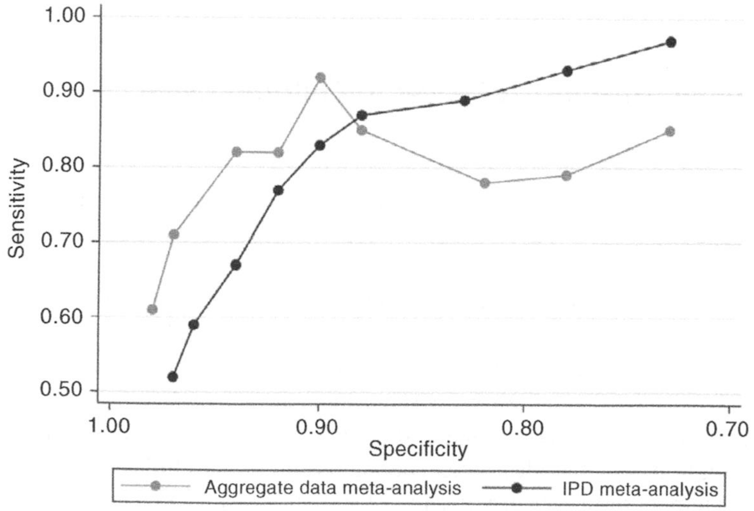

The black points denote IPD meta-analysis results based on all 13 studies, whilst the grey points denote an IPD meta-analysis of 3 studies (threshold 14), 4 studies (thresholds 7, 8, 9, 13 and 15), 5 studies (threshold 11), 6 studies (threshold 12), or 11 studies (threshold 10).

Figure 15.1 Summary receiver operating characteristic (ROC) curves for the diagnostic accuracy of the Patient Health Questionnaire-9 (PHQ-9) produced by a meta-analysis of IPD from 13 studies,[15] either restricting each study to use the subset of thresholds reported in the original study publications (grey points) or allowing all studies to use all thresholds (black points). The points shown correspond to PHQ-9 threshold values of 7 to 15, from right to left. *Source:* Richard Riley. Figure derived using data reported by Levis et al.[15]

depression. The maximum total PHQ-9 score is 27, and higher scores represent increased severity of depressive symptoms. Their IPD meta-analysis allows all studies to contribute results for all thresholds from 7 to 15, and this leads to a well-defined monotonically increasing curve; that is, sensitivity decreases and specificity increases as the threshold value increases. In contrast, when restricting each study to only contribute results at the threshold(s) reported in that study's publication, the summary curve is not monotonically increasing and is thus improper; for example, the summary sensitivity sometimes increases as the threshold value increases, due to different sets of studies (and thus different sets of participants) contributing to each threshold. An extended version of this IPD meta-analysis project will serve as a motivating example throughout this chapter.[16]

Another major advantage of IPD is that it facilitates the modelling of participant-level characteristics. In particular, diagnostic tests may perform better for some individuals than others, and so conventional meta-analysis results relating to some 'average' individual may be insufficient. Rather, IPD allows meta-analysts to assess if and how participant-level covariates modify test accuracy (Section 15.3.7), in a similar way to how IPD allows treatment-covariate interactions to be modelled at the participant level in a meta-analysis of randomised trials (Chapter 7). Comparisons and combinations of tests can also be considered more easily by having IPD.[17]

15.1.3 Scope of This Chapter

In this chapter, we provide a guide to conducting an IPD meta-analysis of test accuracy studies. We consider each of the key steps involved, and our main focus is on evaluating the accuracy of a single index test, although extension to test comparisons is considered in Section 15.6. We begin by introducing a further motivating example (diagnosis of fever in children), which will be used throughout the chapter alongside the aforementioned IPD meta-analysis of Levis et al. examining the PHQ-9.[16]

15.2 Motivating Example: Diagnosis of Fever in Children Using Ear Temperature

Craig et al. systematically reviewed thermometry studies comparing temperatures taken via the ear and rectum in children,[23] and one objective was to assess the accuracy of infrared ear thermometry for diagnosing fever.[24] Twenty-three studies (including a total of 4098 children) were identified, each of which provided published aggregate data regarding sensitivity and specificity. Most studies defined fever as being a temperature $\geq$ 38.0 °C (Table 15.3), consistent with clinical guidelines for diagnosing fever in children. The studies included children already in hospital or attending an Accident and Emergency (A&E) department,[23] and so the observed prevalence of fever was high, around 50%. Rectal temperature was the reference standard, as it is a well-established method of measuring temperature in children, and it guides clinical decisions and fever definition.[25] However, measuring ear (tympanic) temperature is clearly less invasive than measuring rectal temperature, and so ear measurement would be preferable if its diagnostic accuracy was adequate.

Heterogeneity was apparent across studies in, amongst other factors, different types of ear and rectal measurement devices, the proportion of infants and the thresholds used to define test positivity (Table 15.3).[26] However, 16 of the 23 studies also provided their IPD, which contained the actual ear and rectal temperature values for each child, with 11 of the 16 also providing the age of each child (Table 15.3). This serves as a motivating example throughout the chapter, as the availability of IPD helps to standardise the choice of thresholds and allows the assessment of how measurement device and age (including infant status) modify diagnostic accuracy.

Table 15.3 Summary of 23 studies used by Riley et al. in an IPD meta-analysis to examine the accuracy of ear temperature for diagnosis of fever[26]

First author	IPD?	Total with fever and test positive r_{11i}	Total with fever n_{1i}	Total without fever and test negative r_{00i}	Total without fever n_{0i}	IPD for age?	Threshold value for rectal/ear temperature (°C)*	Rectal thermometer device type	Ear thermometer device type
Bernardo	Y	0	3	33	35	Y	38.0/38.0	Electronic	CoreCheck
Brennan	Y	150	203	155	167	N	38.0/38.0	Electronic	FirstTemp
Davis	Y	9	18	46	48	Y	38.0/38.0	Electronic	FirstTemp
Green	Y	8	9	12	12	Y	38.0/38.0	Electronic	FirstTemp
Hoffman, i	Y	30	42	56	58	Y	38.0/38.0	Electronic	FirstTemp
Hoffman, ii	Y	36	62	32	34	Y	38.0/38.0	Electronic	CoreCheck
Hoffman, iii	Y	41	42	44	55	Y	38.0/38.0	Electronic	Thermoscan
Hooker, i	Y	10	15	24	24	Y	38.0/38.0	Electronic	FirstTemp
Hooker, ii	Y	75	99	78	81	Y	38.0/38.0	Mercury	Thermoscan
Lanham	Y	53	103	74	75	N	38.0/38.0	Electronic	FirstTemp
Loveys, i	Y	12	30	44	46	N	38.0/38.0	Electronic	LightTouch Pedi-Q
Loveys, ii	Y	37	47	74	93	N	38.0/38.0	Electronic	LightTouch Pedi-Q
Nypaver	Y	282	425	445	453	Y	38.0/38.0	Electronic	FirstTemp
Petersen-Smith	Y	9	10	214	222	Y	38.0/38.0	Mercury	FirstTemp
Rhoads	Y	7	27	38	38	Y	38.0/38.0	Electronic	FirstTemp
Robinson	Y	1	2	13	13	N	38.0/38.0	Probe	CoreCheck
Akinyinka	N	77	105	259	273	N	37.5/37.5	Mercury	Thermoscan
Greenes	N	53	109	193	195	N	38.0/38.0	Electronic	FirstTemp

(*Continued*)

Table 15.3 (Continued)

First author	IPD?	Total with fever and test positive r_{11i}	Total with fever n_{1i}	Total without fever and test negative r_{00i}	Total without fever n_{0i}	IPD for age?	Threshold value for rectal/ear temperature (°C)*	Rectal thermometer device type	Ear thermometer device type
Muma	N	48	87	136	136	N	38.0/38.0	Electronic	FirstTemp
Selfridge	N	16	18	75	84	N	38.1/37.6	Mercury	FirstTemp
Stewart	N	57	59	20	20	N	38.0/38.0	Electronic	FirstTemp
Terndrup	N	91	178	105	125	N	37.9/37.9	Electronic	FirstTemp
Wilshaw	N	16	16	60	104	N	38.0/38.0	Mercury	Ototemp Pedi-Q

* 38.0°C was chosen when IPD were available, but other thresholds could have been chosen if desired. When IPD were not available, the threshold closest to 38.0°C with accuracy results available was chosen. NA = not available as IPD for age not provided. Y = yes, N = no.

Source: Table is adapted from Table 1 of Riley et al.,[26] used with permission, © 2008 Wiley

15.3 Key Steps Involved in an IPD Meta-Analysis of Test Accuracy Studies

The key steps of an IPD meta-analysis project for examining test accuracy are now described. The processes for initiation, planning and delivery are very similar to those described in Part 1 of this book for IPD meta-analyses of randomised trials to examine treatment effects. Thus, Part 1 should must be viewed as complementary reading to this chapter. Also, the described steps are not necessarily linear and may overlap; in particular, data extraction, IPD retrieval and cleaning, and risk of bias assessments may occur simultaneously and be an iterative process.

15.3.1 Defining the Research Objectives

Clearly defining the research objectives for the IPD meta-analysis project is essential, as they underpin subsequent steps such as defining inclusion and exclusion criteria, searching for relevant studies, assessing each study's eligibility (whether its setting and participants are applicable to the research question), and so forth. The objectives should be identified with the involvement of key stakeholders (including patients) and framed within the context of a clinical pathway (e.g. current diagnostic pathway where the screening or diagnostic tests are needed) so that the potential role(s) of the test and downstream consequences of test errors (false negatives and false positives) are understood.

There are three main components of a test accuracy research question: *population* (including clinical presentation and any prior testing), *index test*(s) and *target condition*(s). The index test is the actual test we wish to evaluate, and an IPD meta-analysis might consider and compare several index tests. Most index tests are 'new', in the sense that they aim to improve upon current diagnosis, for example to replace an existing test (replacement), to be used before the existing test (triage) or to be used after the existing test (add-on).[27] An index test may be simultaneously assessed for more than one of these roles.

For IPD meta-analysis projects that focus on a single index test, usually the main objectives are to summarise: (i) the average test accuracy of the index test (i.e. how it performs across all relevant populations and settings), (ii) the extent of any between-study heterogeneity (e.g. whether test accuracy varies across studies), and (iii) whether test accuracy is modified by particular participant (e.g. age) or study characteristics (e.g. primary or secondary care). In the fever example (Section 15.2), a main objective was to summarise the accuracy of a single index test (ear temperature) for diagnosing fever (target condition) in children presenting in hospital and A&E settings (population), and to investigate whether test accuracy is associated with ear thermometer mode (different offsets by manufacturers to obtain adjusted temperatures) and participant-level characteristics.

Sometimes, comparison of the index test with other competing tests may be an important objective (Section 15.6). For example, the objective of the breast cancer screening IPD meta-analysis project by Phi et al. was comparative;[10] using biopsy or follow-up as the reference standard, the accuracy of MRI alone and that of MRI combined with mammography were compared to mammography alone to determine the change in sensitivity and specificity for screening women $\geq$50 years who have BRCA1/2 mutations.

15.3.2 Searching for Studies with Eligible IPD

Strategies to identify studies relevant for IPD retrieval should aim to minimise the risk of missing relevant studies. Unfortunately, searching for existing DTA studies is challenging due to a lack of indexing in electronic databases and inconsistent terminology used in study articles. Given these challenges, we recommend that IPD meta-analysis projects seek the help of an information specialist for assistance in developing the search strategy. The target condition and index test(s) are key terms of the search, but sometimes the reference standard, population and setting may also be used. It may be appropriate to limit by time period if the index test or reference standard became available at a specific time-point. For example, Levis et al. searched MEDLINE, PsycINFO and Web of Science but restricted their search to 2000 onwards because the PHQ-9 (their test of interest) was published in 2001.[16] Note that relevant studies may be unpublished, or may be published but focus on an alternative research question. Contacting and engaging experts in the field (e.g. as part of the IPD meta-analysis collaborative group, Chapter 3) may also reveal additional studies or data sources. For example, in addition to searching electronic databases, Craig et al. contacted study investigators and suppliers of clinical thermometers for details of additional studies.[23] In addition, an existing data source may be eligible even if not linked to a particular study (e.g. IPD from a routinely collected dataset may sometimes be useful).

Each of the studies (and data sources) identified from the searches should then be classed as either relevant or not, according to the pre-defined eligibility criteria based on the population, index test(s) and target condition(s), and other relevant aspects such as the reference standard and study design. The IPD meta-analysis project may specify stricter eligibility criteria than used in some of the original studies; however, such studies can still be included if obtaining IPD would allow selection of subsets of their participants that are eligible.

15.3.3 Extracting Key Study Characteristics and Information

Before seeking IPD from a study (or data source) deemed relevant, it is helpful to extract key characteristics and results for each study from their publication(s). Such information facilitates assessment of risk of bias (Section 15.3.4) and may even reveal that some studies do not meet the inclusion criteria after all. The expertise of the research team (including project and patient advisory group if available) should be used to ensure collection of only relevant and essential information, to avoid an overwhelming list of items. Key information includes the study time period, location, design (including how participants were selected, the reference standard and its timing, any methods of measurement), sample size (and any number lost to follow-up), clinical setting (e.g. recruitment setting, point of index test on diagnostic pathway, any prior tests), and inclusion and exclusion criteria. Characteristics of the index test (e.g. type of ear thermometer device), reference standard, and definition of the target condition (e.g. threshold for diagnosis of fever) should also be collected. Test accuracy results (or two-by-two tables, as shown in Table 15.1) might also be extracted, especially if later the IPD meta-analysis researchers will check that the IPD provided replicates the results extracted from the paper. If applicable, data on inconclusive (e.g. intermediate, indeterminate or unevaluable) test results should also be extracted in order to quantify how often they occur. Failure to report inconclusive test results can lead to misleading conclusions about test accuracy and the clinical utility of a test (Section 15.3.4).[28]

15.3.4 Evaluating Risk of Bias of Eligible Studies

The methodological quality of IPD should be examined for each eligible study (and data source), using the revised version of the QUADAS (Quality Assessment of Diagnostic Accuracy Studies) tool, QUADAS-2.[29,30] This tool was designed to assess the quality of published test accuracy studies when undertaking a conventional meta-analysis of aggregate data, but is still highly relevant for IPD meta-analysis. We suggest QUADAS-2 be considered for each study before IPD are obtained (for example, to identify studies at high risk of bias that may be deemed low priority for IPD retrieval) and then updated as necessary after IPD are obtained, cleaned and checked.

QUADAS-2 addresses both a study's internal validity (risk of bias) and external validity (applicability to the IPD meta-analysis research question). The risk of bias assessment focuses on flaws in study design and conduct that may result in invalid estimates of a test's accuracy (e.g. bias arising from selective recruitment of participants), whilst the applicability assessment focuses on variation from the eligibility criteria for the IPD meta-analysis research question's (e.g. recruitment from a specialist hospital setting when the research question is about test accuracy in a community setting). Applicability is essentially a further assessment of whether a study (and its participants) actually meets the eligibility criteria for the IPD meta-analysis research question.

The QUADAS-2 tool consists of four domains: patient selection, index test, reference standard, and flow and timing. The flow and timing domain addresses risk of bias only, whilst the other three domains address both risk of bias and applicability concerns. Within each domain, there are signalling questions that aid judgements about risk of bias (judged high, low or unclear).[29] As the QUADAS-2 tool is generic, IPD meta-analysis projects will need to tailor the scoring of each signalling question and domain to their particular research question, and might even include additional signalling questions if necessary. For example, in their IPD meta-analysis project, Levis et al. included an additional signalling question within the reference standard domain that was specific to their particular research question.[16] Some questions within QUADAS-2 may not be as relevant for IPD meta-analysis projects as for aggregate data meta-analyses. In particular, the question "If a threshold was used, was it pre-specified?" is irrelevant if the IPD provided is in a format that allows the IPD meta-analysis researchers to choose their own thresholds.

Due to poor and incomplete reporting, quality assessment of test accuracy studies is challenging based on published information alone. A major advantage of IPD meta-analysis projects is being able to refine and update risk of bias classifications after receiving the IPD itself and through discussion with IPD providers. IPD may lead to a different risk of bias and applicability classification than initially considered when using the reported information from that study. For instance, regarding flow and timing, in the IPD meta-analysis of Levis et al., relevant primary studies often used a wide range of time intervals between PHQ-9 assessment and the reference standard (diagnostic interview), raising concerns about risk of bias and lack of applicability; however, when using the IPD from such studies the subset of participants with reasonable time intervals could be selected, thereby alleviating these concerns.

Particular attention should be given to the handling of participants for which information about either the test result or the true condition status is inconclusive. For example, a study may have omitted participants who had unclear test results. Such studies may be at high risk of bias if the participants excluded differ systematically from those included in the analysis. Again, with IPD this concern may be reduced if such participants can be reinstated to the analysis.[28] For example, in their IPD meta-analysis of computed tomography angiography (CTA) for diagnosis of obstructive coronary artery disease in patients with stable chest pain, Haase et al. included all participants in their primary analysis irrespective of whether they had evaluable or unevaluable CTA examinations.[31] They applied a worst-case scenario in which unevaluable CTA results were considered false positive if coronary angiography was negative, and considered false negative if coronary angiography was positive.

Risk of bias classifications can be summarised graphically or in a table, and the findings incorporated into the results, discussion and conclusions of the IPD meta-analysis project's publication. In their projects, Levis et al. provide supplementary tables summarising the judgements for each study,[16] whilst Haase et al. provide summary tables and figures across all studies in addition to the results of individual studies.[31]

15.3.5 Obtaining, Cleaning and Harmonising IPD

The process for inviting investigators of eligible studies (and data sources) to provide their IPD and collaborate is similar to that described in Chapters 3 and 4, including the set-up of data-sharing agreements. To facilitate harmonisation of IPD and consistency across studies, study investigators should be provided with a structured data request form with clear definitions of the variables of interest. For studies that used thresholds to dichotomise index test and/or reference standard results in original study publications, it should be made clear that continuous data (for test and reference standard values) are required for the IPD meta-analysis project, to avoid constraints on which thresholds can be examined. It may be helpful to differentiate between essential and desirable items when requesting data. For example, Schuetz et al. classified the participant and study characteristics requested from the corresponding investigators of eligible studies into mandatory and additional items.[32] IPD should be requested alongside a corresponding dataset dictionary, containing details about how to translate the labels and coding within the provided IPD (to minimise subsequent back and forth between the IPD meta-analysis team and the IPD providers).

Upon receipt of the IPD, it is helpful to quickly check that basic information (such as mean age, proportion male, two-by-two tables) match those reported within the original study publication, to flag any immediate concerns that the IPD provided is not as anticipated. Regardless, a potentially long process (often between one and two years, depending on the number of eligible studies) will be required to obtain and clean the IPD for each eligible study, including checking for errors and omitted variables, and resolving any queries with the study investigators. Chapter 4 gives greater details about this process.

15.3.6 Undertaking IPD Meta-Analysis to Summarise Test Accuracy at a Particular Threshold

We now introduce IPD meta-analysis models that summarise a test's sensitivity and specificity. We assume a positive or negative test result is available for all participants (i.e. there are no inconclusive test results; we return to this issue in Section 15.3.8), and that the test result is a binary variable (positive or negative). Thus, ordinal or continuous tests are converted to a binary result using a chosen threshold; we assume one particular threshold is of interest, as in the fever example where test positives are defined by an ear temperature $\geq 38.0\ °C$. Extension to more complex situations such as multiple thresholds and comparative test accuracy are considered in Sections 15.4 to 15.6.

We concentrate on the one-stage bivariate meta-analysis framework of Chu and Cole,[4] which improves upon the two-stage approach of Reitsma et al.[2] One-stage IPD meta-analysis models are preferred in the context of test accuracy, as a two-stage approach may give considerable bias in the summary sensitivity and specificity estimates,[2,4,33,34] because the meta-analysis will often contain many studies with few false positives or false negatives (Chapter 8 discusses this issue). We do not consider the aforementioned HSROC model; this is useful in aggregate data meta-analysis when studies use different thresholds, but IPD should allow a two-by-two table to be obtained for the same threshold(s) in every study.

15.3.6.1 Bivariate IPD Meta-Analysis to Summarise Sensitivity and Specificity

Let there be $i = 1$ to S studies that perform a test on n_{1i} participants truly with the condition and n_{0i} participants truly without the condition, as established by the chosen reference standard. The test classifies each participant as either positive or negative. Let y_{1ik} be the test response (1 = positive, 0

= negative) of participant k in study i who truly has the condition, where $k=1$ to n_{1i}, and let y_{0ij} be the test response (1 = negative, 0 = positive) of participant j in study i who truly does not have the condition, where $j = 1$ to n_{0i}. Thus y_{1ik} and y_{0ij} are equal to 1 if the test response is correct, and 0 otherwise.

Adapting the multivariate meta-analysis framework of Chapter 13, a one-stage bivariate IPD meta-analysis can be used to synthesise the y_{1ik} and y_{0ij} (or equivalently the r_{11i} and r_{00i} of the two by two table of Table 15.1), and estimate the summary sensitivity and specificity of the test.[4 34] This approach models the independent* Bernoulli distributions of y_{1ik} and y_{0ij} within studies (or, equivalently, the independent binomial distributions of r_{11i} and r_{00i}), and allows for potential between-study heterogeneity in the true sensitivity and true specificity, and their between-study correlation:

$$\begin{aligned}
&y_{1ik} \sim \text{Bernoulli}(p_{1i}) \\
&y_{0ij} \sim \text{Bernoulli}(p_{0i}) \\
&\begin{pmatrix} \text{logit}(p_{1i}) \\ \text{logit}(p_{0i}) \end{pmatrix} \sim N\left(\begin{pmatrix} \beta_1 \\ \beta_0 \end{pmatrix}, \begin{pmatrix} \tau_1^2 & \tau_{10} \\ \tau_{10} & \tau_0^2 \end{pmatrix}\right)
\end{aligned} \tag{15.1}$$

Model (15.1) specifies there is a true sensitivity and true specificity in each study, modelled on the logit scale (i.e. $\log(p/(1-p))$), with an average logit sensitivity and logit specificity of β_1 and β_0, respectively, between-study heterogeneity of τ_1^2 and τ_0^2, and between-study covariance of τ_{10}.The corresponding between-study correlation is $\tau_{10}/\tau_1\tau_0$, which may be induced by the causes of heterogeneity across studies (e.g. change in measurement method, clinical setting, country, time period), even when the same threshold is used in every study. Setting τ_{10} to zero may be sensible, for example, if there are convergence issues during estimation, or if between-study correlation is not anticipated or is estimated poorly.[35,36] Model (15.1) is then equivalent to fitting separate meta-analyses for sensitivity and specificity. It is straightforward to include study-level covariates (e.g. measurement device, country) in model (15.1) that may explain heterogeneity.

In a frequentist framework, model (15.1) can be fitted using maximum likelihood estimation, for example using the NLMIXED procedure in SAS, the *melogit* or *meqrlogit* commands in Stata,[37] or the *glmer* function with the *lme4* package in R,[4,38,39] which fit generalised mixed models by maximizing an approximation to the likelihood integrated over the random effects. Different integral approximations are available, such as adaptive Gaussian quadrature, which requires a number of quadrature points to be specified, with increasing estimation accuracy as the number of points increases, but at the expense of an increased computational time. As maximum likelihood estimation tends to give downwardly biased variance estimates, a Bayesian framework can be applied, for example using Markov chain Monte Carlo (MCMC) estimation in software packages such as JAGS, WinBUGS, R or SAS. This additionally requires specification of prior distributions for the unknown parameters.[40,41] Copula approaches have also been suggested for modelling the between-study correlation.[42–44]

15.3.6.2 Examining and Summarising Heterogeneity

Fitting model (15.1) produces estimates of the summary sensitivity and specificity, obtained by $\exp(\hat{\beta}_1)/[1 + \exp(\hat{\beta}_1)]$ and $\exp(\hat{\beta}_0)/[1 + \exp(\hat{\beta}_0)]$ respectively, and their corresponding 95% confidence intervals (or their joint confidence region). If there are multiple thresholds, reference standards, and measurement methods of interest in the IPD meta-analysis project, model (15.1) needs to

* Independent because they relate to different sets of participants, i.e. those with and without the target condition.

be applied separately for each subgroup (i.e. threshold, reference standard, measurement method) of interest. For example, Levis et al. summarise the accuracy of the PHQ-9 test when applying a bivariate meta-analysis separately for each threshold from ≥7 to ≥15 to define test positivity, and for each of three categories of diagnostic interviews used as reference standards for classifying major depression status (the Mini International Neuropsychiatric Interview (MINI), semi-structured, and fully structured excluding MINI).[16] For formally estimating differences in test accuracy across subgroups of studies, model (15.1) should be extended to include study-level covariates (which define the subgroups), which then becomes a bivariate meta-regression (Section 15.3.7).

Even when applied in particular subgroups of studies, heterogeneity will often remain and so it is important to summarise it appropriately, for example by presenting an approximate prediction region for the true sensitivity and specificity in a new population,[2,45] or by calculating the probability that *both* sensitivity and specificity will be above clinically acceptable values. For example, if both sensitivity and specificity need to be at least 90% for the test to be considered useful in practice, there should be a large probability that this criterion will be met in populations represented by the studies in the meta-analysis. This requires us to model the joint predictive distribution of sensitivity and specificity in a new study. If parameters were known, then based on model (15.1) this distribution would be:

$$\begin{pmatrix} \text{logit}(p_{1i})_{\text{new}} \\ \text{logit}(p_{0i})_{\text{new}} \end{pmatrix} \sim N\left(\begin{pmatrix} \beta_1 \\ \beta_0 \end{pmatrix}, \begin{pmatrix} \tau_1^2 & \tau_{10} \\ \tau_{10} & \tau_0^2 \end{pmatrix}\right) \tag{15.2}$$

When using a Bayesian framework to fit model (15.1),[46] values of $\text{logit}(p_{1i})_{\text{new}}$ and $\text{logit}(p_{0i})_{\text{new}}$ can be sampled from the their joint predictive (posterior) distribution to make inferences, which will naturally account for the uncertainty in all parameters in the model. In a frequentist framework, a bivariate *t*-distribution with $k - 2$ degrees of freedom might be used to approximate the joint predictive distribution, which extends the frequentist use of a univariate *t*-distribution to derive a prediction interval for a single measure.[46,47] Further research on this is required, alongside consideration of whether a normal between-study distribution is appropriate.[48]

15.3.6.3 Combining IPD and non-IPD Studies

IPD may only be available from a proportion of studies in the meta-analysis.[49] Other relevant studies not providing their IPD will usually provide two-by-two tables (Table 15.1), which can be used to partially reconstruct their IPD; that is, y_{1ik} and y_{0ij} values can be derived to collectively mirror the totals in the table. This allows non-IPD studies to be combined with IPD studies when fitting model (15.1). This process of reconstructing IPD for binary outcome data is described in Chapter 6. However, it does not resolve all the limitations of not having the original IPD. In particular, for continuous tests, the threshold(s) used in reported two-by-two table(s) may be limited, and not cover the full set of thresholds of interest in those studies which do provide their IPD (Section 15.4). Also, without the original IPD, it is difficult to standardise participant inclusion and exclusion criteria, and information on inconclusive test results may be unknown. Therefore, findings from an analysis combining IPD studies and non-IPD studies should always be considered as a supplement to the main analysis including only IPD studies.

15.3.6.4 Application to the Fever Example

We used Bayesian estimation to fit model (15.1) to the 16 IPD studies using a threshold of ≥ 38.0 °C for ear temperature (index test) and rectal temperature (reference standard) (Table 15.3). We also undertook an analysis additionally incorporating the four non-IPD studies that used these thresholds; this gives similar results to the IPD-only analysis, with a summary sensitivity of 0.71 (95% CrI: 0.57 to 0.84) and a summary specificity of 0.97 (95% CrI: 0.94 to 0.99). The summary specificity is high, so those without fever are usually correctly classed as negative (< 38.0 °C). However, the summary sensitivity is low, indicating that many children with fever are not classed as positive (≥38.0 °C). Further, large between-study heterogeneity ($\hat{\tau}_1^2 = 1.32$ for logit sensitivity, $\hat{\tau}_0^2 = 1.64$ for logit specificity) limits interpretability and emphasises the importance of making the studies more homogeneous in their characteristics. Interestingly, even though the same threshold is used in all studies, there is a strong negative between-study correlation of −0.77.

To reduce heterogeneity and improve interpretability, a separate meta-analysis was considered for subsets of studies with similar characteristics. For example, model (15.1) was applied to the subset of 11 studies (involving 2323 children from 8 IPD and 3 non-IPD studies) that evaluated the accuracy of a FirstTemp branded ear thermometer against an electronic rectal thermometer (Table 15.3). This gave a summary sensitivity of 0.65 (95% CrI: 0.51 to 0.77) and a summary specificity of 0.98 (95% CrI: 0.96 to 0.99), and these results suggests that many children with fever are not classed as positive by an ear temperature test. Also, there remains considerable between-study heterogeneity in both sensitivity and specificity, despite using the same ear thermometer manufacturer (FirstTemp), a consistent threshold (38.0 °C) and a common reference standard (rectal temperature) in all 11 studies. This is illustrated by the wide 95% prediction region within Figure 15.2, and corresponding wide 95% prediction intervals for sensitivity (0.21 to 0.94) and specificity (0.89 to 1) in a new population. Direct probabilistic statements can also be made by sampling from the (joint) predictive distribution for a new set of sensitivity and specificity (based on model (15.2)), shown in Figure 15.3. For example, in a new population similar to those included in the meta-analysis, the probability that sensitivity will be over 80% is 0.19, and the probability that specificity will be over 80% is 0.99. The joint probability that both sensitivity and specificity in a new population will be > 80% is just 0.18 (Figure 15.2). Hence, if sensitivity and specificity above 80% is deemed the minimum acceptable, there is less than a one in five chance that ear temperature will be adequate within a new population.

15.3.6.5 Bivariate Meta-Analysis of PPV and NPV

A potential criticism of model (15.1) is that it focuses on summarising sensitivity and specificity, which are not immediately applicable within clinical practice as they provide the probability of a particular test result conditional on knowing an individual's true condition state. In practice, healthcare professionals manage individuals whose true condition status is unknown, and so they need the individual's probability of having the condition, conditional on the test result (i.e. they require PPV and NPV, Table 15.2). Such probabilities depend on the condition's prevalence, which may vary across studies included in the IPD meta-analysis due to changes in the study populations (e.g. case-mix) and other factors. This may lead to the condition's prevalence being correlated with sensitivity and specificity across studies,[50] and motivates a trivariate meta-analysis model that jointly synthesises the condition's prevalence, sensitivity and specificity (Section 15.5.2).[43,51,52] A trivariate model produces summary results for sensitivity, specificity and prevalence which can then be translated to predicted probabilities (PPV and NPV) by using Bayes' theorem.[45]

A more direct modelling option is a bivariate meta-analysis of PPV and NPV.[5] This has the same specification as for model (15.1), but requires a change in coding: k now denotes a test positive participant and y_{1ik} equals 1 if they truly have the condition (and 0 otherwise), and j denotes a test negative participant and y_{0ij} equals 1 if they truly do not have the condition (and 0 otherwise). Now p_{1i} and p_{0i} represent the true PPV and NPV in study i, respectively, such that the meta-analysis

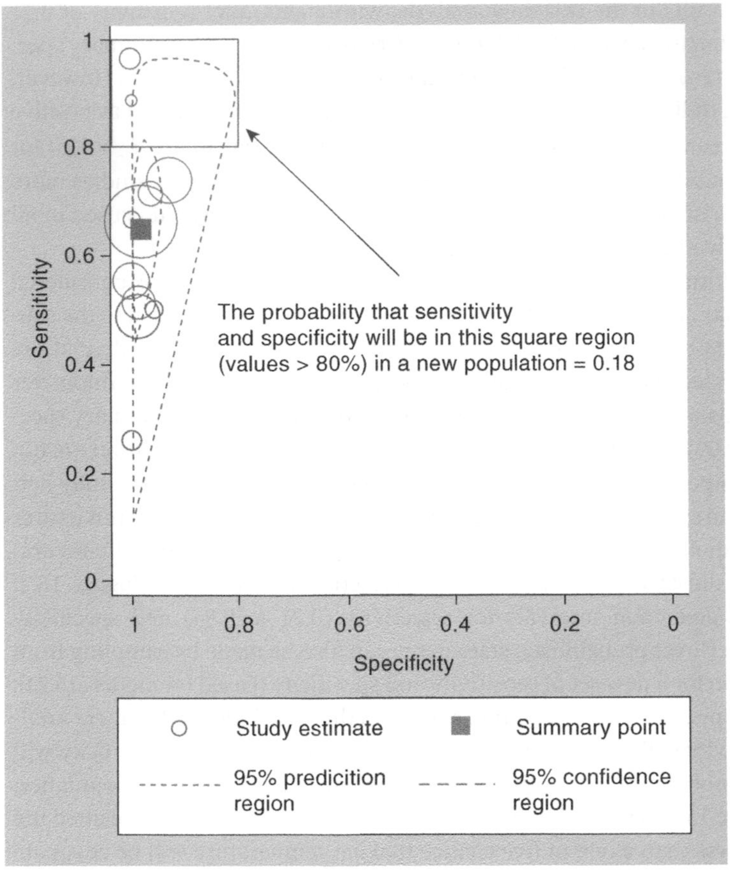

Figure 15.2 Confidence and prediction regions following application of model (15.1) to the fever data. *Source:* Figure taken from Figure 1 of Riley et al., reproduced with permission, © 2015 Wiley.

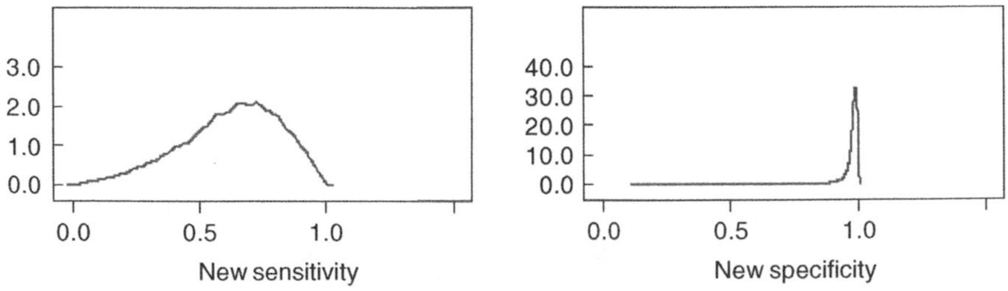

Figure 15.3 Predictive (posterior) distributions for the true sensitivity and true specificity of the FirstTemp ear temperature device in a new population, derived from Bayesian estimation of model (15.1) assuming the joint predictive distribution of model (15.2). *Source:* Richard Riley.

estimates the average logit-PPV and logit-NPV (i.e. β_1 and β_0), and the corresponding between-study heterogeneity (τ_1^2 and τ_0^2), and between-study covariance (τ_{10}).

When this approach was applied to the fever example, using the 11 studies that used the FirstTemp ear thermometer and electronic rectal thermometer, the summary PPV is 0.97 (95% CI: 0.94 to 0.98), which suggests that when ear temperature is $\geq$38.0 °C, there is a large probability of truly having fever. However, the summary NPV is 0.76 (95% CI: 0.72 to 0.81), suggesting that about 24 of every 100 children who have an ear temperature <38.0 °C will actually have fever. The latter is concerning if a negative test would be used, for example, to send a child home from hospital untreated.

Heterogeneity in PPV and NPV is likely and so prediction intervals (and posterior distributions) for PPV and NPV in a new setting are useful to disseminate the uncertainty in their actual values.[45] A bivariate meta-analysis of PPV and NPV makes most sense when the condition's prevalence is similar in the included studies. Otherwise, to include studies with different prevalences, Riley et al. suggest including (logit) prevalence as a study-level covariate within the bivariate meta-analysis of PPV and NPV, in order to allow PPV and NPV to be derived (predicted) conditional on the (logit) prevalence of the condition of a particular population.[45] Alternatively, a trivariate meta-analysis of PPV, NPV, and (logit) prevalence is possible.[52] For either approach, a cross-validation approach can be used to check the calibration of the model's predicted PPV and NPV values against the observed PPV and NPV values in new studies.[45] This is closely linked to an approach called 'internal-external cross-validation' which is used to validate the predictive performance of a risk prediction model using IPD meta-analysis (Chapter 17).[53]

Note that either the trivariate meta-analysis of sensitivity, specificity and prevalence, or the bivariate meta-analysis of PPV and NPV, require all included studies to have representative samples of the target population (e.g. based on consecutive or random recruitment); otherwise, the summary estimates of prevalence, PPV and NPV are likely to be biased.

15.3.7 Examining Accuracy-covariate Associations

Alongside the standardisation of threshold values across studies, a key motivation for an IPD meta-analysis of test accuracy studies is to estimate whether participant-level covariates (such as age and sex) modify test accuracy. If a test works better for some individuals than others, then it may be appropriate to use it only on the subset of individuals who benefit most. Let z_{ik} and z_{ij} refer to one particular participant-level covariate observed for both participants with (k) and without (j) the condition. Given IPD for each study, model (15.1) can be extended to assess the association of this covariate with diagnostic accuracy, which we label the accuracy-covariate associations. As described for treatment-covariate interactions in Chapter 7, the one-stage model specification must carefully separate out within-study and across-study relationships.[26] Participant-level covariates may vary both within studies (e.g. the age of participants varies within studies) and across studies (e.g. the mean age of participants varies across studies). Of key interest is the *within-study* association between test accuracy and covariate values; i.e. the sensitivity-covariate association, γ_{1W} say, and the specificity-covariate association, γ_{0W} say (where W emphasises this is a *within-study* relationship). These must be separated from the *across-study* associations, which quantify how the mean covariate value in each study (e.g. mean age) is associated with the underlying sensitivity and specificity across studies; i.e. the effect of $\bar{z}_{ik}$ on underlying mean logit sensitivity across studies, γ_{1A}, and the effect of $\bar{z}_{ij}$ on underlying mean logit specificity across studies, γ_{0A} (where A emphasises this is an *across-study* relationship). These across-study associations may explain the between-study variation as specified in model (15.1) through τ_1^2 and τ_0^2, but may differ from the within-study associations due to *aggregation bias*, which arises due to study-level confounding. For example, assume that there is no genuine accuracy-age association within studies, but that test accuracy (based on all study participants) is influenced by the setting of primary or emergency care, which changes across studies but not within studies. In this situation, the estimated within-study accuracy-age associations cannot be influenced by care setting if the setting is fixed for all participants in the same study. However, if the mean age is higher (or lower) in emergency care study settings compared to primary care study settings, the estimated across-study association may suggest a relationship between mean age and overall test accuracy, due to unaccounted confounding by care setting.

15.3.7.1 Model Specification Using IPD Studies

Within-study and across-study associations can be separated by including z_{ik} centered about its mean $\bar{z}_{ik}$ and by including z_{ij} centered about its mean $\bar{z}_{ij}$ in the within-study likelihood (Bernoulli component), whilst including separate terms for $\bar{z}_{ik}$ and $\bar{z}_{ij}$ to explain between-study variability (meta-regression component), as follows:[26]

$$
\begin{aligned}
&y_{1ik} \sim \text{Bernoulli}(p_{1i}) \\
&\text{logit}(p_{1i}) = \alpha_{1i} + \gamma_{1W}(z_{ik} - \bar{z}_{ik}) \\
&y_{0ij} \sim \text{Bernoulli}(p_{0i}) \\
&\text{logit}(p_{0i}) = \alpha_{0i} + \gamma_{0W}(z_{ij} - \bar{z}_{ij}) \\
&\begin{pmatrix} \text{logit}(p_{1i}) \\ \text{logit}(p_{0i}) \end{pmatrix} \sim N\left(\begin{pmatrix} \lambda_1 + \gamma_{1A}\bar{z}_{ik} \\ \lambda_0 + \gamma_{0A}\bar{z}_{ij} \end{pmatrix}, \begin{pmatrix} \tau_1^2 & \tau_{10} \\ \tau_{10} & \tau_0^2 \end{pmatrix} \right)
\end{aligned}
\tag{15.3}
$$

The key parameters of interest in model (15.3) are γ_{1W} and γ_{0W}, which summarise how a one-unit increase in the participant covariate value (z_i) changes the logit sensitivity and logit specificity, respectively. The γ_{1W} and γ_{0W} are assumed common (i.e. their true values are the same in every study), but between-study heterogeneity can be allowed by including further random effects; that is, by replacing γ_{1W} with $\gamma_{1Wi} \sim N\left(\gamma_{1W}, \tau^2_{\gamma_{1W}}\right)$ and γ_{0W} with $\gamma_{0Wi} \sim N\left(\gamma_{0W}, \tau^2_{\gamma_{0W}}\right)$. Frequentist or Bayesian approaches can be used to fit the model, as described previously. The same principles to including covariates also apply when extending a bivariate meta-analysis of PPV and NPV as introduced in Section 15.3.6.5.

Model (15.3) considers a single covariate that is either continuous or binary, but extension to multiple covariates and other types (e.g. ordinal) is possible. For continuous covariates, model (15.3) assumes a linear association, but non-linear effects can alternatively be specified using restricted cubic splines or fractional polynomials. However, these must be used cautiously in one-stage IPD meta-analyses such as model (15.3) because the mean covariate value may differ importantly across studies which, due to centering the covariate at its mean, makes the non-linear trends have a different reference point in each study; subsequently, the summary non-linear trend will be hard to interpret. Chapter 7 discusses this issue in detail and recommends a two-stage approach to synthesising non-linear relationships defined by restricted cubic spline functions with knot positions forced the same in each study. This may also be useful here, perhaps focusing on the larger studies that allow a reasonable estimate of the within-study associations in situations without sparse data.

The parameters γ_{1A} and γ_{0A} summarise how a one-unit increase in the mean covariate value ($\bar{z}_i$) in a study changes the overall logit sensitivity and logit specificity, respectively, across studies. Even if not of interest, it is important to include $\bar{z}_{ik}$ and $\bar{z}_{ij}$ in the meta-regression component, as otherwise the magnitudes of within-study association and ecological bias (the difference in the within-study and across-study associations) are constrained to be equal (Section 7.4.2 gives further details on this), which may lead to bias in the estimated within-study associations. This advice corrects a previous recommendation that the meta-regression component in model (15.3) could be removed.[26]

Additional study-level covariates (e.g. measurement device) can also be included in the meta-regression component if desired.[26]

15.3.7.2 Combining IPD and Aggregate Data

Note that, unlike model (15.1), it is difficult to include non-IPD studies within model (15.3), as values of the participant-level covariate (z_i) are difficult to reconstruct from only aggregate data. The key exception is when a two-by-two table is reported for each category of a categorical variable (e.g. sex). However, if a non-IPD study provides the estimated within-study associations directly (i.e. $\hat{\gamma}_{1W}$ and $\hat{\gamma}_{0W}$), alongside their variances ($\text{var}(\hat{\gamma}_{1W})$ and $\text{var}(\hat{\gamma}_{0W})$), then we can simultaneously fit two models: one for the IPD studies and one for the non-IPD studies, with shared parameters. For example, assuming the within-study associations are common, we could fit:

IPD studies:

$$\begin{aligned}
&y_{1ik} \sim \text{Bernoulli}(p_{1i}) \\
&\text{logit}(p_{1i}) = \alpha_{1i} + \gamma_{1W}(z_{ik} - \bar{z}_{ik}) \\
&y_{0ij} \sim \text{Bernoulli}(p_{0i}) \\
&\text{logit}(p_{0i}) = \alpha_{0i} + \gamma_{0W}(z_{ij} - \bar{z}_{ij}) \\
&\begin{pmatrix} \text{logit}(p_{1i}) \\ \text{logit}(p_{0i}) \end{pmatrix} \sim N\left(\begin{pmatrix} \lambda_1 + \gamma_{1A}\bar{z}_{ik} \\ \lambda_0 + \gamma_{0A}\bar{z}_{ij} \end{pmatrix}, \begin{pmatrix} \tau_1^2 & \tau_{10} \\ \tau_{10} & \tau_0^2 \end{pmatrix} \right)
\end{aligned} \tag{15.4}$$

Non-IPD studies:

$$\begin{aligned}
&\hat{\gamma}_{1W} \sim N(\gamma_{1W}, \text{var}(\hat{\gamma}_{1W})) \\
&\hat{\gamma}_{0W} \sim N(\gamma_{0W}, \text{var}(\hat{\gamma}_{0W}))
\end{aligned}$$

The parameters γ_{1W} and γ_{0W} are specified in both the IPD and non-IPD models, and so estimated using both the IPD and aggregate data. The approach works because γ_{1W} and γ_{0W} have practically no correlation with other paramcter estimates in the IPD model, due to the centering of the covariate about its mean in the within-study likelihood and the inclusion of the mean covariate values in the meta-regression component. As mentioned, extension to allow for between-study heterogeneity in the within-study associations is straightforward. A limitation of model (15.4) is that $\text{var}(\hat{\gamma}_{1W})$ and $\text{var}(\hat{\gamma}_{1W})$ are assumed known, but actually they may be estimated with large uncertainty when non-IPD studies are small, and this may lead to worse estimation properties than had IPD been known for all studies (such that the assumption of known variances could have been avoided by using the one-stage model (15.3)).

15.3.7.3 Application to the Fever Example

Returning to the fever example, it is of interest whether diagnostic accuracy of ear temperature is different for infants (< 1 year of age) and non-infants, as alternatives to rectal temperature devices are perhaps more important for non-infants, due to their increased emotional awareness. Eleven IPD studies provided age (Table 15.3) across a range of measurement devices, which allows an assessment of the accuracy-infant association both within studies and across studies. Model (15.3) was fitted in a frequentist framework using maximum likelihood estimation, with age as a binary participant-level covariate, such that z_{ik} and z_{ij} were 1 for infants and 0 for non-infants, respectively, and $\bar{z}_{ik}$ and $\bar{z}_{ij}$ were the proportion of infants in the fever and non-fever groups, respectively.

The estimates of within-study associations are close to zero and do not provide any evidence that either the sensitivity-infant association ($\hat{\gamma}_{1W}$= 0.10, 95% CI: −0.25 to 0.45) or the specificity-infant association ($\hat{\gamma}_{0W}$= 0.12, 95% CI: −0.59 to 0.83) are important, though confidence intervals are quite wide. The across-study association estimates are very different; for example, $\hat{\gamma}_{0A}$ is equal to 0.87, which is about seven times larger than $\hat{\gamma}_{0W}$, emphasising the importance of separating out within-study and across-study information. The discrepancy is even larger when rectal and ear temperature device types are included as additional study-level covariates in the meta-regression component.[26]

Comparing test accuracy of infants and non-infants may seem clinically intuitive, but statistically this dichotomisation loses power to detect genuine accuracy-age associations, and so we also examined age as a continuous covariate. Assuming a linear association, there was no clear evidence of a within-study association between participant age and test accuracy, though further research may consider potential non-linear relationships.

15.3.8 Performing Sensitivity Analyses and Examining Small-study Effects

Sensitivity analyses are often needed and ideally should be pre-specified in the IPD meta-analysis protocol. For example, sensitivity analyses may involve repeating the IPD meta-analysis after applying a more stringent inclusion criteria, such as including only studies of a certain design, with a particular reference standard measurement, or at low risk of bias. The handling of participants with inconclusive test results may also be examined which, as previously mentioned in Section 15.3.3, is an important issue that is often ignored.[28] For example, inconclusive test results might be omitted from the main analysis, but then including in the sensitivity analysis assuming they were all test positives or all test negatives, or as otherwise deemed appropriate.

As discussed for IPD meta-analysis of randomised trials in Chapter 9, issues of publication bias, availability bias, and selection bias may lead to small-study effects (the tendency for smaller studies to give different, usually greater, test accuracy estimates than larger studies). There is only limited evidence of the impact of small-study effects on meta-analyses of test accuracy studies.[54] Publication bias is a major threat, but (unlike randomised trials examining treatment effects) it may not be linked to statistical significance of *p*-values, since most test accuracy studies evaluate a single test and focus on estimation of accuracy rather than hypothesis testing.[55] Selective publication based on observed test accuracy results may still occur and lead to some studies being missed (and hence their IPD not sought) for the IPD meta-analysis project (although the network of researchers contributing to the IPD meta-analysis project might reduce this concern). Availability bias might be reduced by inclusion of published two-by-two tables from studies that do not provide their IPD but use the same threshold(s) chosen for the IPD studies. Selection bias can be reduced by seeking IPD from all identified studies (or all those at low risk of bias).

Statistical methods discussed in Chapter 9 for assessing small-study effects in funnel plots are not appropriate. Deeks et al. propose a method for detecting small-study effects in test accuracy meta-analysis.[55] However, this method has low power when there is between-study heterogeneity in test accuracy, which is usually expected. Therefore, to examine small-study effects, we recommend IPD meta-analysis researchers simply compare how their test accuracy conclusions change after exclusion of smaller studies (with the definition of 'small' ideally pre-defined in the protocol).

15.3.9 Reporting and Interpreting Results

Clear and transparent reporting of an IPD meta-analysis of test accuracy studies is essential. The PRISMA-DTA checklist is the PRISMA extension for reporting systematic reviews and meta-analyses of diagnostic accuracy.[56] However, PRISMA-DTA does not address issues specific to the IPD approach, and thus we suggest also using relevant aspects of the PRISMA-IPD checklist as an adjunct.

Reporting and dissemination of results should include a careful interpretation of the findings and their implications in terms of the consequences of false positive (e.g. overdiagnosis or overtreatment) and false negative (missed cases) results. Previous research has highlighted poor understanding of test accuracy measures amongst healthcare professionals and others.[57–59] Illustrating test accuracy using natural frequencies in text or in visual aids may facilitate improved understanding. Whiting et al. provide a worked example for deriving these frequencies using prevalence, sensitivity and specificity.[58] The calculations can be done for a range of plausible prevalence values and tabulated. Levis et al.[16] present nomograms of predictive values, derived by applying sensitivity and specificity estimates from their meta-analysis to hypothetical major depression prevalence values of 5% to 25%. To further aid understanding and assist clinicians, they also provide a web-based tool (www.depressionscreening100.com/phq) for estimating the expected number of positive screens and true and false screening results. There may be a dependence between the underlying prevalence of the condition, sensitivity and specificity, and ideally this should be accounted for when making predictions of sensitivity and specificity for a given prevalence (Section 15.5.2).[45,52] Similarly, the translation of test accuracy meta-analysis results to predictive probabilities (PPV and NPV) requires careful consideration (Section 15.3.6.5).[5,45]

Any limitations of the IPD meta-analysis project, including issues related to obtaining the IPD, risk of bias, applicability concerns, and heterogeneity should be reflected in the discussion. For example, a limitation stated by Levis et al. was the inability to include IPD from 14 of 69 published eligible datasets (20% of eligible datasets and participants).[16] Any important limitations should be considered when drawing conclusions. For more guidance on interpretation, we recommend the *Cochrane Handbook for Systematic Reviews of Diagnostic Test Accuracy*, as their guidance remains applicable even when IPD are used.[60]

15.4 IPD Meta-Analysis of Test Accuracy at Multiple Thresholds

Sometimes it is of interest to evaluate and compare the accuracy of an ordinal or continuous test at multiple thresholds. For example, in their IPD meta-analysis project to examine the accuracy of the PHQ-9 to detect major depression, Levis et al. compared the standard threshold of 10 with other threshold choices.[16] There are various options for analysing tests with multiple thresholds in an IPD meta-analysis, some of which are now described.

15.4.1 Separate Meta-Analysis at Each Threshold

The simplest way to model multiple thresholds is to apply a separate meta-analysis model at each threshold. Generally this is our recommended approach (especially if the IPD allows results for all thresholds to be evaluated in all studies), as it is straightforward and allows the application of the previously described methods for meta-analysis. As mentioned, Levis et al. appliedy a separate bivariate meta-analysis model (15.1) at each PHQ-9 threshold from 5 to 15. Their summary meta-analysis results are displayed in Figure 15.4, with 'cross hairs' added to display 95% confidence intervals for sensitivity and specificity at each threshold.[61] Assuming sensitivity and specificity are equally important, the investigators conclude that the standard threshold score of 10 gives the best summary meta-analysis results, both overall and for subgroups.

15.4.2 Joint Meta-Analysis of All Thresholds

By performing meta-analysis at each threshold separately, the monotonic ordering of summary results (i.e. sensitivity and specificity should decrease and increase, respectively, as the threshold increases) is not enforced across thresholds. This is because the relationship of test accuracy results

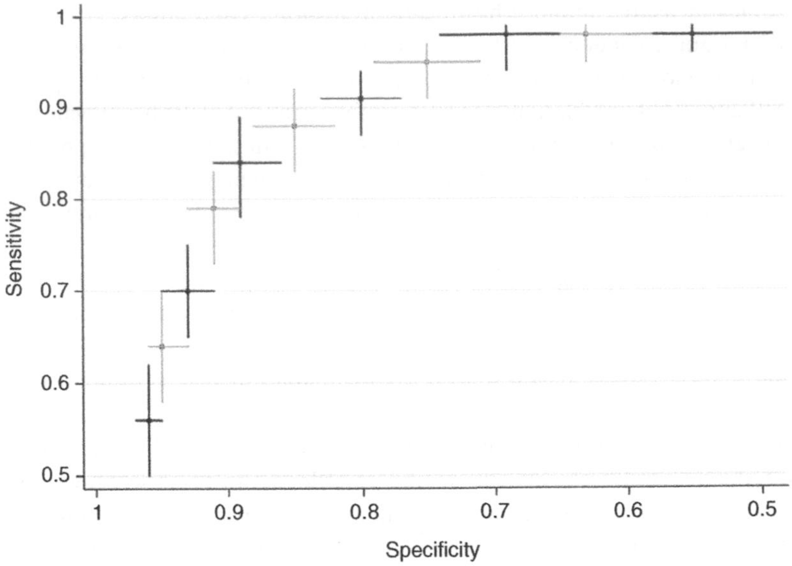

Figure 15.4 Results of an IPD meta-analysis of 29 studies (6725 participants, with 924 cases), summarising sensitivity and specificity at various thresholds of the PHQ-9 test for diagnosis of major depression, with semistructured interview as the reference standard. Each 'cross hair' denotes the summary sensitivity and specificity at a particular theshold and coresponding 95% confidence intervals. Threshold values correspond to a PHQ-9 value of 15 (far left) to 5 (far right). *Source:* Richard Riley, produced using data extracted from Levis et al. [16]

across neighbouring thresholds (both within studies and across studies) is ignored. In our experience, this is rarely an issue in the IPD meta-analysis setting, as usually all studies enable results for all thresholds. For example, the summary curve for the PHQ-9 test in Figure 15.4 is well-defined. Occasionally it may be an issue if there is more heterogeneity at some thresholds than others. But, the main concern is when some studies do not provide IPD, and their aggregate data from only a subset of thresholds are included alongside the IPD studies. This leads to discrepant numbers of studies included in the meta-analysis at each threshold and a potentially ill-defined summary ROC curve (as in Figure 15.1).

To address this, a number of options have been proposed.[12,14,62–67] Here, we consider two approaches: parametric modelling of the actual distribution of continuous test values, and a multinomial approach after dividing the continuous test into categories defined by clinically relevant thresholds.

15.4.2.1 Modelling Using the Multinomial Distribution

Rather than modelling the distribution of a test's continuous values, the test's values can be categorised by using a series of relevant thresholds and then the corresponding multinomial distribution modelled in each study. This approach was proposed by Hamza et al.,[12] with the underlying sensitivity and specificity at each threshold allowed to vary across studies, and the focus on estimating a summary (perhaps linear) relationship across studies between threshold value and each of logit specificity and logit sensitivity. This sophisticated approach often suffers from convergence issues, and it may be hard to accommodate non-IPD studies that provide aggregate data for only a subset of thresholds of interest. Hamza et al. note: "the total number of different thresholds across all studies is the limiting factor in our approach. If it is too large, the number of parameters might be too large to estimate and the likelihood method may not work properly."[12] Restricting the number of thresholds to five or less may be helpful. When all studies provide all thresholds, the benefit of this approach (over and above applying meta-analysis model (15.1) at each threshold separately) appears to be minimal.[68]

15.4.2.2 Modelling the Underlying Distribution of the Continuous Test Values

Unlike the Hamza et al approach, the underlying distribution of the continuous test could be modelled directly in each study. For example, Steinhauser et al. considered normal or log normal distributions to model test values in groups with and without the condition,[62] and combined them to produce summary distributions for each. This is appealing, as the summary distributions immediately enable the summary sensitivity and specificity to be calculated at any threshold of interest. For example, assume that higher values indicate a higher risk of the condition; then, for the group with the condition, the area of the distribution to the right of the threshold gives sensitivity; for the group without the condition, the area of the distribution to the left of the threshold gives specificity. This approach also naturally enforces a monotonically increasing (decreasing) relationship between summary specificity (sensitivity) values and threshold values.

However, the underlying distribution of the continuous test is often not truly known, and will differ for groups with and without the condition, as well as across studies. Key inferences are often made toward the tails of a distribution, for which there may be less information, and therefore the chosen parametric distribution may have a strong impact on results. To illustrate this, consider an IPD meta-analysis of the eight fever studies that used a FirstTemp ear device and an electronic rectal device. Figure 15.5 provides histograms of the ear temperature value for fever and non-fever participants. In many studies the observed distribution approximately reflects a normal distribution, with different means and standard deviations across groups and studies. Therefore, we produced a summary normal distribution by using a two-stage multivariate meta-analysis approach (Chapter 13). In the first stage, the estimate and variance of the mean and ln(standard deviation) of the ear test values in the fever and non-fever groups were estimated in each study separately. These were then combined (accounting for their correlation), using REML estimation of a bivariate random-effects meta-analysis, to estimate a summary mean and summary ln(standard deviation) for each of the fever and non-fever groups, which defined summary normal distributions from which sensitivity and specificity are derivable at any threshold (Figure 15.6). For example, at a threshold of 38.0 °C for ear temperature, the summary sensitivity is 0.77 and the summary sensitivity is 0.88. Unfortunately, these results are heavily influenced by the normality assumption. Compare results to those from a bivariate meta-analysis (model (15.1)) of sensitivity and specificity for a threshold of 38.0 °C; this method requires no assumptions for the underlying distribution of ear temperature values, and gives sensitivity and specificity estimates of 0.63 and 0.98, respectively, which are very different from those when assuming normality.

Therefore, parametric approaches that strictly enforce a particular shape should be used with caution. To address this concern, Jones et al. suggest a Bayesian approach that allows a Box-Cox transformation when modelling the distribution of the underlying continuous test,[69] which provides more flexibility to model the observed relationship between threshold value and test accuracy. Their approach also allows the incorporation of non-IPD studies providing only a subset of thresholds.

Benedetti et al. used a subset of the PHQ-9 IPD meta-analysis dataset to compare accuracy results estimated using the Steinhauser and Jones methods (which analyse all thresholds together by making parametric assumptions about the continuous test distribution),[70] and those from the conventional bivariate model (15.1) (which analyses each threshold separately but avoids making parametric assumptions about the continuous test distribution). They compared results when

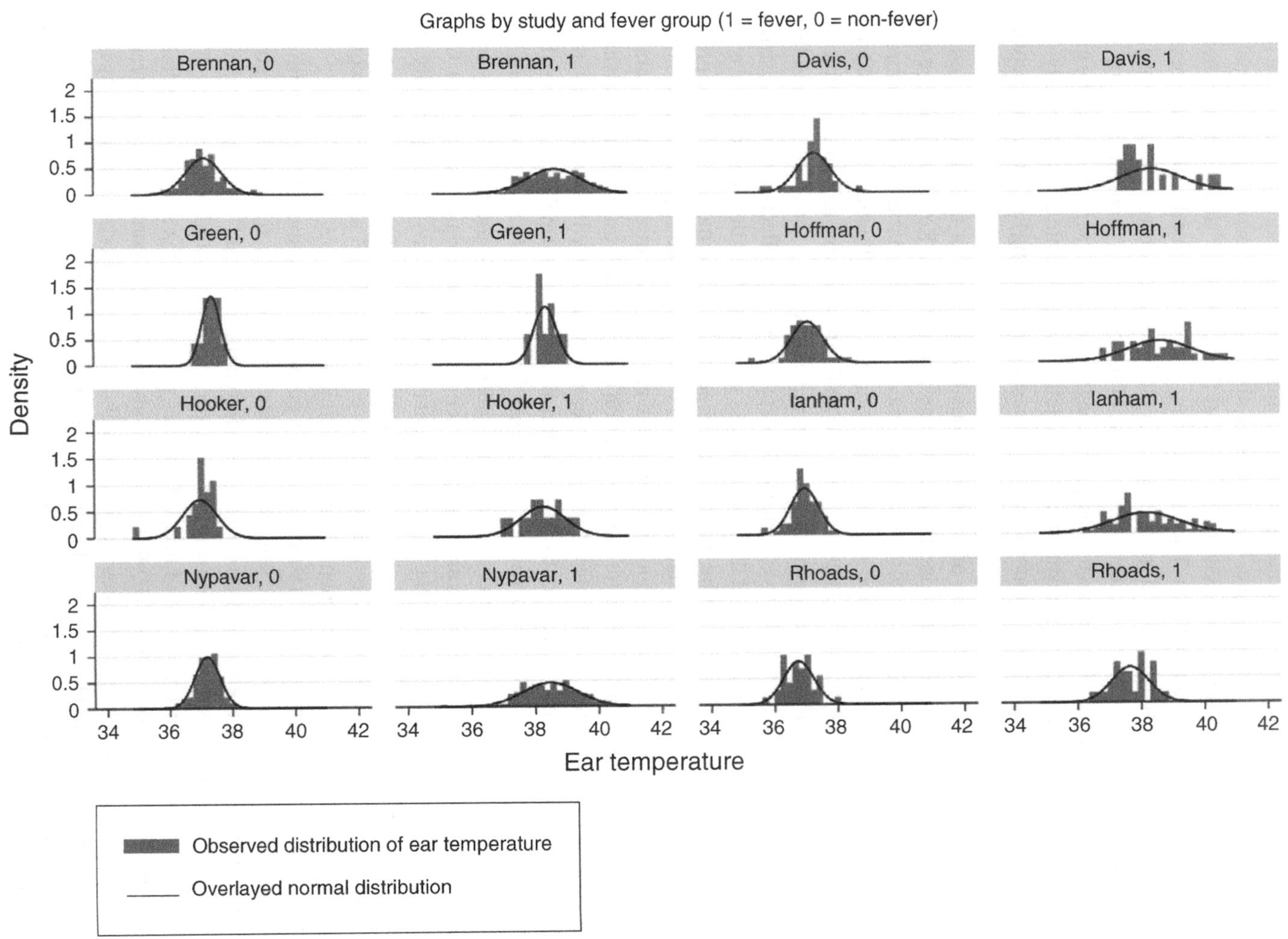

Figure 15.5 Histograms showing the observed distributions of ear temperature values in the fever and non-fever groups of eight IPD studies that used a FirstTemp ear device and an electronic rectal device. Source: Richard Riley, created based on data from Riley et al.[26]

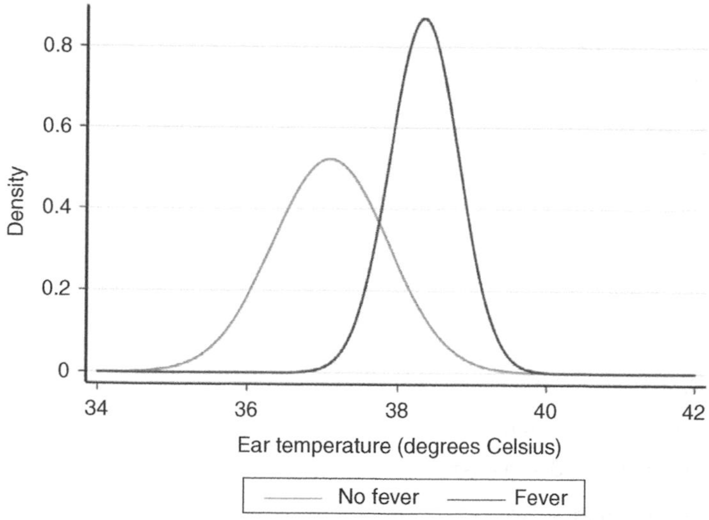

Figure 15.6 Summary normal distribution for the fever and non-fever groups based on assuming ear temperature values are normally distributed (though with different means and variances) for fever and non-fever children in each of eight IPD studies that used a FirstTemp ear device and an electronic rectal device (reference standard). These summary distributions can be used to derive sensitivity and specificity for any threshold of interest on the *x*-axis, as described in Section 15.4.2.2. *Source:* Richard Riley, created based on data from Riley et al.[26]

assuming all thresholds are available in all studies, and when using only those thresholds reported in study publications. When some thresholds are missing, widths of confidence or credible intervals for summary sensitivity and specificity are narrower when using the Steinhauser method and, especially, the Jones method than compared to the bivariate model. This gain in precision likely arises because the Jones and Steinhauser methods analyse all thresholds simultaneously and make stronger assumptions about the underlying distribution of test values. Also, even with some missing thresholds, the summary ROC curves estimated via the Jones and Steinhauser methods were quite close to the ROC curve from a bivariate analysis based on all thresholds from all studies (Figure 15.7), although there were still notable differences at extreme threshold values (potentially where the choice of parametric distribution is most influential).

Further research is needed to evaluate the Jones and Steinhauser methods in other empirical and simulated datasets, and also with comparison to other options to deal with missing thresholds,[14,65] including a multiple imputation approach proposed by Ensor et al.[64] and the time-to-event models for interval censored data proposed by Hoyer et al.[66,67] Currently we recommend using the bivariate model if all thresholds of interest are available in all studies (typically the situation when just using IPD studies), but to additionally consider one of the other methods in situations where some studies have missing thresholds (e.g. when also including non-IPD studies).

15.5 IPD Meta-Analysis for Examining a Test's Clinical Utility

Sensitivity and specificity characterise the performance of a medical test, but neither captures the clinical consequences of using the test to inform medical decisions.[71] Therefore, when used to direct clinical decision-making (e.g. as part of a clinical decision rule to initiate treatment or decide who is

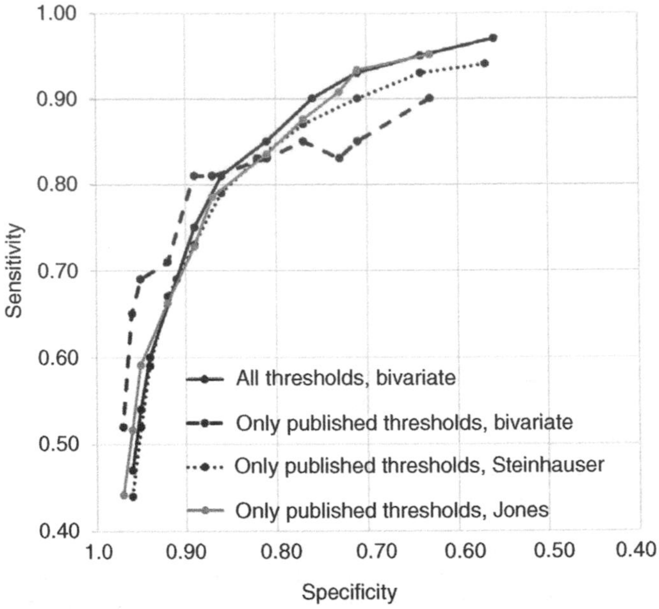

Figure 15.7 Summary ROC curves when applying the conventional bivariate model (which analyses each threshold separately), the Steinhauser method and the Jones method (which each analyse all thresholds simultaneously) to a subset of the PHQ-9 IPD meta-analysis dataset of Levis et al.[16] The bivariate model was applied to the IPD, with all thresholds provided by all studies. Then, pretending full IPD were unavailable, the three methods were applied assuming each study's IPD only enabled thresholds reported in their original study publication. *Source:* Brooke Levis.

admitted to hospital), a test should also be evaluated for its overall benefit on clinical outcomes and healthcare. This can be examined using measures of clinical utility, which are now introduced in general, before outlining how to summarise them using IPD meta-analysis.

15.5.1 Net Benefit and Decision Curves

The overall consequences of using a test for clinical decisions can be measured using the net benefit, which requires only the weighing of the benefits (e.g. improved patient outcomes) against the harms (e.g. worse patient outcomes, additional costs).[72,73] This approach essentially puts benefits and harms on the same scale by specifying an exchange rate, a clinical judgement of the relative value of benefits and harms associated with using the test to determine clinical decisions.[72] It requires the research team to choose a risk threshold p_t, such that if an individual's predicted risk of the condition is $\geq p_t$ there will be a clinical action (e.g. onset of treatment, referral to specialist, etc). For example, Van Calster et al. consider a risk threshold value of $p_t = 0.1$ to inform the need for biopsy after screening individuals for prostate cancer,[74] such that those with a predicted risk of 0.1 or above receive biopsy, but those with a predicted risk <0.1 do not. Based on the chosen risk threshold, the net benefit is the difference between the number of true positive (*TP*) results and the number of false positive (*FP*) results, relative to the total sample size (*N*), and weighted by a factor $\frac{p_t}{1-p_t}$. The weighting factor is essentially the odds of the condition at the chosen risk threshold value (the probability of the condition divided by the probability of not having the condition), which can equivalently be considered to represent an acceptable harm to benefit ratio. For example, a chosen risk threshold of $p_t = 0.1$ (i.e. a risk of 10 in 100) is equivalent to assuming a harm-to-benefit ratio of 1:9 (or 10/90) is acceptable. In other words, the chosen p_t should reflect where the expected benefit of clinical action is equal to the expected benefit of avoiding clinical action.[73]

Net benefit (NB_{p_t}) at risk threshold p_t can be written formally as:

$$NB_{p_t} = \frac{TP}{N} - \left(\frac{FP}{N} \times \frac{p_t}{1-p_t}\right) = \frac{TP - \left(FP \times \frac{p_t}{1-p_t}\right)}{N}$$
$$= (\text{sensitivity} \times \text{prevalence}) - \left((1-\text{specificity}) \times (1-\text{prevalence}) \times \frac{p_t}{1-p_t}\right) \tag{15.5}$$

where TP and FP are the true and false positives, respectively, at the chosen threshold value p_t.

Positive values of the net benefit indicate the test has clinical utility, as the benefits outweigh the harms. The maximum possible value of the net benefit is the condition's prevalence; therefore, it is bounded below 1, and will be close to zero when the prevalence is low. It is helpful to multiply the net benefit by 1000, so it can be interpreted as *the additional number of true cases identified for treatment (or another clinical action like referral or biopsy) without increasing the number treated unnecessarily per 1000 individuals*. The net benefit is zero if the benefit compensates the harm, and negative if harm surpasses benefit. Some researchers prefer to use the standardised net benefit,[75] which is the net benefit divided by the condition's prevalence, as then the maximum value is always 1.

Often the exact choice of risk threshold is unclear and so (standardised) net benefit should then be examined across a range of plausible p_t values.[73,76,77] The obtained net benefit values can be displayed on a decision curve,[72,73] and compared to those based on other competing tests and strategies (e.g. treatment is applied to all or applied to none). The basic interpretation of a decision curve is that the test or strategy with the highest net benefit at a particular threshold probability has the highest clinical value.[72] It is wrong to use the plot to guide the choice of risk threshold to direct clinical decisions;[75] rather, the graph should be interpreted as a sensitivity analysis over a range of plausible decision thresholds chosen a priori by clinical experts in the field.

15.5.2 IPD Meta-Analysis Models for Summarising Clinical Utility of a Test

Wynants et al. show how IPD meta-analysis can be used to summarise the net benefit of a test at a given risk threshold for clinical action,[78] using a trivariate meta-analysis of sensitivity, specificity and prevalence. Suppose IPD from $i = 1$ to S studies are available, which is used to create a two-by-two table, as shown in Table 15.1 (for continuous tests, using the same threshold value to define test positive and test negative in each study). Without the inclusion of participant-level covariates, we can assume a binomial distribution for the number of participants with the condition, the number of true positives, and the number of true negatives in each study. Across studies, the true study-specific prevalence (prev$_i$), sensitivities (Se$_i$), and specificities (Sp$_i$) are assumed normally distributed on the logit scale with means γ_1, γ_2, and γ_3:

$$\begin{aligned} n_{1i} &\sim \text{Binomial}(n_i, p_i) \\ r_{11i} &\sim \text{Binomial}(n_{1i}, \text{Se}_i) \\ r_{00i} &\sim \text{Binomial}(n_{0i}, \text{Sp}_i) \end{aligned}$$
$$\begin{pmatrix} \text{logit}(\text{prev}_i) \\ \text{logit}(\text{Se}_i) \\ \text{logit}(\text{Sp}_i) \end{pmatrix} \sim N\left[\begin{pmatrix} \gamma_1 \\ \gamma_2 \\ \gamma_3 \end{pmatrix}, \boldsymbol{\Omega}\right], \boldsymbol{\Omega} = \begin{pmatrix} \tau_1^2 & \rho_{12}\tau_1\tau_2 & \rho_{13}\tau_1\tau_3 \\ \rho_{12}\tau_1\tau_2 & \tau_2^2 & \rho_{23}\tau_2\tau_3 \\ \rho_{13}\tau_1\tau_3 & \rho_{23}\tau_2\tau_3 & \tau_3^2 \end{pmatrix} \tag{15.6}$$

The variance-covariance matrix $\mathbf{\Omega}$ contains the between-study variances in the logit prevalence (τ_1^2), the logit sensitivity (τ_2^2), and the logit specificity (τ_3^2), and their between-study correlations (e.g. ρ_{12}). After frequentist estimation of model (15.6), or by sampling from the posterior distribution as part of the Bayesian estimation process, the summary net benefit at the chosen risk threshold (p_t) can now be derived from γ_1, γ_2, γ_3, and p_t, as follows:

$$\begin{aligned}\text{Summary } NB_{p_t} &= (\text{sensitivity} \times \text{prevalence}) \\ &\quad - \left((1-\text{specificity}) \times (1-\text{prevalence}) \times \frac{p_t}{1-p_t}\right) \\ &= \frac{\exp(\gamma_2)}{1+\exp(\gamma_2)} \times \frac{\exp(\gamma_1)}{1+\exp(\gamma_1)} \\ &\quad - \left(\left(1-\frac{\exp(\gamma_3)}{1+\exp(\gamma_3)}\right) \times \left(1-\frac{\exp(\gamma_1)}{1+\exp(\gamma_1)}\right) \times \frac{p_t}{1-p_t}\right)\end{aligned} \tag{15.7}$$

As for summary sensitivity, specificity and prevalence, the Bayesian framework will provide samples from the posterior distribution of the summary NB_{p_t} in order to make inferences. The summary NB_{p_t} can also be plotted across a range of clinically relevant p_t values, to form a summary decision curve and its 95% credible interval. A 95% prediction interval for NB_{p_t} in a new study can also be calculated.[78]

The summary NB_{p_t} of a test is usually compared to the net benefit of treat all,

$$NB(\text{treat all})_{p_t} = \text{prevalence} - \left((1-\text{prevalence}) \times \left(\frac{p_t}{1-p_t}\right)\right) \tag{15.8}$$

and to the net benefit of treat none (NB(treat none)), which equals zero irrespective of p_t.

Both NB_{p_t} and $NB(\text{treat all})_{p_t}$ are dependent on the prevalence; therefore, it is helpful to also calculate the summary or predicted NB_{p_t} and $NB(\text{treat all})_{p_t}$ conditional on a particular prevalence. This can be achieved easily in the Bayesian framework by sampling from posterior distributions after fixing a particular prevalence value.

Also useful is to calculate the probability that the test is clinically useful,

$$\text{P(test is best strategy)} = \text{P}\left(NB_{p_t} > \max\left(NB(\text{treat all})_{p_t}, 0\right)\right) \tag{15.9}$$

and this can also be calculated after conditioning on a chosen prevalence. Furthermore, if there are competing tests, then the net benefit of the multiple tests can be compared, and the probability of each one being the best strategy can be computed. A summary decision curve can also be obtained for a test by displaying its summary NB_{p_t} values obtained from equation 15.7 after a separate trivariate meta-analysis (model (15.6)) at each risk threshold value in the plausible range of interest.

Extension of the above methods to include study-level and participant-level covariates follows in the same way as described for the bivariate models, allowing net benefit and decision curves to be summarised for particular settings, subgroups and participant characteristics, as necessary. However, where multiple covariates are of interest in addition to test results, it will usually be better to develop and validate a diagnostic prediction model, and then evaluate the clinical utility of risk predictions from this model (Chapter 17).

15.5.3 Application to the Fever Example

Wynants et al. applied the trivariate meta-analysis of model (15.6) to the 11 studies that evaluated the accuracy of a FirstTemp branded ear thermometer in relation to an electronic rectal thermometer (Table 15.3).[78] Based on an ear temperature threshold of $\geq$38.0 °C, they obtained a summary sensitivity of 0.65, and a summary specificity of 0.98, with considerable between-study heterogeneity, especially in sensitivity and prevalence. Do these results suggest that using ear thermometry to diagnose fever is clinically useful? On the one hand, we want to avoid missing serious infectious diseases in young children and stress the harm of a false negative classification. In this case, sensitivity is important, and the low summary estimate of 0.65 is concerning. On the other hand, we want to avoid overtreatment of fever and unnecessary hospitalization costs, when the child can be safely taken care of at home. In this case, specificity is important and the summary value of 0.98 is promising, although with heterogeneity across settings. To make statements regarding the likely clinical usefulness of ear thermometry in a new population, a summary of the net benefit is helpful.

Wynants et al. calculated the NB_{p_t} of using an ear thermometer at three risk thresholds for illustrative purposes:[78] 0.2, 0.5, and 0.8. A risk threshold of 0.2 indicates that we would be willing to diagnose four healthy children with fever to detect one true positive case, and the estimated summary $NB_{0.2}$ following a trivariate meta-analysis is 0.30 (95% CrI 0.19 to 0.42). This suggests that the net benefit of this diagnostic test is equivalent to the benefit of correctly classifying a net number of 30 children with fever per 100 patients, and no false positive classifications. Due to the heterogeneity in prevalence and test accuracy, of more relevance is a 95% prediction interval, which reveals there is a 95% probability that $NB_{0.2}$ will be between 0.03 and 0.68 in a new study. For a new study with a prevalence of fever of 50%, the estimated summary $NB_{0.2}$ is 0.32 and prediction interval of 0.12 to 0.47, which is narrower because it is calculated conditional on prevalence, which restricts the likely values of NB_{p_t} in the new setting. If we compute the NB_{p_t} at higher risk thresholds, indicating equal or lower perceived harms for false negatives than for false positives, the summary NB_{p_t} is lower. This reflects the increasing correction for the number of false positives.

Using equation 15.9, at $p_t = 0.2$ (i.e. a harm ratio of 1:4) there is a 44% chance that using an ear thermometer is clinically useful in any new setting and a 34% chance that this strategy is clinically useful in a setting with a known prevalence of fever of 0.50. However, assuming that false positive and false negative diagnoses are equally bad ($p_t = 0.5$), there is a 97% chance that using an in-ear thermometer is clinically useful in any new setting and a 99.9% chance that this strategy is clinically useful in a setting with a known prevalence of fever of 0.50. At $p_t = 0.8$, the probability of usefulness in any new setting is 95%, and the probability of usefulness in a new setting with a prevalence of 0.50 is 99%. Wynants et al. provide the decision curve,[78] which shows that the summary NB_{p_t} of ear thermometry is below the summary NB_{p_t} of treating all patients up to risk threshold 0.23. For higher risk thresholds, the summary NB_{p_t} of using an ear thermometer is higher than the summary NB_{p_t} of both treat all and treat none strategies. An illustration of a decision curve is given in Section 17.8.2.

15.6 Comparing Tests

IPD meta-analysis projects may also want to compare the accuracy of competing tests that can be used at the same point in the healthcare pathway.[79] Ideally, this requires the synthesis of IPD from comparative (head-to-head) test accuracy studies, which compare the accuracy of two or more index tests in the same study population by giving participants all index tests (paired or within-subject design) or by randomly allocating the tests to participants (randomised design), in addition to verification with the reference standard. Such studies *directly* compare index tests being evaluated, and ideally include all the index tests of interest to the IPD meta-analysis project, so that direct comparisons can then be made for each pair of tests.

Comparative studies of all index tests will often be scarce, and so the inclusion of other studies that examine the accuracy of just one or a subset of index tests is sometimes considered. Such studies should be included with caution, however, as they introduce indirect comparisons (across studies) of the relative accuracy of competing tests. In other words, as a different set of studies is available for each index test, the comparison of tests is no longer based on like-with-like comparisons at the participant-level. Then, the difference in accuracy is prone to study-level confounding, for example due to study differences in case-mix variation, reference standards and measurement methods.[79] Such indirect comparison of test accuracy is similar to naïve (unadjusted) indirect comparisons of treatments where the results of individual arms of randomised trials are compared across trials (thus breaking randomisation). Further, unlike meta-analysis of randomised trials where the *relative* effects of comparator treatments are modelled (e.g. risk or odds ratios), in meta-analysis of test accuracy studies the sensitivity and specificity of each test are usually modelled, rather than relative or absolute differences in sensitivity and specificity between tests.

The validity of including indirect comparison relies on the different sets of studies for each test being similar, on average, in characteristics that may affect test accuracy. Availability of IPD may help to improve the similarity of studies providing direct and indirect evidence, for example by standardising the reference standards, choice of thresholds, and inclusion/exclusion criteria. However, in a case study using IPD, differences between direct and indirect comparisons persisted, even after adjusting for differences in threshold, reference standard and participant characteristics.[80] Therefore, the results of any indirect comparisons should be carefully interpreted, taking into account the possibility that differences in test performance may be confounded by clinical and/or methodological factors across studies. The quality and strength of the evidence of test comparisons should be clearly addressed in the discussion and conclusions of the IPD project.

15.6.1 Comparative Test Accuracy Meta-Analysis Models

Comparative meta-analysis is an active area of ongoing research and several network meta-analysis models are emerging.[65,81–83] A simple approach is to extend the bivariate model (15.1) by adding test type as a study-level covariate in the meta-regression component. This framework is flexible, as it allows different types of comparative studies (randomised or within-subject design), inclusion of any number of tests, and different numbers of studies per test. For example, if there are T tests of interest, one of the tests is chosen as the reference group to which the remaining $T-1$ tests are compared. The $T-1$ indicator variables are added (one for each of the other tests) in the meta-regression component, denoted by z_{it} (= 1 for test t and 0 otherwise), as follows:

$$
\begin{gathered}
y_{1ikt} \sim \text{Bernoulli}(p_{1it}) \\
y_{0ijt} \sim \text{Bernoulli}(p_{0it}) \\
\begin{pmatrix} \text{logit}(p_{1it}) \\ \text{logit}(p_{0it}) \end{pmatrix} \sim N\left(\begin{pmatrix} \lambda_1 + \sum_{t=1}^{T-1} \gamma_{1t} z_{it} \\ \lambda_0 + \sum_{t=1}^{T-1} \gamma_{0t} z_{it} \end{pmatrix}, \begin{pmatrix} \tau_1^2 & \tau_{10} \\ \tau_{10} & \tau_0^2 \end{pmatrix}\right)
\end{gathered}
\tag{15.10}
$$

Here, y_{1ikt} is the value of test t (1 = positive, 0 = negative) of participant k in study i who truly has the condition, where k= 1 to n_{1i}, and y_{0ijt} is the test response (1 = negative, 0 = positive) of participant j in study i who truly does not have the condition, where j = 1 to n_{0i}. Thus y_{1ikt} and y_{0ijt} are equal to 1 if the classification of test t is correct, and 0 otherwise. The parameters λ_1 and λ_0 denote the summary logit-sensitivity and logit-specificity, respectively, for the test chosen as the reference group ($t = T$). Also, γ_{1t} and γ_{0t} denote the difference in logit sensitivity and logit specificity, respectively, for test t compared to the reference group test. Comparisons of other pairs of tests can be found by taking linear combinations of these parameters. Participant-level covariates might also be added akin to that described for model (15.3).

Model (15.10) is a simplified example of a comparative test accuracy IPD meta-analysis model. It assumes that the between-study variance of logit sensitivity and logit specificity (and their between-study correlation) is the same for every test. This assumption can be relaxed, though doing so may lead to estimation problems, especially when tests have few studies available. The model also assumes test results from the same participant are independent. To address this, Trikalinos et al. extend model (15.10) to more appropriately model within-subject study designs.[84] However, the number of model parameters grows rapidly with each additional test, leading to potential estimation issues.[63,84] Note that even when all studies provide all tests measured in all participants, model (15.10) may still allow some indirect evidence to contribute toward the findings, especially when the heterogeneity is constrained to be equal for all tests.

15.6.2 Applied Example

Phi et al. used model (15.10) to compare three options for screening women with BRCA1/2 mutations for breast cancer.[10] They included IPD from six prospective cohort studies of women with BRCA1/2 mutations that each compared mammography and MRI for breast cancer screening, and had at least one year of follow-up after the last screening round to confirm absence of disease. IPD allowed the investigators to consider the combination of MRI and mammography, as well as each of MRI and mammography in isolation, and to compare tests over all women, and for subgroups defined by age < 50 and ≥ 50 years. They found that across 437 women aged ≥ 50 years, combining MRI and mammography significantly increased sensitivity (summary estimate 0.94; 95% CI: 0.78 to 0.99) compared to using mammography alone (summary estimate: 0.38, 95% CI: 0.22 to 0.57), with a p-value of < 0.001 for the difference. The combination also had a higher summary sensitivity estimate than MRI alone (summary estimate 0.84; 95% CI: 0.62 to 0.95), but the confidence interval was wide, suggesting further research is needed to clarify the true difference. They conclude that women with BRCA1/2 mutations may still benefit from MRI screening after reaching age 50 years.

15.7 Concluding Remarks

IPD meta-analysis projects to summarise test accuracy have the potential to improve the quality and interpretability of test accuracy results for clinical practice. Researchers embarking on such projects should consider the various steps and issues outlined in this chapter, which focused on evaluating or comparing tests defined by one overall piece of information, such as temperature or PHQ-9 score. Decisions in healthcare are often based on multiple pieces of information (e.g. test results in combination with age, sex, family history, and blood pressure) and thus require multivariable modelling. Also, estimates of sensitivity and specificity are not immediately applicable to clinical decision-making, and translation to predicted probabilities is preferred; these issues can be addressed by developing and validating diagnostic prediction models, as described in Chapter 17.

16

IPD Meta-Analysis for Prognostic Factor Research

Richard D. Riley, Karel G.M. Moons, and Thomas P.A. Debray

Summary Points

- A prognostic factor is any variable associated with the risk of future health outcomes.
- Primary studies to identify prognostic factors are abundant, but often have conflicting findings and variable quality. This motivates systematic reviews and meta-analyses to identify, evaluate and summarise the evidence for whether particular factors are prognostic.
- Meta-Analysis based on published aggregate data are severely limited, especially by poor reporting of primary studies and inappropriate analyses, including use of cut-points to categorise continuous variables and lack of adjustment for existing prognostic factors.
- IPD meta-analyses can help overcome these problems. In particular, by standardising the inclusion/exclusion criteria; harmonising the set of adjustment factors; and analysing continuous factors on their original scale whilst allowing for potential non-linear trends.
- Such IPD meta-analyses require a clear research question framed using a PICOTS system, and a transparent search undertaken for eligible studies and datasets. Initiating a collaborative network of researchers may help identify relevant IPD from studies currently unpublished.
- Before obtaining IPD, researchers should extract relevant information from each study, to help decide on their inclusion and whether IPD should be sought. Items from the CHARMS-PF checklist may be used to guide this process.
- The applicability and risk of bias of IPD from identified studies can be checked, using items from the QUIPS and PROBAST tools.
- IPD meta-analyses should primarily aim to summarise the adjusted prognostic effect of a particular factor, to establish the factor's added prognostic value after adjustment for established prognostic factors.
- Two-stage and one-stage IPD meta-analysis approaches are possible, and usually yield similar results. Advantages of the two-stage approach include being more computationally feasible and naturally avoiding aggregation bias, whilst having flexibility to include studies that differ in design (e.g. case-control, cohort, case-cohort, etc.)
- Non-linear trends can be examined in either one-stage or two-stage IPD meta-analyses, for example using fractional polynomials or splines; in the two-stage approach, this requires a multivariate meta-analysis in the second stage to summarise the non-linear shape.
- Small-study effects (potential publication bias) can be examined on a funnel plot, which is most convenient after a two-stage IPD meta-analysis.
- REMARK and PRISMA-IPD guide the reporting of IPD meta-analysis for prognostic factors.

Individual Participant Data Meta-Analysis: A Handbook for Healthcare Research, First Edition.
Edited by Richard D. Riley, Jayne F. Tierney, and Lesley A. Stewart.

16.1 Introduction

Many IPD meta-analysis projects are being initiated to identify *prognostic factors*, which are characteristics associated with an increased likelihood of particular (adverse) health outcomes in populations with an *existing* disease (e.g. cancer, Alzheimer's or osteoporosis) or within a particular health condition (e.g. pregnancy, being scheduled for surgery, being submitted to intensive care).[85] For example, prognostic factors for recurrence and mortality in cancer patients include tumour grade, stage of disease, and various genetic and biological variables (biomarkers). Other names for prognostic factors include *predictors* and *prognostic variables, indicators, or determinants.* IPD meta-analysis projects are also being set up to identify *risk factors*, which traditionally refer to aetiological characteristics that increase the likelihood of future disease occurrence in otherwise healthy populations. For example, risk factors for cardiovascular disease include age, body mass index, blood pressure, ethnicity and family history.[86] In this chapter, we focus on IPD meta-analysis projects to identify prognostic factors, though nearly all the issues and methods described also apply to investigations of risk factors.

Different values (or categories) of a prognostic factor are associated with a better or worse prognosis, and thus values of such factors in an individual can inform patient counselling and clinical management (e.g. treatment decisions, monitoring strategies). For example, tumour grade is a prognostic factor in breast cancer patients, as a higher grade is associated with a greater rate of cancer recurrence or mortality,[87,88] and this may motivate different (more aggressive) treatment strategies in higher grades. Moreover, patient advice and clinical decisions are increasingly informed by multiple prognostic factors in combination (e.g. via a multivariable prediction model, Chapter 17), such as tumour grade alongside an individual's age, family history, co-morbidities, and frailty. Other potential applications of prognostic factors include refining disease definitions and subtypes; improving the design and analysis of randomised and observational studies that examine the effects of therapeutic or preventive treatments (as prognostic factors are potential confounders in this setting); and even providing targets for the development of new treatments.[88] The latter is motivated by prognostic factors that are likely to be causally related to the outcome, and thus modifying their values may directly lower future outcome risk or improve future outcome values. Examining causality is complex,[85] and this chapter focuses solely on using IPD meta-analysis to estimate prognostic associations, not to infer causality.

16.1.1 Problems with Meta-Analyses Based on Published Aggregate Data

> *"The considerable variability in results reported within the prognostic marker categories, the poor quality of studies and the lack of studies for some categories have made it difficult to provide clear conclusions as to which markers might offer the most potential as prognostic parameters for localised prostate cancer. These reasons also meant that it was not possible to quantitatively synthesise the results."*[89]

Within each disease field, multiple studies exist that investigate prognostic factors for a particular outcome; often these report very different estimates about the magnitude (and even direction) of the factor's prognostic effect.[88] This creates confusion about which factors are genuinely prognostic. Hence, meta-analysis should be an important research tool to resolve the debate, at least in principle. Sadly, a conventional aggregate data meta-analysis of published prognostic factor studies is problematic and rarely provides conclusive answers.[88] The issue is the primary studies themselves,[90–93] which are often poorly designed,[94,95] badly analysed,[96,97] and poorly reported,[98–100] and even labelled a 'playground' for researchers looking for significant *p*-values and quick publications to further academic careers.[91,101,102] For example, in cancer prognostic factor studies, Kyzas and colleagues conclude that "investigators may tend to conduct opportunistic studies on the basis of specimen availability rather than on thoughtful design."[103] Hemingway et al. refer to this as a "what's in the freezer?" approach,[102] in which the investigator argues: "given the data we already have, what abstract can be produced to allow a junior colleague to present at a conference?"

A major challenge for meta-analysis of aggregate data is obtaining appropriate effect estimates from study publications, in particular *adjusted* risk ratios, odds ratios, or hazard ratios. These respectively quantify how changes in a particular factor's values are associated with the change in the absolute risk, odds, or rate of the outcome, after adjusting for other (established) prognostic factors. In other words, adjusted effects measure the added prognostic value of a particular factor over and above other factors. As studies will often have different follow-up lengths and include censored observations, adjusted *hazard ratios* (rather than odds ratios) are preferable as these account for the time to event or end of follow-up. Many primary studies fail to report even unadjusted effect estimates for the factors of interest,[98] or fail to give standard errors or confidence intervals of any effect estimates that are reported. To help meta-analysts address this, Parmar et al., Tierney et al., and Perneger et al. describe how to obtain unadjusted hazard ratio estimates (and their variances) when they are not reported directly.[104–106] Even with such indirect estimation methods, not all results will be obtainable. For example, in a systematic review of prognostic factors in neuroblastoma,[98] the methods of Parmar et al. were used to obtain 204 hazard ratios estimates and their confidence intervals, but this represented only 35.5% of the prognostic factor results sought. Further, the indirect methods mainly help retrieve *unadjusted* and not adjusted prognostic factor effects.

A related problem is that published prognostic factor studies often exhibit small-study effects (Chapter 9), whereby smaller studies tend to show stronger effects (or more promising results) than larger studies. Evidence suggests this will often be due to publication bias or selective reporting. For example, Kyzas et al.[107] evaluated 1575 articles on different prognostic factors for cancer, and staggeringly found that nearly all suggest significant findings, with 98.5% reporting statistically significant results or elaborating on non-significant trends. Simon concludes that: "The literature is probably cluttered with false-positive studies that would not have been submitted or published if the results had come out differently."[92] This relates to the "what's in the freezer?" approach to prognostic factor research,[102] which perpetuates quick but poor-quality studies that are ultimately not replicated in new data.

Another notable problem is that primary studies usually categorise continuous factors (such as age, blood pressure, and most biomarker values) at arbitrary cut-points, even though it is well-documented that this is best avoided as it loses power and is biologically implausible.[97,108,109] In particular, researchers often dichotomise a continuous variable to create two groups of participants based on a chosen cut-point; those participants with values above the cut-point are usually classed as high (or abnormal) and participants below the cut-point are usually classed as low (or normal). Yet, dichotomisation is similar to throwing away about one third of the data,[108,110] loses the opportunity to examine non-linear prognostic effects, and leads to data dredging for 'optimal' p-values.[97] It also leads to different cut-points across studies and thus between-study heterogeneity. There are a multitude of other potential causes of heterogeneity across primary prognostic factor studies, including different methods of measurement (for the factors and/or outcomes of interest), different lengths of follow-up, and different sets of adjustment factors.

For all these reasons, the main conclusion from a meta-analysis of aggregate data may "be the realisation that there is little good quality information in the literature ... providing the justification for a well-designed prospective study."[111] However, new prospective cohort studies are expensive and time-consuming, and, rather, the collection of IPD from existing studies may overcome many of these difficulties.

16.1.2 Scope of This Chapter

In this chapter, we outline the potential advantages of IPD for meta-analysis of prognostic factor studies, and provide guidance on the key steps involved in such projects: from defining the research question to data collection, risk of bias assessment, and statistical methods for IPD meta-analysis. The chapter builds on our previously published work,[21,85,112] and throughout we provide illustrated examples and highlight potential challenges.

16.2 Potential Advantages of an IPD Meta-Analysis

Many of the potential advantages of having IPD for meta-analysis of prognostic factor studies are similar to those discussed for randomised trials and diagnostic test studies in previous chapters. However, some specific benefits for the prognostic factor setting are important to emphasise, as follows.

16.2.1 Standardise Inclusion Criteria and Definitions

IPD allows greater standardisation of the participant inclusion and exclusion criteria, so that subsequent meta-analysis results about prognostic effects are applicable to those populations and settings of interest to the researcher. IPD also allows standardisation of how outcomes are defined, so that subsequent meta-analysis results are more interpretable. For example, IPD from multiple randomised trials and observational studies enabled the IMPACT (International Mission for Prognosis and Analysis of Clinical Trials) consortium to standardise summaries of the Glasgow Coma Scale (i.e. the outcome) at six months following a traumatic brain injury; in particular, to examine the odds of each category of the outcome scale, and avoid categorisations used in the original study publications.[113] Likewise, factors of interest can be defined more consistently. For example continuous variables, such as BMI, age and most biomarkers, can be kept on their continuous scale, rather than being forced to retain (arbitrary) categorisations used in study publications.

IPD also allows specific characteristics of participants to be better identified (e.g. ethnic groups, treatments received, particular measurement methods for outcomes or factors, etc), so that prognostic effects can be broken down to relevant subgroups, settings and aspects of current care. For example, IPD allowed the IMPACT collaborators to summarise the distribution of the Glasgow Coma Scale at six months for participants with and without secondary insults of hypoxia, hypotension, and hypothermia.[114] Similarly, IPD allowed Trivella et al. to examine the prognostic effect of microvessel density (MVD) on overall survival in participants with non-small-cell lung carcinoma,[115] separately for each of two methods for measuring MVD: the Chalkey method or the 'all-vessels' method.[115] We will use this example throughout the chapter.

16.2.2 Standardise Statistical Analyses

A major advantage of IPD is the ability to standardise statistical analysis within each study. In particular, IPD allows adjusted prognostic effect estimates to be derived; enables a more consistent, and potentially even the same, set of adjustment factors to be used in each study; and allows continuous factors to be analysed on their original scale rather than using the categorisations applied in the original study publications. Let us return to the example of Trivella et al.,[115] who obtained IPD from 17 published and unpublished studies, involving a total of 3200 participants, to examine whether MVD counts (a measure of angiogenesis) is a prognostic factor for overall survival in patients with non-small-cell lung carcinoma. A two-stage IPD meta-analysis was applied to summarise the prognostic effect of MVD (described further in Section 16.3.6.1), for each measurement method separately (Figure 16.1), adjusting for age and stage of disease in every study. MVD was analysed on a continuous

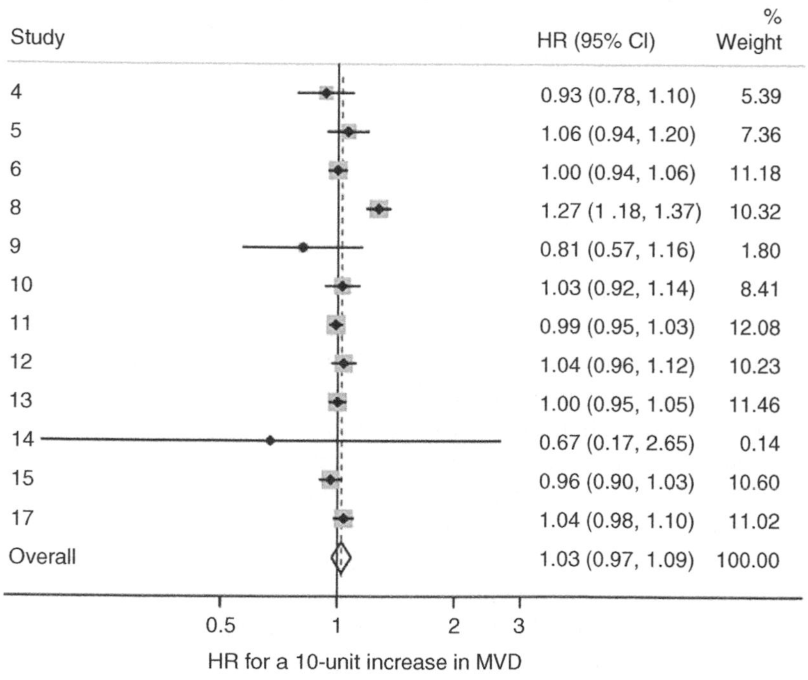

All hazard ratios (HRs) show the prognostic effect of a 10 count increase in MVD adjusted for stage and age. Summary results are derived using a two-stage IPD meta-analysis. In the first stage, a multivariable Cox regression model was used to obtain a log HR estimate and its standard error for MVD, adjusted for stage and age (as a continuous variable). In the second stage, we applied a random-effects model (using REML estimation, as recommend in Chapter 5) to pool the log HR estimates, with the Hartung-Knapp-Sidik-Jonkmann approach used to derive 95% confidence intervals. Study ID numbers correspond to those in the Trivella et al. paper.

Figure 16.1 Forest plot showing the study estimates and IPD meta-analysis results of Trivella et al. for the prognostic effect of microvessel density (MVD) in regard to mortality in patients with non-small-cell lung carcinoma, with MVD measured by the all-vessels method.[115] *Source:* Richard Riley, produced using data reported from the publication of Trivella et al.[115]

scale, assuming a linear association with the outcome. For the all-vessels measurement method, and in relation to a 10-count increase, the summary adjusted HR is 1.03 (95% CI: 0.97 to 1.09), providing no clear evidence that MVD has prognostic value. This contradicts the results of an earlier meta-analysis using published aggregate data that concluded MVD was a prognostic effect.[116] The IPD meta-analysis was more reliable as it utilised unpublished studies, analysed MVD on its original and continuous scale, and adjusted for stage and age in all studies. It was also more interpretable for clinical practice, as it was able to consider each method of measurement separately.

16.2.3 Advanced Statistical Modelling

Unlike published aggregate data, IPD provides the opportunity to check model assumptions and undertake more advanced modelling.[117–120] For example, IPD allows examination of non-linear prognostic effects, interactions between two or more factors, and proportional hazards (non-constant hazard ratios). IPD may even allow modelling of measurement error, time-dependent relationships, multiple events per participant, and survival and longitudinal data jointly.

Without IPD it is hard to examine the relationship between a continuous factor and outcome risk, because extracted aggregate data will often be inconsistent across studies (Section 16.1.1). For example, some studies assume a linear effect, some a non-linear effect, and others – usually the majority – compare arbitrary categories of the continuous factor. When studies report results for three or more categories, an aggregate data meta-analysis can model the trend in the factor-outcome association across categories as a function of 'exposure' level (e.g. mid-point or median of factor values in each category).[121–125] However, some additional knowledge of the factor's underlying distribution is usually needed to help define the exposure level, as the chosen value can impact upon the results,[123] and the categorisation can only reduce power to detect genuine relationships. This is entirely avoided when IPD are available.

For example, Gasparrini et al. show how to use a two-stage IPD meta-analysis to summarise a potential non-linear prognostic relationship between a continuous factor and an outcome,[126] often referred to as 'dose-response' relationship. In the first stage they estimate a spline function in each study separately (using the same knots at fixed locations in each study) and then, in the second stage, perform a multivariate meta-analysis of all the parameter estimates, to produce a summary spline (non-linear) function (Section 16.3.6.2 details this multivariate meta-analysis further). They apply the approach to examine whether there is a relationship between environmental temperature and non-accidental mortality rates, and look at data from 20 US cities ('studies') between 1987 and 2000. Splines were modelled using four interior knots (at −4.7, 6.0, 16.7, and 24.8 degrees Celsius) and two boundary knots (at −18.3 and 29.2 degrees Celsius), and adjustment was made for two variables: elapsed time and day of the week. The study-specific and summary meta-analysis results are shown in Figure 16.2(a). The summary curve indicates that mortality rate is largest at the extreme temperature values, and lowest around the reference temperature of 20 degrees. There is a steep rise in the relative mortality rate at the temperature increases above about 25 degrees, but a more gradual rise of the temperature decreases below about 18 degrees. The spread of *estimated* study-specific curves in Figure 16.2(a) is a consequence of both within-study sampling error (chance) and between-study heterogeneity. Figure 16.2(b) reveals the *shrunken* (also known as best linear unbiased predictions, BLUP) study-specific curves, which are derived post-estimation of the multivariate model. Their spread is much narrower, as the variation across shrunken curves reflects only between-study heterogeneity.

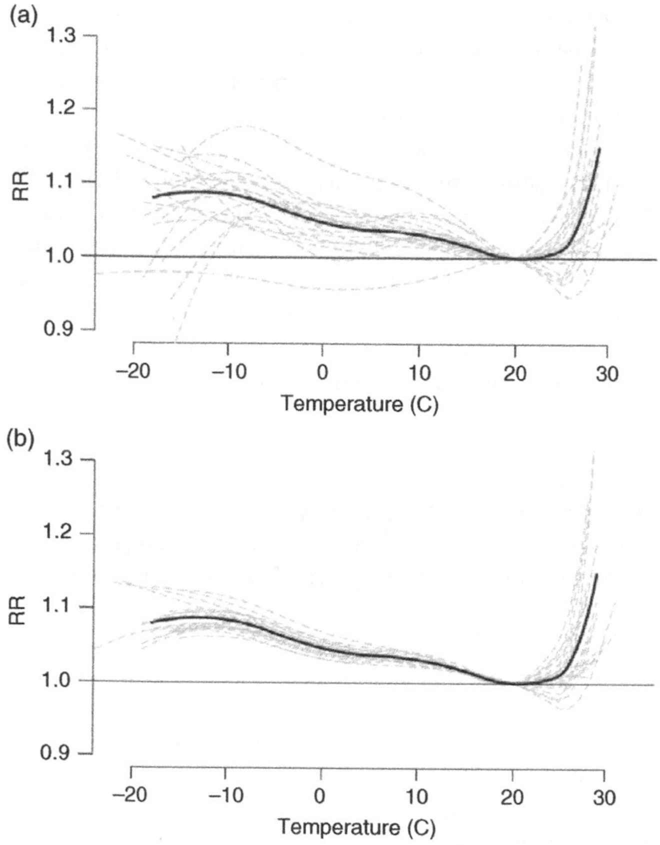

RR = relative rate at that temperature versus the reference temperature of 20 degrees
C = degrees Celsius.

Figure 16.2 Non-linear prognostic relationship between temperature and relative rate (RR) of accidental mortality in 20 US cities ('studies'), with a temperature of 20 degrees the reference group, as reported by Gasparrini et al.[126] *Source:* Gasparrini et al.,[126] © 2012, John Wiley & Sons.

16.3 Key Steps Involved in an IPD Meta-Analysis of Prognostic Factor Studies

We now describe the key steps involved in IPD meta-analysis projects to examine prognostic factors. Many aspects are the same as described in Parts 1 and 2 of this book for IPD meta-analysis of treatment effects, and so we particularly focus on the additional nuances that are specific to the prognostic factor setting.

16.3.1 Defining the Research Question

A fundamental step is to define the research question. IPD meta-analyses of prognostic factor studies fall within the remit of type 2 of the PROGRESS (prognosis research strategy) framework,[127] as they aim to summarise the prognostic value of a particular factor (or each of multiple factors) within a particular clinical population for relevant health outcomes and time-points. Some IPD meta-analysis projects have a broad or exploratory focus, for example to examine a wide-range of potential prognostic factors, but a more specific focus is preferable, in terms of examining the (adjusted) prognostic value of a small set of pre-defined factors.

CHARMS (checklist for critical appraisal and data extraction for systematic reviews of prediction modelling studies) provides guidance for formulating a research question.[128] Although CHARMS was developed,[128] and further refined,[129] for reviews of prediction model studies, it can also be used to define and frame the question for reviews of prognostic factor studies, including IPD meta-analyses. CHARMS, and related guidance,[128,129] proposes a modification of the traditional PICO system (population, index treatment, comparison, and outcome) used in systematic reviews evaluating treatment effects (as described in Chapters 3 and 4). The modification is called PICOTS, because it also considers timing and setting. The PICOTS system for the aforementioned Trivella et al. IPD meta-analysis project is shown in Box 16.1.

Box 16.1 Six items to help define the question for IPD meta-analysis projects aiming to examine prognostic factors, abbreviated as PICOTS,[112,128] and applied to the project of Trivella et al. to examine microvessel density (MVD) as a prognostic factor in non-small-cell lung carcinoma.[115]

- **Population:** *define the target population in which the prognostic factor(s) under review are to be used.*
  MVD project: patients with stages I–III primary non-small-cell lung carcinoma (NSCLC) with complete surgical resection (complete removal of the tumour).
- **Index factor:** *define the prognostic factor(s) under review.*
  MVD project: MVD count (a measure of angiogenesis).
- **Comparators:** *if applicable, define the other comparator prognostic factors.* For example, a typical prognostic factor review aims to investigate the prognostic value of a particular index factor adjusted for other (i.e. comparator) prognostic factors, and sometimes the review may aim to compare the prognostic value of a certain index factor to one or more other (i.e. comparator) prognostic factors
  MVD project: the focus was on the added prognostic value of MVD count; i.e. its prognostic effect after adjusting for the established prognostic factors of stage of disease and age.
- **Outcome:** *define the outcome(s) for which the prognostic ability of the factor(s) under review are of interest.*
  MVD project: overall survival defined as the number of days a patient survived from the date of surgery to the date of last follow-up or death by any cause.
- **Timing:** *define at what time-points the prognostic factors are to be used and over what time period the outcome(s) are predicted.*
  MVD project: prognostication was at the point of complete anatomical resection of NSCLC. All-cause mortality at two years and beyond (included datasets must have had some patients with at least two years of follow-up after surgery).
- **Setting:** *define the intended role or setting of the prognostic factor(s) under review.*
  MVD project: MVD is measured only after surgical excision of the tumour. A tumour section is examined under the microscope to determine the number of vessels in carefully chosen areas of the tumour (hot spots). MVD count may help inform prognosis and thus facilitate patient counselling and clinical decision-making.

Source: Richard Riley.

In the context of prognostic factor IPD meta-analysis projects, the P of population and O of outcome remain largely the same as in the original PICO system, whereas the I refers to the index prognostic factor(s). The C needs careful thought. It is usually not defined by reference values of the factor itself, especially as most prognostic factors are continuous, such as age, BMI, blood pressure, and leucocyte count (and so do not have a reference group as such). Rather, C usually refers to other comparator prognostic factors. For example, a typical prognostic factor review aims to investigate the prognostic value of a particular index factor adjusted for other (i.e. comparator) prognostic factors, and sometimes the review may aim to compare the prognostic value of a certain index factor to one or more other (i.e. comparator) prognostic factors. Only when the index factor is categorical, and its unadjusted prognostic effect is of interest, might C refer to the reference category of the index factor itself. For example, if the index factor is a comorbidity (present or absent) and is studied in isolation, then the I might be considered as one category (e.g. comorbidity present) and the C taken as the other reference category (e.g. comorbidity absent).

The T denotes timing and refers to two concepts of time: (i) at what time-point the prognostic factors under review are to be measured/assessed (i.e. the time-point at which prognosis information is required) and (ii) over what time period the outcome(s) are predicted by these factors. The S refers to setting, which is the clinical setting or context in which the index prognostic factor(s) are to be used; this is important, as the prognostic value of a factor may change across healthcare settings.

16.3.1.1 Unadjusted or Adjusted Prognostic Factor Effects?

An important component of IPD projects addressing prognostic factors is whether unadjusted or adjusted factor effects (or both) are summarised. The crude (unadjusted) prognostic effect of a factor may completely disappear after adjustment for other factors and is therefore rather uninformative, especially since prognostication in healthcare is rarely based on a single factor but rather on the information of multiple factors.[130] In addition, unadjusted prognostic effects may be highly dependent on population characteristics and are therefore prone to substantial between-study heterogeneity. For this reason, we recommend focusing on estimating *adjusted* prognostic effects, as these reveal whether a factor contributes or adds prognostic value over and above (i.e. adjusted for) the contribution of established prognostic factors. This is sometimes referred to as a factor having 'independent' prognostic value. Most clinical settings have established prognostic factors that are routinely measured (e.g. stage of disease). Therefore, for index factors of interest within the IPD meta-analysis, it is important to understand whether they contribute additional prognostic information to those already established as prognostic.

We recommend that IPD meta-analysis projects pre-define the core set of established prognostic factors for the outcome of interest (e.g. age, gender, smoking, disease stage, etc.), that represents the desired minimal set of adjustment factors. A consensus process, gathering views from health professionals and researchers in the field, may be required to agree on this set based on current prognostication of the clinical population of interest. Ultimately, if one or more identified studies do not have IPD that contain this minimal set of adjustment factors, it might be considered lower priority for inclusion and IPD retrieval than others that do (dealing with missing adjustment factors is considered further in Section 16.3.6.6 and Chapter 18).

An example from the IMPACT collaboration is given in Figure 16.3, as shown by Riley et al.[88] This forest plot shows an IPD meta-analysis of six studies, aiming to establish whether glucose level is prognostic of unfavourable six-month outcome (defined by a Glasgow Outcome Score of 1, 2 or 3) following traumatic brain injury. The unadjusted summary odds ratio of 1.14 (95% CI: 1.11 to 1.18) suggests that glucose level is a prognostic factor, as the odds of the unfavourable outcome increase

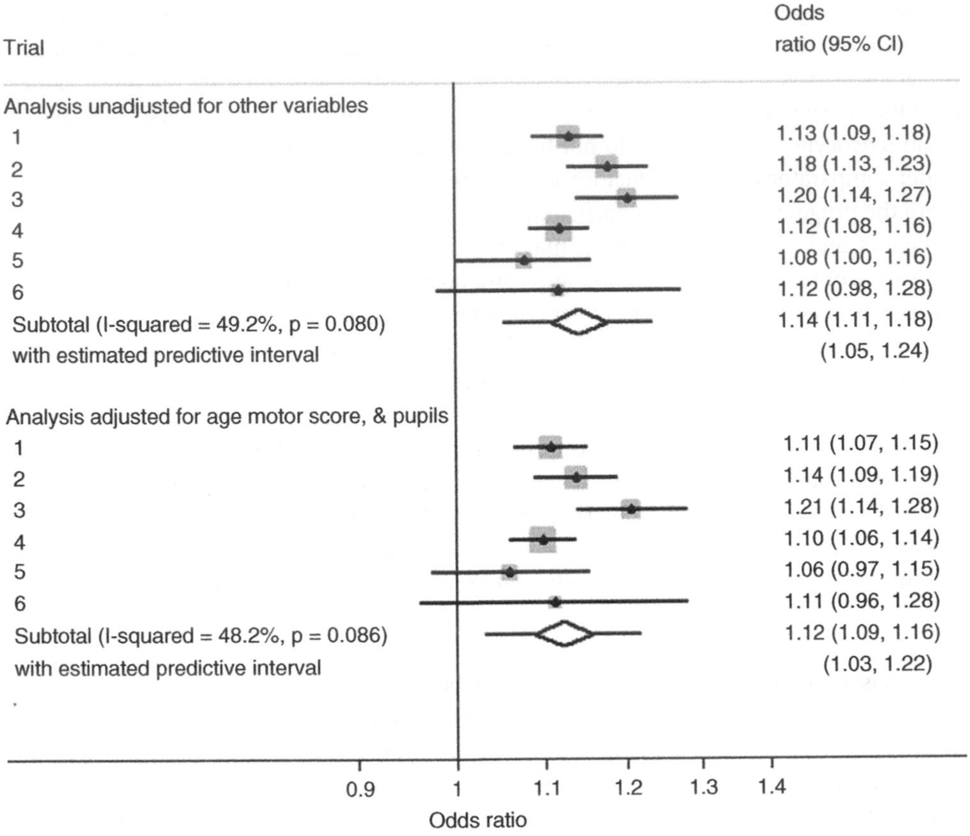

Figure 16.3 IPD meta-analysis to examine whether glucose is a prognostic factor in traumatic brain injury,[113–133] before and after adjustment for other prognostic factors. *Source:* Richard Riley, using data from the IMPACT collaboration.[113,133]

as glucose levels increase (odds ratio > 1). More importantly, the prognostic association remains after adjusting for age, motor score and pupillary reactivity, a set of prognostic factors known to be important for risk prediction in this field,[131,132] and available in all datasets. The summary adjusted odds ratio of 1.12 (95% CI: 1.09 to 1.16) suggests that glucose provides additional prognostic value over and above these established prognostic factors often used in practice.

16.3.2 Searching and Selecting Eligible Studies and Datasets

A careful process is required to identify relevant primary studies that are eligible for inclusion in the IPD meta-analysis project, according to the pre-defined PICOTS framework. Crucially, relevant IPD may exist from studies that were not originally designed to examine the prognostic effect of particular factors. In particular, randomised trials focused on examining treatment effects may provide a rich resource, as they usually record many variables at baseline, and so their IPD can be used to examine the prognostic effects of these variables. Indeed, such IPD may be larger and of better quality than IPD from published studies actually labelled as prognostic factor research.

Sometimes IPD meta-analysis projects only consider obtaining IPD from existing studies that are immediately accessible to them. For example, Green et al. used IPD meta-analysis to examine prognostic factors across different regional musculoskeletal pain sites, and only included IPD from seven randomised therapeutic trials carried out within the Arthritis Research UK Primary Care Centre at Keele University.[134] Generally, such a convenience-driven approach is not recommended, due to the threat of selection bias. However, it may be adequate if the available datasets are high-quality and comprehensive in the sense that they represent all index and comparator (adjustment) factors, participants come from the target population of interest, and outcome measures are of interest. Relevant IPD may also exist in datasets without any corresponding publications such as registries and electronic-healthcare record databases.

Usually, it is preferable to incorporate a systematic review for identifying the potentially available studies, and thus incorporate a formal search strategy. It is essential to define the study inclusion and exclusion criteria based on the PICOTS structure, as it determines the study search and selection strategy. Broad search and selection filters are typically required, combining terms related to prognosis research (such as prognostic, predict, predictor, factor, independent, adjusted, covariate) with terms related to the individual PICOTS items, notably for the population(s), index factor(s) and outcome(s) of interest.[135] Such a broad search comes at the (often considerable) expense of retrieving many irrelevant records. Geersing et al.[136] validated various existing search strategies for prognosis studies and also suggest a generic filter for identifying studies of prognostic factors,[135,137,138] which extends the work of Ingui, Haynes and Wong.[135,137,138] When tested in a single review of prognostic factors, this generic filter had a number needed to read (NNR) of 569 to identify one relevant article, emphasising the difficulty in targeting prognostic factor articles. The NNR might be considerably reduced in situations where names of specific prognostic factors and/or patient populations are added to the filter. Even then, care is still needed to be inclusive, as multiple terms are often used for the same meaning; for example, biomarker MYCN is also referred to as n-myc and nmyc, amongst other names.[139]

As mentioned, relevant IPD may also come from studies that did not originally focus on prognostic factor questions. Hence, relevant studies may not even mention that particular factors or outcomes were measured. For example, in the IPD meta-analysis of Green et al.,[134] the included IPD were from published randomised trials that aimed to examine a range of interventions for musculoskeletal pain conditions. Nevertheless, as they also recorded many participant characteristics at baseline, the IPD provided a valuable opportunity to examine potential prognostic factors defined by these characteristics. This emphasises the importance of establishing an IPD collaborative group (Chapter 3), where researchers in the field are encouraged to join and provide any relevant IPD (published or unpublished). For example, the Trivella et al. project was the first IPD meta-analysis conducted by the Prognosis in Lung Cancer project, which was an international collaborative study group specifically set up to obtain IPD from all available datasets that allow examination of potential prognostic factors in non-metastatic, surgically treated non-small-cell lung carcinoma. This led to 17 datasets being identified that met the PICOTS system in Box 16.1, including IPD of three datasets from unpublished studies.

Once the search is complete, each potentially relevant study or dataset must be screened for whether it meets the eligibility criteria for the IPD meta-analysis project based on the defined PICOTS system. The IPD meta-analysis project may specify stricter eligibility criteria than used in some of the original studies; however, such studies can still be included if obtaining IPD would allow selection of subsets of their participants that are eligible.

Table 16.1 Selected items of the CHARMS-PF* checklist to be extracted when identifying and considering studies or datasets for inclusion in an IPD meta-analysis project to examine prognostic factors, as proposed by Riley et al.[112]

Domain	Key items
Source of data	Source of data (e.g. cohort, case-control, randomised trial participants, or registry)
Participants	Participant eligibility and recruitment method (e.g. consecutive participants, location, number of centres, setting, inclusion and exclusion criteria)
	Participant descriptions
	Details of treatments received, if relevant
	Study dates
Outcome(s) to be predicted	Definition and method for measurement of outcome(s)
	Was the same outcome definition (and method for measurement) used in all participants?
	Type of outcome(s) (e.g. single or combined endpoints)
	Was the outcome(s) assessed without knowledge of the candidate prognostic factors (i.e. blinded)?
	Were candidate prognostic factors part of the outcome (e.g. when using a panel or consensus outcome measurement)?
	Time of outcome(s) occurrence or summary of duration of follow-up
Prognostic factors (including index and adjustment factors)	Number and type of prognostic factors (e.g. obtained from demographics, patient history, physical examination, additional testing, disease characteristics)
	Definition and method for measurement of prognostic factors
	Timing of prognostic factor measurement (e.g. at patient presentation, at diagnosis, at treatment initiation, end of surgery)
	Were prognostic factors assessed blinded for outcome, and for each other (if relevant)?
	Handling of prognostic factors in the modelling (e.g. continuous, linear, non-linear transformations or categorised)
Sample size	Was a sample size calculation conducted and, if so, how?
	Number of participants and number of outcomes/events
	Number of outcomes/events in relation to the number of candidate prognostic factors (events per variable)
Missing data	Number of participants with any missing value (in the prognostic factors and outcomes)
	Number of participants with missing data for each prognostic factor of interest

* Some domain and items within the original CHARMS-PF tool have been removed, as they are not relevant for IPD meta-analysis projects, or can be addressed by the IPD meta-analysis researchers themselves (e.g. in the data management or analysis phase).

Source: Table adapted from items within Table 1 of Riley et al.[112], with permission, © 2019 BMJ Publishing Group Ltd.

16.3.3 Extracting Key Study Characteristics and Information

For each study (or dataset) selected as eligible, it is necessary to extract or obtain information that will inform subsequent summaries, such as a subsequent risk of bias assessment. The CHARMS-PF checklist provides guidance about which study-level data should be retrieved (Table 16.1),[112] including fundamental information such as the dates, setting, study design, definitions of start-points, outcomes, follow-up length, and prognostic factors; usually there is large heterogeneity across studies in these aspects. The extracted information allows construction of summary tables of study characteristics. In addition, more specific information is needed to inform proper risk of bias assessments, such as methods of measurement of the outcomes and factors of interest (including both index and comparator factors). Note that CHARMS-PF was designed for systematic review and meta-analysis of prognostic factors using published aggregate data, therefore not all items and domains are relevant to an IPD meta-analysis projects. In particular, the Analysis, Results and Interpretation domains, and items relating to the handling of missing data and continuous variables, have been removed from Table 16.1, as they can be addressed by having and analysing the IPD itself.

16.3.4 Evaluating Risk of Bias of Eligible Studies

As described in Chapter 4, evaluating the quality of IPD requires the use of risk of bias tools and is an ongoing process. Classifications typically begin before IPD collection based on the information extracted from study publications, and are then refined and updated after IPD are obtained. To examine risk of bias in IPD meta-analyses of prognostic factors, the first four domains from QUIPS are relevant,[140] as are the first three domains within PROBAST covering participant selection, prognostic factors and outcomes.[141,142] Chapter 17 discusses PROBAST in detail. Additional guidance for risk of bias assessment may also be found from general tools examining the quality of observational studies[143,144] and the REMARK guideline for reporting of primary prognostic factor studies.[145,146]

16.3.5 Obtaining, Cleaning and Harmonising IPD

The process of obtaining, cleaning and harmonising IPD is the same as that described in Chapters 3 and 4 for IPD meta-analyses of randomised trials. A list of challenges and complexities encountered in the prognostic setting is provided by Trivella et al.[147] and Marmarou et al.,[113] though most are akin to those from randomised trials.

Often it will be sensible to restrict IPD retrieval to those studies classified at low risk of bias (as based on the information in study publications, i.e. before IPD collection). This is especially sensible when resources are limited and there are time constraints (e.g. due to short deadlines for funding reports), or when faced with an abundance of small, low-quality studies. Sadly, this will often be the case, and so the IPD meta-analysis researchers should pre-specify (in their protocol) the criteria for deciding how to restrict IPD retrieval to a subset of high-quality studies. A potential downside is that risk of bias classifications may change upon receipt of IPD from a particular study or dataset (e.g. if it allows re-inclusion of relevant participants previously excluded, or a more standardised outcome definition).

IPD are unlikely to be available from all studies and datasets requested (Chapter 9). Abo-Zaid et al.[21] reviewed nine IPD meta-analyses of prognostic factors that each used a literature review to identify relevant studies for IPD retrieval. All nine projects failed to obtain IPD from all studies desired, with reasons including non-response to e-mails, IPD no longer available, and lack of resources to participate. The percentage of studies providing IPD ranged from 32% to 88%, and five of the nine projects obtained IPD from 60% or less of the requested studies.

16.3.6 Undertaking IPD Meta-Analysis to Summarise Prognostic Effects

When summarising prognostic effects, statistical approaches for IPD meta-analysis should adhere to the high standards required (though rarely met) in primary studies[85,88] – in particular, to analyse continuous factors on their continuous scale, thereby avoiding the use of arbitrary cut-points to categorise them;[97,109,108,148] to examine non-linear relationships, for example using fractional polynomials or a spline approach; [96,149] to focus on effect estimates and confidence intervals, rather than just *p*-values;[98] to examine a factor's prognostic value adjusted for existing prognostic factors; and to examine potential time-dependent prognostic effects (i.e. non-constant hazard ratios).

A common mistake is to only consider unadjusted (univariable) prognostic effects,[98] even though a main objective should be to establish if a factor adds prognostic value over established factors. Even when researchers do perform multivariable analyses, they typically incorporate a selection procedure (such as based on *p*-values from univariable analyses) to identify a final set of adjustment factors to include in the multivariable analysis. This is not sensible, as the aim is to identify factors that add prognostic value to those already established prognostic factors. Therefore, adjustment for such established prognostic factors is needed (regardless of their statistical significance) and should be pre-specified. In this way, the findings will build explicitly on existing knowledge. Hence item 17 in the REMARK reporting guidelines:[145,150] "Among reported results, provide estimated effects with confidence intervals from an analysis in which the marker and standard prognostic variables are included, regardless of their statistical significance." Treatment should also be included as an adjustment factor in datasets where treatments vary across participants and influence prognosis.[151]

We now outline approaches to IPD meta-analysis, focusing on obtaining adjusted prognostic factor effect estimates. As unexplained between-study heterogeneity is expected, a random-effects modelling framework is essential.[47]

16.3.6.1 A Two-stage Approach Assuming a Linear Prognostic Trend

A two-stage IPD meta-analysis approach to examine prognostic factors is very similar to that described in Chapter 5 for examining treatment effects. The main difference is that adjustment for other variables is more essential, and added complexity arises when dealing with continuous factors (rather than a binary treatment variable). Consider the Trivella et al. example from Figure 16.1, where the prognostic value of MVD adjusted for age and disease stage is of interest. This example uses survival analysis methods in the first stage, but the general principles also apply to situations involving binary or continuous outcomes. Assuming linear effects of age and MVD, in the first stage we can use maximum likelihood estimation to fit a Cox regression model to the IPD in each study separately:

$$h_{ij}(t) = h_{0i}(t)\exp\left(\theta_{1i}\text{MVD}_{ij} + \beta_{1i}\text{age}_{ij} + \beta_{2i}\text{stage2}_{ij} + \beta_{3i}\text{stage3}_{ij}\right) \tag{16.1}$$

Here, $h_{ij}(t)$ is the hazard rate over time, t, for participant j in study i; $h_{0i}(t)$ is the baseline hazard (i.e. for those in stage 1 with zero MVD and age values); and θ_{1i}, β_{1i}, β_{2i} and β_{3i} denote the study-specific log hazard ratios (i.e. the adjusted prognostic effects) for MVD, age, stage 2, and stage 3, respectively.

In the second stage, as the focus is on the prognostic effect of MVD (and not the entire regression model), we can apply a conventional random-effects meta-analysis to pool just the prognostic effect estimates (i.e. the $\hat{\theta}_{1i}$) for MVD,

$$\hat{\theta}_{1i} \sim N(\theta_{1i}, s_{1i}^2)$$
$$\theta_{1i} \sim N(\theta_1, \tau^2) \tag{16.2}$$

where s_{1i}^2 is the variance of $\hat{\theta}_{1i}$ (as estimated from the first stage but assumed known in this second stage) and τ^2 is the between-study variance of the true adjusted prognostic effects of MVD. This is the same random-effects meta-analysis model that was introduced in Chapter 5 when combining treatment effect estimates. As discussed in that chapter, there are a variety of estimation methods for this model, and we generally recommend restricted maximum likelihood (REML) estimation followed by Hartung-Knapp Sidik-Jonkman confidence interval derivation. This provides $\hat{\theta}_1$, which denotes the summary (average) adjusted prognostic effect of MVD; the corresponding $\exp(\hat{\theta}_1)$ denotes the summary hazard ratio comparing to participants who differ in MVD by one unit, after adjusting for age and stage. Heterogeneity can also be summarised by $\hat{\tau}^2$ and prediction intervals for the prognostic effect in a new study.[46]

As each study is analysed separately, the two-stage framework allows different sets of adjustment factors in each study. However, this will ultimately make it hard to interpret the summary prognostic effect estimates from meta-analysis. As mentioned, we recommend that the IPD meta-analysis project team pre-specify a minimum set of adjustment factors to always be included, so at least there is a clear base to build from.

We previously illustrated the importance of analysing continuous factors on their continuous scale (Figures 16.1 and 16.2), but a challenge is when continuous factors are provided on their continuous scale in some IPD but on a categorised scale in other IPD. For example, Rovers et al.[152] note that "some predictor and outcome variables (e.g. fever and pain) might have been more informative if analysed on a continuous scale. Some trials did measure these items on a continuous scale but, because others did not, we needed to recode these items as dichotomous variables." Rather than reverting to the categorised scale entirely, we recommend including an IPD meta-analysis of the subset of studies providing continuous values; indeed – due to the aforementioned loss of information from categorisation – this subset of studies may still have the largest power to detect genuine prognostic relationships.

In principle, non-IPD studies can be included in the second stage (model (16.2)), provided they provide comparable type of aggregate data to that generated from the IPD studies in the first stage. However, such aggregate data are unlikely to be available for non-IPD studies, due to the aforementioned problems of categorisation of continuous factors, lack of adjustment for established factors, and so forth, within published prognostic factor studies. Note that if studies have small numbers of participants or outcome events, it is important to apply Firth's correction when analysing the IPD in each study, to reduce small sample bias in the prognostic effect estimates.[153]

16.3.6.2 A Two-stage Approach with Non-linear Trends Using Splines or Polynomials

Rather than adjusting for age in the first stage, an alternative is to fit the Cox regression model with age as the time scale (rather than time since study entry), so that $h_0(t)$ summarises the hazard rate over different ages.[154] A related issue is that the effect of age and other continuous adjustment factors may be non-linear, and so adjusting for them assuming linear trends (as in model (16.1)) may be sub-optimal. Similarly, there may be a non-linear prognostic effect for the continuous index factor of interest, and assuming linearity may distort its actual association with the outcome. These issues can be addressed by an IPD meta-analysis that allows for non-linear trends (of the index and adjustment factors) via splines or polynomials.[155–157]

16.3.6.2.1 Using Splines to Model Non-linear Trends

Our general preference is an IPD meta-analysis of spline functions, as proposed by Gasparrini et al.[126] Firstly, consider that in the first stage of our IPD meta-analysis examining MVD as a prognostic factor, we modify model (16.1) to include a restricted cubic spline function for both age and MVD, with cubic relationships allowed across four internal knots and a linear relationship before and after these internal knots. The knot positions are fixed to be the same in each study (age in years: 47, 60, 66, and 75; MVD count: 2, 19, 50, 131), based on the 5th, 35th, 65th and 95th percentile values observed in the *entire* IPD meta-analysis dataset.[158] We can now fit the following Cox model to each study separately:

$$h_{ij}(t) = h_{0i}(t)\exp\begin{pmatrix}\theta_{1i}\text{MVD}_{ij}{}^{S1} + \theta_{2i}\text{MVD}_{ij}{}^{S2} + \theta_{3i}\text{MVD}_{ij}{}^{S3} + \beta_{1i}\text{age}^{S1} \\ + \beta_{2i}\text{age}^{S2} + \beta_{3i}\text{age}^{S3} + \beta_{4i}\text{stage2}_{ij} + \beta_{5i}\text{stage3}_{ij}\end{pmatrix} \tag{16.3}$$

Here, the superscript $S1$, $S2$ and $S3$ terms denote three spline transformations of the original variable corresponding to the four chosen knots. Once the model is fitted, the parameter estimates for MVD can now be summarised in a multivariate meta-analysis, whilst accounting for their within-study and between-study variances and correlation. Other parameters in model (16.3) are nuisance parameters, and thus do not need to be included in the multivariate meta-analysis, which eases computational burden.

Multivariate meta-analysis models are explained in detail in Chapter 13. In our example, we require a trivariate meta-analysis as there are three MVD parameters to synthesise per study $(\hat{\theta}_{1i}, \hat{\theta}_{2i}, \hat{\theta}_{3i})$, and this produces three summary estimates $(\hat{\theta}_1, \hat{\theta}_2, \hat{\theta}_3)$ which define the average relationship between MVD and the log-hazard rate across studies. The summary spline curve for MVD is shown in Figure 16.4, alongside results when assuming a linear trend or a quadratic trend.

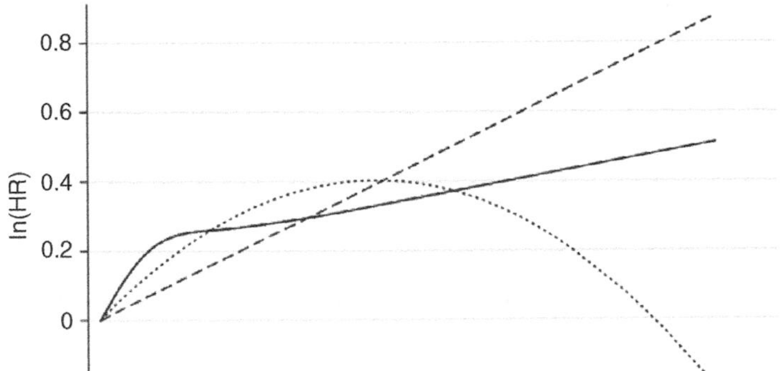

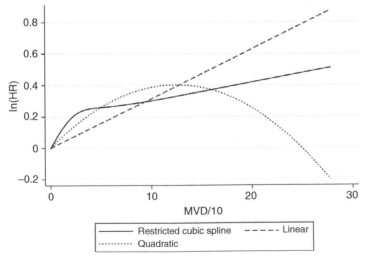

Figure 16.4 Summary of the relationship between MVD and mortality rate, according to a two-stage IPD meta-analysis assuming either a restricted cubic spline, a quadratic trend, or a linear trend. *Source:* Richard Riley, using data from Trivella et al.[115]

The summary spline function suggests a steep increase in the hazard ratio (i.e. the adjusted prognostic effect of MVD), as MVD increases from 0 to about 50 counts, before then having a linear and more gradual increase thereafter. This is perhaps more biologically plausible than a linear trend, as the impact of larger MVD values may be less dramatic once MVD levels are already high. For the quadratic relationship the hazard ratio decreases after about 150 counts, which also does not seem intuitive.

There is some evidence to support the non-linear spline shape ($\hat{\theta}_1 = 0.11; p = 0.10; \hat{\theta}_2 = -0.70, p = 0.02; \hat{\theta}_3 = 1.10; p = 0.03$), but the confidence intervals are wide and considerably overlap a log hazard ratio of zero (Figure 16.5); there is also large between-study heterogeneity, especially for θ_{2i} (between-study standard deviation = 2.01) and θ_{3i} (between-study standard deviation = 2.99). Recall that there was also no clear evidence for a prognostic association assuming a linear trend (Figure 16.1). Hence, after allowing for potential non-linearity, there remains no clear evidence that MVD (when measured by the all-vessels method) is a prognostic factor in non-small-cell carcinoma, and further research is still warranted to resolve the uncertainty.

Gasparinni et al. discuss the choice of knots in the spline function.[126] The choice may not be straightforward when the range of factor values varies considerably across studies. One option is to use knot positions based on fixed percentile values, but then the corresponding factor values will differ across studies, thus losing interpretability of the summary curve at the meta-analysis level. An alternative is for each study to only estimate those parts of the spline for the ranges that data are available. Studies with a limited or narrow range of factor values will then yield missing parameters values for some of the spline function (e.g. in the MVD example of model (16.3), a study may only estimate θ_{1i} and θ_{2i}, but not θ_{3i}). Such missing parameter estimates can easily be accommodated in the multivariate meta-analysis used in the second stage (see discussion on missing outcomes in Chapter 13), thereby allowing all studies to contribute toward the summary spline curve.

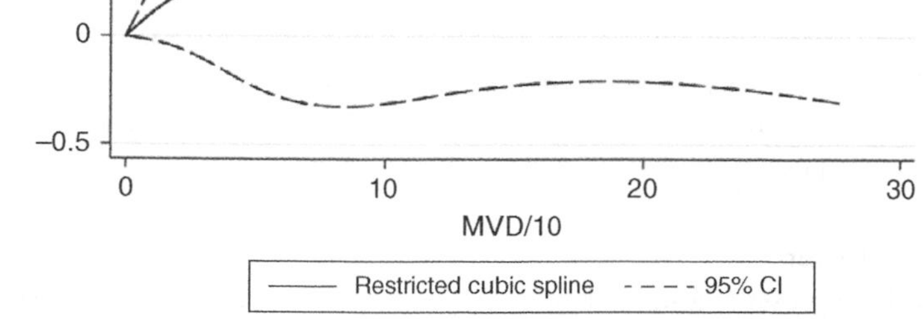

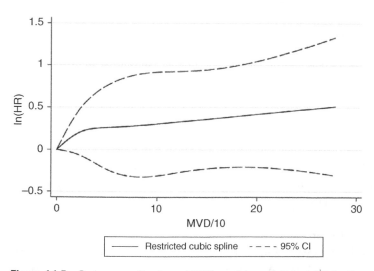

Figure 16.5 Summary estimate and 95% confidence interval (CI) for the relationship between MVD and mortality rate, according to a two-stage IPD meta-analysis assuming a restricted cubic spline. *Source:* Richard Riley, using data from Trivella et al.[115]

16.3.6.2.2 Using Polynomials to Model Non-linear Trends

Rather than a multivariate meta-analysis of spline functions to summary non-linear trends, White et al. propose a method to combine (fractional) polynomial functions.[155] This requires the same polynomial function to be specified in each study (e.g. a quadratic trend). Knowing what the correct function should be, however, is challenging. It is wrong to test for a particular trend in each study separately, as this defeats the purpose of meta-analysis; genuine relationships are more likely identified at the meta-analysis level, as the combined sample size and number of events increases the statistical power. Abo-Zaid gave an applied example that shows when examining the prognostic value of glucose in traumatic brain injury, there is no statistically significant evidence against a linear trend within each of four studies; however, after combining IPD there is significant evidence to support a quadratic rather than linear trend.[159]

Sauerbrei and Royston suggest a two-stage 'metacurve' approach that combines common or study-specific curves based on fitting (potentially different) polynomials in each study,[157] using a point-wise weighted averaging of functions (implemented using the package *metacurve* in Stata). Using theoretical arguments, White et al. show that the two methods differ most when covariate distributions differ across studies,[155] and simulations suggest that the multivariate meta-analysis approach of polynomial functions is more efficient when the polynomial is correctly specified, but *metacurve* is more robust to model misspecification. In general, however, the differences between the methods may not be important in practice. A limitation of *metacurve* is that it does not account for correlation between different parts of the curve, and therefore is less efficient; a downside of the multivariate meta-analysis of polynomials is that the same polynomial function is required in each study. To address this, the aforementioned multivariate meta-analysis of (restricted) cubic spline functions is appealing, as it accounts for correlation (and thus improves efficiency) whilst allowing study-specific non-linear trends. A downside of splines, however, is that the summary trend is more complex to express mathematically than a polynomial function.

White et al. also show how categorisation of the continuous factor, for example into 10 or 20 equally sized groups (if sample size allows) is a good way to initially examine and visualise the (non-linear) trend in the summary prognostic association over covariate values.[155] A summary effect is obtained for each group (relative to the reference group), via a univariate or multivariate meta-analysis, and these are then plotted. Their application suggests a U-shaped relationship between the prognostic effect of BMI for subsequent cardiovascular disease (Figure 16.6), which can then be modelled properly using, for example, splines or fractional polynomials.

16.3.6.2.3 Modelling Interactions

The prognostic effect of an interaction between two factors may also be of interest. If one or both of these factors are continuous, a multivariate meta-analysis of splines or polynomial functions could again be useful, to summarise the overall function of the two factors and their interaction.[160,161] This was already illustrated in Chapter 7, in the context of a treatment-covariate interaction in an IPD meta-analysis of randomised trials.

16.3.6.3 Incorporating Measurement Error

Many prognostic factors, such as blood pressure and most biomarkers, are measured with error. As the variation due to this error is typically unknown, measurement error is rarely modelled when examining the prognostic effect of a factor. As a consequence, and especially when the variation is large, prognostic factor associations are often distorted. For example, sometimes they are downwardly biased (e.g. hazard ratios and odds ratios closer to 1) and/or too precise.[162] For instance, in a single study, Crowther et al.[163] investigated the prognostic value of SBP (as a continuous

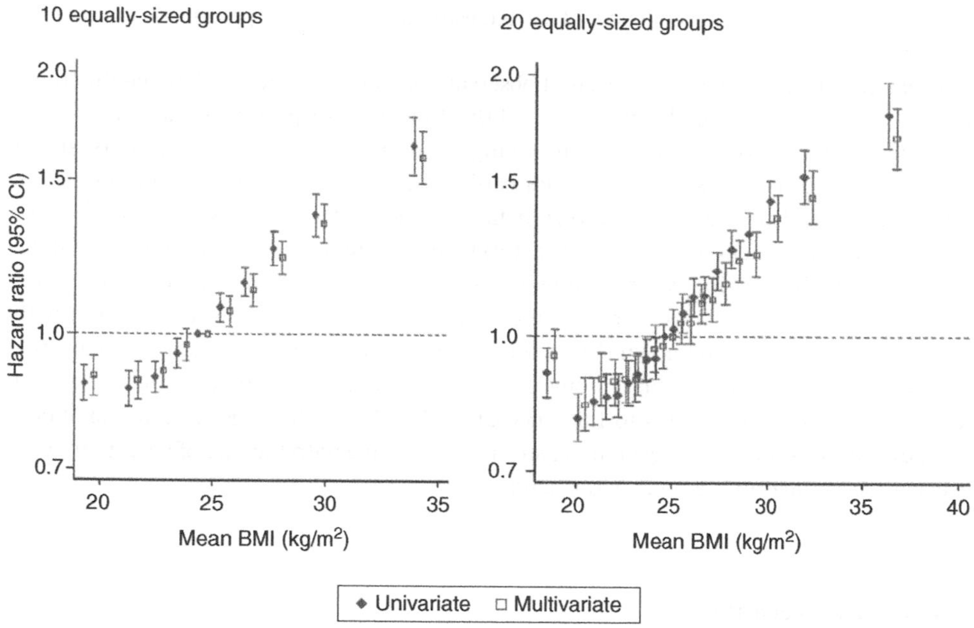

Figure 16.6 Prognostic effect of BMI for subsequent cardiovascular disease, across 10 or 20 categories of BMI containing equally sized groups, relative to the reference group of a mean BMI of 25. As reported by White et al.[155] *Source:* Figure reproduced from Figure 4 of White et al.,[155] with permission, © 2018 Wiley.

variable) for stroke in patients with diabetes. The hazard ratio comparing two participants with SBP one mmHg apart was smaller and more precise when ignoring measurement error (HR = 1.11; 95% CI: 1.05 to 1.17) than when allowing for it (HR = 1.20; 95% CI: 1.11 to 1.30). However, measurement error does not always attenuate prognostic effect estimates,[164] and the impact will depend on many issues, including whether the error is consistent across the range of a factor's values, and whether the outcome and adjustment factors are also prone to error.[165] Dealing with measurement error is especially important when aiming to establish causality of an association, as then one needs to model the underlying relationship between the true factor value and outcome risk, rather than between the observed (measured with error) factor value and outcome risk. Keogh and White discuss approaches for dealing with measurement error in single studies, for example using regression calibration and multiple imputation.[166]

If repeated measurements of a factor are taken in a small time period, and available in the IPD provided, then the variability can be measured and measurement error accounted for when estimating prognostic effects in the first stage of the IPD meta-analysis, using approaches beyond the scope of this book.[162,165–168] For example, if MVD_{ij} is measured with error in model (16.1), then we might specify that observed MVD_{ij} values are drawn from a particular distribution (e.g. normal with a mean and variance either estimated with the IPD or using external information). A related issue is when considering repeated measurements over a longer time period,[166] and whether a longitudinal profile of factor values is prognostic. In such situations, a joint longitudinal and survival model will often be helpful in the first stage of the IPD analysis, to estimate prognostic effects whilst simultaneously allowing for measurement error and censoring over time.[120,169] Adjustment in measurement error in adjustment factors is also important, as otherwise this can even lead to distorted estimates of the true prognostic effect of the factor of interest.

A notable example is the IPD meta-analysis of observational studies conducted by the Emerging Risk Factors Collaboration (ERFC),[170] who gathered IPD from 116 prospective studies and over 1.2 million participants. One particular analysis, involving 31 studies and 154,311 participants, aimed to examine whether fibrinogen is a risk factor for cardiovascular disease (CVD). Thompson et al. describe a range of sophisticated two-stage IPD meta-analysis methods for this situation.[117] They estimated that, after adjustment for known risk factors (age, sex, smoking, total cholesterol, systolic blood pressure and body mass index), the summary hazard ratio per 1 g/l increase in fibrinogen is 1.38 (95% CI: 1.31 to 1.45), and thus there is strong evidence that fibrinogen is a risk factor, with prognostic values over and above known risk factors. There was no evidence for a non-linear association. However, after allowing for measurement error in fibrinogen and some of the adjustment factors, the HR increased dramatically to 1.86 (95% CI: 1.66 to 2.06). This suggests that the underlying (average) value of fibrinogen is even more strongly associated with the rate of CVD than originally revealed when measurement error was ignored.

16.3.6.4 A One-stage Approach

The two-stage approach to IPD meta-analysis can mirrored by one-stage IPD meta-analysis models. As mentioned in Chapter 8, one-stage and two-stage methods usually give very similar results when their assumptions and estimation methods are similar.[171] Nevertheless, adopting a one-stage framework is potentially more convenient when comparing different non-linear relationships (e.g. choosing between various fractional polynomial terms) and examining overall model fit. It also allows the consideration of generalised additive models,[172] another approach to modelling smooth functions of covariates (outside the scope of this book). Furthermore, if outcome events are rare, then one-stage models might be preferred on the basis of using a more exact likelihood, and that estimation of prognostic effects and non-linear relationships in single studies is too restricted or even biased.[153] A downside of one-stage modelling is that, due to the multiple parameters (e.g. intercepts, adjustment terms, etc) and potentially multiple random effects, it may be prone to estimation problems (Chapter 6) and introduce aggregation bias (Chapter 7). Also, when studies are few, a one-stage meta-analysis model for binary or time-to-event outcomes that incorporates random effects may suffer from downward bias in between-study variance estimates from maximum likelihood estimation (Chapter 6).[173]

In a one-stage IPD meta-analysis it is also important to center covariates by their study-specific means, to avoid aggregation bias and potentially improve maximum likelihood estimation performance.[173,174] For example, we applied a one-stage IPD meta-analysis to examine the prognostic effect of one-year increase in age in women with breast cancer, for the outcome of mortality. We fitted a one-stage IPD meta-analysis model in a Cox regression framework using maximum likelihood estimation (as described in Chapter 6), whilst allowing for heterogeneity in the prognostic effect of age. When coding age on its original scale the summary hazard ratio was 1.011 (95% CI: 1.007 to 1.014; $p < 0.001$), with the between-study variance estimated to be zero. However, when using the 'study-specific centering' coding (where participant values of age are centered by the mean value in the participant's study), the summary hazard ratio was lower (1.007) and the 95% CI was wider (0.999 to 1.105; $p = 0.065$), due a larger estimate of $\hat{\tau}^2$ (0.0001). Thus the prognostic effect of age is more uncertain than initially observed when using the original age coding. Note that, unless the means in each study are very similar, centering of covariates makes it difficult to examine non-linear prognostic associations, as one-unit deviations away from the mean correspond to different points on the non-linear curve, and so a summary curve would not be interpretable.

Further difficulties (for both one-stage and two-stage approaches) are when some studies do not have all the adjustment factors of interest (Section 16.3.6.6), when some study-specific terms are hard to estimate due to zero or few events, or when there is perfect prediction (i.e. separation of events and non-events) across patterns of covariates values,[175] which may require data augmentation or penalisation techniques to address it.[176,177] Hence, there are pros and cons to both one-stage and two-stage methods. Unless most studies are small (i.e. data are sparse), in general the two-stage approach is more convenient and practical for IPD meta-analysis of prognostic factors. For example, let us revisit the two-stage analysis of model (16.3) following by a multivariate meta-analysis of the MVD spline function. Then, the equivalent one-stage Cox model must allow for a separate baseline hazard per study (not assumed proportional across studies); adjust for a study-specific restricted cubic spline for age (with four knots positioned as described earlier); adjust for study-specific terms for stage 2 and 3; allow a restricted cubic spline term for MVD (with four knots as described earlier), and include random effects on all three MVD terms, defined by a trivariate distribution with means of zero and an unstructured covariance matrix.

$$h_{ij}(t) = h_{0i}(t)\exp\begin{pmatrix} \theta_{1i}\mathrm{MVD}_{ij}{}^{S1} + \theta_{2i}\mathrm{MVD}_{ij}{}^{S2} + \theta_{3i}\mathrm{MVD}_{ij}{}^{S3} \\ + \beta_{1i}\mathrm{age}^{S1} + \beta_{2i}\mathrm{age}^{S2} + \beta_{3i}\mathrm{age}^{S3} + \beta_{4i}\mathrm{stage2}_{ij} + \beta_{5i}\mathrm{stage3}_{ij} \end{pmatrix}$$

$$\begin{pmatrix} \theta_{1i} \\ \theta_{2i} \\ \theta_{3i} \end{pmatrix} \sim N\left(\begin{pmatrix} \theta_1 \\ \theta_2 \\ \theta_3 \end{pmatrix}, \begin{pmatrix} \tau_1^2 & \tau_{12} & \tau_{13} \\ \tau_{12} & \tau_2^2 & \tau_{23} \\ \tau_{13} & \tau_{23} & \tau_3^2 \end{pmatrix}\right) \tag{16.4}$$

This one-stage model is complex, and requires estimation of over 50 main parameters plus three between-study variances and three between-study covariances; thus, it is difficult to specify and fit in statistical software packages, and we failed to do so. In contrast, the two-stage approach (i.e. Cox model in each study, followed by multivariate meta-analysis of MVD parameter estimates) is computationally feasible and produces results within 30 seconds.

16.3.6.5 Checking the Proportional Hazards Assumption

IPD also allows researchers to check the proportional hazards assumption; that is, whether the hazard ratio for a particular factor is a constant over time. In a two-stage IPD meta-analysis, this can be achieved by pooling (e.g. in a random-effects meta-analysis akin to model (16.2)) study-specific estimates of the interaction between time and the prognostic effect of a factor; in a one-stage analysis, this could be included directly after study-specific centering of the prognostic factor to avoid aggregation bias. In their two-stage IPD meta-analysis of the effect of fibrinogen, Thompson et al. found no evidence of a non-constant HR over the 20-year follow-up period,[117] as the pooled interaction between the log hazard ratio and time was close to zero with a wide confidence interval (0.002, 95% CI: –0.007 to 0.010). Ideally, non-linearity of the interaction would also be examined.

16.3.6.6 Dealing with Missing Data and Adjustment Factors

A common problem facing IPD meta-analysis of existing observational studies is missing data for particular outcomes, index factors, or adjustment (comparator) factors of interest. Missing data can be *partially* missing data and *systematically* missing data. Partially missing data refers to when a factor (or outcome) is recorded within a study's IPD for some participants but not for others. This can be handled by applying multiple imputation within each study separately.[178,179] Systematically missing data is when a factor is not recorded at all within a study. This is a particular issue for adjustment factors, with some studies in the IPD meta-analysis having a more complete set of adjustment factors than others.[180] Systematically missing data is harder to handle, and imputation requires the borrowing of information across studies.[180–184] These issues are discussed in Chapter 18. A related issue is when the scale of measurement changes across studies (for either outcomes or factors), such that standardisation may be essential in order for any synthesis to be possible, or imputation to one particular scale.[185]

16.3.7 Examining Heterogeneity and Performing Sensitivity Analyses

As applies to all meta-analyses, it is important to quantify and report the magnitude of heterogeneity in IPD meta-analyses examining prognostic factors, for example via the estimate of τ^2 (the between-study variance),[186] or an approximate 95% prediction interval indicating the potential true prognostic effect of a factor in a new population (Chapter 5).[46,47] A visual summary of predicted trends in the studies included in the meta-analysis is also helpful. Figure 16.2(b) shows the between-study heterogeneity in the aforementioned trend between temperature and risk of accidental mortality, by plotting the shrunken study-specific curves following the multivariate meta-analysis of spline estimates.[126]

Meta-regression can be used to examine the potential (study-level) causes of heterogeneity, with the caveat that observed associations may be prone to low power and study-level confounding. For example, Gasparrini et al. used multivariate meta-regression to identify that the effect of hot temperature is, on average, higher in more northern cities ('studies') within their IPD, with a steep rise in the risk of accidental mortality after about 20 degrees.[126]

Sensitivity analyses are also important, for example removing any IPD considered at unclear or high risk of bias; removing IPD with factor/outcome measurements that are non-standard or unclear; and, for non-linear trends, changing the number (and/or position) of the knots in a spline function, or the assumed polynomial relationship. In the aforementioned MVD example, changing the number and/or position of knots did not make a noticeable difference to the summary curve.

16.3.8 Examining Small-study Effects

Chapter 9 discussed ways to examine small-study effects using funnel plots and tests of asymmetry. To illustrate this in the prognostic factor setting, Figure 16.7 provides a contour-enhanced funnel plot of the 31 studies included in the aforementioned IPD meta-analysis of Thompson et al.,[117] who evaluated the effect of fibrinogen and the rate of CVD. Hazard ratios shown are adjusted for age. Interestingly, there does seem to be some visual suggestion of small-study effects,[187] with smaller studies to the bottom right of the plot more prominent than those toward the bottom left (Debray's test: $p = 0.10$).[188] If publication-related biases are the cause of this slight asymmetry, then IPD from studies with hazard ratios close to (or less than) 1 are potentially missing, which would make the summary IPD meta-analysis result upwardly biased in favour of fibrinogen. Asymmetry may alternatively be due to other reasons, such as the play of chance or genuine differences in prognostic effects between smaller and larger studies; so the presence of small-study effects does not necessarily imply publication bias. Nevertheless, the example illustrates that – even in one of the largest and comprehensive IPD meta-analyses in existence – publication-related biases remain a slight threat.

Publication-related biases are likely less of a threat when the IPD retrieved comes from studies that had a different primary objective than examining prognostic factors. For example, the IMPACT

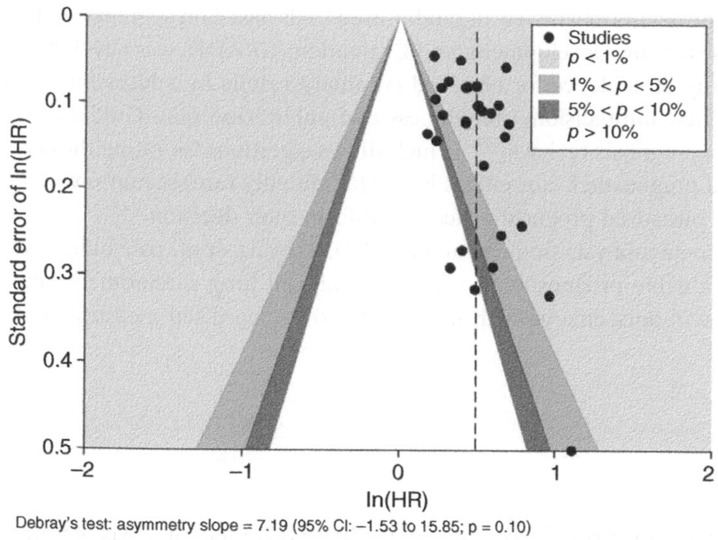

Figure 16.7 Contour-enhanced funnel plot of the 31 studies included in the meta-analysis shown within Thompson et al.,[117] evaluating the effect of a 1 g/l increase in fibrinogen on rate of CVD, adjusted for age. The dashed line shows the summary estimate of the hazard ratio (HR) obtained from a random-effects meta-analysis of the adjusted ln(HR) estimates from each study; the shaded regions reveal the p-value in each study relating to the test against the null hypothesis that the ln(HR) is zero. *Source:* Richard Riley, using data extracted from Thompson et al.[117]

collaboration retrieved most of their IPD from randomised trials examining treatment effects, which routinely record many variables at baseline (e.g. to summarise participant characteristics at baseline) and these are potential prognostic factors; any selective reporting of such trials is based on the treatment effects and not the prognostic effects of the baseline variables. Reassurance is given by Marmarou et al., who note that "part of the requirements for ABIC (the American Brain Injury Consortium) and EBIC (the European Brain Injury Consortium) when taking on a traumatic brain injury study is that the data should ultimately be made available for use in academic projects such as IMPACT."[113] For such reasons, Abo-Zaid did not identify any concerns of small-study effects in meta-analyses conducted by the IMPACT collaboration.[159] In the Trivella et al. IPD meta-analysis examining the prognostic effect of MVD,[115] publication-related biases were not a concern (Debray's test: $p = 0.69$) because "centre selection was unrelated to the findings of any research done at the centres, or to whether the centre had published their findings", and IPD from unpublished studies were obtained.

16.3.9 Reporting and Interpreting Results

To guide reporting of IPD meta-analyses of prognostic factor studies, we recommend adhering to REMARK.[145,146] These guidelines are aimed at improving the reporting of primary prognostic factor studies in cancer, but are still a good starting point for IPD meta-analyses of prognostic factors, in any clinical field, and are complemented by the reporting guidelines of MOOSE and PRISMA-IPD (Chapter 11).[189,190]

Interpretation and translation of summary meta-analysis results is an important part of reporting, and should include some discussion about if and how the prognostic factors identified may be useful in practice (i.e. translation of results to clinical practice), and what further research is necessary.

For interpreting the *certainty* of the results of a review of randomised trials based on aggregate data, Grades of Recommendation, Assessment, Development, and Evaluation (GRADE) was developed. This approach scores the certainty of evidence for obtained summary results by addressing five domains: risk of bias, inconsistency, imprecision, indirectness and publication bias. Guidance is emerging for adapting GRADE to prognosis reviews,[191,192] including suggestions for rating the certainty of evidence for unadjusted prognostic factor effects in the (admittedly rare) scenario where clinicians require a single easily measured prognostic factor to inform their decision.[193]

When interpreting their IPD meta-analysis findings about MVD, Trivella et al. conclude: "At present, that MVD can play a valuable prognostic part in non-small-cell lung carcinoma seems unlikely", and a clearer picture will only emerge with improved and standardised measurement techniques in primary studies.[116]

16.4 Software

Several statistical software packages are currently available to facilitate IPD meta-analysis of prognostic factor studies. When adopting a two-stage meta-analysis approach, the default R package *stats* provides functions for standard regression modelling in the first stage. In small samples, *logistf* (logistic regression) or *coxphf* (Cox regression) can be used to adopt the Firth bias correction. When considering modelling of non-linear effects, researchers may use *mfp* or *rms* for multivariable fractional polynomials or restricted cubic splines, respectively. In the second stage, the (multivariate) meta-analysis of (nonlinear) prognostic factor associations can then be implemented using *metafor*, *mvmeta* and several other packages (see https://cran.r-project.org/web/views/MetaAnalysis.html for more details).

In Stata, *ipdmetan* can be used to perform a two-stage IPD meta-analysis of a linear prognostic effect.[194] To model non-linear prognostic effects, the two stages of a multivariate meta-analysis can be implemented using the package *mvmeta*, which includes *mvmeta_make*.[176,177] In the first stage, *mfp* can be used to fit multivariable fractional polynomials, or *mkspline* used to create spline terms; the non-linear associations can be fitted and stored using *mveta_make*. In the second stage, multivariate meta-analysis can be used to combine non-linear associations via *mvmeta*.

When adopting a one-stage meta-analysis approach, it is common to use generalized linear mixed models (Chapter 6). Many of these models can be extended to include non-linear trends via fractional polynomials, splines, or generalised additive models. For instance, in R, the packages *splines*, *gamm4* and *mgcv* can be used to add non-linear terms to a mixed effects regression model (e.g. estimated using the package *lme4*). Also, *lmeSplines*, *sme*, *mgcv* and *pammtools* may be useful.

Finally, the presence of selective reporting and publication bias can be evaluated in R using several packages, including *metamisc*, *meta* and *metafor*. In Stata, this can be achieved using the packages *metabias* and *confunnel*, for example.

16.5 Concluding Remarks

Most meta-analysis projects aiming to identify prognostic factors would benefit from using IPD, and this chapter provides a guide for researchers embarking on such an endeavour. As shown in our examples, IPD meta-analysis projects have considerable advantages and can lead to novel findings. Some challenges may still exist, such as missing adjustment factors in some studies and differences in study measurement methods for outcomes or factors. To improve projects further, we encourage a more prospective approach to IPD meta-analysis of prognostic factor studies.[195] Enabling this requires research groups to collaborate at the onset of their work, to ensure their new studies are high-quality and comparable (e.g. in terms of the factors assessed, outcomes recorded, and methods of measurement) so that, upon completion, they can be immediately pooled in an IPD meta-analysis. Reductions in heterogeneity and methodological challenges are then expected compared to a retrospective IPD meta-analysis, which may speed up the identification of genuine prognostic factors.

During this chapter we focussed on using IPD meta-analysis to examine prognostic factors. Our proposed steps are very similar when examining risk factors (i.e. factors in healthy individuals associated with future outcome risk). Clearly the distinction between risk and prognostic factors is almost artificial, as both aim to summarise a factor-outcome relationship, ideally adjusted. To many, the key difference is that risk factor research is usually focused more on establishing causality (i.e. the factor causes the outcome), for which more detailed consideration of issues such as adjustment for confounding, measurement error and biological mechanisms is warranted.

Occasionally researchers may aim to compare the adjusted prognostic value of multiple prognostic factors, for example, to conclude whether the summary adjusted hazard ratio of factor A is larger than that for factor B. Researchers should restrict comparisons of the adjusted prognostic value of two or more index factors to those IPD studies that measured them both. When there are different scales and distributions of each factor (e.g. continuous or binary), a simple comparison of the prognostic effect sizes (e.g. hazard ratio for factor A versus hazard ratio for factor B) may not be straightforward or sufficient. How index factors add value in terms of improvement in risk classification, predictive performance, and clinical utility is also important.[72,78,196–198] Often this needs to be considered in the context of clinical prediction models, which are the focus of the next chapter.[78,129,199]

17

IPD Meta-Analysis for Clinical Prediction Model Research

Richard D. Riley, Kym I.E. Snell, Laure Wynants, Valentijn M.T. de Jong, Karel G.M. Moons, and Thomas P.A. Debray

Summary Points

- IPD meta-analysis projects offer novel opportunities for the development and validation of clinical prediction models that aid the management of individuals in terms of diagnosis and prognosis.
- Careful steps are required to identify, obtain and clean IPD from relevant studies or data sources.
- Before obtaining IPD, a data extraction phase is helpful to obtain relevant information from each study, to help researchers decide on their inclusion and whether IPD should be sought. Items from the CHARMS checklist should be used.
- The eligibility and risk of bias of IPD from identified studies can be checked, using items from the PROBAST tools, both before and after IPD retrieval.
- For existing models, an IPD meta-analysis may allow their performance to be externally validated across different populations, subgroups and settings.
- Performance can be evaluated using univariate and multivariate meta-analysis models that summarise either calibration and discrimination of model predictions or clinical utility in terms of net benefit. It is important to summarise not only average performance, but also heterogeneity in performance, and so random-effects meta-analysis models are required.
- Often existing models show poor predictive performance when tested or applied in other populations or settings than those used for model development. In this situation, IPD meta-analysis may allow researchers to update or tailor the existing model equation to improve performance in particular populations or settings.
- Sometimes IPD meta-analysis may be needed to develop an entirely new model. Then, suitable methods for model development are required, such as penalised estimation to adjust for overfitting. Generalisability of the model's predictive performance can be examined using an approach called internal-external cross-validation.
- IPD meta-analysis methods for prediction model research are also applicable to other datasets involving clustering, including those from electronic healthcare records.
- The TRIPOD-CLUSTER statement should be adhered to when reporting results from IPD meta-analysis projects for clinical prediction model research.

Individual Participant Data Meta-Analysis: A Handbook for Healthcare Research, First Edition.
Edited by Richard D. Riley, Jayne F. Tierney, and Lesley A. Stewart.

17.1 Introduction

Clinical prediction models are needed to inform an individual's current health state and whether they are at risk of adverse outcomes in the future. A diagnostic prediction model estimates an individual's probability that an outcome (e.g. disease) is already present, whereas a prognostic prediction model estimates an individual's probability that an outcome (e.g. death) will occur in the future (e.g. within six months).[85,130,158,200–203] Related names for clinical prediction models include risk models, prognostic scores, and clinical decision rules. They are typically developed using a multivariable regression framework. This provides an equation to estimate an individual's probability of having or developing an outcome based on his/her values of multiple factors (predictors), including basic current information (e.g. age, gender, BMI), previous events (e.g. medical and family history), physical examination (e.g. blood pressure) and clinical measurements from such as imaging, electrophysiology, and biomarkers within blood, urine and genetic information. Thus, unlike Chapter 16, which focused on the prognostic value of a *single* factor (e.g. in terms of odds ratio or hazard ratio estimates), clinical prediction models utilise multiple factors ('predictors') in combination, and focus on estimates of absolute outcome probability.

Box 17.1 gives the typical format of prediction models equations derived using a logistic or Cox regression framework, which involve an intercept or baseline hazard term combined with multiple predictor effects (corresponding to log odds or hazard ratios). Well-known examples are the Framingham risk score and QRISK2,[86,204] which estimate the 10-year risk of developing cardiovascular disease; the Nottingham Prognostic Index, which predicts the 5-year survival probability of a woman with newly diagnosed breast cancer;[205,206] and the Wells score for predicting the presence of pulmonary embolism.[207,208]

In this chapter we describe the opportunities and challenges involved in prediction model research using IPD meta-analysis. We begin by outlining the various types of prediction model research, and then describe the importance and conduct of IPD meta-analysis projects for each type. This includes external validation of existing models, comparison of multiple models, and development of new models. Throughout we emphasise the importance of evaluating prediction model performance in terms of calibration, discrimination and clinical utility, and the need to examine heterogeneity in performance across studies, settings and subgroups of interest.

17.2 IPD Meta-Analysis for Prediction Model Research

17.2.1 Types of Prediction Model Research

In 2009 the *BMJ* published a series of four articles to guide those undertaking prediction model research,[200,210–212] and further recommendations were made in the 2013 PROGRESS series and related textbook.[85,88,127,130,213] These all emphasise three fundamental components of prediction model research: *model development* (including internal validation), *external validation*, and model *impact evaluation*. Model development is the process that leads to the final prediction equation (Box 17.1), and involves many aspects detailed extensively elsewhere,[85,158,210,214,215] such as the study design, sampling of study participants, data collection, definition and measurement of predictors and outcomes, handling of continuous predictors and missing data, specification of the baseline risk (hazard rate), adjustment for overfitting using penalisation (shrinkage) techniques, and internal validation to examine and adjust for optimism. External validation uses new participant-level data, external to that used for model development, to examine whether the model's

Box 17.1 Typical format of prediction models developed using IPD from a single study.

i) **Diagnostic or short-term prognostic prediction models**

Where the aim is to predict outcome presence (for a diagnostic prediction model) or outcome occurrence in a relatively short time period (e.g. for a prognostic prediction model of mortality within 30 days), researchers typically use logistic regression to develop their prediction model. Let the jth participant's response Y_j be defined by 0 for those without the outcome (no event) or 1 for those with the outcome (event). Then a logistic regression model is of the form:

$$Y_j \sim \text{Bernoulli}\left(p_j\right)$$

$$\ln\left(\frac{p_j}{1-p_j}\right) = \alpha + \beta_1 x_{1j} + \beta_2 x_{2j} + \beta_3 x_{3j} + \ldots + \beta_k x_{kj}$$

Here p_j is the probability of having/developing the outcome, $\ln\left(\frac{p_j}{1-p_j}\right)$ is the log-odds of the disease or outcome, the intercept term α is the baseline log-odds (where 'baseline' refers to participants whose x values are all zero), each x term denotes values of included predictors (e.g. x_1 could be the age of the patient in years, x_2 could be 1 for males and 0 for females, and so on), and each β denotes the change in log-odds (or the log-odds ratio) for each one-unit increase in the corresponding predictor (e.g. β_1 is the increase in the log-odds for each one-year increase in age, and β_2 is the increase in the log-odds for a male compared to a female, and so on). The predicted outcome probability for a new individual (that is, the probability that $Y_j = 1$ conditional on the individual's predictor values and the fitted regression equation) are denoted by $\hat{p}_j$, and obtained by inputting their predictor values into the equation and back-transforming to the probability scale:

$$\hat{p}_j = \frac{\exp\left(\hat{\alpha} + \hat{\beta}_1 x_{1j} + \hat{\beta}_2 x_{2j} + \hat{\beta}_3 x_{3j} + \ldots + \hat{\beta}_k x_{kj}\right)}{1 + \exp\left(\hat{\alpha} + \hat{\beta}_1 x_{1j} + \hat{\beta}_2 x_{2j} + \hat{\beta}_3 x_{3j} + \ldots + \hat{\beta}_k x_{kj}\right)}$$

ii) **Prognostic prediction models over a longer period of time**

Survival models are needed when outcome probability is to be predicted at multiple times and/or when some participants are censored before a key time-point (e.g. when predicting mortality risk by 10 years, some participants in the development dataset may be lost to follow-up before 10 years). In particular, a Cox regression model or a parametric survival model can be fitted, which is typically of the form

$$h_j(t) = h_0(t)\exp\left(\beta_1 x_{1j} + \beta_2 x_{2j} + \beta_3 x_{3j} + \ldots + \beta_k x_{kj}\right)$$

Here $h(t)$ is the hazard rate of the outcome at time t, the intercept term $h_0(t)$ is the baseline hazard rate (where 'baseline' refers to participants whose x values are all zero), the x terms denote values of included predictors, and each β denotes the change in log hazard rate (i.e. the log hazard ratio) for each one-unit increase in the corresponding predictor. The predicted probability of the outcome occurring by time t for a new individual is denoted by $1-\hat{S}_j(t)$, and obtained by inputting their predictor values into the equation and back-transforming to the probability scale:

$$1 - \hat{S}_j(t) = 1 - \hat{S}_0(t)^{\exp\left(\hat{\beta}_1 x_{1j} + \hat{\beta}_2 x_{2j} + \hat{\beta}_3 x_{3j} + \ldots + \hat{\beta}_k x_{kj}\right)}$$

where $S_0(t)$ is the cumulative baseline survival probability until time t (where 'baseline' refers to participants whose x values are all zero).

Source: Figure adapted from Figure 1 of Riley et al.,[209] with permission,

predictions are reliable (i.e. accurate enough) in participants from population(s) where the model may be applied.[130,216,217] Model impact studies evaluate, ideally using a randomised trial design, whether implementing and using a prediction model in practice actually improves patient outcomes (and is cost-effective) compared to settings where the model is not used. For example, improvements may arise due to enhanced patient management decisions (including treatment and monitoring decisions) for individuals according to their predicted outcome probabilities from the model.

Unfortunately, most prediction research focuses on model development, whilst model validation and, in particular, model impact studies are far less frequent.[130,218–220] This leads to a plethora of proposed models in all medical domains and settings, with very little evidence about which models are reliable and under what circumstances. Confusion then ensues: promising models are often quickly forgotten,[221] and, of more concern, many models may be used or advocated without appropriate examination of their performance in other participants and settings.[222]

17.2.2 Why IPD Meta-Analyses Are Needed

Box 17.2 gives examples of why IPD meta-analyses are needed for prediction model research.[223–229] In particular, a shortage of (external) validation studies is often attributed to the lack of data available besides that used for model development. An IPD meta-analysis project directly addresses this concern, as it allows researchers to immediately validate their developed prediction model on multiple occasions (e.g. in each study included in the IPD meta-analysis project), and to check whether model predictions are sufficiently accurate across different locations, settings, and subgroups (case-mix). Ideally, a model's predictive performance will be acceptable on average, and also acceptable across the different subgroups, populations and settings available in the IPD meta-analysis dataset.[209] However, often model performance is heterogeneous and may be inadequate in some situations. Then, rather than simply discarding the entire model outright, an IPD meta-analysis enables model updating strategies to be evaluated, such as recalibration of the model's intercept or predictor effects to tailor them to the populations, settings or subgroups where the original model's performance was inadequate.[230] IPD meta-analysis also allows the benefit of adding a novel predictor to an existing model to be examined across the included studies,[199] for example in terms of clinical utility,[78] or measures of calibration, discrimination and goodness-of-fit.[199,231] When developing an entirely new model, a major advantage of an IPD meta-analysis project (compared to a single model development study) is the larger sample size with increased outcome events,[53] thereby reducing the potential for overfitting and improving the robustness of predictions in new individuals. An example of the above advantages of IPD meta-analysis in prediction model research is the IMPACT consortium which developed a prediction model for mortality and unfavourable outcome in traumatic brain injury by sharing IPD from 11 studies (8,509 participants), with validation of the developed model then performed using IPD from another large study (6,681 participants).[132]

Without IPD, meta-analysis requires the use of aggregate data (from publications or study investigators), but this is problematic for prediction model research. For example, when externally validating an existing model, IPD allows the researcher to apply the model's equation and estimate predictive performance directly. Without IPD, meta-analysis requires suitable study aggregate data that quantifies a model's predictive performance, but key measures (e.g. calibration statistics, confidence intervals) are often missing, such that methods to indirectly estimate them are needed.[129] Development of a new prediction model is also severely restricted without IPD, as when using aggregate data the researcher would require parameter estimates (and their variances and

Box 17.2 Examples of IPD meta-analyses in prediction model research.[223–229]

- When a single (previously published) prediction model is available, an IPD meta-analysis may aim to:
  - Validate and summarize the model's performance across various other study populations, settings and domains. For example, Geersing and colleagues used an IPD meta-analysis to examine the predictive performance of the Wells rule for diagnosing deep venous thrombosis (DVT) across different subgroups of suspected DVT patients.[223]
  - Tailor (update) the model to specific populations or settings. For instance, Majed and colleagues evaluated whether the calibration of the Framingham risk equation for coronary heart disease and stroke improved by applying model adjustments tailored to different settings.[224]
  - Examine the value of adding a specific predictor (e.g. biomarker) to the model, in terms of improvement in predictive performance across different study populations, settings and domains. For example, an IPD meta-analysis was performed to summarise the added value of common carotid intima-media thickness (CIMT) in 10-year risk prediction of first-time myocardial infarctions or strokes in the general population, above that of the Framingham risk score.[225]
- When various competing prediction models are available that were developed for the same target population or the same outcome across various study populations, an IPD meta-analysis may aim to:
  - Compare the models' performance across various study populations, settings and domains. For instance, an IPD meta-analysis was used to validate and compare all non-invasive risk scores for the prediction of developing type 2 diabetes in participants from the general population.[226]
  - Combine the most promising models and adjust them to specific study populations, settings and domains. This approach is illustrated by Debray and colleagues, who validated and updated all existing diagnostic models for predicting the presence of DVT across different settings, and proceeded to combine them into a single meta-model.[227,228]
- Finally, when no existing prediction models are available, an IPD meta-analysis can be used to develop and directly validate a new prediction model using the IPD from all relevant studies. An example is the development of the prognostic PHASES score for prediction of risk of rupture of intra-cranial aneurysms in patients with aneurysms but without any treatment.[229]

Source: Richard Riley.

correlations) from each of multiple studies that fit exactly the same model equation, which is highly unlikely.

As described in Chapters 2 to 4, availability of IPD also enhances risk of bias assessments (i.e. quality assessments of the conducted study and collected data), helps to standardise inclusion criteria, follow-up times and outcome/predictor definitions across studies, and enables examination of subgroups and multiple time-points. Relevant IPD for prediction model research may also be obtainable from studies that originally had a different purpose (e.g. a randomised trial to examine a treatment effect[151]), and thus allows greater utilisation of existing research data.

Alongside the potential advantages, methodological challenges may also arise for IPD meta-analyses for prediction model research,[19–21] and these are similar to those challenges detailed in

Chapter 16 for prognostic factor research. In particular, missing values of predictors or outcomes are likely in some participants, and some predictors may even be systematically missing, which occurs when a predictor is not measured for any participants in one or more studies (Chapter 18). Between-study heterogeneity is also likely, for example in the outcome definition, methods of predictor measurement, the length of follow-up, the timing of predictor measurement, and the quality of available datasets.

17.2.3 Key Steps Involved in an IPD Meta-Analysis for Prediction Model Research

Many of the steps within IPD meta-analysis projects for prediction model research are akin to those described within previous chapters, including Chapters 3 and 4, and Chapter 16 on prognostic factor research. Some steps are the same as when doing a systematic review and meta-analysis using aggregate data.[129] A brief summary of key steps is now provided, but we note that the steps are not necessarily linear, and some (e.g. risk of bias and eligibility assessments) will often be updated after obtaining IPD.

17.2.3.1 Define the Research Question and PICOTS System

A crucial step is to define the prediction model research question (Box 17.2) and outline an associated PICOTS system (population, index model, comparator, outcome, timing and setting). An example is given in Box 17.3.[129] This step is mandatory for the next step, to identify the primary studies or even simply the available datasets that are eligible for inclusion in the IPD meta-analysis project.

17.2.3.2 Identify Relevant Existing Studies and Datasets

The identification of potentially relevant studies should be done via a systematic search. Typically broad search and selection filters are required, combining terms related to prediction research (such as diagnostic, prognostic, prediction, model, score, tool, etc.) with domain- or disease-specific terms (such as the name of the prediction model and the targeted disease or patient population).[135] Aside from published studies of prediction models, relevant IPD may also come from other published studies, such as randomised trials or those using registries or electronic-healthcare databases. Relevant IPD may even be available from cohort studies or routinely collected databases without any corresponding publications. Such issues were discussed for prognostic factor research (Chapter 16). Therefore, the IPD meta-analysis project team need a broad perspective of the potentially relevant IPD. This further motivates establishing a collaborative group, where researchers in the field are encouraged to join and ultimately provide any relevant IPD (regardless of whether it corresponds to a published or unpublished study) containing key predictors and outcomes of interest.

17.2.3.3 Examine Eligibility and Risk of Bias of IPD

In the third step, after potentially relevant IPD are identified, it is fundamental for the quality of the IPD to be examined. A dataset being large does not imply it is of high quality; *actually, the opposite may be true*. Many existing datasets that can be used for prediction model research were collected for other purposes (e.g. randomised trials) or contain routinely recorded information (e.g. e-health records), which may suffer from more problems than a prospectively planned study specifically designed to address a prediction model question. Furthermore, even though a high-quality dataset is available, it may not be applicable to the research question or population of interest (i.e. it does not meet eligibility criteria). Researchers must therefore undertake comprehensive data quality and eligibility checks before including a particular dataset in their IPD meta-analysis project. For this

Box 17.3 The PICOTS system to help define the research question for IPD meta-analysis projects aiming to develop, validate or update prediction models, as illustrated using a systematic review and meta-analysis by Debray et al.[129] of the predictive performance of the EuroSCORE model to predict short-term mortality in patients who underwent coronary artery bypass grafting (CABG).

- Population: define the target population in which the prediction model will be used.
  - In the Debray review, the population of interest comprised patients undergoing CABG.
- Index model: define any existing prediction model that is of primary interest (e.g. for external validation or updating of a particular existing model), or whether a new prediction model will be developed.
  - In the Debray review, the focus was on external validation of the previously developed prognostic EuroSCORE model.
- Comparator (i.e. alternative/competing model): when developing a new model or validating a particular existing model (the defined index models), one may want to compare to another existing model for the target population.
  - In the Debray review, no alternative prognostic models were considered.
- Outcome: define the exact outcome(s) of interest for which the index model under review is supposed to (help) predict.
  - In the Debray review, the outcome was defined as all-cause mortality.
- Timing: This includes defining two time-points: (i) the time-point(s) at which the index model is to be used (so-called prediction time zero or the startpoint), and (ii) the time-point (or time period) at (or over which) the outcome probability is to be predicted.
  - In the Debray review, the EUROSCORE model was validated for its predictive ability when used just before the cardiac surgical procedure, and for predictions of all-cause mortality at 30 days.
- Setting: define the intended role or setting of the prediction model under review.
  - In the Debray review, the originally intended use of the EuroSCORE model was to perform preoperative risk stratification in secondary- and tertiary-care patients scheduled for cardiac surgery to predict short-term all-cause mortality, to determine which patients may need extra perioperative and postoperative surveillance or management.

Source: Figure adapted from Box 1 in Debray et al.,[129] with permission, © 2017 BMJ Publishing Group.

purpose we recommend using the PROBAST tool (Prediction model Risk Of Bias Assessment Tool: www.probast.org). PROBAST includes three signalling questions for examining a study's applicability to the research question, and these can be used to help classify concerns about whether IPD are eligible for the IPD meta-analysis project:[141,142]

- Is there concern that the included participants and setting do not match the IPD meta-analysis research question (as defined in Box 17.3)?
- Is there concern that the definition, assessment or timing of predictors in the model do not match the research question?
- Is there concern that the outcome, its definition, timing or determination do not match the research question?

Table 17.1 Domains and signalling questions within the first three domains of the PROBAST tool (Prediction model Risk Of Bias Assessment Tool).[141,142], which may be used to examine the quality of IPD from each study or dataset contributing to the IPD meta-analysis project for prediction model research.

Domain 1: Participant selection
1.1 Were appropriate data sources used, e.g. cohort or RCT for prognostic prediction model research, or cross-sectional study for diagnostic prediction model research?
1.2 Were all inclusions and exclusions of participants appropriate?*

Domain 2: Predictors
2.1 Were predictors defined and assessed in a similar way for all participants?
2.2 Were predictor assessments made without knowledge of outcome data?
2.3 Are all predictors available at the time the model is intended to be used?

Domain 3: Outcome
3.1 Was the outcome determined appropriately?
3.2 Was a pre-specified or standard outcome definition used?
3.3 Were predictors excluded from the outcome definition?
3.4 Was the outcome defined and determined in a similar way for all participants?
3.5 Was the outcome determined without knowledge of predictor information?
3.6 Was the time interval between predictor assessment and outcome determination appropriate?

* Availability of IPD may reduce this concern. For example, it may allow the re-inclusion of participants previously discarded from a study's original analysis; or it may allow a subset of participants to be identified which (compared to the full dataset) more closely match the intended population of interest for risk prediction. However, IPD will not overcome any inappropriate exclusion of participants from a study's original sampling frame.

Source: Table presents the first three domains of PROBAST freely available at http://www.probast.org/. The PROBAST domains were originally published by Wolff et al. and Moons et al.,[141,142] © 2019 The American College of Physicians.

In addition, PROBAST provides a comprehensive checklist for examining a study's risk of bias.[141,142] This includes four domains: Participant Selection, Predictors, Outcome, and Analysis. Each domain contains signalling questions phrased so that "yes" indicates absence of bias. The first three domains are relevant to IPD meta-analysis projects (Table 17.1), and can be used to determine whether the IPD to be received (from a particular study or dataset) is at low, high or unclear risk of bias.

To help apply PROBAST, and thus decide upon eligibility and bias classifications, it is useful to obtain (extract) detailed information about each study or dataset potentially providing their IPD. Elements of the CHARMS checklist are helpful for this purpose,[128] as shown in Table 17.2, and the required information may be extracted from study publications or associated reports, or obtained from study investigators or database holders directly. Risk of bias and eligibility decisions should be refined and updated after IPD are received, as the IPD itself may reveal new information (e.g. about follow-up lengths, predictor and outcome measurements, etc) (Chapter 4).

17.2.3.4 Obtain, Harmonise and Summarise IPD

A potentially lengthy process may be needed to actually obtain, clean and harmonise the IPD that was identified (from previous steps) of sufficient quality and applicable to the IPD meta-analysis research question. We refer the reader to Chapter 4 for more details. After harmonisation, the IPD for each study (or data source) should be summarised, for example in terms of setting, dates, length of follow-up, and average participant characteristics, so that any heterogeneity across datasets (e.g. in case-mix) can be captured.

Table 17.2 Selected items from the CHARMS checklist to be extracted when identifying, appraising (e.g. for applicability and risk of bias) and considering studies (or datasets) for inclusion in an IPD meta-analysis project for prediction model research.[128]

Domain	Key items
Source of data	Source of data (e.g., cohort, case-control, randomised trial participants, or registry data)
Participants	Participant eligibility and recruitment method (e.g., consecutive participants, location, number of centres, setting, inclusion and exclusion criteria)
	Participant description
	Details of treatments received, if relevant
	Study dates
Outcome(s) to be predicted	Definition and method for measurement of outcome
	Was the same outcome definition (and method for measurement) used in all patients?
	Type of outcome (e.g., single or combined endpoints)
	Was the outcome assessed without knowledge of the candidate predictors (i.e., blinded)?
	Were candidate predictors part of the outcome (e.g., in panel or consensus diagnosis)?
	Time of outcome occurrence or summary of duration of follow-up
Candidate predictors	What predictors (e.g., demographics, patient history, physical examination, additional testing, disease characteristics) are available?
	Definition and method for measurement of candidate predictors
	Timing of predictor measurement (e.g., at patient presentation, at diagnosis, at treatment initiation)
	Were predictors assessed blinded for outcome, and for each other (if relevant)?
Sample size	Number of participants and number of outcomes/events
	Number of outcomes/events in relation to the number of candidate predictors (events per variable)
Missing data	Number of participants with any missing value (include predictors and outcomes)
	Number of participants with missing data for each predictor

Source: Table presents items from the CHARMS checklist published by Moons et al.,[128] with permission,

17.2.3.5 Undertake Meta-Analysis and Quantify Heterogeneity

Using the harmonised IPD, statistical methods for IPD meta-analysis can be applied to address the research question of interest. This forms the focus of the remainder of this chapter, beginning with IPD meta-analysis methods to externally validate an existing model.

17.3 External Validation of an Existing Prediction Model Using IPD Meta-Analysis

Before considering the development of a new model, IPD meta-analysis projects should aim to externally validate the predictive performance of any existing models. As predictive performance can be measured in many ways, this section begins by describing the key measures and their interpretation in a single study. Then, we extend to the IPD meta-analysis setting, by introducing appropriate statistical methods for meta-analysis that allow for between-study heterogeneity in performance.

17.3.1 Measures of Predictive Performance in a Single Study

17.3.1.1 Overall Measures of Model Fit

Overall performance of a prediction model for a continuous outcome is quantified by R^2, the proportion of the total variance of outcome values that is explained by the model, with values closer to 1 preferred. Often this is multiplied by 100, to give the percentage of variation explained. Generalisations of R^2 for binary or time-to-event outcomes have also been proposed, such as the Cox-Snell R^2,[232] Nagelkerke's R^2,[233] O'Quigley's R^2,[234] Royston's R^2,[196] and Royston and Sauerbrei's R^2_D.[197] Another overall measure of fit is the mean-squared error of predictions (also known as the Brier score[235]). In Section 17.8 we also introduce the net benefit measure, to summarise the overall benefit of using the prediction model to inform decision-making.[72,73]

17.3.1.2 Calibration Plots and Measures

Calibration examines the agreement between predicted and observed outcome values (for linear regression models) or between predicted and observed outcome probabilities (for logistic and time-to-event regression models). It should be examined across the whole spectrum of predicted values or probabilities, and at each relevant time-point (for time-to-event models). Fundamentally, calibration should be visualised graphically, using calibration plots. For binary or time-to-event outcomes, a calibration plot should display observed versus predicted probabilities (e.g. across tenths of predicted probability[211]) and include a smoothed non-linear curve generated using a loess smoother or splines.[211,236] It is helpful to add the distribution of the predicted probability values underneath the calibration plot, to show the spread of expected risk in the dataset at hand. Examples are given later in the chapter (e.g. Figure 17.9). For time-to-event outcomes, it is also helpful to display observed and predicted survival curves over time for, say, four or five groups defined by categories of the linear predictor (i.e. by categorising values of $\hat{\beta}_1 x_{1j} + \hat{\beta}_2 x_{2j} + \hat{\beta}_3 x_{3j} + \ldots + \hat{\beta}_k x_{kj}$).[237]

Figure 17.1 illustrates various types of (mis)calibration for a prediction model based on logistic regression for a binary outcome.[85] Calibration can also be quantified by statistical measures including the calibration slope (ideal value of 1), calibration-in-the-large (ideal value of 0), and the observed/expected ratio (O/E, ideal value of 1) or conversely the E/O ratio (Box 17.4). Such measures should be reported with confidence intervals, and derived for the dataset as a whole and, ideally, also for relevant subgroups. Another option is the Estimated (ECI) or Integrated (ICI) Calibration Index, which respectively measure an average of the squared or absolute differences between predicted probabilities from the model and observed probabilities from a calibration curve.[238,239] Calibration should not be quantified using the Hosmer-Lemeshow test,[240] as this requires arbitrary grouping of participants which can influence the calculated p-value, and does not quantify the actual magnitude of any miscalibration.

17.3.1.3 Discrimination Measures

Discrimination refers to how well a model's predictions separate between two groups of participants: those who have (or develop) the outcome and those who do not have (or do not develop) the outcome. Therefore it is most relevant for prediction models of binary and time-to-event outcomes, and not continuous outcomes. The range of observed probabilities on a calibration plot (e.g. separation of mean observed probability across groups defined by tenths of predicted probabilities)

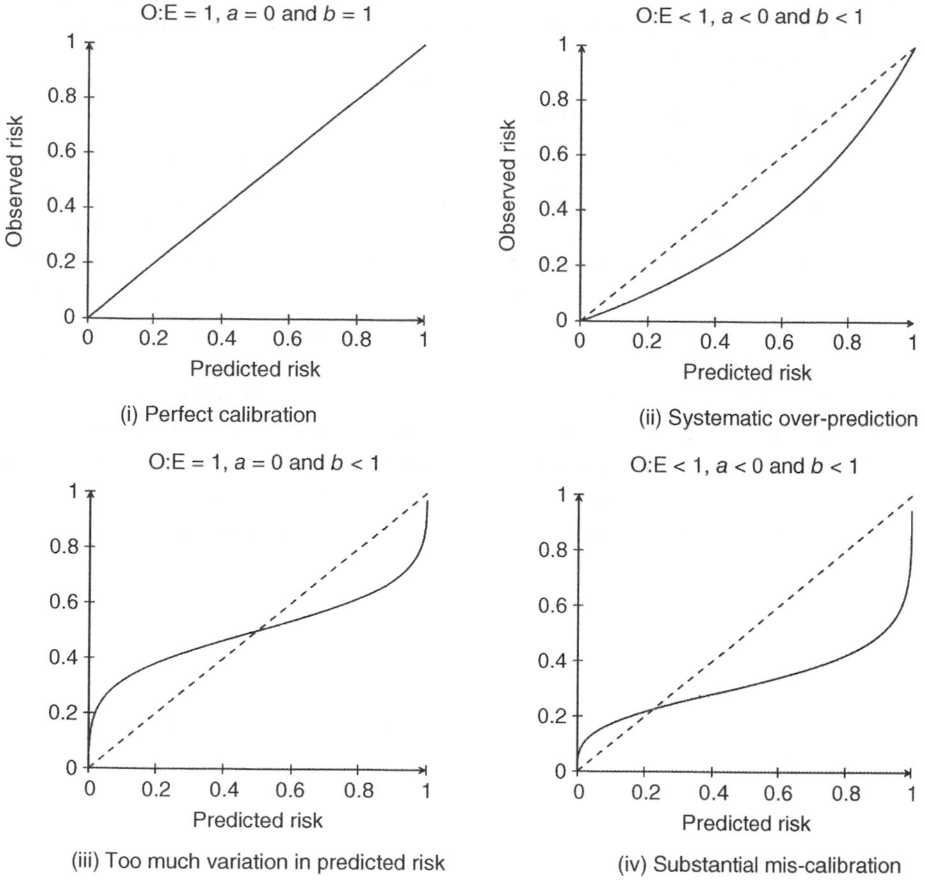

Figure 17.1 Examples of the calibration performance of a logistic regression prediction model for a binary outcome as examined in a single study. O:E = ratio of observed versus expected probability (risk). a = calibration-in-the-large, as calculated on the logit scale; b = calibration slope, as calculated on the logit scale. Note that in (ii), the calibration slope is 1 on the logit scale, but becomes curved when presented on the risk scale shown. *Source:* Richard Riley.

hints at the discrimination performance, as the more separated the probability groups then the better the model discriminates.

Discrimination is formally measured by the concordance (C) statistic (index),[158,241] and a value of 1 indicates the model has perfect discrimination, whilst a value of 0.5 indicates the model discriminates no better than chance. For binary outcomes, it is equivalent to the area under the receiver operating characteristic (ROC) curve. It gives the probability that for any randomly selected pair of participants, one with and one without the outcome, the model assigns a higher probability to the participant with the outcome. Generalisations of the C statistic have been proposed for time-to-event models, most notably Harrell's C statistic.[241,242] This is the proportion (ranging also from 0.5 to 1) of all possible pairs of study participants in which the participant with the higher predicted survival probability actually survived longer than the other participant.[241] The following pairs cannot be ordered and therefore are not included in the calculation of Harrell's C statistic: (i) pairs in which both participants are censored before outcome occurrence, (ii) pairs in which both participants have the outcome at the same time, or (iii) pairs in which one participant is censored at an

Box 17.4 Explanation of some key measures for calibration of a prediction model with binary or time-to-event outcomes

Observed/Expected number of outcomes (O/E)

O/E summarises the overall calibration. For binary outcomes, it provides the ratio of the total observed to have the outcome in a certain time period over the total expected to have the outcome in that same period. Thus an ideal value is 1. Values less than 1 indicate the model is over-predicting the total number of outcomes in the population, whilst values above 1 indicate the model is under-predicting the total number of outcomes in the population. For time-to-event outcomes, mean observed and expected probabilities at a specified time-point can be used instead of total numbers of outcomes to account for censoring. Sometimes, in addition to looking at O/E across the entire dataset, O/E is reported for groups of predicted probability (for example, by tenths of predicted probability). The O/E ratios then also give an indication of the shape of the calibration slope. Note also that sometimes the E/O ratio is presented; under-prediction then occurs for values below 1 and over-prediction for values above 1. For continuous outcomes, an analogous measure of the O/E ratio is the mean predicted outcome value compared to the mean observed outcome value.

Calibration-in-the-large

Calibration-in-the-large is closely related to the overall O/E statistic,[203] but less intuitive to interpret. For binary outcomes, it can be estimated by fitting a logistic model for the probability of the outcome (p_j) with participants' linear predictor value from the developed model (i.e. $LP_j = \hat{\alpha} + \hat{\beta}_1 x_{1j} + \hat{\beta}_2 x_{2j} + \hat{\beta}_3 x_{3j} + \ldots + \hat{\beta}_k x_{kj}$) as a single covariate (offset term),

$$\text{logit}\left(p_j\right) = \alpha + 1\left(LP_j\right) \tag{17.1}$$

where the estimate of α is the estimate of calibration-in-the-large.[203] Calibration-in-the-large should be close to zero for a well calibrated model. Importantly, calibration-in-the-large may be zero and O/E may be 1 even when there is still substantial miscalibration; that is, on average predictions may appear well calibrated, but there can be under-prediction in some predicted probability ranges which cancels out over-prediction (or vice versa) in other ranges, hence stressing the need for always providing calibration plots in combination with these calibration statistical measures.

Calibration slope

The calibration slope is one measure of agreement between observed and predicted probability of the outcome across the whole range of predicted probabilities.[158,203] When a model is developed using traditional estimation techniques (e.g. unpenalised maximum likelihood estimation), the observed calibration slope will always be 1 in the development dataset. However, upon validation in new data, it may often deviate from 1. A slope < 1 indicates that in some probability ranges (which can directly be viewed from the calibration plot) the model predictions are too extreme (i.e. predictions close to 1 are too high, and predictions close to 0 are too low) and a slope > 1 indicates that model predictions are too narrow (i.e. predictions close to 1 are too low, and predictions close to 0 are too high). A calibration slope < 1 is often observed in external validation studies, consistent with a lack of adjustment for over-fitting (optimism) of the model when it was developed.

To estimate the calibration slope, a model must be fitted in the validation dataset in a similar way as above for the calibration-in-the-large. For binary outcomes, it can be estimated using a logistic regression model with the logit of the observed probability of the outcome (p_j) regressed against the linear predictor (LP_j) value as single covariate: $\text{logit}(p_j) = \alpha + \beta LP_j$. Then, $\hat{\beta}$ is the estimated calibration slope. The calibration slope is derived using the *LP* for each participant and does not require grouping.

Note that systematic over- or under-prediction is still possible even when the calibration slope is 1, and thus it is important to consider *both* O/E (or calibration-in-the-large) and calibration slope to better assess calibration performance, always alongside calibration plots. Similarly for time-to-event outcomes, the magnitude of the baseline hazard ($h_0(t)$) may not be appropriate, even if the calibration slope is 1.

Source: Richard Riley.

earlier time than the other participant's outcome occurrence time. The *C* statistic will usually depend on the length of follow-up. Different variants of the concordance statistic are Efron's estimator, Uno's estimator, and Gönen and Heller's estimator.[242] For survival models, the *C* statistic can be calculated overall or at each of multiple time-points.[243] Case-mix-adjusted *C* statistics are also available, and discussed in Section 17.3.2.

Another discrimination measure is Somer's D, which equals $(C - 0.5)/0.5$, and the discrimination slope, which is defined as the mean probability for participants with the outcome minus the mean probability for participants without the outcome,[244] and ranges from 0 (no discrimination) to 1 (perfect discrimination). For time-to-event outcomes Royston's *D* statistic is also useful,[197] as it is interpreted as the log hazard ratio comparing low- and high-risk groups, where these two equally sized groups are defined by dichotomising at the median value of the linear predictor (i.e. $\hat{\beta}_1 x_{1j} + \hat{\beta}_2 x_{2j} + \hat{\beta}_3 x_{3j} + \ldots + \hat{\beta}_k x_{kj}$) from the developed model. Higher values for the *D* statistic indicate greater discrimination.

17.3.2 Potential for Heterogeneity in a Model's Predictive Performance

Single external validation studies often use one local dataset that is too small to properly estimate a model's predictive performance.[236,245] For binary or time-to-event outcomes, recommendations suggest that at least 100 events and 100 non-events are needed,[236,245,246] but often this will only be attainable by combining IPD from multiple studies or datasets. Further, unlike a single study, IPD meta-analysis datasets enable predictive performance of a model to be examined across multiple settings, populations and subgroups of interest,[199,217,247,248] and any *heterogeneity* in model performance to be quantified. Therefore, IPD meta-analysis projects can more fully assess the transportability or generalisability of a prediction model for intended use.[217]

17.3.2.1 Causes of Heterogeneity in Model Performance

There are a number of potential causes of heterogeneous model performance across different settings and populations,[19,53,248] which may occur in isolation or in combination. A major reason is different case-mix variation, which is similar to the spectrum effect,[249,250] a term used to describe variation in test accuracy performance across different populations and subgroups. Here, case-mix refers to the distribution of predictor values, of other relevant participant or setting characteristics (such as treatment received), and of the outcome prevalence (for diagnostic models) or incidence (for prognostic models). Differences in case-mix variation may not only occur between different settings and populations, but also between studies with major differences in design or eligibility criteria (e.g. randomised trial, routinely collected data, etc).[251]

Case-mix variation can lead to genuine differences in the performance of a prediction model, even when the true (underlying) predictor effects are consistent (that is, when the effect of a particular predictor on outcome probability is the same regardless of the study population).[248] It is, for instance, well known that prediction models developed in secondary care usually have a different performance when they are applied in a primary care setting, as the prevalence or incidence of the outcome and/or the distribution of predictor values will be different.[252] For example, the Wells score is a diagnostic prediction model for deep vein thrombosis (DVT), which was developed in secondary-care outpatients. However, Oudega et al.[253] showed that it does not adequately rule out DVT in primary-care patients, as 12% of patients in the low-probability group truly had DVT compared to 3% in the original secondary-care setting. The higher prevalence is due to a change in the selection and definition of patients with suspected DVT, leading to a different distribution of predictor values and case-mix variation in primary care compared to secondary care. Many performance measures (such as mean-squared error, Brier score and C statistic) are dependent on outcome occurrence and/or case-mix. For instance, the range of the Brier score varies according to outcome incidence, and the C statistic depends on the distribution of the linear predictor (in the events and non-events groups).

The magnitude of predictor effects (denoted by β in Box 17.1) may also depend on the case-mix itself. For example, in the cancer field a biomarker's prognostic effect may vary (interact) with particular subgroups, such as the stage of disease or the treatment received, and it may also be non-linear. However, such interactions and non-linear trends are often missed (or mis-specified) when developing a prediction model. Further, a biomarker is often measured differently (e.g. using equipment from different manufacturers, or using a different assay or technique), recorded at a different time-point (e.g. before or after surgery), or quantified differently (e.g. using a different cut-point to define high and low values) across settings. The magnitude and distribution of measurement error in predictors may also be inconsistent.[164,254,255] Many other clinical, laboratory and methodological differences may also exist across different validation settings, including differences in local care, applied treatment or management strategies, clinical experience, disease and outcome definitions, and follow-up lengths, amongst others. All these problems may lead to heterogeneity in predictor-outcome effects and thus in the predictive performance of prediction models.[88,93] Subsequently, a developed model including predictor effects from one population may not perform well in a different population where the magnitude of predictor effects are different due to the change in case-mix, and use of different clinical, laboratory and methodological standards.

Another key reason for variation in a model's predictive performance is heterogeneity in the outcome prevalence or incidence across different populations and settings. This may be caused, for example, by different standards of care and administered treatment strategies across regions and countries, different outcome definitions and measurement, or different starting points (e.g. earlier diagnosis of disease in some populations due to a screening programme).[127] This leads to differences in the required intercept or baseline hazard rate (as defined in Box 17.1) across populations and settings, such that a developed model (which contains a single intercept or a single baseline hazard rate) is not transportable from one population or setting to another, leading to predicted probabilities that are systematically too low or too high. An example is shown in Figure 17.1(ii). Such systematic miscalibration is a major motivation for so-called model updating or tailoring,[230] where the aim is to update the model's intercept or baseline hazard (and sometimes also the predictor effects) to recalibrate predictive performance to the new population.

17.3.2.2 Disentangling Sources of Heterogeneity

To disentangle the possible sources of heterogeneity in prediction model performance, Debray et al. recommend quantifying the relatedness between the development and validation samples.[217] This allows for the isolation of changes in performance that can only be attributed to the use of invalid model parameters (e.g. regression coefficients), and thus to assess which types of model revision may be necessary.

Benchmark values can also be calculated to help quantify model performance across heterogeneous sets of studies.[248] For instance, the case-mix corrected C statistic indicates the discrimination performance under the condition that the model predictions are statistically correct in the validation sample.[256] It can be obtained by simulating the outcome with the case-mix of the validation sample, using the coefficients of the model being validated. A second type of benchmark value is the refitted C statistic, which can be obtained by refitting the model in the validation sample. The refitted C statistic provides an upper bound for the performance, which would be obtained if the coefficients from the development population were exactly equal to those in the validation population. Finally, a third type is the standardised C statistic (de Jong et al., in preparation), where the weights of concordant pairs are defined according to a propensity score model predicting sample membership. The standardised C statistic quantifies the model's discrimination performance for a particular case-mix distribution, and therefore allows the (genuine) transportability of model coefficients to be examined. Extensions of the standardised performance have also been proposed for calibration-in-the-large and the calibration slope. The original development study can be used as the reference sample for standardization, but other studies could be chosen depending on what best reflects the target population. An example is shown in Section 17.3.3.3.

17.3.3 Statistical Methods for IPD Meta-Analysis of Predictive Performance

17.3.3.1 Two-stage IPD Meta-Analysis

To perform an IPD meta-analysis of an existing model's predictive performance, a two-stage approach is most straightforward. In the first stage, for each study separately, the researcher applies the prediction model's original equation to each participant in the dataset, to obtain the predicted outcome probability (or linear predictor value) for each participant in that dataset. Accordingly, by comparing these predicted values with the observed outcome frequencies, the researcher can then estimate the model's predictive performance for each study separately, using aforementioned statistics such as the (conventional or standardised) C statistic, the D statistic, the O/E ratio, and the calibration slope, alongside their variances. For prognostic models, these measures might be derived overall and at multiple time-points of interest for prediction.

In the second stage, for each performance measure separately (and potentially for each time-point separately), a conventional meta-analysis model can be used to synthesise the estimates

Table 17.3 Relevant statistics to be estimated in the first stage of a two-stage IPD meta-analysis of a model's predictive performance.

Research question	Relevant statistics	Appropriate scale for meta-analysis
What is the calibration performance of a prediction model?	Calibration slope; calibration-in-the-large; E/O or O/E ratio	Original; original; $\log_e$
What is the discrimination performance of a prediction model?	*C* statistic; Royston's D statistic	Logit; original

across studies, as described in Chapter 5. It is imperative to allow for potential between-study heterogeneity (Section 17.3.2), and so we suggest using a random-effects meta-analysis model.[46,47] In external validation study i let $\hat{\theta}_{ik}$ be the estimate of the kth performance statistic of interest and let s_{ik}^2 be its variance (assumed known). Then a conventional (univariate) random-effects meta-analysis can be written as:

$$\begin{aligned} \hat{\theta}_{ik} &\sim N\left(\theta_{ik}, s_{ik}^2\right) \\ \theta_{ik} &\sim N\left(\theta_k, \tau_k^2\right) \end{aligned} \tag{17.2}$$

This assumes the $\hat{\theta}_{ik}$ are normally distributed about the ith study's true validation performance, θ_{ik}, and that the θ_{ik} are also normally distributed with an average of θ_k and a between-study standard deviation of τ_k.

Table 17.3 summarises the best scale to use for meta-analysis of statistics commonly used to summarise predictive performance of prediction models. For example, a meta-analysis of C statistics is best done on the logit scale (i.e. $\ln(C/(1-C))$,[257] such that the corresponding summary estimate then provides the average logit C statistic, which can then be back-transformed to the C statistic scale. Similarly, confidence and prediction intervals are derived on the logit scale, and then back-transformed to the C statistic scale. For some measures, non-parametric bootstrapping may be needed to obtain variances of the performance estimates on the desired scale.

As mentioned in Chapter 5, there are many different frequentist methods that can be used for estimation of random-effects meta-analysis models. We recommend restricted maximum likelihood (REML),[177] with a subsequent confidence interval for the average performance, θ_k, obtained by the Hartung-Knapp-Sidik-Jonkman (HKSJ) approach or – if it leads to a wider interval – the standard confidence interval approach.[258–260] With the addition of prior distributions for unknown parameters, a Bayesian approach to estimation is also recommended, for example using Gibbs sampling (Chapter 5).

On its own, the estimated average performance ($\hat{\theta}_k$) is an incomplete summary because it does not adequately summarise the consistency in performance across studies. Estimates such as I_k^2 (the fraction of the total variation in study estimates that is due to between-study heterogeneity),[261] and in particular, $\hat{\tau}_k^2$ (the estimated between-study variance) are also helpful.[186] However, when evaluating performance statistics of a prediction model, we are examining its generalisability across a range of populations that may differ in terms of their setting and case-mix variation.[217] Thus, consistency is best expressed by a $100(1-\alpha)\%$ prediction interval for the performance of the model in a single (new) population.[46,47] For a particular performance measure (e.g. calibration slope), k, an approximate prediction interval is derived by:[46]

$$\hat{\theta}_k \pm t_{\alpha,S-2}\sqrt{\hat{\tau}_k^2 + \mathrm{var}(\hat{\theta}_k)} \tag{17.3}$$

Here, $\mathrm{var}(\hat{\theta}_k)$ is the estimated variance of summary estimate $\hat{\theta}_k$, and $t_{\alpha,\, S-2}$ is the $100(1 - \frac{\alpha}{2})\%$ percentile of the t-distribution for $S - 2$ degrees of freedom (S = number of studies), and α is typically taken to be 0.05 to give a 95% interval. The prediction interval thus indicates a range for the expected performance of the model in a new study population, similar to those included in the meta-analysis. Chapter 5 discusses the limitations of prediction intervals, and alternatives to equation (17.3).[262,263]

To examine study-level covariates that explain between-study heterogeneity in predictive performance, model (17.2) can be extended to a meta-regression that includes study-level covariates to explain between-study heterogeneity, such as treatment policies, country, year of investigation, and length of follow-up. This may help identify populations, settings and situations where model performance is satisfactory and others where it is inadequate, to inform the model's generalisability.[217] The limitations of meta-regression are discussed in Chapters 5 and 7.

We now consider three applied examples of a two-stage IPD meta-analysis to summarise predictive performance of an existing prediction model.

17.3.3.2 Example 1: Validation of Prediction Models for Cardiovascular Disease

Pennells et al. used IPD from the Emerging Risk Factors Collaboration, which comprises participant records from over 2.2 million participants in 125 prospective (mainly cohort) studies of major cardiovascular disease (CVD) outcomes and cause-specific mortality in predominantly Western populations.[199] They focused on prognostic models for prediction of coronary heart disease (CHD), defined as first nonfatal myocardial infarction or coronary death, and used a two-stage IPD meta-analysis to examine the discrimination performance of a Cox model containing conventional predictors, defined by a linear predictor of:

$$\begin{aligned}&(0.068 \times \text{age}) + (0.576 \times \text{smoker}) + (0.012 \times \text{systolic blood pressure})\\ &+ (0.584 \times \text{diabetic}) + (0.221 \times \text{total cholesterol}) - (0.756 \times \text{HDL cholesterol})\end{aligned} \tag{17.4}$$

Their IPD meta-analysis contained 37 cohort studies involving 165,856 participants without a history of cardiovascular disease, among whom 8,806 incident CHD events occurred over an average of 9.8 years of follow-up. In the first stage of the IPD meta-analysis, study-specific estimates and standard errors of the model's C statistic and D statistic were produced. These are presented in their web appendix, and we used them to apply a random-effects meta-analysis (model (17.2)) for each predictive performance measure separately. REML estimation was used, with HKSJ derived confidence intervals. Both analyses reveal considerable between-study heterogeneity, reflected by wide 95% prediction intervals of approximately 0.58 to 0.85 for the C statistic (Figure 17.2), and 0.39 to 2.09 for the D statistic. Thus in some settings the model has only small discrimination, whereas in others it is very large. This is hidden when focusing only on the summary (average) results, such as the summary C statistic of 0.71 (95% CI: 0.69 to 0.74).

Meta-regression shows that studies with a larger standard deviation of linear predictor values (i.e. more variability in predicted probabilities across participants) have better discrimination performance (Figure 17.3(a)). This is sensible, as populations with more variability in their predicted probabilities will represent a more diverse set of individuals (wider range of CVD risks closer to 0 and 1), and thus – as the standard deviation of the linear predictor increases – the model more easily separates between those with and without the outcome.[217] Conversely, as the mean of the linear predictor increases, the discrimination decreases (Figure 17.3(b)). This suggests less

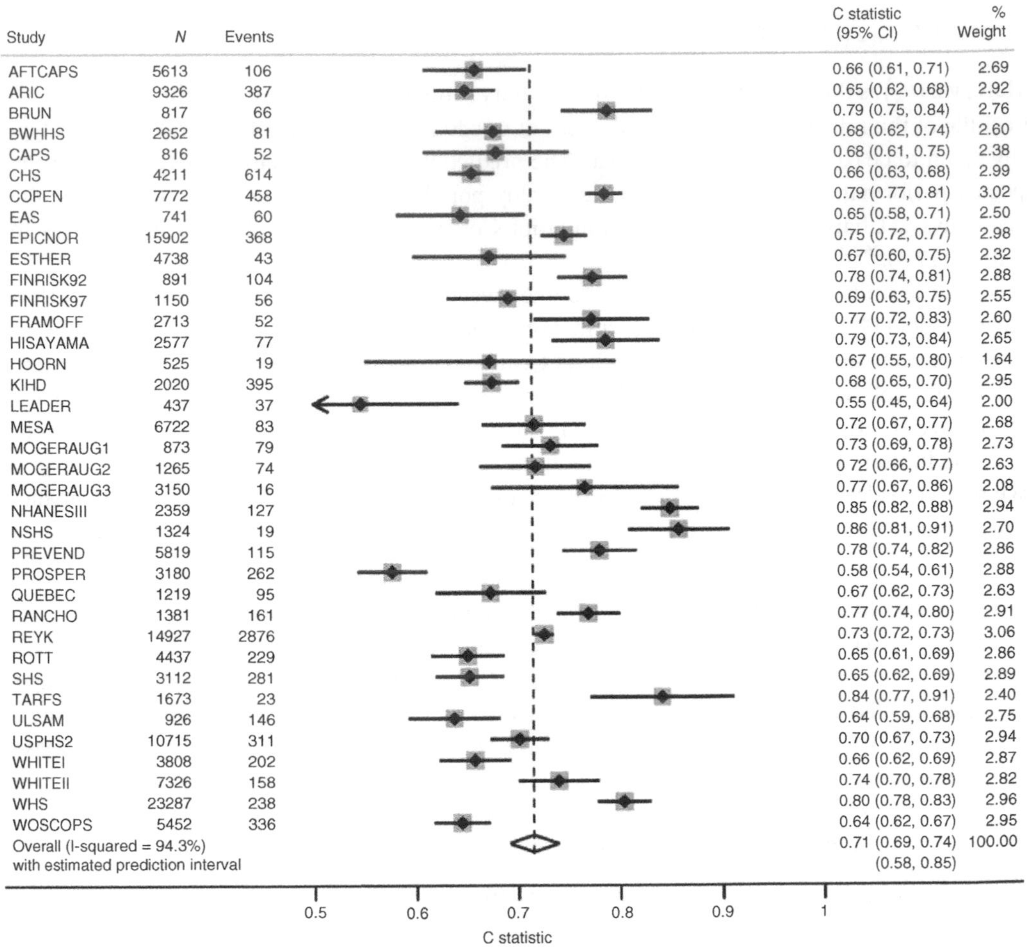
Study N Events
C statistic (95% CI)
% Weight
AFTCAPS 5613 106 0.66 (0.61, 0.71) 2.69
ARIC 9326 387 0.65 (0.62, 0.68) 2.92
BRUN 817 66 0.79 (0.75, 0.84) 2.76
BWHHS 2652 81 0.68 (0.62, 0.74) 2.60
CAPS 816 52 0.68 (0.61, 0.75) 2.38
CHS 4211 614 0.66 (0.63, 0.68) 2.99
COPEN 7772 458 0.79 (0.77, 0.81) 3.02
EAS 741 60 0.65 (0.58, 0.71) 2.50
EPICNOR 15902 368 0.75 (0.72, 0.77) 2.98
ESTHER 4738 43 0.67 (0.60, 0.75) 2.32
FINRISK92 891 104 0.78 (0.74, 0.81) 2.88
FINRISK97 1150 56 0.69 (0.63, 0.75) 2.55
FRAMOFF 2713 52 0.77 (0.72, 0.83) 2.60
HISAYAMA 2577 77 0.79 (0.73, 0.84) 2.65
HOORN 525 19 0.67 (0.55, 0.80) 1.64
KIHD 2020 395 0.68 (0.65, 0.70) 2.95
LEADER 437 37 0.55 (0.45, 0.64) 2.00
MESA 6722 83 0.72 (0.67, 0.77) 2.68
MOGERAUG1 873 79 0.73 (0.69, 0.78) 2.73
MOGERAUG2 1265 74 0 72 (0.66, 0.77) 2.63
MOGERAUG3 3150 16 0.77 (0.67, 0.86) 2.08
NHANESIII 2359 127 0.85 (0.82, 0.88) 2.94
NSHS 1324 19 0.86 (0.81, 0.91) 2.70
PREVEND 5819 115 0.78 (0.74, 0.82) 2.86
PROSPER 3180 262 0.58 (0.54, 0.61) 2.88
QUEBEC 1219 95 0.67 (0.62, 0.73) 2.63
RANCHO 1381 161 0.77 (0.74, 0.80) 2.91
REYK 14927 2876 0.73 (0.72, 0.73) 3.06
ROTT 4437 229 0.65 (0.61, 0.69) 2.86
SHS 3112 281 0.65 (0.62, 0.69) 2.89
TARFS 1673 23 0.84 (0.77, 0.91) 2.40
ULSAM 926 146 0.64 (0.59, 0.68) 2.75
USPHS2 10715 311 0.70 (0.67, 0.73) 2.94
WHITEI 3808 202 0.66 (0.62, 0.69) 2.87
WHITEII 7326 158 0.74 (0.70, 0.78) 2.82
WHS 23287 238 0.80 (0.78, 0.83) 2.96
WOSCOPS 5452 336 0.64 (0.62, 0.67) 2.95
Overall (I-squared = 94.3%) 0.71 (0.69, 0.74) 100.00
with estimated prediction interval (0.58, 0.85)
0.5
0.6
0.7
0.8
0.9
1
C statistic

Figure 17.2 Forest plot showing study-specific and IPD meta-analysis results for the *C* statistic of a prognostic prediction model for CVD occurrence based on conventional predictors and using the study-specific estimates originally presented by Pennells et al.[199] Meta-Analysis here was performed on the original *C* scale, as this was the scale of the standard error of *C* statistic estimates reported by Pennells et al. *Source:* Richard Riley, with figure produced using data extracted from the publication of Pennells et al.[199]

discrimination in more high-risk populations. A meta-regression including both mean and standard deviation of the linear predictor as covariates explains nearly all the between-study variability for either the *C* statistic or the D statistic. For example, for the D statistic the fitted meta-regression is

$$\hat{D}_i = 2.17 + (1.23 \times SD_i) - (0.32 \times MEAN_i) + u_i + e_i$$

$$u_i \sim N(0, 0.0006) \qquad e_i \sim N\left(0, \mathrm{var}\left(\hat{D}_i\right)\right)$$

where SD_i and $MEAN_i$ are the standard deviation and mean of the linear predictor, respectively, in study i, and their coefficients have corresponding p-values <0.0001. The value of 0.0006 is the residual between-study variance ($\hat{\tau}^2$), which is considerably smaller than the value of $\hat{\tau}^2 = 0.17$ without covariates.

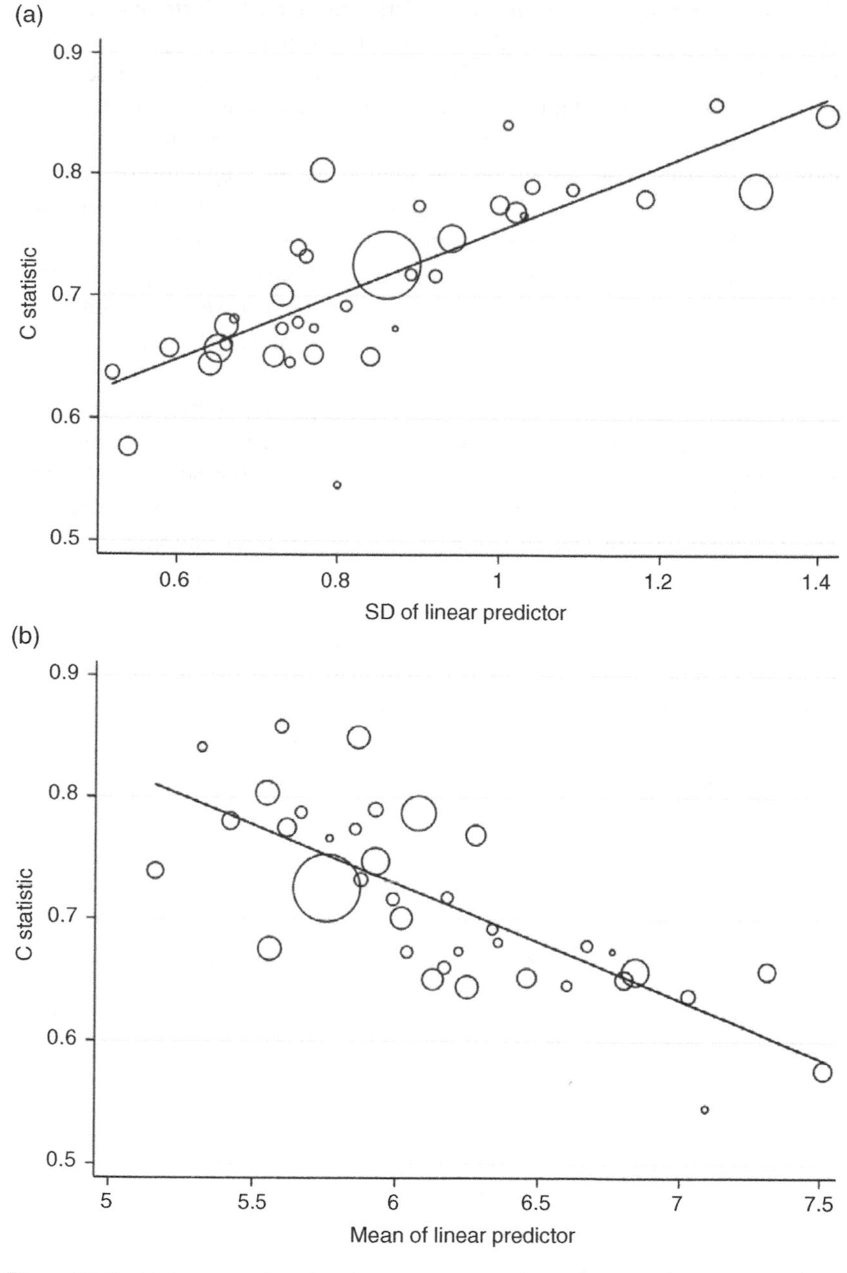

Figure 17.3 Meta-regression showing a strong association between the observed *C* statistic in each study and (a) the standard deviation of the linear predictor, and (b) the mean of the linear predictor. Based on study-specific results presented by Pennells et al.,[199] with the size of each study's circle proportional to the precision of their estimated *C* statistic (i.e. studies with more precise estimates have larger circles). *Source:* Richard Riley, with figure produced using data extracted from the publication of Pennells et al.[199]

17.3.3.3 Example 2: Meta-Analysis of Case-mix Standardised Estimates of Model Performance

Rather than trying to explain heterogeneity in model performance using meta-regression with study-level covariates defining case-mix, a potentially better approach is to meta-analyse case-mix *standardised* estimates of performance. Standardisation may reduce heterogeneity that is a result of case-mix variation, such that meta-analysis results are then specific to the chosen (reference) target population used for standardisation (de Jong et al., in preparation). That is, by meta-analysing standardised estimates of model performance, any remaining heterogeneity in performance only reflects the use of invalid model coefficients, thereby highlighting whether local updating of model coefficients is necessary for that target population. Simpler models (with fewer predictors) tend to be more prone to heterogeneity caused by case-mix differences, whereas more complex models (with more predictors) are generally more affected by invalid coefficients.

For example, we used IPD from 12 studies to validate eight existing prediction models for calculating the risk of actual DVT in patients suspected of DVT. The eight models differed in the number of included predictors (ranging from one to eight), and the coefficients of each model equation are shown in Table 17.4. All eight models were validated in each of the 12 validation studies, and model performance was quantified using unstandardised and case-mix standardised estimates of the *C* statistic, calibration slope and calibration-in-the-large. Then, for each performance measure separately, random-effects meta-analysis model (17.2) was applied to summarise average performance and to quantify any between-study heterogeneity. For calculation of the standardised predictive performance measures in each study, a propensity score weighting approach was taken in regards to the target population defined by that in the development sample.

The meta-analysis results are shown in Figure 17.4. Summary estimates of the *C* statistic were similar regardless of whether the usual (i.e. unstandardised) or standardised measure was used.

Table 17.4 Coefficients of eight prediction models for diagnosing DVT in patients suspected of DVT. All models were developed from the same data, and hence coefficient values are similar.

	Estimated logistic regression coefficients for each prediction model								
Model	**Intercept**	**D-dimer**	**Cdif**	**OC**	**Gender**	**notraum**	**Vein**	**Malign**	**Surg**
1	−3.39	2.58							
2	−3.84	2.42	1.11						
3	−3.90	2.44	1.13	0.40					
4	−4.25	2.46	1.15	0.72	0.72				
5	−4.87	2.49	1.17	0.72	0.73	0.68			
6	−4.95	2.47	1.16	0.70	0.72	0.66	0.52		
7	−4.93	2.44	1.14	0.72	0.70	0.64	0.52	0.53	
8	−5.02	2.43	1.15	0.76	0.71	0.67	0.53	0.50	0.42

Empty cells indicate the coefficients for the respective predictor is assumed zero. D-dimer = D-dimer test results (0 = normal, 1 = abnormal), Cdif = calf difference (0 for < 3 cm, 1 for >= 3 cm), OC = oral contraceptive or HST use (0 = no, 1 = yes), gender (0 = female, 1 = male), notraum = absence of leg trauma (0 = leg trauma present, 1 = leg trauma absent), vein = vein distension (0 = no, 1 = yes), malign = presence of malignancy (0 = no, 1 = yes), surg = recent surgery or bedridden (0 = no, 1 = yes).
Source: Richard Riley.

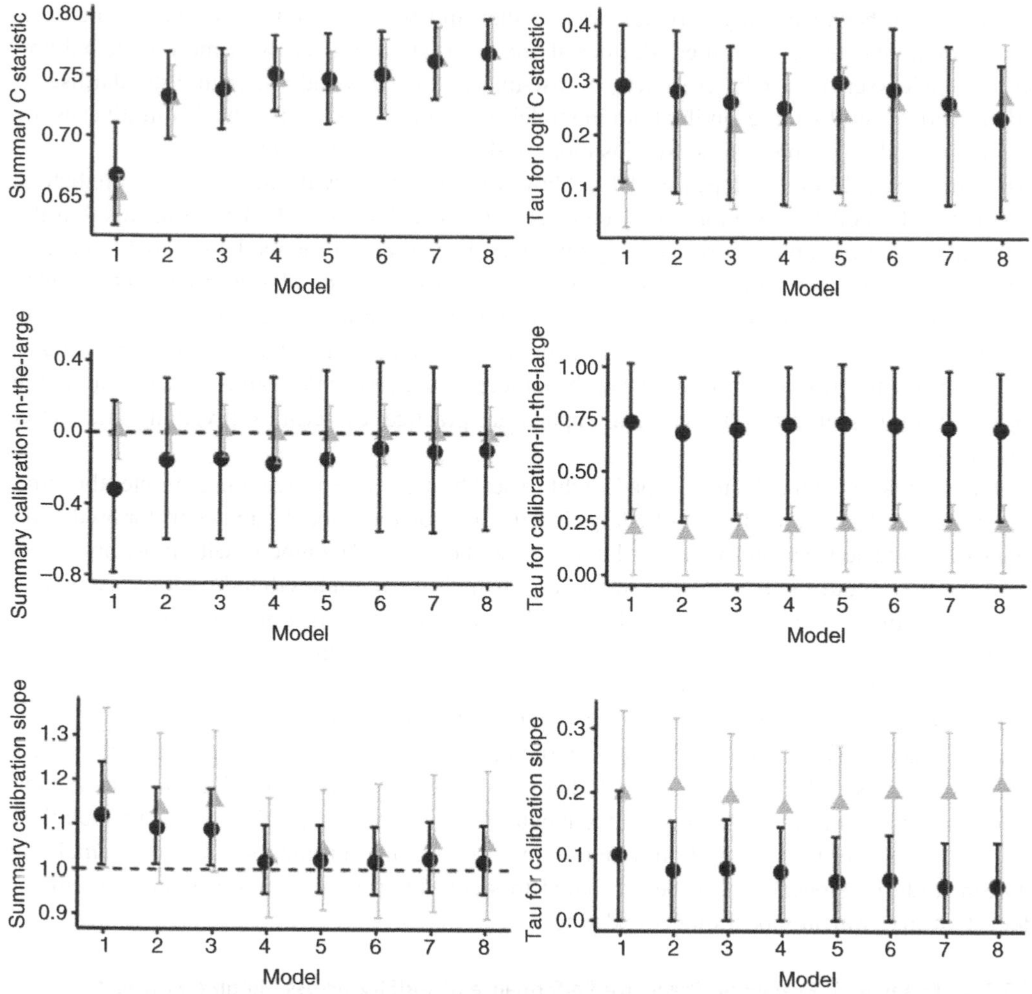

Figure 17.4 Summary estimates (and 95% CIs) of standardised and unstandardised performance for each of eight prediction models (defined in Table 17.4) for diagnosis of DVT in patients with suspected DVT, as obtained from a random-effects meta-analysis of performance estimates from 12 validation studies providing IPD. Circles: unstandardised performance estimates. Triangles: case-mix standardised performance estimates. Tau = estimated between-study standard deviation in performance. Tau is measured on the logit scale for the *C* statistic. *Source*: Valentijn de Jong.

This implies that *on average* there were no major effects of case-mix differences on discrimination performance between target population and validation samples. However, heterogeneity estimates did differ considerably. For instance, for model 1 (which included only one predictor), the between-study standard deviation (τ) of the unstandardised logit *C* statistic is estimated to be 0.30, which suggests that predictions from this model may have limited transportability across the included validation studies unless the model's predictor effects are updated to each study. However, when using the standardised logit *C* statistic, the estimated τ decreases to 0.11. This shows that much of the between-study variation in discrimination performance can be attributed to differences in case-mix, rather than the use of invalid model coefficients. That is, when standardising to the target population, the between-study variation was smaller and so local model updating of predictor effects may no longer be warranted. Further, it appears that the models with more included predictors were less sensitive to heterogeneity in case-mix, as their unstandardised and standardised *C* statistic were generally more similar than in models with fewer predictors. This is intuitive, as the inclusion of additional predictors explains more of the case-mix variability.

The summary calibration slopes are 1.1 or above for the models with three or fewer predictors, but closer to 1 when four or more predictors were included (Figure 17.4). This confirms that the inclusion of additional predictors generally improves the validity of the model's regression coefficients in the target population. Interestingly, for all models the standardised calibration slope values are larger than the unstandardised values, and there is more between-study heterogeneity after standardisation. This implies that the model coefficients genuinely differed between studies with the same case-mix distribution (that of the target population), which raises concerns about the calibration of model predictions when applied in practice to settings involving the target population.

Before standardisation, all models had slight miscalibration on average; for example, the summary unstandardised calibration-in-the-large is 0.30 for prediction model 1 and −0.08 for prediction model 8, and the between-study standard deviation is about 0.75. The models with more predictors have better unstandardised calibration-in-the-large, which again implies that the additional predictors help explain case-mix differences. After standardisation to the target population, the summary calibration-in-the-large is close to zero for all models, and between-study standard deviation is reduced to about 0.25 (Figure 17.4). Hence, for the target population, miscalibration-in-the-large appears less of a concern than when transporting to other populations.

In conclusion, this example shows the importance of using case-mix standardised performance estimates when using IPD from multiple studies to validate a prediction model. In particular, compared to just using unstandardised estimates, it helps focus results on a particular target population, and removes the impact of study differences in case-mix distributions so that any remaining between-study heterogeneity can be attributed to study differences in intercepts and predictor effects that may warrant local model updating.

17.3.3.4 Example 3: Examining Predictive Performance of QRISK2 across Multiple Practices

An excellent description of dealing with clustered datasets within prediction modelling is given by Wynants et al.[264,265] Alongside IPD meta-analysis datasets, some single-study datasets also contain clustering. For example, a multi-centre study contains clustering of participants within centres,[266] and a study using electronic health records studies will have participants clustered within practices, hospitals, or countries.[209] For example, QRISK2 was developed using e-health data from the QRESEARCH database using over 1.5 million patients (with over 95,000 new cardiovascular events) from 355 randomly selected general practices,[86] with external validation carried out by independent investigators in an additional 1.6 million patients from a further 364 practices.[267] Across clusters, case-mix and outcome prevalence or incidence are likely to vary. Such clusters can be viewed as 'studies' and then IPD meta-analysis techniques used to examine a model's predictive performance in each cluster, and not just on average across all clusters combined. Wynants et al. quantified that 64% of cardiovascular prediction models published since 2000 and included in the Tufts registry utilised a dataset containing multi-centres;[268] in a random sample of 50 of these, 39 ignored clustering and only one used an IPD meta-analysis approach to quantify performance, which is a wasted opportunity.

To illustrate the role of IPD meta-analysis with clustered data, Riley et al. externally validated QRISK2 using IPD from 364 general practices,[209] and performed a two-stage IPD meta-analysis to summarise the C statistic. In the first stage the logit C statistic and its corresponding standard error were estimated in each practice separately, and in the second stage these were combined across practices using random-effects model (17.2). This gave a summary (average) C statistic of 0.83 (95% CI: 0.826 to 0.833), but with large between-practice heterogeneity, reflected by a wide 95% prediction interval for the true C statistic in a new practice (0.76 to 0.88). More recently, Li et al. examined between-practice heterogeneity in the calibration performance of the QRISK3 model in 392 general practices (including 3.6 million patients) from the Clinical Practice Research Datalink.[269,270] Baseline risk substantially varied between practices, however there was very little between-practice heterogeneity in the combined effect of included predictors (calibration slope near 1). For this reason, further updates of the QRISK3 model might consider even more predictors to explain heterogeneity in baseline risk (CVD incidence).

Following such IPD meta-analysis, the use of forest plots to display cluster-specific and meta-analysis results is often impractical given the large number of clusters. An alternative approach to visualise any variability in model performance at the cluster level is to present plots of performance estimates versus their precision (or sample size or number of events).[271] Such plots are often called funnel plots, and the extremes of the funnel help reveal particular general practices where the model is performing much better, or much worse, than on average. The presence of heterogeneity can also be visualized by constructing bee swarm plots, where performance estimates at the cluster level are displayed as separate closely packed dots. For instance, Li et al. used bee swarm plots to visualize heterogeneity in calibration performance of QRISK3 across various risk strata and predictor values.[269]

17.3.3.5 One-stage IPD Meta-Analysis

A one-stage IPD meta-analysis to summarise a prediction model's predictive performance is potentially preferable when the outcome prevalence or incidence is low and/or studies are small (Chapters 6 and 8). By analysing the IPD in a single step and incorporating more exact within-study distributional assumptions (e.g. Bernoulli or Poisson), a one-stage approach avoids assuming study-specific estimates are normally distributed with known variances (as done in the second stage of the two-stage approach), which is likely to be inappropriate when studies are small or outcomes are rare. For example, to validate predicted probabilities from a binary outcome prediction model, one-stage models could be fitted to estimate the calibration slope, calibration-in-the-large, and O/E statistic.[45] This requires random effects on key parameters. For example, equation (17.1) could be fitted with a random effect on the intercept to allow for between-study heterogeneity in the calibration-in-the-large. To summarise the calibration slope in a one-stage IPD meta-analysis, the researcher could fit:

$$\begin{aligned} &Y_{ij} \sim \text{Bernoulli}\left(p_{ij}\right) \\ &\text{logit}\left(p_{ij}\right) = \alpha_i + \theta_i LP_{ij} \\ &\theta_i \sim N\left(\theta, \tau_\theta^2\right) \end{aligned} \qquad (17.5)$$

Here, LP_{ij} is the linear predictor value for participant j in study i as derived from the existing prediction model. Of key interest is θ, the summary (average) calibration slope across studies, and τ_θ^2, the between-study variance of the calibration slope. One-stage approaches have also been proposed for (derivations of) the C statistic.[272]

17.4 Updating and Tailoring of a Prediction Model Using IPD Meta-Analysis

"When data is heavily clustered, center-specific predictions offer the best predictive performance at the population level and the center level."[264]

External validation of an existing prediction model may incorporate updating or tailoring of the prediction model equation, which is often needed to improve the performance in the setting or population at hand.[203,212,230,273,274] As mentioned, miscalibration is common for predictions obtained from models in settings that differ from that of the development sample. A common updating approach is recalibration, where one or more terms (parameter estimates) in the model equation are changed to better fit the populations and settings of the validation datasets.[230,275] In an IPD meta-analysis situation, this may be done either globally (i.e. a term is changed by the same amount for all populations and settings) or locally (i.e. a term is allowed to change by a different amount for each population and setting). A common strategy is to change the model's intercept or (especially for parametric survival models) the magnitude of the baseline hazard, and this can often substantially improve performance. More intricate updating options include changing the shape of the baseline hazard, adjusting a model's entire linear predictor by a uniform scaling factor, or by modifying a subset of predictor effects.

An IPD meta-analysis also allows different updating or tailoring strategies to be formally evaluated and compared. The goal is to identify a strategy that, for each performance measure, has excellent performance on average (indicated by $\hat{\theta}_k$); small values of between-study standard deviation (indicated by $\hat{\tau}_k$); and a narrow prediction interval that suggests consistently good performance across relevant populations or settings. Understanding the potential causes of heterogeneity in prediction model performance is helpful to identify meaningful updating or tailoring strategies. In particular, the model may substantially benefit from recalibration if its parameters (e.g. intercept term) are invalid in new settings or populations. Conversely, more substantial revisions are required if variation in model performance is mainly caused by differences in case-mix. For this reason, prior to evaluating different updating strategies, it is recommended to validate the model(s) of interest and to inspect the presence of case-mix effects (as described in Sections 17.3.3.2 and 17.3.3.3).[217,248,251]

We now illustrate the concept of model updating and tailoring through two applied examples of mortality risk prediction in breast cancer patients.

17.4.1 Example 1: Updating of the Baseline Hazard in a Prognostic Prediction Model

Ensor et al. used an IPD meta-analysis of seven studies to examine the performance of a prognostic model for mortality risk in breast cancer patients.[276] The model was developed using a dataset from the Netherlands, but a two-stage IPD meta-analysis was used to examine the generalisability of the model to IPD from other countries. In most countries there was notable miscalibration of predictions over time. For example, using model (17.2) to combine study-specific estimates of the log expected/observed (E/O) event risk at three years post-surgery, the summary E/O is 0.93 (95% CI: 0.87 to 1.00), suggesting slight under-prediction of risks on average. Furthermore, the heterogeneity is large, reflected by a wide 95% prediction interval for E/O in a single country of 0.73 to 1.20.

However, after applying a simple local recalibration of the magnitude (not shape) of the baseline hazard in each country, the overall calibration is substantially improved at all time-points. For example, at three years E/O is 0.99 (95% CI: 0.97 to 1.00), and the heterogeneity in E/O across

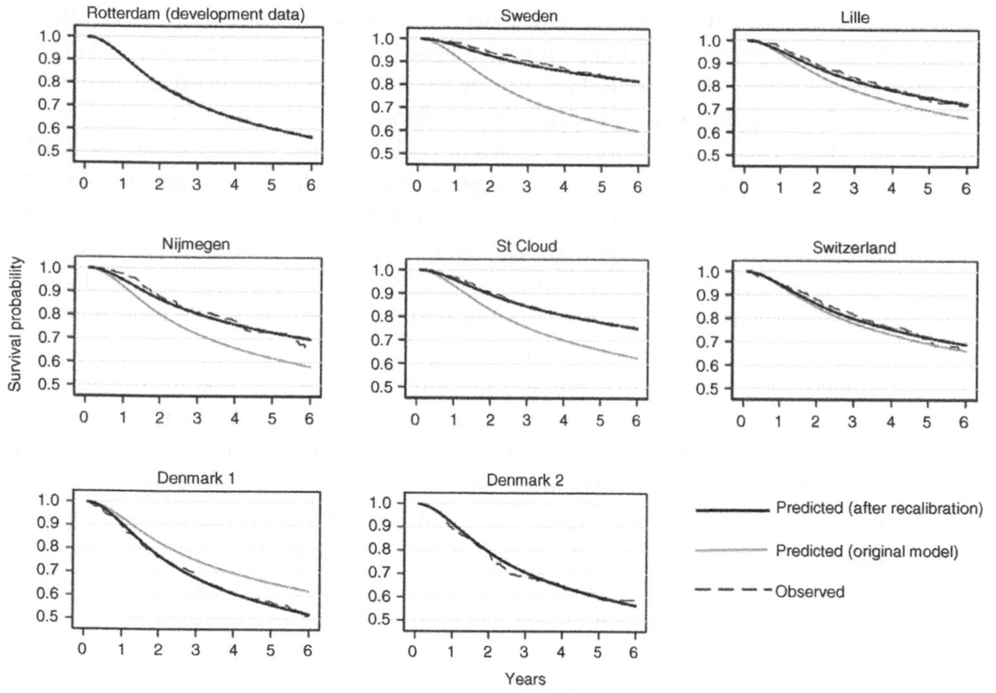

Figure 17.5 Overall calibration performance of a prognostic model for breast cancer mortality using IPD from seven external validation studies (countries), before and after local recalibration of the magnitude (not shape) of the baseline hazard in the developed model, as demonstrated by Ensor et al.[276] *Source:* Richard Riley, adapting figures reported by Ensor et al.[276] with permission.

studies is completely removed. This is illustrated by the observed and predicted survival curves in Figure 17.5, which only show close agreement after recalibration of the model. Therefore, as long as country-specific baseline hazard terms are used, the model is expected to have excellent overall calibration when applied to the different countries represented by the IPD meta-analysis. Further evaluations are needed to check calibration performance within subgroups, for example defined by categories of the linear predictor or by particular participant-level characteristics (e.g. gender, age).

17.4.2 Example 2: Multivariate IPD Meta-Analysis to Compare Different Model Updating Strategies

Snell et al. used IPD from eight cohort studies (relating to eight different countries) to evaluate an existing prognostic model for the risk of mortality over time in women recently diagnosed with breast cancer.[277] For validation, there were 7,435 participants (ranging from 69 to 3,242 participants per study) and 2,043 events, and across the eight studies the maximum and median follow-up durations were 120 and 86.3 months, respectively. The existing model contained seven predictors, and external validation assessed Harrell's *C* statistic, Royston's D statistic, and also the overall calibration, defined akin to the calibration slope in Box 17.4 but with the baseline hazard forced to be the same as in the developed model. Thus, the overall calibration represents an amalgamation of calibration-in-the-large and calibration slope in this example. Study-specific estimates of the three performance measures were obtained, and bootstrapping was used to estimate their within-study variances and correlations.

Within-study correlations were all positive, and generally moderate to large, emphasising that a multivariate meta-analysis may be useful to jointly synthesise the three measures (rather than performing a separate meta-analysis for each). Multivariate meta-analysis is described in Chapter 13, and Snell et al. describe its application to prediction model peformance.[277,278] Results of a trivariate meta-analysis of *C*, D and overall calibration are shown in Table 17.5. The average *C* statistic is 0.71 and a 95% prediction interval for *C* is 0.66 to 0.76, suggesting the model has a range of moderate discrimination values across countries. The summary overall calibration was almost perfect (0.99, 95% CI: 0.83 to 1.58), but there is again large between-country heterogeneity evidenced by wide 95% prediction interval for the calibration slope of 0.41 to 1.58 (Figure 17.6(a)). This signals that the model's calibration performance may be quite poor in particular settings. Calibration plots per study are also essential, but are not shown here for brevity.

Snell et al. extended their work by examining if the model's overall calibration performance improved with local recalibration of the baseline hazard function in each country;[277] that is, although the model's predictor effects were not modified, the baseline hazard of the developed model was re-estimated (in terms of both magnitude and shape) for each country. There was a substantial improvement in the breast cancer model performance (Figure 17.6(b)): heterogeneity was substantially reduced, and the updated 95% prediction interval for the overall calibration was 0.93 to 1.08, which is narrow and close to 1. Therefore, for this model local recalibration of the baseline hazard is recommended before application, which will require the use of local data.

Following a multivariate meta-analysis, joint inferences are possible. For example, the joint probability for a *C* statistic ≥ 0.7 and an overall calibration between 0.9 and 1.1 is 0.67 after local recalibration (Table 17.5); Snell et al. show how this can be depicted by a joint prediction ellipse.[277] This criteria is used for illustration, and should not be taken as a blanket rule for defining 'good' predictive performance, as other factors might be considered (e.g. calibration plots, clinical utility, etc).

17.5 Comparison of Multiple Existing Prediction Models Using IPD Meta-Analysis

IPD meta-analysis projects may provide an opportunity to compare the predictive performance of two or more existing prediction models for the same outcome and target population(s). We illustrate this with two examples.

17.5.1 Example 1: Comparison of QRISK2 and Framingham

Due to their larger sample sizes, IPD meta-analysis projects allow competing prediction models to be compared overall and in relevant subgroups. This is similar to the use of other big datasets containing clustering. For example, an external validation study of QRISK2 and the Framingham risk score in a large e-health records dataset containing clustering by assessed model calibration across all participants (by tenth of predicted probability) and also within particular age groups.[279] For example, on average across the entire sample of 1.1 million women, both models exhibit good overall calibration between predicted and observed 10-year CVD risk, with a summary E/O at 10 years of 1.01 for QRISK2 and 1.03 for the Framingham risk score (Figure 17.7, panel (a)). However, checking predictive performance by five-year age groups (Figure 17.7, panel (b)) reveals that Framingham over-predicts the 10-year CVD risk in women aged 40 to 64 years and under-predicts risk in women aged 70 to 74 years; in contrast, QRISK2 appears to accurately predict 10-year CVD risk across all age groups. Further work could also examine between-practice heterogeneity in the

Table 17.5 Trivariate random-effects meta-analysis results for calibration (as measured by the overall calibration*) and discrimination performance (as measured by the *C* and D statistic) of the prediction model for breast cancer mortality, before and after recalibration.

Strategy for applying the prediction model to the IPD in each validation study (country)	Validation statistic	Pooled estimate (95% CI)	95% prediction interval	I-squared	Estimate of τ	Joint probability of 'good'** predictive performance in a new population
(1) No recalibration: Implement prediction model using the baseline hazard in the developed model	Overall calibration	0.994 (0.835 to 1.153)	0.411 to 1.577	98%	0.224	0.22
	C statistic	0.711 (0.691 to 0.732)	0.662 to 0.761	43%	0.017	
	D statistic	0.332 (0.212 to 0.452)	−0.080 to 0.745	88%	0.157	
(2) Recalibration: Implement model after magnitude (but not shape) of baseline hazard re-estimated in each validation study (country)	Overall calibration	1.003 (0.971 to 1.036)	0.927 to 1.080	35%	0.026	0.67
	C statistic	0.711 (0.690 to 0.733)	0.657 to 0.766	49%	0.019	
	D statistic	0.328 (0.215 to 0.442)	−0.056 to 0.713	87%	0.146	

* The overall calibration is defined akin to the calibration slope in Box 17.4 but with the baseline hazard forced to be the same as in the developed model. Thus, the overall calibration represents an amalgamation of calibration-in-the-large and calibration slope.

** Defined by a *C* statistic $\geq$0.7 and an overall calibration between 0.9 and 1.1. This criteria is used for illustration, and should not be taken as a blanket criteria to define good performance, as this depends on context and potential use.

Source: Table adapted from Table 3 of Snell et al.,[277] with permission, © 2016 Elsevier (CC-BY 4.0).

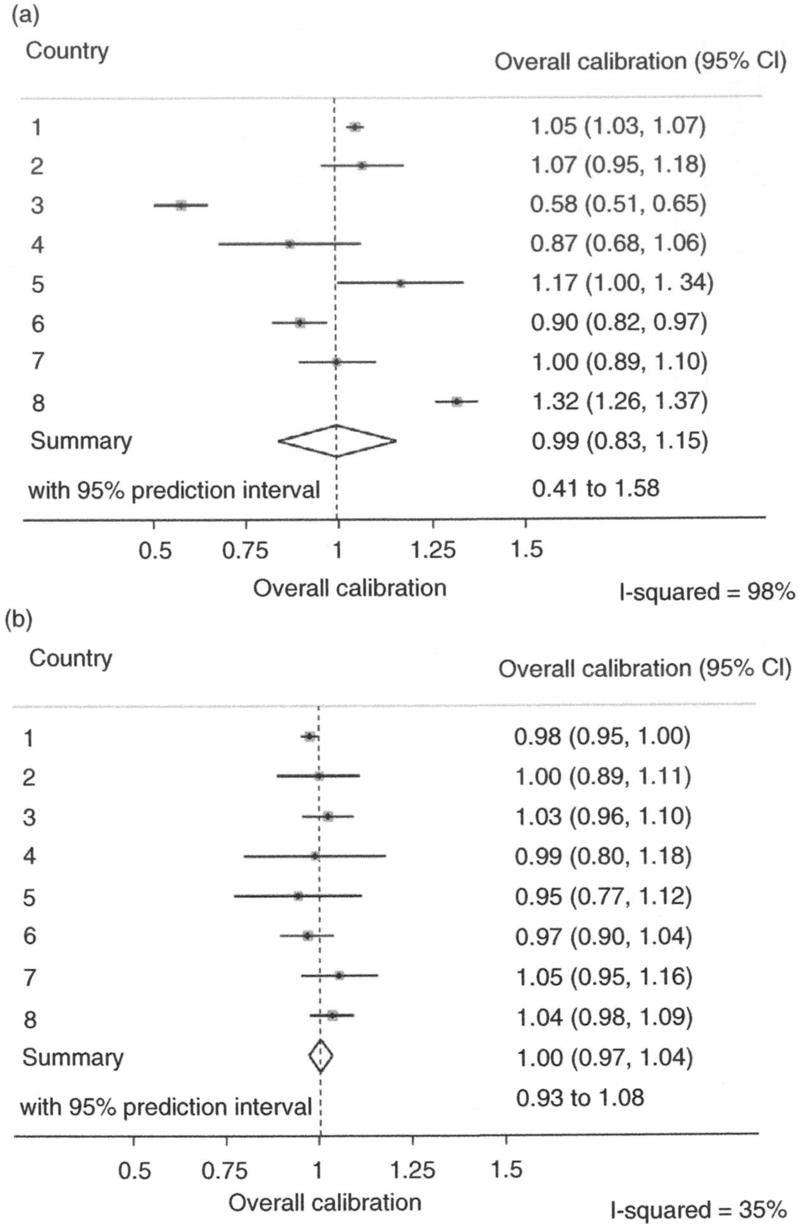

* Overall calibration should ideally be 1; it provides an overall measure of the discrepancy in the magnitude of the baseline hazard and the discrepancy in the effect of the model's linear predictor.

Figure 17.6 Overall* calibration performance of a prediction model for mortality in breast cancer patients evaluated before and after recalibration of the baseline hazard rate in each country. *Source:* Richard Riley, adapted from Figure 6 of Riley et al.,[209] with permission, © 2016 BMJ Publishing Group (CC-BY 4.0).

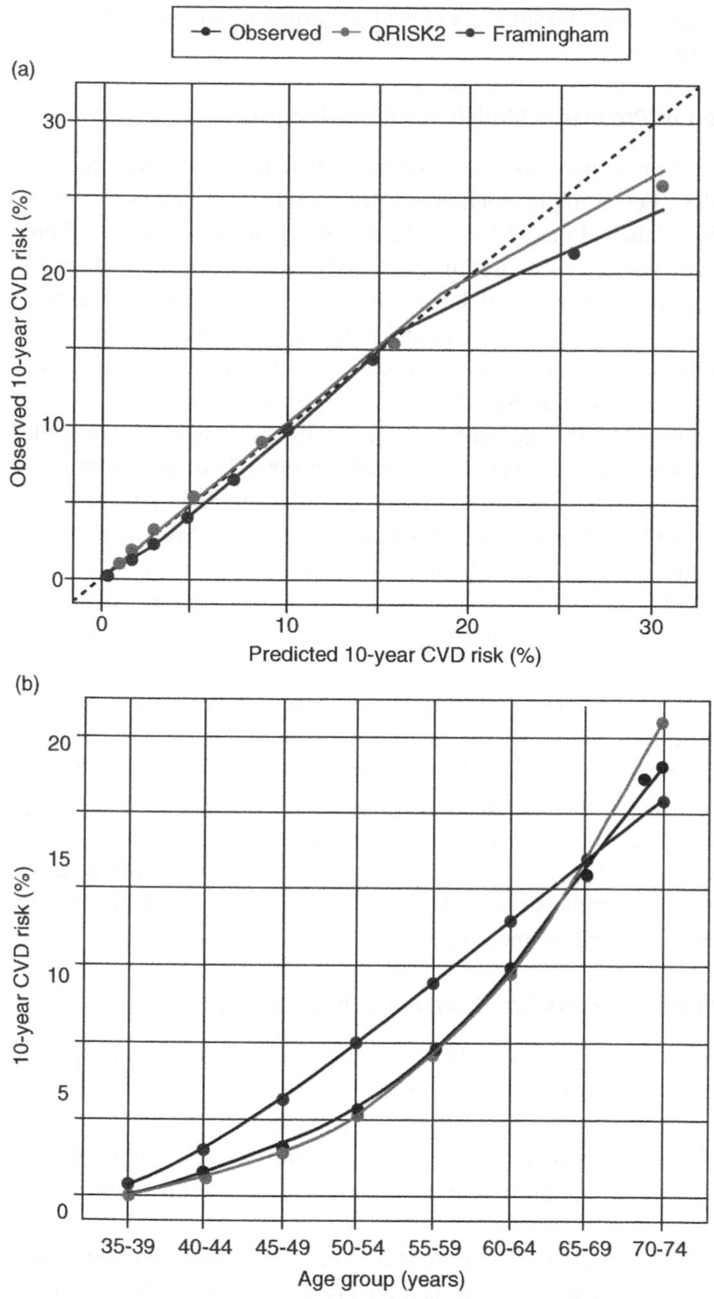

Figure 17.7 Calibration of QRISK2 and the Framingham risk score in women aged 35 to 74 years averaged across multiple practices in a large validation dataset of 1.1 million women: shown by smoothed calibration curves and (a) within tenths of predicted risk and (b) within eight age groups; dotted lines denote perfect calibration. *Source:* Richard Riley, adapted from Figure 4 of Riley et al.,[209] with permission, © 2016 BMJ Publishing Group (CC-BY 4.0).

calibration performance for each age group, and similarly look at performance within categories of other important subgroups (e.g. ethnicity).

17.5.2 Example 2: Comparison of Prediction Models for Pre-eclampsia

The previous example compared two prediction models, but often an IPD meta-analysis project will need to validate many more models. For example, Snell et al. used an IPD meta-analysis to externally validate 24 prediction models (labelled model 1 to model 24 for simplicity) for onset of pre-eclampsia in UK participants.[280] The number of studies in which each model was validated ranged from one to eight, with total number of events (over all datasets included) ranging from 9 (for models predicting early pre-eclampsia) to 5716 events (for a model predicting late pre-eclampsia).

A two-stage IPD meta-analysis was used to summarise the predictive performance of each model (Section 17.3.3.1), and the results are now summarised. The average calibration slope is < 1 for the majority of prediction models (Figure 17.8); though confidence intervals are wide, the general picture suggests that the prediction models suffer from overfitting and optimism. In other words, models generally have predictions that are extreme (too high and/or too low) compared to the observed risks in the validation datasets. Most models also had heterogeneity in the calibration slope. To illustrate the general concern about poor calibration, Figure 17.9 presents calibration plots (with loess smoothed calibration curves) for models predicting late-onset pre-eclampsia in each study that had more than 100 events. Most plots show large differences between predicted and observed risks across the entire range of predicted risk.

The discrimination of the models ranges from a summary *C* statistic of 0.49 for model 12 to 0.91 for model 16; however, 95% confidence intervals are generally wide, due to few studies per meta-analysis and less than 100 events in total for most models. For models that could be validated in datasets with a total of more than 100 events, their *C* statistics were mostly between 0.6 and 0.7.

Given these findings, Snell et al. recommend that models 1 to 24 are not suitable for use in practice,[280] and other models are needed that (i) include additional predictors to improve discrimination, (ii) are developed using larger sample sizes, and (iii) adjust for overfitting during model development (e.g. using penalisation estimation methods).

17.5.3 Comparing Models When Predictors Are Unavailable in Some Studies

A common problem when comparing prediction models head-to-head using IPD meta-analysis is that not all predictors are available in all studies (i.e. some predictors are systematically missing in some studies); then, as in the previous example, different sets of studies are used to validate different models. This makes it difficult to directly compare the predictive performance of multiple models, and simply restricting to only studies that provide all predictors may leave only a few studies (or even none).

To address this, an extended multivariate IPD meta-analysis could be used to deal with both multiple performance statistics and multiple models, as long as there are some studies that allow multiple models to be compared directly. In the first stage, each study provides estimates of each of the multiple performance statistics for each model it can validate. Then, in the second stage, the multivariate meta-analysis synthesises all study performance estimates simultaneously, accounting for their within-study and between-study correlation. This provides an overall summary of predictive performance for each model, and allows a ranking of models according to their (joint) predictive performance (e.g. ranked according to the probability that their *C* statistic will be above 0.7, their calibration slope will be between 0.9 and 1.1, and their O/E will between 0.9 and 1.1).[277] Under a missing at random assumption, the framework can handle performance statistics being unavailable

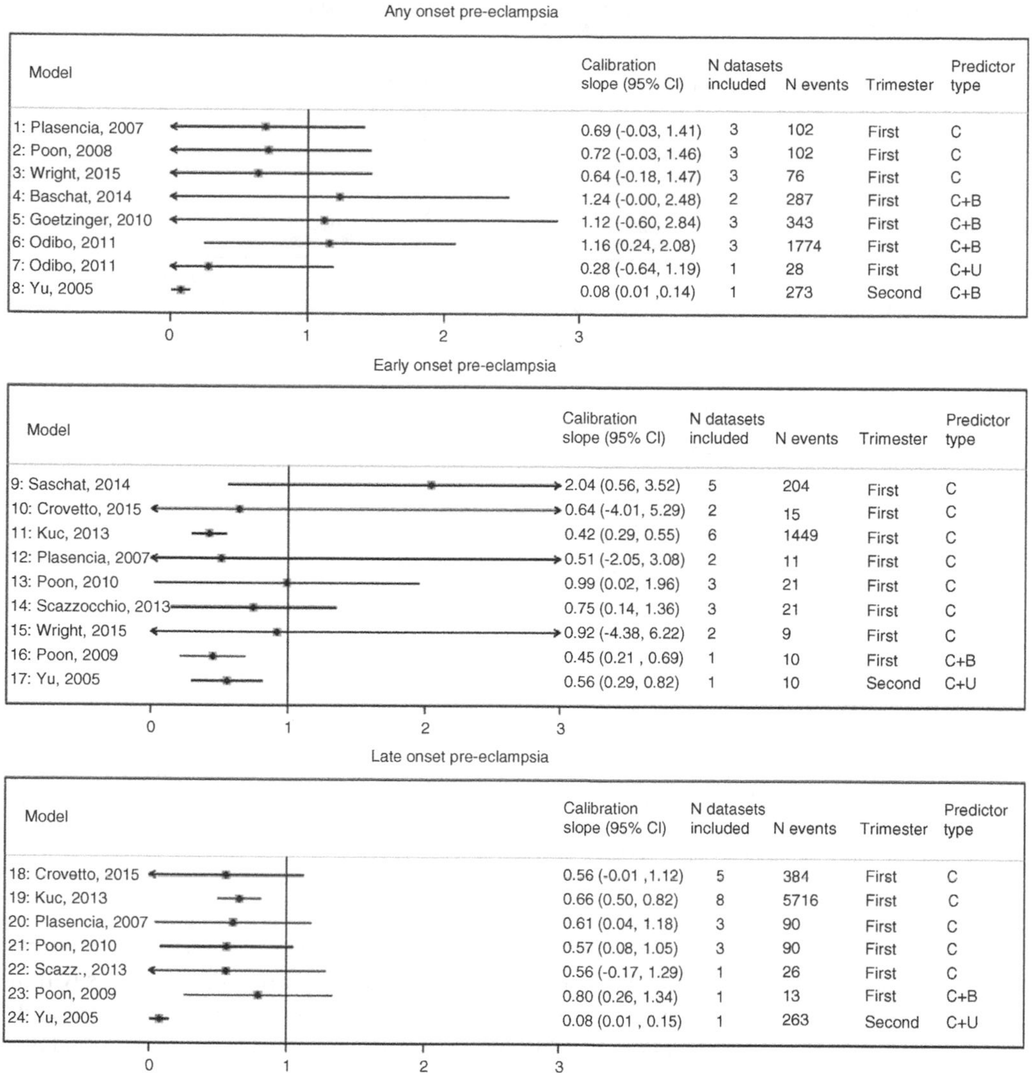
Any onset pre-eclampsia
Model
Calibration slope (95% CI)
N datasets included
N events
Trimester
Predictor type
1: Plasencia, 2007 0.69 (-0.03, 1.41) 3 102 First C
2: Poon, 2008 0.72 (-0.03, 1.46) 3 102 First C
3: Wright, 2015 0.64 (-0.18, 1.47) 3 76 First C
4: Baschat, 2014 1.24 (-0.00, 2.48) 2 287 First C+B
5: Goetzinger, 2010 1.12 (-0.60, 2.84) 3 343 First C+B
6: Odibo, 2011 1.16 (0.24, 2.08) 3 1774 First C+B
7: Odibo, 2011 0.28 (-0.64, 1.19) 1 28 First C+U
8: Yu, 2005 0.08 (0.01 ,0.14) 1 273 Second C+B
0 1 2 3
Early onset pre-eclampsia
Model
Calibration slope (95% CI)
N datasets included
N events
Trimester
Predictor type
9: Saschat, 2014 2.04 (0.56, 3.52) 5 204 First C
10: Crovetto, 2015 0.64 (-4.01, 5.29) 2 15 First C
11: Kuc, 2013 0.42 (0.29, 0.55) 6 1449 First C
12: Plasencia, 2007 0.51 (-2.05, 3.08) 2 11 First C
13: Poon, 2010 0.99 (0.02, 1.96) 3 21 First C
14: Scazzocchio, 2013 0.75 (0.14, 1.36) 3 21 First C
15: Wright, 2015 0.92 (-4.38, 6.22) 2 9 First C
16: Poon, 2009 0.45 (0.21 , 0.69) 1 10 First C+B
17: Yu, 2005 0.56 (0.29, 0.82) 1 10 Second C+U
0 1 2 3
Late onset pre-eclampsia
Model
Calibration slope (95% CI)
N datasets included
N events
Trimester
Predictor type
18: Crovetto, 2015 0.56 (-0.01 ,1.12) 5 384 First C
19: Kuc, 2013 0.66 (0.50, 0.82) 8 5716 First C
20: Plasencia, 2007 0.61 (0.04, 1.18) 3 90 First C
21: Poon, 2010 0.57 (0.08, 1.05) 3 90 First C
22: Scazz., 2013 0.56 (-0.17, 1.29) 1 26 First C
23: Poon, 2009 0.80 (0.26, 1.34) 1 13 First C+B
24: Yu, 2005 0.08 (0.01 , 0.15) 1 263 Second C+U
0 1 2 3

Figure 17.8 Forest plot of summary calibration slopes for different prediction models for pre-eclampsia, based on results presented by Snell et al.[280] Predictor type: C = clinical characteristics, B = biomarkers, U = ultrasound variables. *Source:* Kym Snell, created using results originally presented by Snell et al.,[280] with permission.

for some models in some datasets. This set-up is akin to a network meta-analysis of multiple treatments (Chapter 14). However, in a network of prediction models, so-called inconsistency (differences in direct and indirect evidence for a model's predictive performance) are likely, especially when there are changes in the case-mix variability in studies that do (direct) and do not (indirect) evaluate a particular prediction model. To reduce inconsistency, it may help to include case-mix covariates in the multivariate meta-analysis, such as the mean and standard deviation of the linear predictor. Also, as the multivariate model will require estimation of many parameters, simplifications may be necessary to aid convergence, in particular regarding the specification of the between-study covariance matrix.

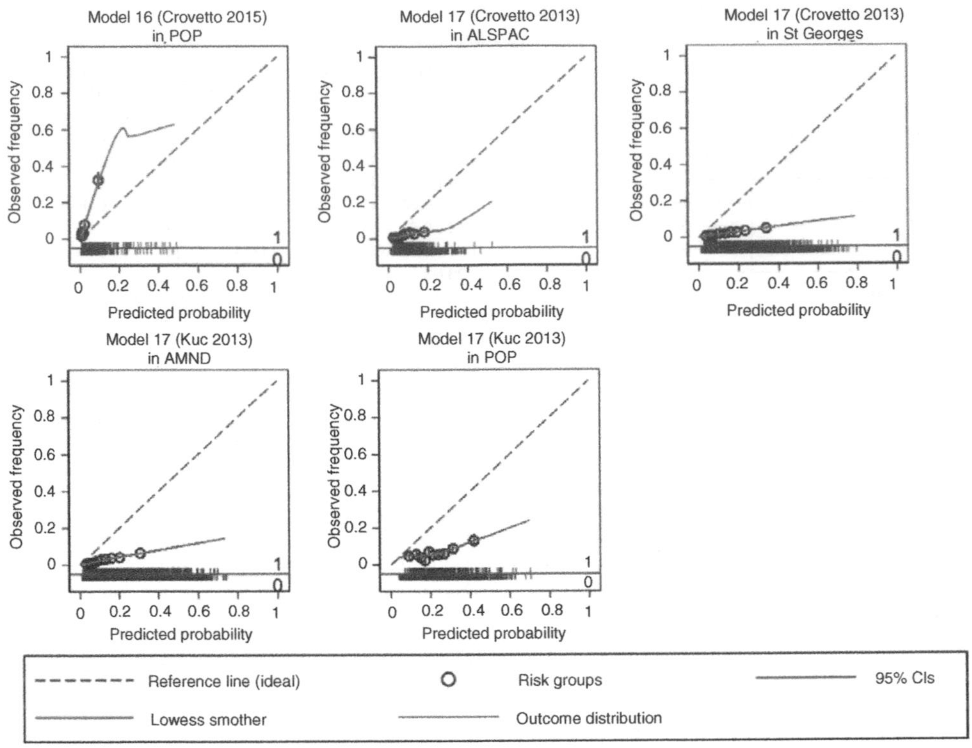

Figure 17.9 Calibration plots for models predicting late-onset pre-eclampsia using first trimester clinical characteristics and biochemical markers in those studies in the IPD meta-analysis that had over 100 outcome events and 100 non-events, extending the results presented by Snell et al.[280] *Source:* Kym Snell, recreating figures originally shown in Snell et al.[280] with permission.

An alternative approach is to impute values of systematically missing predictors using multiple imputation, based on all studies combined whilst accounting for clustering of participants within studies and allowing for potential heterogeneity across studies.[281,282] Again, this allows more studies to contribute to each model validation. Multiple imputation is considered in Chapter 18, for both systematically and partially missing predictors.

17.6 Using IPD Meta-Analysis to Examine the Added Value of a New Predictor to an Existing Prediction Model

IPD meta-analysis projects may allow the added value of a new predictor (e.g. a novel biomarker) to be examined. For example, Pennells et al. extended their aforementioned IPD meta-analysis to evaluate the contribution of C-reactive protein (CRP) concentration toward the risk prediction of CVD when added to conventional predictors.[199] The added value of CRP could be evaluated in terms of its adjusted prognostic effect (i.e. the adjusted hazard ratio) as outlined in Chapter 16. Consider the change in discrimination performance (C statistic or D statistic) when adding log CRP to the model (assuming a linear trend). We applied a two-stage IPD meta-analysis, where study-specific estimates of differences in C statistics were obtained and then pooled using random-effects model (17.2). Results suggest a slight increase in discrimination performance when adding CRP; the summary C statistic increases by 0.005 (95% CI: 0.003 to 0.006). Furthermore, unlike the C statistic itself (Figure 17.2), there is no heterogeneity in the change in C statistic across studies. Pennells et al. attributed this to the similarity in the distribution of log CRP across studies and to homogeneity in the hazard ratio for log CRP across studies.[199] What constitutes a useful improvement in the C statistic is difficult to define and context-specific. Other measures of model performance are also important to consider. In particular, we suggest examining the change in the Cox-Snell generalised R^2 statistic, which is a measure of overall model fit (proportion of variance explained) and based on the likelihood ratio statistic.[232] It is also important to evaluate the impact of adding a new predictor to the model's net benefit, in order to examine clinical utility (Section 17.8).[72,78,283]

Note that recalibration of an existing prediction model's coefficients (e.g. intercept and/or predictor effects) may be more essential than adding a new predictor. For example, Tzoulaki et al. show that the value of novel markers added to the Framingham risk score is almost null when the coefficients of the Framingham risk score are re-estimated before examine the added value of particular markers in the same dataset.[231]

17.7 Developing a New Prediction Model Using IPD Meta-Analysis

Sometimes there may not be an existing prediction model, or the IPD meta-analysis may show that existing models perform poorly, even after recalibration. In this situation, researchers will want to use the IPD meta-analysis dataset to develop a new model. To address this, in this section we consider some of the issues involved in prediction model development using IPD meta-analysis.

17.7.1 Model Development Issues

The development of a prediction model always requires careful planning and suitable statistical methods. Guidance for model development within single datasets (i.e. non IPD meta-analysis settings or situations without clustering) is provided in various textbooks,[85,130,158,203] series of articles[200,210–212] and by the TRIPOD (Transparent Reporting of a multivariable prediction model for Individual Prognosis or Diagnosis) group.[201,202] Such guidance remains highly relevant for prediction model development in IPD meta-analysis or clustered data settings, and key recommendations are given in Box 17.5. In particular, a suitable sample size is needed,[284–286] and important issues include choosing an appropriate modelling framework (e.g. multivariable linear or logistic regression, or a multivariable survival model); dealing with missing data; estimating the baseline hazard in survival models; handling of continuous outcomes and predictors;[287] dealing with complexities such as censoring and competing risks;[288,289] selecting predictors for inclusion; assigning weights per predictor; internal validation to quantify and adjust for optimism (due to overfitting); use of penalisation and shrinkage techniques to adjust for overfitting; production of a final model equation, and quantifying the (optimism-adjusted) predictive performance of the model (e.g. in terms of discrimination and calibration). Some additional issues also arise for the IPD meta-analysis setting, as described in the following sub-sections.

17.7.1.1 Examining and Handling Between-study Heterogeneity in Case-mix Distributions

A major advantage of IPD meta-analysis projects is that they increase the available case-mix variability,[19] thereby facilitating the development of prediction models that might be generalisable across the different settings and populations identified as applicable for the research question (Section 17.2.3). The variability of participant characteristics typically increases by combining

Box 17.5 General recommendations for IPD meta-analysis projects aiming to develop a prediction model

- Define the research question using the PICOTS system defined in Box 17.3.
- Register the study and publish a protocol describing data sources, participant inclusion (startpoint) criteria, predictor and outcome definitions, and (intended) strategy for data analysis.
- Select available IPD from datasets and studies that are representative of the target population(s) and setting(s) defined by the completed PICOTS system. Ideally, use data from well-designed and conducted, preferably prospective, cohort studies or, if not feasible, from some other type of existing datasets such as from a biobank, electronic-health records, or completed randomised trials.
- Examine the quality (risk of bias) and eligibility (applicability to the IPD meta-analysis research question) of the IPD obtained, using the PROBAST tool, that consider participant recruitment, predictor measurement, and outcome recording. Potentially restrict model development to the higher-quality IPD studies.
- Use IPD with clearly defined outcomes and time-points (e.g. in relation to the startpoint at which predictions are made, and time horizon for predictions) that are meaningful to the targeted individuals and healthcare professionals.
- Identify relevant candidate predictors *a priori* (e.g. based on previous evidence and availability in the IPD), including any relevant treatments that are administered (in routine care).
- Use a clear definition of each predictor and outcome, and ensure they are valid and reliably measured in each IPD study being used.
- In advance of model development, explore study differences in case-mix variability and potential causes of this.
- Use an IPD meta-analysis model appropriate to the outcome data of interest (e.g. logistic regression for a binary outcome, survival model for a time-to-event outcome), and deal with loss to follow-up appropriately (e.g. censor participants at their drop-out time if non-informative).
- Handle clustering of participants within studies, for example by including random effects on the intercept or baseline hazard, or by stratifying intercepts/baseline hazards by study, to allow for between-study heterogeneity in baseline risk. Potentially also allow for heterogeneity of predictor effects.
- Consider whether some parameters might only be estimated by the IPD from a subset of studies; for example, the intercept for use (in the final model) might be based on the IPD from cohort studies that reflect the target population.
- Handle continuous predictors appropriately (i.e. avoid categorisation), ideally by considering potential non-linear trends using, for example, restricted cubic splines or fractional polynomials.
- Handle missing data appropriately by considering methods that account for the missing data mechanism (e.g. using multiple imputation to impute partially missing predictors within studies, and potentially systematically missing predictors across studies).
- Reduce the potential for overfitting (i.e. producing models that are overly tailored to the data at hand, hence yielding predictions that are too extreme in new datasets) by:
  - Ensuring a sufficiently large sample size (and numbers of events) for model development according to the criteria of Riley et al.; ideally use all selected IPD studies to build the model.

- Reducing the number of candidate predictors in advance of predictor-outcome analysis (e.g. based on previous evidence, and by removing some predictors from a set of highly correlated predictors);
- Avoiding univariable screening to select candidate predictors for the multivariable model;
- Applying penalised estimation techniques (e.g. uniform shrinkage, lasso, elastic net, ridge regression), that penalise (shrink) predictor effect estimates to reduce overfitting;
- Include all candidate predictors in the final model, regardless of their statistical significance, or incorporate predictor selection within a penalisation method such as lasso or elastic net.

• Use internal validation methods that adopt resampling techniques, such as bootstrapping or cross-validation, to quantify the optimism in the model's apparent performance in terms of calibration and discrimination.
• Derive optimism-adjusted estimates of calibration and discrimination performance.
• Summarise the model's predictive performance on average across all studies, but also for each study separately, for example by using internal-external cross-validation and meta-analysis of predictive performance.
• Report the study process and findings (e.g. full regression model, model performance) according to the TRIPOD-CLUSTER statement, including exactly how to use the model to make predictions in practice (e.g. what intercept to use, and whether any local recalibration is recommended).

Source: Richard Riley.

studies with different (often more narrow) target populations, patient eligibility criteria or sampling procedures (e.g. IPD from randomised trials). However, a key problem when combining IPD from studies with differences in case-mix distributions is that certain model parameters (e.g. intercept term, predictor effects) may not generalise well across the included populations. For instance, it is possible that a predictor's effect is (approximately) linear within a certain range of predictor values, but non-linear across a wider range. Similarly, studies that adopt very strict eligibility criteria (e.g. randomised trials) may yield an intercept term that substantially differs from those obtained in broader populations (e.g. from routine care registry data). Conversely, when differences in case-mix distributions are the result of differences in sampling procedures, it is possible that certain model parameters are not intended to generalize. For instance, the intercept term from a case-control study reflects the ratio of sampled cases and non-cases, rather than the genuine baseline risk in a certain population. Similar issues may arise when including data from cross-sectional or case-cohort studies.

Although differences in case-mix distributions do not necessarily impact the validity of a developed prediction model, it is important to understand the possible sources of case-mix variability before embarking on model development using IPD meta-analysis. Possible options include:[217,248,251]

• Comparing the distribution of participant-level variables (outcome and candidate predictors) across studies. This approach does not take into account the possible correlation between variables.

- Using the IPD from all studies to fit a (global) prediction model including a core set of predictors, then comparing the distribution of the linear predictor between studies.
- Using the IPD from all studies to fit a multinomial model to predict study membership based on a core set of candidate predictors.[217] The *C* statistic of this membership model then indicates whether or not there is discrimination in the case-mix of included studies (and, possibly, in terms of their baseline risk).

It is also important to examine any study differences in the definitions or measurement methods for predictors or outcomes, as this may also lead to an increased variability in the *observed* case-mix distributions, and affect the generalizability of model parameters. For instance, Luijken et al. show that predictor measurement heterogeneity can substantially influence the (discrimination and calibration) performance of a prediction model, even to the extent that the prediction model may no longer be considered clinically useful.[255,290]

Where case-mix differences are a concern, it may be possible to harmonise datasets (e.g. predictor and outcome definitions) to some extent, for example by standardising variables or by transforming or imputing to a particular scale. Sometimes removing IPD from particular studies may be warranted, to help ensure more homogenous set of populations, settings and variable measurement methods. However, this is usually a last resort, as by the model development phase the harmonised IPD should already been classed as eligible (i.e. applicable for the target populations), and so excluding a subset of IPD may lead to narrower applications in practice, as well as reducing sample size for model development. Therefore, we recommend the decision to exclude IPD from a subset of studies is best decided after examinations of model performance based on all studies, by using the cross-validation approach described in Section 17.7.2.

In the next section, we focus on the statistical modelling of heterogeneity in baseline risk and predictor effects when estimating the prediction model. Such heterogeneity may be the result of variability in case-mix distributions across studies, and dictates the extent to which predicted probabilities from the developed model are likely to generalise across different settings and populations.[264] Ideally, there would be no heterogeneity as the goal is to create a single model equation that is immediately applicable to all the populations and settings of potential use. To improve homogeneity, it may be tempting to include only those predictors with homogenous effects across studies. However, a predictor with a heterogeneous effect may still be important; for example, its effect may be strong in all studies but vary in magnitude, and therefore excluding it will lead to lower discrimination performance (e.g. reduce the *C* statistic). Removing predictors may also increase between-study heterogeneity in the baseline risk.

17.7.1.2 One-stage or Two-stage IPD Meta-Analysis Models

As for other IPD meta-analysis applications, the prediction model equation can be estimated by using either a one-stage or a two-stage approach. The former will usually be more convenient, as the one-stage framework (Chapter 6) naturally leads to a full model equation containing the parameter estimates needed for making predictions in new individuals (e.g. it produces a regression equation based on summary estimates of the predictor effects and the intercept or baseline hazard terms). A two-stage approach requires a multivariate meta-analysis to jointly combine all the different parameter estimates across studies, whilst accounting for any within-study and between-study correlation (Chapter 13).

17.7.1.3 Allowing for Between-study Heterogeneity and Inclusion of Study-specific Parameters

For either the one-stage or two-stage approach, a particular issue for model development is how to handle potential between-study heterogeneity in baseline risk and predictor effects.[266] For example, random effects could be included for some parameters (e.g. intercept and/or particular predictor effects) within one-stage IPD meta-analysis models, as described for generalised linear mixed models and frailty survival models in Chapter 6. Then predictions in new individuals could be based on using the average (summary) parameter estimates, or preferably by integrating over entire distributions of the random effects.[291] Briefly, the latter strategy can be achieved by calculating the linear predictor using draws from the random effects distribution(s), and taking the average of the resulting predictions.

Alternatively, some model parameters (e.g. intercept and predictor effects) could be stratified by study, leading to study-specific terms in the developed prediction model equation. For example, Westeneng et al. performed a meta-analysis with IPD from 14 specialized amyotrophic lateral sclerosis (ALS) centres in Europe to develop a prognostic model for predicting survival in patients with ALS.[292] They used a one-stage IPD meta-analysis approach, fitting a Royston-Parmar survival model to the entire set of data from 11,475 participants,[293] and assumed that the baseline hazard and all predictor effects were common to all ALS centres ('studies'). However, because the resulting model showed some evidence of miscalibration upon validation, study-specific baseline hazard functions were reported to enable health professionals to tailor model predictions to their own population. Thus their final prediction model was of the form

$$1 - \hat{S}_j(t) = 1 - \hat{S}_{0i}(t)^{\exp\left(\hat{\beta}_1 x_{1j} + \hat{\beta}_2 x_{2j} + \hat{\beta}_3 x_{3j} + \ldots + \hat{\beta}_k x_{kj}\right)}$$

where $S_{0i}(t)$ is the cumulative baseline survival probability until time t (where 'baseline' refers to participants whose x values are all zero) in study i.

The use of study-specific terms raises issues, however. Firstly, it increases the number of parameters to estimate, which may increase the problem of model overfitting (Section 17.7.1.7). Secondly, prediction model equations which contain study-specific terms (for either the intercept, baseline hazard or the predictor effects) may be problematic to apply in practice, as new individuals (for whom predicted probabilities are needed) are not actually from a particular study per se. For example, the Westeneng model allows predictions for new patients from the included ALS centres, but it is not immediately clear which $S_{0i}(t)$ should be used when the model is applied elsewhere.

The need for study-specific terms strongly indicates that local recalibration is needed when the model is applied in practice. That is, the study-specific terms in the model need to be replaced with estimates from data local to each population and setting of application, as discussed in Section 17.4. To reduce the need for study-specific terms, and thereby avoid problems of local updating and the need for local data, one option is for the developed prediction model to include additional predictors that remove (or at least substantially reduce) between-study heterogeneity. For example, study-level (or centre-level) characteristics such as level of care (i.e. primary, secondary or tertiary) may be included to explain differences in outcome incidence across studies.[294,295] Similarly, causes of heterogeneity could be explicitly modelled; for example, if measurement methods vary for a particular predictor across studies, a separate effect of the predictor could be included for each method of measurement (i.e. the prediction model equation could include an interaction between the predictor and method of measurement). Then, predictions for a new individual could be made conditional on the actual level of care and predictor measurement method available to that individual.

Note that identifying important study-level covariates may be challenging, and their effect may be poorly estimated if the number of studies is small (e.g. < 10–20). The inclusion of non-linear associations for continuous predictors may also reduce heterogeneity to some extent.

In our experience, it is very difficult to develop a model that works well both on average and also in each study separately. It is aided by the inclusion of strong predictors (both participant-level and study-level covariates) that ensure between-study heterogeneity is minimal, and appropriate modelling of continuous variables. Evidence from prognostic factor research about key predictors is vital (see Chapter 16). However, key predictors might be unknown or not measured in the IPD available, and important between-study heterogeneity will often remain for some parameters, such that local tailoring of a model is needed to ensure it works well in each population and setting of interest. Examples of local recalibration are provided in Section 17.4, and the need for local recalibration after model development can be examined using cross-validation (Section 17.7.2). Further discussion is also provided elsewhere.[19,20,53,209,251,264]

17.7.1.4 Studies with Different Designs

In some situations, IPD may be available from studies with a mixture of designs, such as cohort studies, randomised trials and case-control studies. In such situations, it may be necessary to distinguish the parameters to be estimated by all studies (and thus all designs) and those parameters to be estimated by only a sub-set of studies. For example, although the IPD from case-control and randomised studies may contribute toward the estimation of predictor effects (such as odds ratios), it might not provide reliable information about the baseline risk (i.e. intercept term) in real-world populations. Thus, when finalising the prediction model equation, the intercept might be based solely on that estimated using the subset of IPD from the cohort studies, or even chosen to be from the study that most closely matches the target population. For instance, Steyerberg et al. developed a prognostic model for risk of mortality or unfavourable outcome by six months in patients with traumatic brain injury, using IPD from a mixture of cohort and randomised studies.[132] Their one-stage modelling framework used logistic regression with the intercept stratified by study, and so produced multiple intercepts to choose from. However, for application in practice they chose the intercept estimated from one particular study as "it represented typical proportions of mortality and unfavourable outcome" in the target population.[132]

17.7.1.5 Predictor Selection Based on Statistical Significance

Sometimes variable selection is of interest, to select a subset of predictors for inclusion in the final model. We generally prefer to pre-specify the predictors for inclusion (e.g. based on evidence from systematic reviews of prognostic factors) and fit a model containing all these predictors. Where variable selection is based on *p*-values, an issue is that, due to the larger numbers of participants and events, many candidate predictors investigated may be statistically significant in an IPD meta-analysis, even when they only improve prediction performance by a small amount. Therefore, rather than focusing on statistical significance, a more considered predictor selection process is needed, perhaps based on clinical relevance and magnitude of effect; otherwise, the prediction model equation may include a vast number of predictors unnecessarily. As mentioned, it may also be helpful to ascertain which candidate predictors have heterogeneous effects across studies, for example in order to identify any inconsistencies across studies with respect to the measurement of a predictor that impacts upon subsequent model performance; Wynants et al. suggest the residual intra-class correlation for this purpose.[296] Alternatively, it is possible to perform predictor selection by adopting penalization methods that allow for heterogeneity between studies, for example by using generalized linear mixed models with L1-penalty terms.[297] Because predictor selection can compromise the validity and variance of model predictions, it has been recommended that stability investigations and sensitivity analyses be performed. More guidance on this is provided by Heinze et al.[298]

17.7.1.6 Conditional and Marginal Apparent Performance

Unless penalised estimation techniques have been used (Section 17.7.1.7), usually when examining the *apparent* calibration performance of a prediction model (i.e. the performance in the development dataset), the calibration slope will be 1. However, this may not be the case in a situation involving clustering, depending on whether conditional or marginal predictive performance is of interest, and whether cluster-specific terms are included in the model equation.[264] In particular, after developing a model using the IPD from all studies, the apparent calibration slope in a particular study (i.e. conditional on study) will only be 1 if the prediction model equation contained study-specific estimates for each parameter in the model. If some parameter estimates in the model equation are based on a weighted average across studies (perhaps they even ignored clustering entirely), then the potential deviation from 1 will increase as the between-study heterogeneity in true parameter values increases; consequently, even a meta-analysis of the calibration slopes from each study may not give a summary estimate of 1 in this situation.[264] Conversely, if the prediction model equation does not contain any study-specific terms and ignored clustering, then the apparent calibration slope will be 1 when calculated in the entire IPD meta-analysis dataset (i.e. its marginal performance ignoring clustering by study). However, then the calibration slopes in particular studies are unlikely to be 1 if there is between-study heterogeneity in the true values of model parameters (e.g. intercept and predictor effects).

We generally prefer to focus on conditional estimates, to properly reveal predictive performance in each study;[266] if an overall summary is required, these conditional estimates can then be meta-analysed to quantify the average conditional performance of the model. Note that study-level covariates (e.g. country, level of care) will not contribute to the discrimination performance of the model when it is applied to the IPD in each study separately. That is, estimates of the *C* statistic conditional by study will generally be lower than the marginal *C* statistic as obtained by applying the model to the entire IPD meta-analysis dataset in a single step.

17.7.1.7 Sample Size, Overfitting and Penalisation

Apparent performance of a prediction model (i.e. in the development dataset) is usually optimistic, primarily due to overfitting of predictor effects to the dataset at hand. To reduce overfitting in a single study, researchers should use all their data for model development and perform internal validation using bootstrapping.[299] The same applies to the IPD meta-analysis setting: *use all IPD to develop the model*, and ensure it is large enough to meet the sample size criteria outlined by Riley et al. and van Smeden et al.[284–286,300] Data are precious, and developing a robust prediction model is difficult, so all the data are needed for development. Random resampling techniques such as bootstrapping allow a suitable internal validation (including examination and adjustment of overfitting and optimism) without the need for leaving studies out of the model development, and can account for clustering in the resampling.[301] In the IPD meta-analysis setting, bootstrapping should be done within each study separately, so that a bootstrap sample is obtained for each study with the same size as in the original IPD meta-analysis dataset. Then, study-specific and pooled optimism-adjusted performance statistics can be calculated, as described in Box 17.6.

If overfitting is a concern, penalisation techniques should be used to allow shrinkage of predictor effects to improve the accuracy of a developed model's predictions in new individuals. Penalisation can be embedded within the model development phase, for example by using methods such as

Box 17.6 The bootstrap procedure for internal validation and optimism-adjustment of the predictive performance of a prognostic model,[158,203] extended to the IPD meta-analysis setting.

1) Develop the prediction model using the IPD from all studies; then determine the apparent predictive performance (e.g. *C* statistic, calibration slope, etc in the same IPD) by applying the model in each study separately. The developed model should be applied as intended in practice. In particular, if the prediction model includes study-specific parameters, and these are to be used when applying the model in practice, then use these study-specific parameter values for calculating the risk predictions in each study. Otherwise, if average parameter values are to be used when applying the model, then ensure that the same average values are used when calculating the risk prediction in each study. After application to each study separately, summarise apparent predictive performance across studies by using a random-effects meta-analysis (model (17.2)) for each performance statistic.
2) Generate a bootstrap IPD meta-analysis dataset that has the same number of participants in each study as the original model development dataset. That is, for each study separately, sample participants with replacement from the original IPD for that study, until the bootstrap sample size is the same as that in the original IPD. Merge these bootstrap study samples to form the bootstrap IPD meta-analysis dataset.
3) Develop a prediction model using the bootstrap IPD meta-analysis dataset from step 2; ensure all the same modelling and predictor selection methods are used as in step 1. Then:
   a) Estimate the apparent predictive performance (e.g. *C* statistic, calibration slope) of this bootstrap model on the *bootstrap* IPD in each study separately, and for each performance statistic pool estimates using a random-effects meta-analysis (model (17.2)) to give a summary estimate of the *apparent* performance of the bootstrap model. Again, when making study-specific predictions make sure that the model is applied as intended in practice (see step 1).
   b) Estimate the predictive performance of the bootstrap model in each study separately using the *original* IPD, and for each performance statistic pool estimates using a random-effects meta-analysis (model (17.2)) to give a summary estimate of the *test* performance of the bootstrap model.
4) Estimate the optimism in predictive performance of the bootstrap model by calculating the difference between the summary apparent performance (step 3(a)) and the summary test performance (from step 3(b)). This should be done for each performance statistic of interest (e.g. *C* statistic, calibration slope).
5) Repeat steps 2, 3 and 4 for b times (at least 100), to obtain b estimates of the optimism for each performance statistic of interest.
6) For each performance statistic, average the b estimates of optimism from step 5, and subtract this average optimism value from the pooled apparent performance of the model obtained in step 1; this gives an optimism-adjusted estimate of the model's average performance. For example:

$$\begin{aligned}&\text{optimism-adjusted calibration slope}\\&= (\text{apparent calibration slope for developed model from step 1})\\&\quad - (\text{mean of the } b \text{ optimism estimates of calibration slope obtained from step 5}).\end{aligned}$$

Optimism-adjusted estimates in each study might also be obtained by subtracting from the apparent performance in each study (step 1) the estimated study-specific difference in the bootstrap apparent and bootstrap test performance (from steps 3a and 3b respectively).

Source: Richard Riley, adapting the approach in a single-study setting recommended by Harrell[158] and Steyerberg.[203]

lasso, ridge regression, or elastic net. Alternatively, penalisation can be undertaken after model development by using a uniform shrinkage factor calculated from the internal validation process (Box 17.6). In particular, the optimism-adjusted calibration slope derived from the bootstrap process can be used to shrink predictor effects in the model; for example, if the model's pooled optimism-adjusted calibration slope is 0.9, then the predictor effects in the model can be revised by multiplying their original values by 0.9, and then the model intercept recalculated (holding fixed the revised predictor effects) to ensure overall calibration-in-the-large. Study-specific predictor effects might be better penalised by study-specific optimism-adjustments (Box 17.6), but how to implement this requires further research. Further details of penalisation methods is given elsewhere.[85,158,203]

17.7.2 Internal-external Cross-validation to Examine Transportability

Random resampling methods for internal validation, such as conventional bootstrapping or cross-validation (Box 17.6), allow the researcher to examine reproducibility of the model predictions for new participants from the same populations included in the development dataset. However, it is also possible to generate *non-random* samples in order to examine external validity of the model predictions; that is, to check whether model predictions are likely to be robust in new populations external to those used for model development. In an IPD meta-analysis, a natural choice for generating multiple non-random samples is to split the data by study. This strategy can be implemented through a cross-validation approach, and is known (perhaps confusingly) as internal-external cross-validation.[53,247] Essentially, this method allows the researcher to address the questions "are the IPD studies compatible for developing a single prediction model equation?" and "how might my developed model perform in other settings that potentially differ to those represented by the IPD used to develop the model?" We now describe and illustrate this method.

17.7.2.1 Overview of the Method

Let us assume the IPD comes from S studies, and that all the IPD are used to develop the model using appropriate techniques (including any penalisation), as described in Section 17.7.1. After model development, internal-external cross-validation allows the researcher to examine the potential generalisability of model predictions to new populations. It proceeds by using IPD from all but one of the S studies for model development, with IPD from the remaining study used for external validation; this is repeated a further $S - 1$ times, on each occasion omitting a different study to ascertain external validation performance (e.g. in terms of E/O, calibration slope and C statistic). Each cycle should ensure an adequate sample size for model development,[284–286] and apply appropriate model development methods as used to originally develop the model on all studies;

otherwise, poor performance in the omitted study may simply reflect small sample sizes, overfitting, and sub-standard development techniques.

By this process, internal-external cross-validation produces estimates of predictive performance in each of S cycles, and then meta-analysis can be used to summarise average estimates and the amount of between-study heterogeneity (e.g. by applying random-effects model (17.2) or the multivariate approach described in Section 17.4.2). Empirical Bayes estimates of study-specific performance may also be useful to report.

The study-specific and meta-analysis results may reveal that a developed model works consistently well in other targeted settings and populations not used in model development. Conversely, it might reveal that a developed model has unreliable predictive performance in other settings and populations. To gauge this better, it may help if case-mix differences between the hold-out samples are accounted for in the internal-external cross-validation procedure. In particular, it is possible to estimate case-mix corrected performance statistics in each hold-out sample,[217,248] and to pool these in a random-effects meta-analysis. Then, any observed heterogeneity in case-mix corrected estimates of performance indicate that the prediction model's coefficients may not transport well across different setting and populations (Sections 17.3.2.2 and 17.3.3.3). This infers that model updating or recalibration methods are needed to improve performance in local settings. Even more stringent, it might suggest the IPD from a few studies (e.g. those reflecting a specific population and/or setting) should be removed entirely, as they are not compatible with the IPD from other studies. Then, developing a model in the remaining IPD is more likely to ensure that a more robust model is developed that better generalises and transports to those populations and settings represented by this remaining IPD.[217,230,275]

If IPD are available from studies with different designs, then it may not be appropriate to estimate all performance measures in all studies. For example, when the IPD omitted for validation is from a randomised trial with inclusion criteria that are narrower than in the target population, the calibration-in-the-large (or the E/O statistic) may provide misleading results about the model's performance in new patients. This is because miscalibration on average might be expected if the developed model's intercept was estimated using studies that better reflect the target population, such as observational cohort studies. Similarly, the C statistic also depends on the distribution of participant characteristics in the hold-out study, and may therefore not always reflect meaningful estimates of discriminative performance in the target population if the validation study's population has a different (e.g. narrower) case-mix than the target population.

Note that, if all included studies have a similar case-mix and setting (such that included participants are essentially exchangeable across studies), then internal-external cross-validation corresponds to the traditional cross-validation and assesses model reproducibility (rather than transportability).

17.7.2.2 Example: Diagnostic Prediction Model for Deep Vein Thrombosis

For illustrative purposes, we used IPD from 12 studies to develop a diagnostic model for the risk of having deep vein thrombosis (DVT) in patients who were suspected of having DVT.[223,277] IPD from a total of 10,002 participants were available across the 12 studies (with study sample sizes ranging from 153 to 1768 participants), and 1864 (19%) participants truly had DVT. The prediction model was developed using a one-stage IPD meta-analysis model; that is, a logistic regression, including a separate intercept for each study and three predictors chosen *a priori*: *sex* (male = 1, female = 0), *surgery* (recent surgery or bedridden = 1, no recent surgery or bedridden = 0) and *calf difference* ($\geq$3 cm = 1, <3 cm = 0, with this dichotomisation unfortunately enforced by the format of values provided in the IPD). No heterogeneity in predictor effects was examined and, given the larger number of events (1864) and events per predictor parameter (1864/3 = 621), no adjustment for over-fitting (optimism) was considered necessary (i.e. no penalisation/shrinkage of predictor effects was used).

When developing the prediction model equation, a separate intercept was included for each study. Thus, when using the developed prediction model to estimate the probability of DVT in participants from other datasets (i.e. external to that used for model development), three different strategies were considered for the choice of intercept value to use in the prediction model equation:

- Strategy (1): Use a new intercept estimated from the external dataset itself; essentially this is local recalibration of the baseline risk that requires using new data (external to that for model development) from the local setting.
- Strategy (2): Use the estimated weighted average of the study-specific intercept terms from the IPD meta-analysis dataset that were used to develop the model.
- Strategy (3): Use the estimated intercept for one of the studies used to develop the model that had the most similar prevalence of DVT to the population represented by the external dataset.

To examine predictive performance of the developed model for each of these three strategies, internal-external cross-validation was undertaken with 12 cycles. In each cycle, the IPD from 11 studies were used for model development and the IPD from the remaining study was used for validation of the developed model for each of the three strategies above. The developed model's predictor effect estimates (log odds ratios) are very similar in each cycle (Table 17.6).

In each cycle of the internal-external cross-validation process, and for each strategy separately, we used a two-stage multivariate IPD meta-analysis to summarise the developed model's (derived from 11 IPD studies) performance in the external validation study. In the first stage, estimates and standard errors of four performance measures were calculated after applying the developed model to the external validation study: calibration-in-the-large, calibration slope, the *C* statistic, and the ratio of expected and observed DVT cases (i.e. E/O). Within-study correlations between each pair of performance statistic were also obtained using bootstrapping (Chapter 13).

The multivariate meta-analysis results for each performance measure are shown in Table 17.7, for each of the three implementation strategies. The meta-analysis results for the *C* statistic are practically the same for all strategies, as are those for the calibration slope. This is expected, as the $\beta_1 x_{1i} + \beta_2 x_{2i} + \beta_3 x_{3i}$ component of the logistic regression is not changed within each strategy (minor differences are due to bootstrap sampling error). The average *C* statistic is 0.69 (95% CI: 0.67 to 0.71), with a small amount of between-study heterogeneity ($\hat{\tau} \approx 0.02$), leading to a 95% prediction interval of 0.64 to 0.73 for the *C* statistic in a new population, revealing fairly consistent discrimination performance across studies. The average calibration slope is around 0.98 (95% CI: 0.85 to 1.10), which is close to the ideal value of 1, but between-study heterogeneity is large ($\hat{\tau} \approx 0.16$), reflected by a wide 95% prediction interval for the potential calibration slope in a new setting (e.g. 0.59 to 1.38 for strategy (2)).

Calibration-in-the-large does differ more importantly across the three strategies (Table 17.7), as it is sensitive to the choice of intercept. The meta-analysis results reveal that it is, on average, slightly worse for strategy (1) as there is a small over-prediction in the proportion with DVT (−0.13, 95% CI: −0.19 to −0.08). However, there is almost no heterogeneity in the calibration-in-the-large ($\hat{\tau}$ = 0.008), leading to a narrow 95% prediction interval for the calibration-in-the-large in a new population (−0.20 to −0.07). Using strategy (2) or (3) the average calibration-in-the-large is closer to zero (−0.004 and 0.047, respectively), but comes at the expense of slightly larger between-study heterogeneity ($\hat{\tau} = 0.53$ and 0.27, respectively), leading to wider prediction intervals. For example, for strategy (2) the 95% prediction interval for the calibration-in-the-large in a new population is −1.24 to

Table 17.6 Model parameter estimates for the fitted DVT model obtained in each cycle of the internal-external cross-validation approach to obtain predictor effects and study-specific intercepts.

Study used for external validation	Study-specific intercept ($\hat{\alpha}_i$) Study 1	Study 2	Study 3	Study 4	Study 5	Study 6	Study 7	Study 8	Study 9	Study 10	Study 11	Study 12	Age ($\hat{\beta}_1$)	Sex ($\hat{\beta}_2$)	Calf ($\hat{\beta}_3$)
Study 1	–	1.256	2.528	1.807	2.511	2.316	3.061	1.839	2.165	2.339	2.038	**2.788**	0.372	0.606	1.304
Study 2	2.694	–	2.555	1.823	2.538	2.338	3.080	**1.857**	2.192	2.353	2.059	2.817	0.370	0.624	1.344
Study 3	2.670	1.253	–	1.805	**2.504**	2.312	3.062	1.840	2.157	2.336	2.033	2.779	0.400	0.556	1.286
Study 4	2.604	1.191	2.443	–	2.426	2.245	3.005	**1.785**	2.082	2.289	1.967	2.700	0.366	0.513	1.197
Study 5	2.682	1.265	**2.538**	1.814	–	2.324	3.070	1.849	2.173	2.343	2.045	2.797	0.387	0.579	1.315
Study 6	2.672	1.255	2.529	1.811	**2.508**	–	3.066	1.843	2.161	2.343	2.041	2.783	0.409	0.589	1.277
Study 7	**2.672**	1.255	2.529	1.810	2.509	2.319	–	1.842	2.162	2.342	2.040	2.784	0.401	0.594	1.283
Study 8	2.677	1.260	2.532	**1.812**	2.513	2.321	3.068	–	2.166	2.342	2.042	2.788	0.403	0.572	1.294
Study 9	2.660	1.245	2.515	1.797	2.498	2.304	3.050	1.828	–	2.329	**2.026**	2.777	0.350	0.611	1.300
Study 10	2.677	1.260	2.531	1.809	2.515	2.318	3.066	1.844	2.168	–	2.039	**2.791**	0.381	0.572	1.313
Study 11	2.678	1.261	2.533	1.812	2.515	2.321	3.069	1.847	**2.167**	2.342	–	2.790	0.399	0.565	1.301
Study 12	2.672	1.256	2.528	1.808	2.509	2.317	3.064	1.841	2.162	**2.339**	2.038	–	0.391	0.585	1.293

Bold numbers represent the intercept used for external validation in the excluded study for strategy (3), where the intercept from the study with the closest prevalence was selected. *Source:* Richard Riley and Kym Snell.

Table 17.7 Trivariate meta-analysis results* for the calibration and discrimination performance of the DVT model for each strategy of which intercept value to use when applying the model in new populations.

Strategy	Performance measure	Summary estimate (95% CI)	95% prediction interval
Strategy (1): Develop using logistic regression and implement with intercept estimated in external validation study	Calibration-in-the-large	−0.130 (−0.185 to −0.075)	−0.195 to −0.065
	Calibration slope	0.975 (0.855 to 1.097)	0.597 to 1.353
	Log(Expected/Observed)	0.086 (0.047 to 0.124)	0.041 to 0.128
	C statistic	0.687 (0.670 to 0.704)	0.645 to 0.729
Strategy (2): Develop using logistic regression and implement with average study intercept taken from developed model	Calibration-in-the-large	−0.004 (−0.313 to 0.305)	−1.240 to 1.232
	Calibration slope	0.980 (0.853 to 1.107)	0.585 to 1.375
	Log(Expected/Observed)	0.022 (−0.206 to 0.250)	−0.887 to 0.931
	C statistic	0.687 (0.669 to 0.705)	0.640 to 0.734
Strategy (3): Develop using logistic regression and implement with intercept taken from a study used in development data with a similar prevalence	Calibration-in-the-large	0.047 (−0.120 to 0.214)	−0.584 to 0.678
	Calibration slope	0.976 (0.851 to 1.102)	0.578 to 1.375
	Log(Expected/Observed)	−0.029 (−0.150 to 0.093)	−0.485 to 0.427
	C statistic	0.687 (0.669 to 0.705)	0.640 to 0.734

* A trivariate meta-analysis was fitted to calibration-in-the-large, calibration slope and *C* statistic, and then again for log(Expected/Observed), calibration slope, and C statistic. Perfect negative correlation between calibration-in-the-large and expected/observed within studies prevents all four measures being analysed together (due to collinearity). Results were practically the same for calibration slope and *C* statistic, regardless of the trivariate model fitted. Results also similar if the *C* statistic is modelled on the logit scale.

Source: Table taken from Table 1 of Snell et al.,[277] with permission, © 2016 Elsevier (CC-BY 4.0).

1.23. As anticipated, the results for E/O follow a similar pattern to those for calibration-in-the-large (Table 17.7), with the narrowest prediction interval for strategy (1) and slightly improved average performance for strategies (2) and (3).

Overall, therefore, strategy (1) appears best, as it removes heterogeneity in the calibration-in-the-large and E/O, whilst the discrimination remains practically the same. However, the prediction model would benefit from additional predictors (and the analysis of calf difference on its continuous scale, rather than dichotomised), as currently discrimination is only moderate and there is large heterogeneity in calibration slope. This is confirmed by a joint probability of only 0.03 that strategy (1) will give a C statistic ≥ 0.7 and a calibration slope between 0.9 and 1.1 in a new population. Further work (not shown here) suggests that adding a study-level predictor indicating level of care (i.e. primary versus secondary) may remove much of the heterogeneity.

17.8 Examining the Utility of a Prediction Model Using IPD Meta-Analysis

Calibration and discrimination characterise the predictive performance of a prediction model, but neither captures the consequences of a particular level of discrimination or degree of miscalibration.[71] Prediction models influence individuals' health outcomes or the cost-effectiveness of care when clinical decisions are based on the model's predictions (e.g. of individual outcome probabilities).[212,219] Therefore, when used to direct decision-making, a prediction model should also be evaluated for its overall benefit on participant and healthcare outcomes, also known as its clinical *utility*. For example, for binary or time-to-event outcomes, if the predicted probabilities from a prediction model are above a certain threshold value, then the patient and healthcare professional, in shared decision-making, may be directed to administer a particular treatment, monitoring strategy, or life-style change.

Chapter 15 shows how the benefits, harms and overall impact of a *single* test can be evaluated using IPD meta-analysis (Section 15.5). In particular, a trivariate IPD meta-analysis of sensitivity, specificity and prevalence can be used to summarise the net benefit (*NB*). The same approach can be applied to evaluate the clinical utility of a prediction model, at a particular threshold (p_t) defined by a model's predicted probability.[78,283] For example, it has been suggested that a threshold value of $p_t = 0.08$ is used to inform the continuation of treatment after 30 days following a first venous thromboembolism,[302] such that those with a predicted risk of recurrence of 0.08 or above continue treatment, but those with a risk less than 0.08 should stop (and thus avoid side effects such as bleeding). A threshold below 0.5 indicates that the consequences of a false negative (here, an unexpected recurrence) are worse than the consequences of a false positive (unnecessary preventative treatment). A suggested threshold of $p_t = 0.08$ indicates that the perceived harms of a false negative is 11.5 $(= (\frac{1-0.08}{0.08}))$ times larger than the perceived harm of a false positive. Alternatively, one could say that preventing one recurrence justifies unnecessary preventative treatment of up to 11.5 patients. This 'exchange rate' is used in the calculation of the NB_{p_t}, thus quantifying a model's utility. A decision curve can be used to summarise NB_{p_t} across a range of relevant thresholds.

For prediction models of a binary outcome, the maximum value of NB_{p_t} is the proportion of the target population who have the outcome event (i.e. disease prevalence for diagnostic models, or outcome incidence for prognostic models). It may be helpful to multiply NB_{p_t} by 1000, to give the additional number of true cases (those who truly have an outcome event) identified for treatment, or some other clinical action, without increasing the number treated unnecessarily per 1000 individuals. An example is now provided.

17.8.1 Example: Net Benefit of a Diagnostic Prediction Model for Ovarian Cancer

The International Ovarian Tumour Analysis (IOTA) group developed a prediction model (called 'LR2') to obtain a predicted probability of ovarian cancer presence in those who have at least one persistent adnexal (ovarian, para-ovarian, and tubal) tumour (for which malignant or benign status is unknown) and are considered to require surgery.[303] Their logistic regression model included age and five ultrasound variables: maximal diameter of the largest solid component, irregular internal cyst walls, presence of papillary projections with detectable flow, acoustic shadows, and ascites.

Testa et al. performed a validation study of the predictive performance of the LR2 model,[304] which included 2403 participants from 18 centres (here considered 'studies'). All participants were selected for surgical removal of an adnexal mass and histology was the reference standard to establish whether the tumour was malignant (i.e. cancer) or benign. The observed prevalence of malignancy varied between 15% and 69% across studies. A two-stage IPD meta-analysis of the 18 included studies gave a summary *C* statistic of 0.92 (95% CI: 0.91 to 0.93) for the LR2 model, with little between-study heterogeneity, demonstrating excellent discrimination between benign and malignant tumours. However, the LR2 model tended to underestimate the probability of malignancy in most studies; in the nine largest studies, Testa et al. conclude that "the risk of malignancy was underestimated in seven of the nine (studies), slightly overestimated in one (study) and perfectly calibrated in one (study)".

Despite the general miscalibration, the LR2 model may still have utility. To examine this Wynants et al. used a Bayesian framework to fit the trivariate meta-analysis of sensitivity, specificity and prevalence that was described in Section 15.5.[78] The results are used to calculate the LR2 model's net benefit for 'diagnosing' ovarian cancer when individuals have predicted probabilities greater than or equal to a particular threshold.

17.8.1.1 Summary and Predicted Net Benefit of the LR2 Model

At a risk threshold of 0.05, the summary $NB_{0.05}$ of the LR2 model is 0.27 (95% CrI: 0.21 to 0.34). Hence, at this threshold, the summary net benefit of the LR2 model is equivalent to the benefit of a strategy that correctly detects a net number of 270 cancer cases per 1000 patients, without false positive classifications. The between-study heterogeneity in $NB_{0.05}$ between studies is quite large, as reflected by a 95% prediction interval for $NB_{0.05}$ of 0.05 to 0.66. A more precise prediction of the $NB_{0.05}$ in a new setting may be obtained by conditioning on a known prevalence, as described in Section 15.5.2. For example, regional settings typically have a lower cancer prevalence than university hospitals with a specialized gynaecological oncology unit. For a new setting with a known prevalence of 15%, Wynants et al. calculated a 95% probability that $NB_{0.05}$ will be between 0.12 and 0.14. For a new setting with a known prevalence of 35%, the predicted $NB_{0.05}$ is between 0.29 and 0.33, which suggests there will be between 290 and 330 additional true cases identified for clinical action (treatment) without increasing the number treated unnecessarily per 1000 individuals. As the threshold value increased, the summary NB_{p_t} results for the LR2 model became lower, reflecting that gradually more weight is given to false positive classifications.

17.8.1.2 Comparison to Strategies of Treat All or Treat None

The LR2 model's net benefit results can be compared to those of a 'treat all' strategy. In this clinical context, 'treat all' represents assuming all patients have malignancy and so should proceed to surgery, whereas 'treat none' represents assuming no patients have malignancy and so should not have surgery. Estimation of the trivariate meta-analysis model at $p_t = 0.05$ (i.e. where the perceived harms of false negatives are 19 times larger than the perceived harms of false positives) finds a 69% chance that LR2 is useful in a new study (i.e. it has a highest net benefit than 'treat all' or 'treat none' strategies). When conditioning on a malignancy prevalence of 15%, the probability of usefulness is 99.9 %; if on the other hand the malignancy prevalence is 35%, there is a lower probability that LR2 is useful (75%). This is likely due to the miscalibration of LR2, which seemed to be especially pronounced in studies with a high prevalence.

17.8.2 Decision Curves

A decision curve shows a model's net benefit across a range of relevant thresholds (Section 15.5.1). Figure 17.10 shows the summary decision curve for the LR2 model, which is higher than the summary curves of 'treat all' and 'treat none' strategies at all considered risk thresholds. However, the between-study heterogeneity in decision curves is very large in the LR2 and 'treat all' models, as reflected by the wide prediction intervals. This is mainly caused by between-study heterogeneity in the prevalence of malignancy across studies. The probability that LR2 has the highest clinical utility in new studies is above 90% for risk thresholds between 0.20 and 0.50. Hence, if the clinician's judgement is that a false negative is between four and one times as harmful as a false positive, the LR2 model appears to be a suitable tool to pre-operatively diagnose ovarian cancer. If the clinician

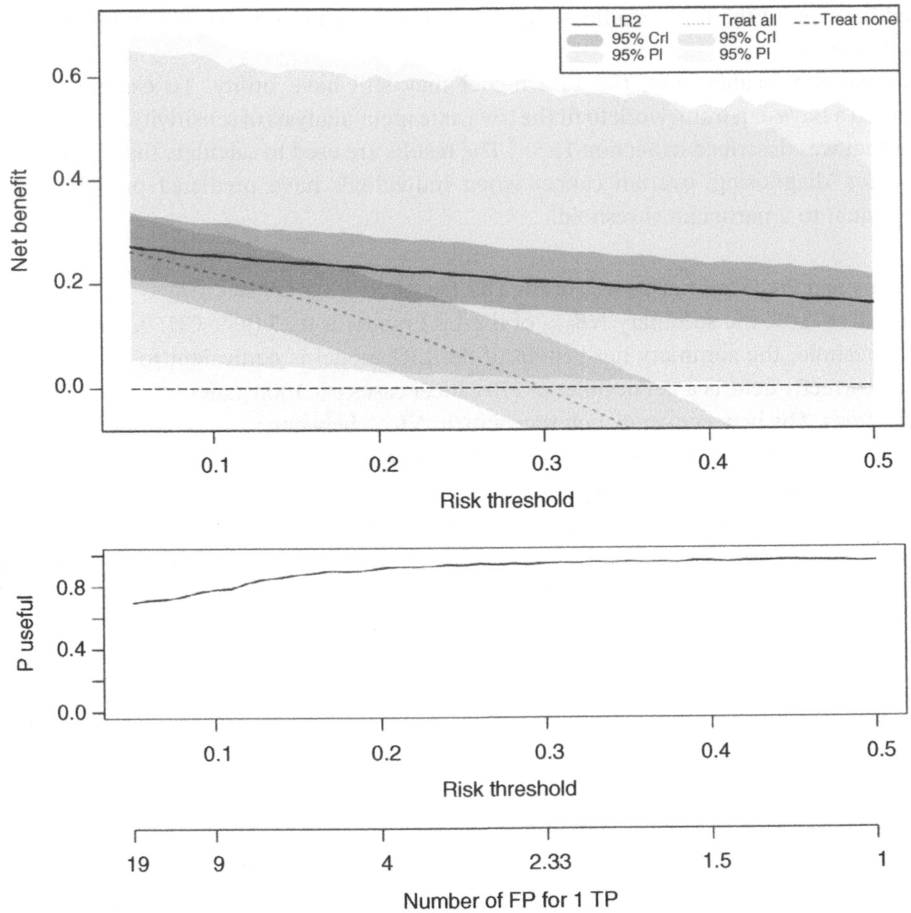

Figure 17.10 Top panel: Summary and predicted decision curves for diagnosing ovarian malignancy using the LR2 model, a 'treat all' or 'treat none' strategy. Middle panel: the probability that using the LR2 model is the most clinically useful strategy (i.e. it has a higher NB_{p_t} than 'treat all' and 'treat none') in a new study. Bottom panel: translation of risk threshold to the number of false positives (FPs) for each true positive (TP). *Source:* Figure adapted from Figure 3 of Wynants et al.,[78] with permission, © 2018 Wiley.

believes that a false negative is 19 times as harmful as a false positive, the probability that the LR2 model is useful in a new setting is 70%, which is still quite high.

17.9 Software

Several statistical software packages are available to facilitate prediction model research. For instance, in R the default package *stats* provides functions for standard regression modelling, and can thus be used to develop multivariable prognostic models. For survival (time-to-event) models, the packages *survival* (Cox regression) and *flexsurv* (Royston-Parmar models) can be used. When considering penalization during model development, researchers may use *rms* or *glmnet* (lasso, elastic net and ridge regression). Alternatively, *logistf* (logistic regression) or *coxphf* (Cox regression) can be used to adopt the Firth bias correction in small samples. When considering modelling of non-linear effects, researchers may use *mfp* or *rms* for multivariable fractional polynomials or restricted cubic splines, respectively. The *rms* package also incorporates functions for survival modelling, penalization, estimation of non-linear effects, and the assessment of (optimism-corrected) model performance. Specific software for prediction model research using an IPD meta-analysis is currently underdeveloped, although methods for meta-analysis of prediction model performance have been implemented in *metamisc*. This package also provides functions to perform internal-external cross-validation and to develop new prediction models with variable selection (and in the future penalization) in heterogeneous data sources such as IPD meta-analyses.

In Stata, many of the regression modelling commands are built in, such as *regress*, *logistic* and *stcox* for linear, logistic and Cox regression models, respectively. The *stpm2* command enables Royston-Parmar models to be fitted and can be installed from the SSC (Statistical Software Components) archive. To model non-linear prognostic effects, multivariable fractional polynomials can be implemented using *mfp*, and *mkspline* used to create spline terms. For model performance, *roctab*, *estat concordance* and *stcstat2* estimate the *C* statistic for logistic, Cox and Royston-Parmar models, respectively, whilst the post-estimation module *fitstat* computes a variety of measures of fit for many kinds of regression models.

Of course, standard meta-analysis packages (such as *admetan* in Stata or *metafor* in R) can be used to combine estimates of predictive performance in the second stage of a two-stage IPD meta-analysis, as discussed in Chapter 5.

17.10 Reporting

As with all IPD meta-analyses, transparent reporting is essential. The TRIPOD statement provides guidance for reporting studies developing, validating or updating a prediction model.[201,202] This has been refined and extended to TRIPOD-CLUSTER,[305] specifically for settings involving datasets with clustering such as IPD meta-analysis and electronic health record data projects (Table 17.8). Key issues to report are the selection and eligibility criteria for participants and data sources, steps taken to prepare the data (including any cleaning, harmonization and linkage), assessments of data quality, accounting for clustering, modelling of heterogeneity, and evaluation of generalizability. Graphical displays presenting model performance are particularly important. For instance, forest and funnel plots can be used to display meta-analyses as shown during this chapter, ideally with calibration plots for the whole dataset and in each cluster separately (Figure 17.9).[53,247]

17.11 Concluding Remarks

Meta-Analysis using IPD from multiple studies provides novel opportunities for prediction model research. In particular, it allows researchers to interrogate and compare the predictive performance of models across multiple settings, populations, and subgroups of interest. Subsequently, if performance is considered unsatisfactory, IPD meta-analysis also enables strategies (such as recalibration) for updating and tailoring the prediction model equation to improve performance to local

Table 17.8 Preliminary version of the TRIPOD-CLUSTER statement extended to situations where a prediction model is developed (D) and/or validated (V) using IPD meta-analyses or electronic health records.[305]

Section / Topic	#	Description
Title and Abstract		
Title	1	Identify the study as developing and/or validating a prediction model, the target population, and the outcome to be predicted.
Abstract	2	Provide a summary of research objectives, setting, participants, data source, sample size, predictors, outcome, statistical analysis, results, and conclusions.
Introduction		
Background and objectives	3a	Explain the medical context (including whether diagnostic or prognostic) and rationale for developing or validating the prediction model, including references to existing models, and the advantages of the study design.
	3b	Specify the objectives, including whether the study describes the development or validation of the model.
Methods		
Participants and data	4a	Describe eligibility criteria for participants and data sources.
	4b	Describe the origin of the data, and how the data were identified, requested and collected.
	5	Explain how the sample size was arrived at.
Outcomes and predictors	6a	Define the outcome that is predicted by the model, including how and when assessed.
	6b	Define all predictors used in developing or validating the model, including how and when measured.
Data preparation	7a	Describe how the data were prepared for analysis, including any cleaning, harmonisation, linkage, and quality checks.
	7b	Describe the method for assessing risk of bias and applicability in the individual clusters (e.g. using PROBAST).
	7c	For validation, identify any differences in definition and measurement from the development data (e.g. setting, eligibility criteria, outcome, predictors).
	7d	Describe how missing data were handled.
Data analysis	8a	Describe how predictors were handled in the analyses.
	8b	Specify the type of model, all model-building procedures (e.g. any predictor selection and penalization), and method for validation.
	8c	Describe how any heterogeneity across clusters (e.g., studies or settings) in model parameter values was handled.
	8d	For validation, describe how the predictions were calculated.
	8e	Specify all measures used to assess model performance (e.g. calibration and discrimination) and, if relevant, to compare multiple models.
	8f	Describe how any heterogeneity across clusters (e.g., studies or settings) in model performance was handled and quantified.
	8g	Describe any model updating (e.g., recalibration) arising from the validation, either overall or for particular populations or settings.
Sensitivity analysis	9	Describe any planned subgroup or sensitivity analysis, e.g. assessing performance according to sources of bias, participant characteristics, setting.

Results		
Participants and datasets	10a	Describe the number and flow of clusters and participants from data identified through to data analysed. A flow chart may be helpful.
	10b	Report the characteristics overall and where applicable for each data source or setting, including the key dates, predictors, treatments received, sample size, number of outcome events, follow-up time, and amount of missing data.
	10c	For validation, show a comparison with the development data of the distribution of important variables (demographics, predictors, and outcome).
Risk of bias	11	Report the results of the risk of bias assessment in the individual clusters.
Model development and specification	12a	Report the results of any across-cluster heterogeneity assessments that led to subsequent actions during the model's development (e.g., inclusion or exclusion of particular predictors or clusters).
	12b	Present the final prediction model (i.e. all regression coefficients, and model intercept or baseline survival at a given time-point) and explain how to use it for predictions in new individuals.
Model performance	13a	Report performance measures (with CIs) for the prediction model, overall and for each cluster.
	13b	Report results of any heterogeneity across clusters in model performance
Model updating	14	Report the results from any model updating (including the updated model equation and subsequent performance), overall and for each cluster.
Sensitivity analysis	15	Report results from any subgroup or sensitivity analysis.
Discussion		
Interpretation	16a	Give an overall interpretation of the main results, including heterogeneity across clusters in model performance, in the context of the objectives and previous studies.
	16b	For validation, discuss the results with reference to the model performance in the development data, and in any previous validations.
	16c	Discuss the strengths of the study and any limitations (e.g. missing or incomplete data, non-representativeness, data harmonisation problems).
Implications	17	Discuss the potential use of the model and implications for future research, with specific view to generalisability and applicability of the model across different settings or (sub)populations.
Other information		
Supplementary information	18	Provide information about the availability of supplementary resources (e.g. study protocol, analysis code, data sets).
Funding	19	Give the source of funding and the role of the funders for the present study.

Source: Thomas Debray.

populations and settings.[217] Sometimes development of an entirely new prediction model is warranted, and then IPD meta-analysis provides larger sample sizes and opportunities to examine generalisability and external validity. Yet there are also challenges, especially dealing with between-study heterogeneity and case-mix variability, and the issue of missing data is given greater attention in the next chapter.

18

Dealing with Missing Data in an IPD Meta-Analysis

Thomas P.A. Debray, Kym I.E. Snell, Matteo Quartagno, Shahab Jolani, Karel G.M. Moons, and Richard D. Riley

Summary Points

- Missing data is a common problem in healthcare research, including IPD meta-analysis projects.
- Complete-case analysis discards participants with missing data, but is generally undesirable, as it is invalid when data are not missing completely at random (MCAR) and leads to a loss of information even when data are MCAR.
- For prognosis and prediction studies, it is usually preferable to assume data are missing at random (MAR), and to adopt multiple imputation methods that impute missing values for a variable conditional on observed values for other variables.
- Multiple imputation can be achieved by explicitly defining a joint distribution of the observed data (joint modelling), or by defining a series of conditional distributions (fully conditional specification, FCS).
- In an IPD meta-analysis, missing data are either sporadically or systematically missing. Sporadically missing data occur when variables are missing for some (but not all) participants in one or more studies. Systematically missing values occur when variables are missing for *all* participants of one or more studies.
- A practical approach to account for sporadically missing values is to perform multiple imputation for each study separately. This avoids borrowing information across studies, and requires systematically missing variables to be dropped.
- The imputation of systematically missing data requires borrowing information across studies and adopting multilevel imputation methods that utilise the FCS or joint model framework. These methods account for the clustering of participants within studies, and allow for between-study heterogeneity on key parameters of the imputation model.
- The choice between multilevel joint models or FCS approaches is context specific, and recommendations are only just emerging.
- It is important that the generation of imputed values is consistent ("congenial") with the analysis of the imputed data.
- In some situations, it is possible to avoid imputing missing values at the participant level, and rather borrow information directly at the study level. In particular, when some studies have a full set of variables and other studies have the same subset of variables, a bivariate meta-analysis can be used to jointly synthesise fully adjusted and partially adjusted results, whilst accounting for their correlation.

Individual Participant Data Meta-Analysis: A Handbook for Healthcare Research, First Edition.
Edited by Richard D. Riley, Jayne F. Tierney, and Lesley A. Stewart.

18.1 Introduction

Missing values of participant-level variables (e.g. covariates, predictors, diagnostic tests, risk and prognostic factors, outcomes) occur in all types of research,[179,306–312] including IPD meta-analysis projects. Such missing data may occur for many reasons, including chance, time pressures, budget and burden constraints, drop-out, and the perceived relevance of recording or collecting certain variables or their likely values. Often researchers perform a complete-case analysis that discards any participants that have a missing value for one or more of the study variables of interest. However, a small number of missing values in each of several variables can result in a complete-case analysis excluded a large number of participants from multivariable models, thereby lowering sample size and reducing precision to estimate effects of interest.[306,307,313,314] In addition, especially in observational research, complete-case analysis can lead to biased estimates of the study associations (e.g. prognostic factors on outcomes) when the participants without any missing values are not representative of the target population.[178] Adding a separate category to denote that a participant-level covariate is missing (i.e. the missing indicator method) also typically leads to biased results in observational research examining etiology, diagnosis and prognosis,[313–315] though may be suitable within the analysis of randomised trials examining a treatment effect (Chapter 5).[315,316] Therefore, more sophisticated methods are required to handle missing data in healthcare research, especially those IPD meta-analyses projects described in previous chapters addressing diagnostic tests, prognostic factors, and prediction models.

In a conventional meta-analysis of aggregate data from published studies, the original study investigators may not have properly accounted for missing data in their study; this may lead to bias in the results from some studies and thus subsequent bias in aggregate data meta-analysis results. In contrast, an IPD meta-analysis project allows the meta-analyst to handle missing data in each study directly, and thus potentially improve upon the missing data methods used by the original study, whilst also ensuring that the same approach is used in every study. In this chapter we provide an overview of different methods for dealing with missing data in an IPD meta-analysis. Dedicated textbooks and articles exist that describe how to deal with missing data in primary research studies, including the following.[178,179,306–316] Our aim is to highlight the specific challenges of dealing with missing data in an IPD meta-analysis context, including how to preserve the clustering of participants within primary studies, whilst allowing for potential between-study heterogeneity. We begin with a motivating example, and then describe the various types of missing data that can occur in an IPD meta-analysis project, and the strategies, statistical approaches and software to deal with each. We generally focus on dealing with missing data in the context of IPD meta-analyses of observational studies, for example for examining prognostic factors or developing prediction models. Most statistical approaches we discuss (e.g. multiple imputation) can also be used to handle missing data in IPD meta-analyses of randomised trials, but further options are discussed in Chapters 5 and 6. Note that we focus on missing values of *participant-level* variables (and not study-level variables), and so the word 'variables' in this chapter refers to covariates or outcomes recorded for participants.

18.2 Motivating Example: IPD Meta-Analysis Validating Prediction Models for Risk of Pre-eclampsia in Pregnancy

A number of prognostic factors ('predictors') are known to be associated with the incidence of pre-eclampsia; for example, a woman has a higher risk if she had pre-eclampsia in a previous pregnancy, or if there is a family history of pre-eclampsia, diabetes, or renal disease. Many multivariable prognostic models have also been published aiming to predict a woman's risk of pre-eclampsia conditional on their values of multiple predictors, mostly within a logistic regression framework, as the outcome is binary (e.g. pre-eclampsia before delivery: yes or no). However, the predictive performance of such models is rarely externally validated (i.e. checked in individuals external to the model development dataset). To address this, the International Prediction of Pregnancy Complication Network (IPPIC) was established comprising over 100 researchers from 25 countries, who contributed IPD from 78 datasets involving 3.6 million pregnancies into a central database.[317] The IPD provided information on multiple variables, including pre-eclampsia outcomes and values of various predictors including maternal characteristics (such as age, medical and family history), biochemical markers, and ultrasound features. Although the combined data was very large, individual studies were originally designed for an array of research questions, resulting in different sets of predictors being available for each study (i.e. most predictors were not recorded in all studies). Furthermore, even when a predictor was recorded within a study, often there were missing values for some participants.

Snell et al. identified IPD from a subset of the studies in the IPPIC network that allowed women from the United Kingdom (UK) to be identified,[318] and used it to externally validate 24 of the previously developed prediction models for any time onset, early onset (<34 weeks gestation) or late onset (≥34 weeks) pre-eclampsia. For example, IPD from five studies (including 7785 women) in the IPPIC network allowed external validation of the predictive performance of a prediction model for late onset of pre-eclampsia developed by Crovetto et al.[319] These five studies, summarised in Table 18.1, had 256 participants with a missing value for at least one variable (outcome or predictor) required to validate the Crovetto logistic regression model (late onset pre-eclampsia is binary: yes or no). The work by Snell et al. serves as a motivating example throughout the chapter.

Table 18.1 Summary of five IPD studies from the IPPIC network that were used to validate the prediction model for onset of late pre-eclampsia proposed by Crovetto et al. (2015),[319] which was a logistic regression model.

Study ID	Type of study	Number of participants	Number (%) with late pre-eclampsia	Number (%) of participants with a missing value for either the outcome or a required predictor in the Crovetto model
1	Prospective cohort	658	26 (4)	4 (<1)
2	Prospective cohort	1045	13 (1)	7 (<1)
3	Randomised trial	316	29 (9)	33 (10)
4	Randomised trial	1554	49 (3)	55 (4)
5	Prospective cohort	4212	263 (6)	157 (4)

Source: Kym Snell.

18.3 Types of Missing Data in an IPD Meta-Analysis

When missing values occur in an IPD meta-analysis dataset, it is important to distinguish between *sporadically* (also known as *partially*) missing data and *systematically* missing data. An IPD meta-analysis project has sporadically missing data when it contains a study with missing values of a variable for some, but not all, participants in that study. For instance, in study 4 of the pre-eclampsia IPD meta-analysis example (Table 18.1), missing values occurred for several predictors including previous pre-eclampsia and family history of pre-eclampsia, as illustrated in Table 18.2.

An IPD meta-analysis project contains systematically missing values when it contains a study that has a missing value of a particular variable for *all* participants in that study. This occurs because studies often have different objectives, and so measure and record different sets of variables (outcomes, predictors, covariates, etc). For instance, in the pre-eclampsia example, IPD were obtained from a mixture of randomised trials and cohort studies, which had different objectives and so recorded different sets of variables. Systematically missing variables included systolic and diastolic blood pressure at trimester 1, which have not been measured for any participants in study 4 (Table 18.2).

18.4 Recovering Actual Values of Missing Data within IPD

The first, and most fundamental, strategy for resolving missing values in an IPD meta-analysis is to contact those study investigators who provided their IPD and to ask them for additional information. In our experience, this has proved very successful. For example, missing values may be located within ancillary files, and dialogue with study investigators may confirm that some missing values actually denote absence of a factor; for example, it may become apparent that a study coded the smoking variable as blank for participants who do not smoke, such that the blank (apparently missing) values can then be replaced with a 'does not smoke' label. Similarly, apparent outliers (i.e. extreme or nonsensical values) may also be resolved and potentially corrected after dialogue with study investigators.

A variable may be systematically missing (i.e. not recorded for any participant) in a study simply as a consequence of the study's inclusion and exclusion criteria. For example, if a trial only recruits female participants, then the sex variable may be missing as otherwise all participants would be coded with the same value (i.e. female). Hence, having a full appreciation of the study inclusion and exclusion criteria is essential. In some situations, systematically missing variables can be calculated from values of other variables that are available in the dataset. For example, BMI can be calculated from height and weight; therefore, even if study investigators do not provide BMI it can be calculated if height and weight are still available. Further details of the process of IPD retrieval, checking and cleaning are described in Chapter 4.

18.5 Mechanisms and Patterns of Missing Data in an IPD Meta-Analysis

Communication with study investigators may not recover all missing values or variables of interest in every study in the IPD meta-analysis. Then, additional strategies are needed to deal with the missing data. The approach to take is context specific, and an important initial step is to consider

Table 18.2 Example of sporadically missing predictors (previous pre-eclampsia and family history of pre-eclampsia) and systematically missing predictors (Trimester 1 (T1) SBP and DBP) in hypothetical data for 10 participants similar to those in study 4 of the pre-eclampsia example of Table 18.1.

Participant ID	Nulliparous	Previous pre-eclampsia	Renal disease	Hypertension	Diabetes	Family history of pre-eclampsia	T1 SBP	T2 SBP	T1 DBP	T2 DBP
1	No		No	No	No	No		116		77
2	No	No	No	No	No			130		81.5
3	Yes	No	No	No	No			109		72.5
4	No	Yes	No	No	No			105		57
5	No		No	No	Yes	No		115.5		68.5
6	Yes	No	No	No	No	No		118.5		73.5
7	Yes	No	No	No	No	No		121		72
8	No	No	No	Yes	No	Yes		125		76
9	No	Yes	No	No	No	No		120		70
10	No	No	No	No	No	No		118.5		80.5

Source: Kym Snell.

the potential missing data mechanism (the underlying cause of missing values) and the pattern of missing data in the IPD meta-analysis dataset, as now described.

18.5.1 Mechanisms of Missing Data

In the IPD of a particular study, the probability that a certain value is missing can be:

- **Identical for all participants**: The data are then said to be *missing completely at random* (MCAR). For instance, it is possible that blood pressure measurements are missing because the automatic sphygmomanometer suddenly broke down. Complete-case analysis only yields valid results when the MCAR assumption holds, but it is inefficient as it reduces the sample size and therefore lowers the precision and statistical power of the analysis.
- **Dependent on other observed variables or information**: The data are then said to be *missing at random* (MAR). For example, the probability of a participant's smoking status being missing may be completely dependent on their values of other observed variables such as disease presence, physical activity, blood pressure, cholesterol level, and body-mass index.
- **Dependent on unobserved information or on the missing value itself**: The data are then said to be missing not at random (MNAR). For example, in a study on social economic status and cardiovascular outcomes, participants with (far) above average incomes may be less likely to report their annual income, in order not to expose this sensitive information, than participants with average incomes; that is, the probability of annual income being missing is dependent on the actual income value itself and cannot be completely informed by values of other observed variables.

As we will describe, it is possible to evaluate whether data are (likely to be) MCAR. However, data are seldom MCAR, and the cause of missingness is often related to other variables observed in the dataset, suggesting that MAR is more appropriate as a default assumption. Then, multiple imputation methods are generally recommended, to give estimates that are less likely to be biased than those from a complete-case analysis. Multiple imputation is also preferred when data are MCAR, as it allows participants with missing values to be retained, thereby improving precision and statistical power. Finally, even when data are suspected to be MNAR, traditional multiple imputation methods may still partially reduce bias or be a useful sensitivity analyses (though more sophisticated methods to perform multiple imputation are available to deal with specific types of MNAR data,[320] which we do not consider in this chapter).

18.5.2 Patterns of Missing Data

Regardless of the amount of missingness, in both primary studies and IPD meta-analyses it is helpful to have a sense of whether participants with any missing data are a completely random subset of those with completely observed data (i.e. data are MCAR). For each study in the IPD meta-analysis, researchers should summarise the distribution (e.g. mean, median and standard deviation for continuous variables) of observed study variables for both the group of participants with observed data and the group with missing data. If the two groups are similar for all study variables, it adds more credence that the data could be MCAR and a complete-case analysis may yield valid results (though less precise, as discussed previously). However, it is much more likely that the two compared groups (those with completely observed data and those with at least one missing value) have a different distribution for their observed variables. Then, there is a strong concern that the participants with complete observations are a selective subset of the original study sample, and that missingness is not MCAR. Then a MAR assumption is more plausible, especially if studies provide many other variables that can be used to inform the missing values. However, regardless of how many other variables are available, and whether participants with and without missing values differ in their distribution of observed study variables, MNAR cannot be ruled out because the reason(s) for missing values may still depend on unobserved information.

18.5.3 Example: Risk of Pre-eclampsia in Pregnancy

Let us return to the pre-eclampsia example (Section 18.2), where the aim was to use IPD from multiple studies to externally validate existing prediction models for pre-eclampsia. Missingness was summarised for each variable in each study of the IPD meta-analysis. For each study separately, summary statistics for observed variables were compared between the participants with completely observed data versus those with at least one missing value.

Table 18.3 shows the comparison for study 2, which contains 1045 women (917 with complete data and 128 with missing data). For most variables, summary statistics were fairly similar across the two groups; for example, the mean age of participants was 30 years in both groups, and the median BMI was around 24 with similar interquartile ranges. However, differences appeared for ethnicity (higher percentage of Asians with missing values) and for parity (higher percentage of women who had a previous birth with missing values). As a consequence, it is possible that performing a complete-case analysis (and therefore excluding participants with any missing values) may lead to a selected group of participants (e.g. with fewer Asian people and fewer parous women); this selection bias may then distort results from the IPD meta-analysis.

Hence, rather than a complete-case-analysis, we assume that data are MAR for study 2 and also the other studies in this IPD meta-analysis. MAR assumes that, although the choice to measure (or to not measure) certain variables in the provided IPD may have been driven by perceived health

Table 18.3 Summary statistics for participants with complete data, and for participants with one or more values missing for variables of interest, in study 2 of the IPD meta-analysis to validate pre-eclampsia prediction models.

	Summary statistics	
Variable	**Complete (*N* = 917)**	**With missing data (*N* = 128)**
Age, mean (SD)	29.9 (5.1)	29.7 (5.6)
BMI, median [IQR]	24.6 [21.6 to 27.3]	23.8 [21.5 to 27.2]
MAP, mean (SD)	87.9 (9.5)	87.2 (10.5)
Ethnicity, %		
White	40	28
Black	10	7
Asian	45	63
Mixed	1	1
Other	3	2
Parity and previous PE, %		
Nulliparous	58	42
Parous but no previous PE	41	54
Previous PE	1	4
Smoking during pregnancy, %	4	2
History of hypertension, %	1	1

NB: This table considers a broader set of variables than those predictors included in the Crovetto prediction model.
Source: Kym Snell.

status or outcome risk, this process is captured by the values of other variables that are routinely collected in each study's IPD. MNAR cannot be ruled out entirely, as missing values may also be dependent on other variables that are not routinely collected, but the MAR assumption should at least partially mitigate the concern of missing data. To deal with data that are MAR in IPD meta-analyses of observational studies, multiple imputation is a preferred analysis strategy (Section 18.6).

18.6 Multiple Imputation to Deal with Missing Data in a Single Study

Consider for now that there are missing values of an important variable within a single study, and that these are associated with values of other observed variables. Then, the missing values may be predicted (and thus replaced or *imputed*) conditional on the observed data, using a process called imputation. When each missing value is imputed on two or more occasions, it is referred to as *multiple imputation*. Multiple imputation conditional on the observed data is an appropriate method to handle missing data, as it usually leads to less bias and more appropriate standard errors of parameter estimates (as compared to complete-case analysis and most other missing data methods) in situations where data are MCAR or MAR;[178,179,306–308,314,315,321,322] it may even perform better than complete-case analysis when data are partially MNAR (i.e. bias in estimates can still be reduced, even if not fully). With multiple imputation, multiple copies of the dataset are created, with the missing values replaced by imputed values conditional on the observed data. Single imputation is generally inappropriate, especially for observational research, as it ignores the uncertainty of imputed values and this leads to artificially precise estimates. Uncertainty arises because (i) the parameters of the imputation method or model are themselves estimated with uncertainty, and (ii) observations are prone to random variation (i.e. there is residual error). The use of multiple imputation enables the uncertainty of imputed values to be propagated during subsequent analysis.

An important component of multiple imputation is the specification and utilisation of a joint distribution of all the variables to be used in the imputation process. The full set of variables must include all those variables that are to be used in the main study analysis (i.e. the planned analysis for that study), but also any other auxiliary variables (including covariates and outcomes) in the dataset that may provide better predictions of the missing values to be imputed. The joint distribution is typically modelled using either a joint modelling approach or by specifying a series of separate conditional distributions, as now described.

18.6.1 Joint Modelling

The general idea of joint modelling multiple imputation is to explicitly define a joint model for all the variables, so that the partially observed data can be used to impute any missing values for the included variables. To introduce the idea, we consider a single dataset containing values of three continuous variables (y_j, x_{1j}, x_{2j}) for j=1 to N participants, where y_j is the outcome of the study's intended main (sometimes called substantive) analysis model, and x_{1j} and x_{2j} are two covariates. Assume also that all three variables have missing values. The simplest joint model is the multivariate normal model:

$$\begin{aligned} y_j &= \beta_0 + \epsilon_{0j} \\ x_{1j} &= \beta_1 + \epsilon_{1j} \\ x_{2j} &= \beta_2 + \epsilon_{2j} \end{aligned} \qquad \begin{pmatrix} \epsilon_{0j} \\ \epsilon_{1j} \\ \epsilon_{2j} \end{pmatrix} \sim N\left(\begin{pmatrix} 0 \\ 0 \\ 0 \end{pmatrix}, \Omega = \begin{pmatrix} \omega_{0,0} & \omega_{0,1} & \omega_{0,2} \\ \omega_{0,1} & \omega_{1,1} & \omega_{1,2} \\ \omega_{0,2} & \omega_{1,2} & \omega_{2,2} \end{pmatrix} \right)$$

Having chosen this imputation model, Bayesian methods are an appealing way to fit the model and use it to impute the missing data. In particular, Gibbs sampling can be used to fit a multivariate normal model, dealing with missing data via a data augmentation algorithm.[323] This consists of repeatedly drawing new values for all the parameters in the model, one at a time, from the relevant conditional distributions, which are analytically derived from the joint distribution itself. The parameters of the model are the main effects $\boldsymbol{\beta}$ and the covariance matrix $\boldsymbol{\Omega}$. In addition, each missing value is treated as an unknown parameter. For example, for a participant j with a missing value for x_{2j}, the imputed value for x_{2j} at iteration t is drawn from the relevant distribution, conditional on observed data and current draws of the other parameters:

$$f\left(x_{2j}\middle|y_j, x_{1j}, \boldsymbol{\beta}_t, \boldsymbol{\Omega}_t\right) \sim N(\mu, \sigma)$$

$$\mu = \beta_{2t} + \begin{pmatrix} \omega_{0,2,t} \\ \omega_{1,2,t} \end{pmatrix}^T \begin{pmatrix} \omega_{0,0,t} & \omega_{0,1,t} \\ \omega_{0,1,t} & \omega_{1,1,t} \end{pmatrix}^{-1} \begin{pmatrix} y_j - \beta_{0t} \\ x_{1j} - \beta_{1t} \end{pmatrix},$$

$$\sigma = \omega_{2,2,t} - \begin{pmatrix} \omega_{0,2,t} \\ \omega_{1,2,t} \end{pmatrix}^T \begin{pmatrix} \omega_{0,0,t} & \omega_{0,1,t} \\ \omega_{0,1,t} & \omega_{1,1,t} \end{pmatrix}^{-1} \begin{pmatrix} \omega_{0,2,t} \\ \omega_{1,2,t} \end{pmatrix}$$

The sampler has to be run until it converges to the stationary distribution. Then, the current draw of the missing values is combined with the observed data to make the first imputed dataset. Each of the remaining required imputed datasets are obtained after running the sampler for an additional number of iterations, in order to guarantee stochastic independence between imputations.

Before running the Gibbs sampler, it is necessary to choose starting values for the model parameters; the more plausible the starting values, the faster the sampler converges. Furthermore, being a Bayesian method, prior distributions must be specified. For imputation under MAR these are usually flat or weakly informative.[324] The joint modelling approach can be extended to include categorical variables by assuming a latent Gaussian variable (rather than directly modelling x or y as Gaussian), and draws of this variable are transformed into discrete values using an appropriate link function.[324,325]

18.6.2 Fully Conditional Specification

The fully conditional specification (FCS) approach (also known as multiple imputation by chained equations, or MICE) is a common method for producing multiple imputations. It imputes missing data on a variable-by-variable basis such that for a given incomplete variable, an appropriate regression model is specified conditional on the remaining variables. For example, the method defines a linear regression model for a continuous variable, a logistic regression model for a binary variable, a multinomial logistic regression model for an unordered categorical variable, and an ordinal regression model for an ordered categorical variable. The predictions from the regression models are then used to generate new, imputed values. It is also possible to define semi-parametric models for the conditional distributions. For instance, predictive mean matching uses regression models to identify participants that resemble the participant with missing values. The imputed value is then randomly sampled from these so-called donors, and therefore is less dependent on the regression modelling assumptions.[326] Other flexible modelling strategies that have been proposed for defining the conditional distributions include recursive partitioning, random forests, and generalized additive models.[327–330]

The FCS approach is an iterative procedure resembling a Markov chain Monte Carlo (MCMC) method. For example, consider the procedure for a single-study dataset with four incomplete variables, y_j, x_{1j}, x_{2j}, and x_{3j}. It starts by an initial imputation, where all missing values are filled in using a random sample from the observed data. Then, the first incomplete variable (y_j) is imputed from the variables x_{1j}, x_{2j}, and x_{3j}. Next, the second incomplete variable (x_{1j}) is imputed from the variables y_j, x_{2j}, and x_{3j} (using the updated imputations of y_j). The process continues until the last variable (x_{3j}) is imputed, resulting in completion of the first cycle. This whole cycle is then iterated a number of times (say 10–20) to stabilize the results. Then, assuming the algorithm has converged to a stationary distribution, the imputation process continues until the required number of multiple imputation datasets is obtained. Although this iterative procedure resembles joint modelling imputation, the main difference here is that conditional distributions are not analytically derived from a (pre-specified) joint distribution. Instead, it is simply assumed that the combination of conditional distributions describes an (unknown) global joint distribution.

When adopting FCS imputation methods, the full conditional distribution of each incomplete variable should be compatible with the global joint distribution of the multivariate missing data. This requirement holds, for instance, when all incomplete variables are normally distributed. The conditional models can then be described by a linear regression, and are compatible with a multivariate normal model. In practice, however, the conditional models are generally incompatible with a joint model. This may influence the results of an analysis from multiply imputed datasets because a joint distribution from which imputations are drawn might not exist, and thus the results might be sensitive to the order of imputations (i.e., which variable was imputed first). Nevertheless, several empirical studies (via simulation) have shown that the incompatibility of the specified conditional models is of little importance in practice.[331,332]

18.6.3 How Many Imputations Are Required?

When generating multiple completed versions of a single-study dataset with missing values by using imputation, researchers have to choose how many datasets to generate. Clearly the more imputations the better, but the flip-side is that large numbers of imputations increase computational time and may not be necessary. The optimal number of imputations depends on a number of factors, including the fraction of information missing, the research question and the parameters of interest for the main analysis.[310] Therefore a blanket answer is difficult, but some rules of thumb have been proposed: a simple one is that 20 copies are enough for most purposes, whilst another is that the number of copies (K) should be greater than or equal to the total percentage of participants with (one or more) missing values in the dataset.[333]

18.6.4 Combining Results Obtained from Each Imputed Dataset

Assume the multiple imputation has produced M imputed (i.e. completed) datasets for a particular study. Then, for each imputed dataset separately, the researcher must undertake their main analysis to estimate the statistics of interest (e.g. prognostic factor effect, prediction model performance). This leads to M estimates of each statistic of interest, as well as M standard errors. For example, in each study within the pre-eclampsia example (Section 18.2), the main analysis is to estimate the performance of a prediction model for risk of developing pre-eclampsia. One measure of interest is the calibration slope (defined in Chapter 17) and so, in a particular study, the researcher would obtain M estimates of the calibration slope. The overall estimate for that study is then the average of these M estimates. To obtain an appropriate standard error for this estimate, it is important to account for the number of imputed datasets (M) and the variation within and between the imputed datasets; Rubin's rules can be used for this purpose.[334] The resulting standard error can be used alongside the overall (average) estimate of the statistic to derive confidence intervals and make inferences for that study.

18.7 Ensuring Congeniality of Imputation and Analysis Models

It is important for the statistical model used for the multiple imputation process to be consistent ("congenial") with the statistical model used for the intended (main) study analysis to be used to obtain statistics of interest (e.g. effect estimates, predictive performance measures), as otherwise substantial bias may arise in the results.[335] This implies that researchers should consider carefully if and how variables should be used to describe the distribution of the observed data, and the model assumptions used during imputation, for example with respect to the chosen link function, functional form, residual error specification, presence of clustering, and so forth. Problems may appear, for instance when the main study analysis intends to investigate non-linear relationships between a particular covariate and outcome, but only linear relationships are assumed during imputation. Non-congeniality may also arise when imputation models ignore the observed outcome, or the potential for interactions, competing events or time-varying effects.

Congeniality of the imputation method is particularly important in an IPD meta-analysis project, as usually the main IPD meta-analysis will preserve clustering of participants within studies and allow for unexplained between-study heterogeneity. Hence, if the clustering of participants within studies and potential between-study heterogeneity is ignored during imputation, the subsequent IPD meta-analysis results may be misleading; for example, between-study variance estimates and thus standard errors of summary results may be diluted. Therefore, clustering and between-study heterogeneity must be incorporated into the imputation model to maintain the congeniality with the subsequent IPD meta-analysis model.[336] We now describe how to do this.

18.8 Dealing with Sporadically Missing Data in an IPD Meta-Analysis by Applying Multiple Imputation for Each Study Separately

For IPD meta-analysis projects that are affected by sporadically missing values only (i.e. there are no studies where values of a key variable are unobserved for all participants), a straightforward solution is to perform multiple imputation separately in the IPD for each study. This approach is also known as within-study imputation and naturally preserves the clustering of participants within studies and any heterogeneity between studies. Multiple imputation can then be achieved as described in Section 18.6, using joint modelling or FCS in each study separately. This yields multiple imputed datasets for each study, which can be analysed in different ways, as shown by Burgess et al. and presented in Figure 18.1.[336]

Assuming the same number of imputed datasets are created for each study, one approach is to combine (stack) the imputed datasets from each study; that is, to stack the first imputed datasets for each study into an IPD meta-analysis dataset, then stack the second imputed datasets for each study into another IPD meta-analysis dataset, and so forth. This produces M imputed versions of the IPD meta-analysis dataset, derived from the M imputed versions of each primary study. Then, each imputed version of the IPD meta-analysis dataset can be analysed separately by performing a one-stage or two-stage IPD meta-analysis, and the M results obtained can be pooled using Rubin's rules to obtain the final meta-analysis results.[336]

An alternative and generally preferable approach is for researchers to first combine the multiply imputed datasets per study. That is, the imputed dataset for each study is analysed separately and so M results are obtained for each study; these are then pooled within each study using Rubin's rules to

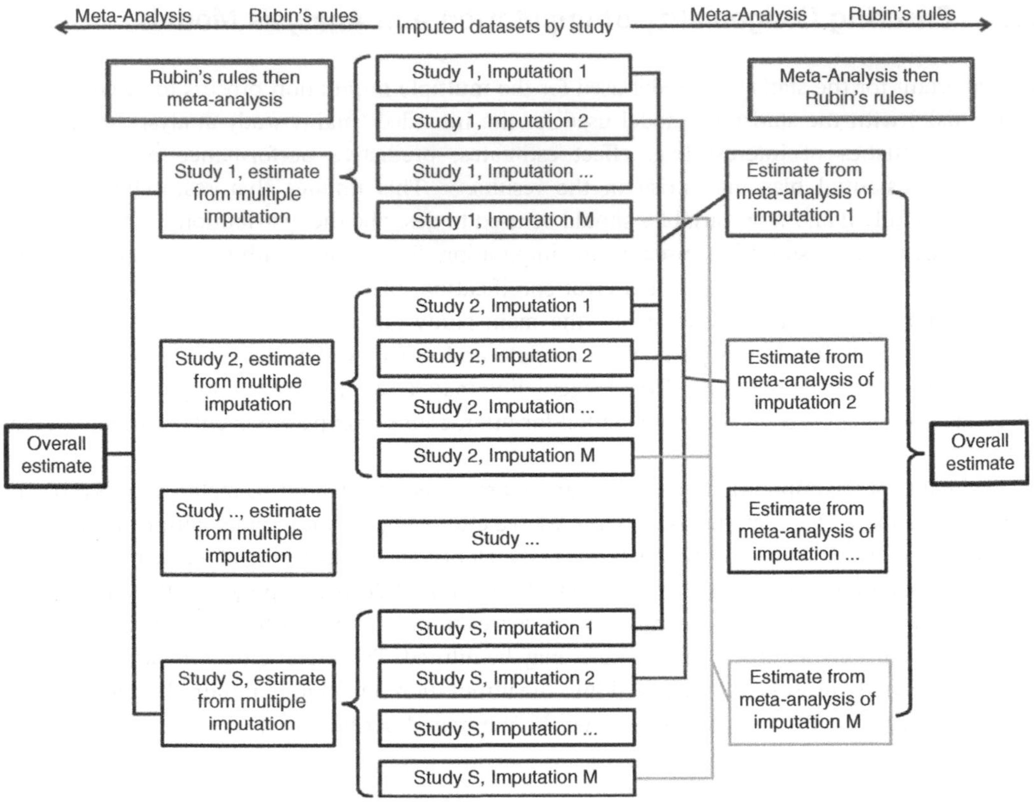

Figure 18.1 Options to analysing multiple imputation datasets in an IPD meta-analysis with sporadically missing values, as proposed by Burgess et al.[336] The 'overall estimate' is the final summary result (e.g. prognostic effect) from the meta-analysis after incorporating multiple imputation. *Source:* Figure taken from Figure 1 of Burgess et al.,[336] with permission, © Wiley 2013.

get a final estimate and standard error for each study. Finally, these study-specific estimates are combined using conventional meta-analysis methods (i.e. the common-effect or random-effects models introduced in Chapter 5 for the second stage of a two-stage IPD meta-analysis) to produce the final meta-analysis results. Simulation studies have demonstrated that this approach is preferable to the method mentioned in the previous paragraph (i.e. applying Rubin's rules of M meta-analysis estimates),[336] as it preserves adequate coverage levels for the estimated associations of interest. When using the other approach, heterogeneity of the meta-analysis results is inflated by random variation across imputations, which in turn leads to coverage that is overly conservative.

Within-study imputation is often the preferred approach for dealing with sporadically missing data in an IPD meta-analysis project, as it can be implemented using traditional software packages and avoids the need to make any specific assumptions about how the associations between the variables vary across studies. However, within-study imputation can become problematic when certain primary studies include very few participants,[309] and becomes obviously unfeasible when important variables are systematically missing in some studies. It also cannot borrow information from study-level covariates, or from participant-level covariates that do not vary within a study. For this reason, multilevel imputation methods may offer an appealing alternative (Section 18.10).

18.8.1 Example: Risk of Pre-eclampsia in Pregnancy

Let us return to our motivating example introduced in Section 18.2, where Snell et al. used IPD meta-analysis to externally validate 24 existing models for predicting pre-eclampsia.[318] To handle the sporadically missing data and preserve any heterogeneity between studies, multiple imputation was applied within each study separately. The decision of how many imputations to use was based on the study with the highest percentage of participants with missing data for any of the variables (predictors or outcomes) missing. Two studies had about 98% of participants with at least one missing value, and therefore 100 imputations were created for all studies with missing data. This was perhaps excessive, and led to long computational times, but was chosen to capture the full uncertainty of imputations.

Consider the external validation of the prediction model of Crovetto et al,[319] which used IPD from the five studies introduced in Table 18.1. A two-stage IPD meta-analysis approach was used to summarise the model's predictive performance. For each study separately, the risk prediction model's linear predictor value (i.e. the model equation's predicted logit risk) was calculated for all participants within each imputation, and this was used to estimate the model's predictive performance in terms of the *C* statistic, expected/observed (E/O) ratio, calibration slope and calibration-in-the-large. For each performance measure separately, the estimates were then pooled across the imputations for each study using Rubin's rules, applying transformations where necessary to improve the normality assumption. For example, the *C* statistic was pooled on the logit scale and E/O was pooled on the natural logarithm scale.[257,337] This produced a final estimate and standard error for each performance measure in each study. These were then summarised across studies using a random-effects meta-analysis with REML estimation, for each performance measure separately, using the same transformations as for pooling across imputations. The Hartung-Knapp-Sidik-Jonkman approach was used to calculate 95% confidence intervals.[259] The analysis is illustrated for the calibration slope in Table 18.4. The summary results show that, on average across the five studies, there is poor calibration of the model's predicted risks and the observed risks, with a summary calibration slope well below 1 (indicative of overfitting during model development, as explained in Chapter 17). There is also considerable between-study heterogeneity, suggesting large variability in the calibration slope across studies. Interestingly, in this example the complete-case results are very similar, although those based on multiple imputation were slightly more precise, due to the additional participants that could be included.

18.9 Dealing with Systematically Missing Data in an IPD Meta-Analysis Using a Bivariate Meta-Analysis of Partially and Fully Adjusted Results

So far we have considered within-study imputation to deal with sporadically missing values only. However, important variables may also be systematically missing in some studies, and this leads to a dilemma when these variables are to be included in the IPD meta-analysis: either throw studies with systematically missing variables away (and thus lose valuable participant data that is observed for other variables) or use methods that allow such studies to be retained by borrowing information across studies about the systematically missing variables. For example, if a particular variable (e.g., a single predictor or outcome) is systematically missing in one study (such that its values are unobserved for all participants), then it cannot be imputed based on that study's data alone; however, if

Table 18.4 A summary of the results at each stage of the multiple imputation process to examine the calibration slope of a prediction model for risk of late-onset pre-eclampsia using IPD from five studies.

Study	Step 1: Calculate calibration slope within each imputation (*M*) for each study: estimate (SE)	Step 2: Pool estimates of calibration slope from step 1 for each study (using Rubin's rules): estimate (SE)	Step 3: Apply random-effects meta-analysis of estimates from step 2 to summarise calibration slope
Study 1	$M = 1$: 0.3661 (0.3067) $M = 2$: 0.3405 (0.3089) $M = 3$: 0.3616 (0.3125) .... $M = 100$: 0.4371 (0.2960)	0.3786 (0.3111)	Summary calibration slope = 0.56 95% CI = −0.01 to 1.12 $I^2 = 92.4\%$ $\tau^2 = 0.18$
Study 2	$M = 1$: 0.5162 (0.2080) $M = 2$: 0.5158 (0.2081) $M = 3$: 0.5165 (0.2081) .... $M = 100$: 0.5162 (0.2080)	0.5159 (0.2082)	
Study 3	$M = 1$: 0.3478 (0.0937) $M = 2$: 0.3687 (0.0963) $M = 3$: 0.3799 (0.0984) .... $M = 100$: 0.3531 (0.0959)	0.3450 (0.0983)	
Study 4	$M = 1$: 0.1961 (0.1207) $M = 2$: 0.2001 (0.1236) $M = 3$: 0.1813 (0.1238) .... $M = 100$: 0.1853 (0.1250)	0.2102 (0.1253)	
Study 5	$M = 1$: 1.2482 (0.0652) $M = 2$: 1.2493 (0.0652) $M = 3$: 1.2485 (0.0652) .... $M = 100$: 1.2494 (0.0652)	1.2478 (0.0652)	

Source: Kym Snell.

we are willing to learn from relationships observed in other studies that do record this and other variables, then the study with the systematically missing variable can still be retained.

A key method for borrowing information across studies is a multivariate IPD meta-analysis. Chapter 13 describes multivariate meta-analysis methods in the context of meta-analysing studies with systematically missing outcomes, where the aim is to borrow strength from other correlated outcomes. For example, some cancer studies may allow prognostic effect estimate to be derived for both overall survival and disease-free survival, but other studies may only allow it to be derived for overall survival. A multivariate meta-analysis can incorporate all these studies in the same analysis, and account for the correlation between overall and disease-free survival effect estimates, so that all studies still contribute toward the disease-free survival result (including those studies for which only overall survival was available). Essentially this approach avoids imputing missing outcome values at the participant level, and rather borrows information at the study level.

The same framework can sometimes be used to deal with systematically missing covariates (predictors, adjustment factors, etc). For example, consider the Fibrinogen Studies Collaboration, which obtained IPD from 31 studies to examine whether plasma fibrinogen concentration is a risk factor for cardiovascular disease (CVD) after adjustment for known risk factors.[180] All

31 studies allowed a *partially* adjusted hazard ratio to be obtained, where the hazard ratio for fibrinogen was adjusted for the same core set of known risk factors, including age, smoking, BMI and blood pressure. However, a more *fully* adjusted hazard ratio, additionally adjusted for cholesterol, alcohol consumption, triglycerides and diabetes, was only calculable in 14 of the 31 studies. By definition, partially and fully adjusted results will be highly correlated, and so a bivariate random-effects meta-analysis can be used to account for this correlation, whilst still incorporating studies that only provide a partially adjusted effect estimate. This enables the researcher to borrow strength (at the study level) from partially adjusted effect estimates ($\hat{\theta}_{\text{iP}}$) in studies where fully adjusted effect estimates ($\hat{\theta}_{\text{iF}}$) are unavailable, and allows all studies to contribute toward the summary estimate of the fully adjusted effect (θ_{F}), which is of key interest. This bivariate model can be written as:

$$\begin{pmatrix} \hat{\theta}_{\text{iP}} \\ \hat{\theta}_{\text{iF}} \end{pmatrix} \sim N\left(\begin{pmatrix} \theta_{\text{iP}} \\ \theta_{\text{iF}} \end{pmatrix}, \boldsymbol{\delta}_{\mathbf{i}} \right) \quad \boldsymbol{\delta}_{\mathbf{i}} = \begin{pmatrix} s_{\text{iP}}^2 & \rho_{\text{Wi(P,F)}} s_{\text{iP}}^2 s_{\text{iF}}^2 \\ \rho_{\text{Wi(P,F)}} s_{\text{iP}}^2 s_{\text{iF}}^2 & s_{\text{iF}}^2 \end{pmatrix}$$
$$\begin{pmatrix} \theta_{\text{iP}} \\ \theta_{\text{iF}} \end{pmatrix} \sim N\left(\begin{pmatrix} \theta_P \\ \theta_F \end{pmatrix}, \boldsymbol{\Omega} \right) \quad \boldsymbol{\Omega} = \begin{pmatrix} \tau_P^2 & \tau_P \tau_F \rho_B \\ \tau_P \tau_F \rho_B & \tau_F^2 \end{pmatrix} \qquad (18.1)$$

The s_{iP} and s_{iF} are the standard errors of $\hat{\theta}_{\text{iP}}$ and $\hat{\theta}_{\text{iF}}$, respectively. For each study that allows both partially and fully adjusted estimates to be derived, bootstrapping of the IPD can be used to estimate their within-study correlation ($\rho_{\text{Wi(P, F)}}$), as described in Chapter 13. If there are sporadically missing values in a study, this can be handled using within-study imputation methods described in Section 18.6. The $\boldsymbol{\Omega}$ represents the between-study variance matrix, containing the between-study variances (τ_P^2 and τ_F^2) and between-study correlation (ρ_B) of the true partially and fully adjusted effects. The bivariate model (18.1) may be difficult to fit when the desired full set of adjustment factors is only available in one or a few studies, and so is not a universal solution to dealing with systematically missing covariates (Section 18.10 gives alternative options), but may be useful in some select situations.

Returning to the fibrinogen example, a standard (univariate) random-effects meta-analysis of just the 14 studies that provided a full set of adjustment factors gives a summary fully adjusted HR of 1.31 (95% CI: 1.22 to 1.42), which indicates that a 1 g/L increase in fibrinogen levels is associated, on average, with a 31% relative increase in the hazard of CVD. However, applying bivariate meta-analysis model (18.1) allows inclusion of all 31 studies (and thus an additional 17 studies and >70,000 participants), and utilises the large correlation (close to +1 both within and between studies) between partially and fully adjusted results. This produces the same 'fully' adjusted summary HR of 1.31, but gives a more precise confidence interval (1.25 to 1.38) due to the extra information gained. The summary 'fully' adjusted HR has a large borrowing of strength statistic (*BoS* of 53%), indicating that the correlated evidence (from the partially adjusted results) contributes 53% of the total weight toward the summary result (Chapter 13 explains the *BoS* statistic), although clinical conclusions are not changed in this particular example.

In another example, Riley et al. used IPD from 10 randomised trials of hypertension patients to examine whether smoking is a prognostic factor for stroke, after adjusting for age, BMI and antihypertensive treatment.[338] All 10 trials produced partially adjusted hazard ratio estimates (i.e. unadjusted for age and BMI, but adjusted for treatment). Additionally, five of the 10 trials produced fully adjusted hazard ratio estimates (i.e. adjusted for age, BMI and treatment). Therefore five trials provided both $\hat{\theta}_{\text{iP}}$ and $\hat{\theta}_{\text{iF}}$ (with within-study correlations between 0.89 and 0.99), whilst the other five trials only provided $\hat{\theta}_{\text{iP}}$. When applying bivariate model (18.1) to all 10 trials the summary fully

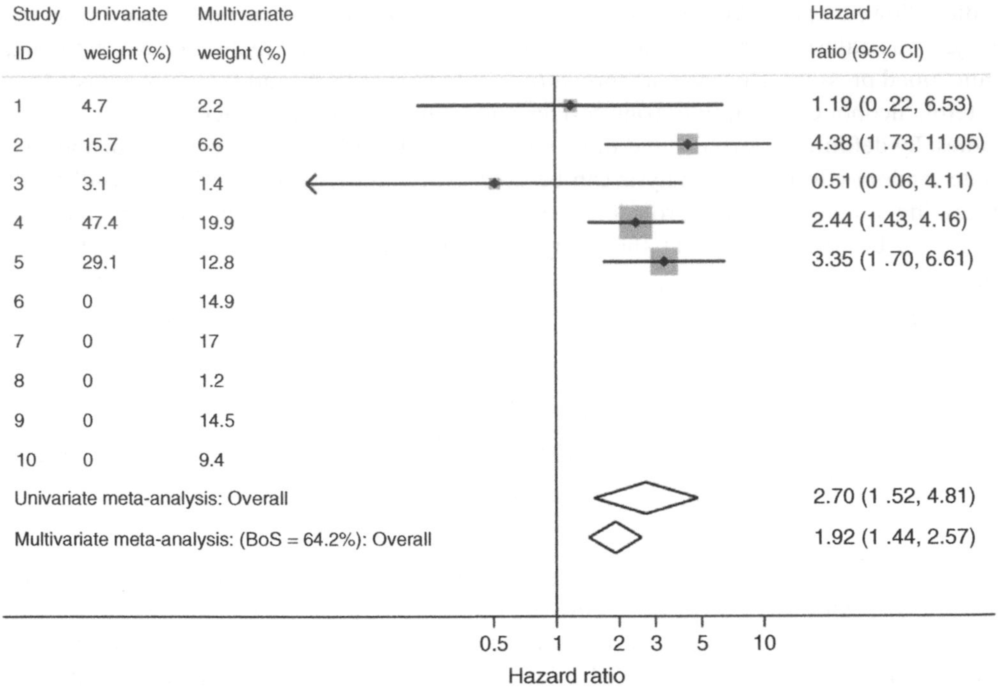
Study ID
Univariate weight (%)
Multivariate weight (%)
Hazard ratio (95% CI)
1 4.7 2.2 1.19 (0 .22, 6.53)
2 15.7 6.6 4.38 (1 .73, 11.05)
3 3.1 1.4 0.51 (0 .06, 4.11)
4 47.4 19.9 2.44 (1.43, 4.16)
5 29.1 12.8 3.35 (1 .70, 6.61)
6 0 14.9
7 0 17
8 0 1.2
9 0 14.5
10 0 9.4
Univariate meta-analysis: Overall 2.70 (1 .52, 4.81)
Multivariate meta-analysis: (BoS = 64.2%): Overall 1.92 (1 .44, 2.57)
0.5
1
2
3
5
10
Hazard ratio

Figure 18.2 IPD meta-analysis of 10 studies examining the prognostic effect of smoking in hypertension patients in regards to the outcome of stroke, as described by Riley et al.[338] The hazard ratio estimated displayed estimate the prognostic factor of smoking after 'fully' adjusting for age, BMI and anti-hypertensive treatment. All three adjustment factors were only available in five of the studies, leading to the displayed univariate meta-analysis results for the adjusted effect of smoking based on these five studies. A multivariate meta-analysis allows all 10 studies to be utilised, as it additionally 'borrows strength' from 'partially' adjusted results (prognostic effect of smoking adjusted just for treatment) available in the other five studies. All models use REML estimation and allow for potential heterogeneity in the effect of smoking. *Source:* Richard Riley.

adjusted hazard ratio for smoking is 1.92 (95% CI: 1.44 to 2.57; $\hat{\tau}_F = 0.18$; $BoS = 64.2\%$); in contrast, a univariate meta-analysis of just the five trials providing fully adjusted results gives a far higher summary hazard ratio of 2.70 (95% CI: 1.52 to 4.81; $\hat{\tau}_F < 0.001$). Thus, in this example, dealing with systematically missing adjustment factors by utilising the correlation between partially and fully adjusted results leads to an important shift (toward the null) in the fully adjusted hazard ratio for smoking. The results are displayed in Figure 18.2.

18.10 Dealing with Both Sporadically and Systematically Missing Data in an IPD Meta-Analysis Using Multilevel Modelling

In the previous sections we discussed how within-study multiple imputation methods can be used to account for sporadically missing data in an IPD meta-analysis, and how a bivariate meta-analysis can be used to deal with systematically missing data when a full set of variables is available in some studies and the same partial set is available in others. Although it is possible to combine these approaches to handle both sporadically and systematically missing values, this strategy may be quite cumbersome to implement and may be impractical when only a few studies provide the fully adjusted result. In addition, even in the absence of systematically missing values, the use of within-study imputation can be problematic. In particular, to ensure the validity of the MAR assumption, it is often necessary to include as many covariates as possible in the within-study imputation model(s). This may not be feasible when studies are relatively small or when they did not measure important variables that explain missingness. Also, when the set of covariates used in the imputation model(s) varies across studies, this may inflate the subsequent between-study heterogeneity observed in the IPD meta-analysis.[339] To address this, multilevel modelling techniques have been proposed to simultaneously impute sporadically and systematically missing data in an IPD meta-analysis. These methods borrow information across studies by implementing random-effects models during imputation, and can be implemented using either the joint modelling or FCS frameworks, as now explained after a further motivating example.

18.10.1 Motivating Example: Prognostic Factors for Short-term Mortality in Acute Heart Failure

The Global Research on Acute Conditions Team (GREAT) network combined IPD from 28 studies to explore prognostic factors associated with short-term mortality in acute heart failure (AHF).[340] Recently, Audigier et al. used the GREAT data to compare various imputation methods, and prepared a simulated version of the IPD meta-analysis with sporadically and systematically missing values.[282] This dataset is freely available from the R package *micemd* and contains information about left ventricular ejection fraction (LVEF), brain natriuretic peptide (BNP) and atrial fibrillation (AFIB), amongst other variables. Since measuring the LVEF requires an ultrasound examination, it is of interest whether more easily measured factors such as BNP and AFIB can be used as a proxy for LVF. Hence, we will use the IPD meta-analysis dataset to examine whether BNP and AFIB are associated with the value of LVEF (which is measured as a percentage). A summary of the IPD is shown in Table 18.5, and it contains both sporadically and systematically missing values for BNP and AFIB.

The complete-case analysis results are depicted in Figure 18.3, using just the 2354 participants from those 17 studies that provided values for each of LVEF, BNP and AFIB. Results were obtained by fitting a one-stage IPD meta-analysis model including BNP and AFIB as covariates, using a linear mixed effects model with correlated random effects for the intercept term and the predictive effect of BNP, and a common prognostic effect of AFIB. There is strong evidence that BNP and AFIB are associated with LVEF; on average a one-unit increase in BNP corresponds to a 10.2% decrease in the LVEF, and the presence of AFIB corresponds to an increase of 3.7% in the LVEF.

We repeated this IPD meta-analysis after multiple imputation of the missing values whilst naively ignoring the presence of clustering. That is, we merged the IPD from all 28 studies (11,685 participants) and used the FCS approach to impute missing values assuming the IPD were obtained from a single study (labelled FCS-naïve in Figure 18.3).[311] We generated 10 imputed datasets and combined the corresponding results using Rubin's rules. Compared to the complete-case analysis, the summary effect estimates for AFBI and BNP are lower after this imputation (Figure 18.3); a one-unit increase in BNP now corresponds to a 9.5% decrease in the LVEF, and the presence of AFIB corresponds to a 2.7% increase. The estimated between-study heterogeneity also changes. For instance, the between-study standard deviation for BNP increased from 0.013 (complete-case analysis) to 0.032 after imputation. However, these findings could be severely affected by the imputation method ignoring clustering, and so more appropriate multilevel imputation methods are required.

Table 18.5 Description of variables and missing data (NA) in the simulated IPD of the GREAT data.

Study	Size	BNP mean ± SD	Percentage of participants with AFIB present	LVEF mean ± SD
1	410	3.008 ± 0.514 (NA = 235)	21% (NA = 1)	0.452 ± 0.186
2	567	2.944 ± 0.473 (NA = 58)	24% (NA = 0)	0.344 ± 0.196
3	210	3.284 ± 0.589 (NA = 5)	NA = 210	0.366 ± 0.183
4	375	2.938 ± 0.478 (NA = 15)	38% (NA = 156)	0.416 ± 0.176
5	107	NA = 107	55% (NA = 0)	0.483 ± 0.168
6	267	NA = 267	40% (NA = 0)	0.413 ± 0.163
7	203	2.413 ± 0.633 (NA = 4)	37% (NA = 0)	0.489 ± 0.214
8	354	3.407 ± 0.457 (NA = 44)	46% (NA = 78)	0.376 ± 0.175
9	137	2.927 ± 0.445 (NA = 0)	50% (NA = 0)	0.380 ± 0.120
10	48	NA = 48	25% (NA = 0)	0.534 ± 0.244
11	208	NA = 208	23% (NA = 0)	0.369 ± 0.162
12	622	NA = 622	44% (NA = 0)	0.374 ± 0.147
13	78	NA = 78	NA = 78	0.273 ± 0.104
14	670	NA = 670	55% (NA = 1)	0.478 ± 0.168
15	1000	2.868 ± 0.698 (NA = 820)	19% (NA = 3)	0.375 ± 0.161
16	1093	NA = 1093	15% (NA = 0)	0.414 ± 0.157
17	18	2.4904 ± 0.912 (NA = 6)	50% (NA = 0)	0.564 ± 0.294
18	1834	2.790 ± 0.551 (NA = 1695)	24% (NA = 7)	0.402 ± 0.165
19	358	2.376 ± 0.597 (NA = 354)	31% (NA = 0)	0.381 ± 0.160
20	54	NA = 54	43% (NA = 1)	0.365 ± 0.209
21	588	2.545 ± 0.424 (NA = 571)	28% (NA = 1)	0.335 ± 0.186
22	651	2.883 ± 0.570 (NA = 478)	37% NA = 11)	0.417 ± 0.162
23	455	3.714 ± 0.483 (NA = 398)	47% (NA = 1)	0.355 ± 0.134
24	294	2.941 ± 0.581 (NA = 237)	20% (NA = 0)	0.332 ± 0.148
25	397	NA = 397	18% (NA = 2)	0.372 ± 0.158
26	295	3.027 ± 0.445 (NA = 194)	27% (NA = 0)	0.433 ± 0.190
27	303	3.036 ± 0.634 (NA = 239)	28% (NA = 0)	0.405 ± 0.160
28	89	2.528 ± 0.493 (NA = 34)	49% (NA = 0)	0.414 ± 0.192
TOTAL	11685	2.942 ± 0.577 (NA = 8931)	30% (NA = 550)	0.396 ± 0.172 (NA = 0)

Source: Thomas Debray, with results calculated from the simulated data of Audigier et al.[282]

18.10.2 Multilevel Joint Modelling

Recall from Section 18.6.1 that in joint modelling multiple imputation, the observed data are modelled according to a multivariate normal distribution, with MCMC sampling used to estimate the parameters of this distribution and, after convergence, to then generate imputations for the missing values. This approach can be extended to simultaneously impute missing values from multiple studies, whilst accounting for the clustering of participants within studies.[341] For example, consider

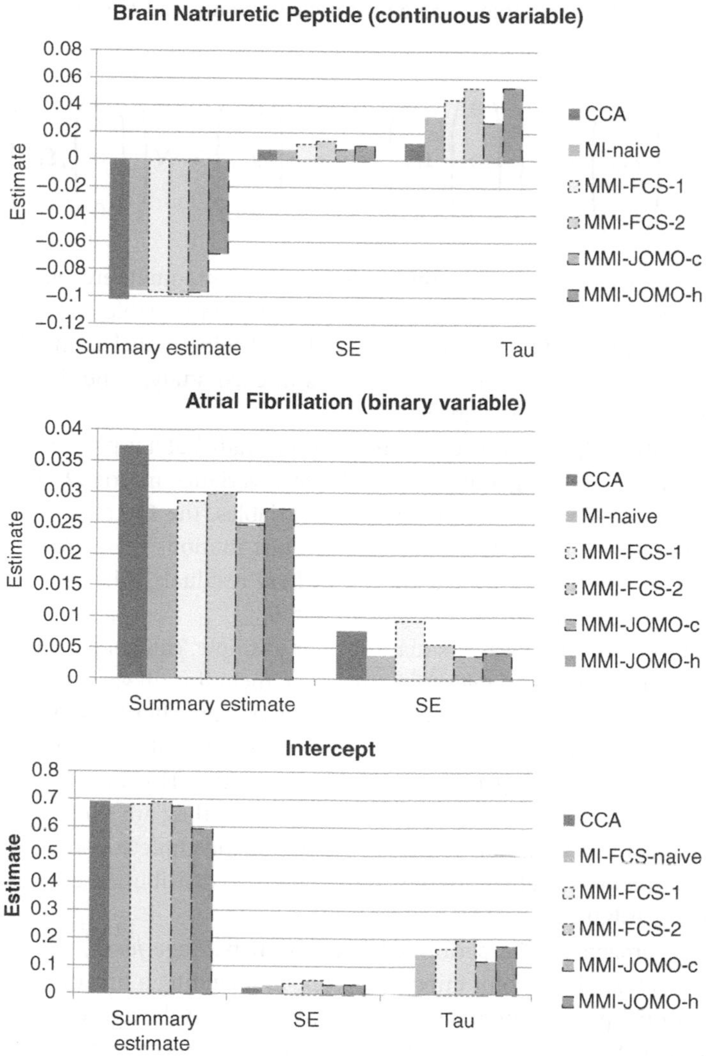

Figure 18.3 Summary results from a one-stage IPD meta-analysis of the GREAT data examining the prognostic effect of brain natriuretic peptide (BNP) and atrial fibrillation (AF) for the outcome of left ventricular ejection fraction (LVEF) for each of various strategies for handling missing data. SE = standard error, Tau = between-study standard deviation, CCA = complete-case analysis, MI-FCS-naïve = multiple imputation using fully conditional specification ignoring clustering, MMI-FCS-2 = two-stage multilevel multiple imputation using fully conditional specification, MMI-FCS-1 = one-stage multilevel multiple imputation using fully conditional specification, MMI-JOMO-c = joint modelling multilevel imputation assuming residual variance matrix is same in each study, MMI-JOMO-h = joint modelling multilevel imputation using a heteroscedastic residual variance matrix *Source:* Thomas Debray, with results calculated from the simulated data of Audigier et al.[282]

the following multilevel joint model for three variables: one continuous outcome and two continuous covariates.

$$\begin{aligned} y_{ij} &= \beta_0 + u_{0i} + \epsilon_{0ij} \\ x_{1ij} &= \beta_1 + u_{1i} + \epsilon_{1ij} \\ x_{2ij} &= \beta_2 + u_{2i} + \epsilon_{2ij} \end{aligned} \qquad \begin{pmatrix} \epsilon_{0ij} \\ \epsilon_{1ij} \\ \epsilon_{2ij} \end{pmatrix} \sim N\left(\begin{pmatrix} 0 \\ 0 \\ 0 \end{pmatrix}, \boldsymbol{\Omega_e}\right) \qquad \begin{pmatrix} u_{0i} \\ u_{1i} \\ u_{2i} \end{pmatrix} \sim N\left(\begin{pmatrix} 0 \\ 0 \\ 0 \end{pmatrix}, \boldsymbol{\Omega_u}\right)$$

Each variable is one of the responses (y_{ij}, x_{1ij}, or x_{2ij}), and the model assumes random intercepts to allow for between-study heterogeneity (and correlation) in the means of each variable, via the unstructured between-study variance matrix ($\boldsymbol{\Omega_u}$).[341] Once the multilevel joint model is fitted, MCMC sampling can be used to impute missing values for variables in each study, conditional on the study-specific random effects and residual variances.

As written, the residual variance matrix ($\boldsymbol{\Omega_e}$) is assumed the same in each study but it is preferable to allow for heteroscedasticity by rather specifying a different variance covariance matrix $\boldsymbol{\Omega_{ei}}$ for each study. In particular, in order to handle systematically missing variables, the $\boldsymbol{\Omega_{ei}}$ also have to be given a distribution, with the conjugate being the inverse-Wishart distribution.[342] Heteroscedasticity better reflects one-stage and two-stage IPD meta-analyses where residual variances are modelled separately in each study, as recommended in Chapters 5 and 6.

The framework can be extended to more complicated situations. For example, categorical variables can be included by means of latent normal variables.[324] Rather than including all variables as responses in a multilevel modelling framework, fully observed variables can alternatively be included as explanatory variables; this has the advantage of making no distributional assumptions for these variables, which can be included assuming a common or random effect. However, when the imputation models include a random slope for the explanatory variables, they are no longer fully congenial with the main IPD meta-analysis model. This is because the incomplete responses then depend on the product of two random variables, for which the marginal distribution cannot properly be modelled by a normal distribution.

The multilevel joint modelling approach can be performed with the R package *jomo*, which allows for the use of a multilevel heteroscedastic joint imputation model, including a mix of continuous and binary variables at both the participant and study levels. We applied the approach to the simulated GREAT data (Table 18.5). Specifically, we generated imputed datasets using the multilevel joint modelling approach with the variables with missing data as responses (BNP, AFIB and five others), and the variables without missing data (gender and LVEF) as explanatory covariates in the imputation model. For each response, we assumed random intercepts and common effects for the two explanatory covariates. Using MCMC estimation, we generated 10,000 burn-in samples to estimate model parameters, and then sampled missing values from the posterior distribution with 5,000 iterations used between imputations to reduce autocorrelation concerns. The results are shown in Figure 18.3 (specifically see the results labelled 'MMI-JOMO'), and still indicate that BNP and AFIB are associated with LVEF, although their estimated regression coefficients are closer to zero than those from the complete-case analysis. They also provide estimates of between-study heterogeneity that are much larger as obtained by complete-case analysis. Allowing for heteroscedastic (rather than common) residual error variances in the studies yielded larger standard errors and between-study heterogeneity estimates (compare results labelled 'MMI-JOMO-h' and 'MMI-JOMO-c').

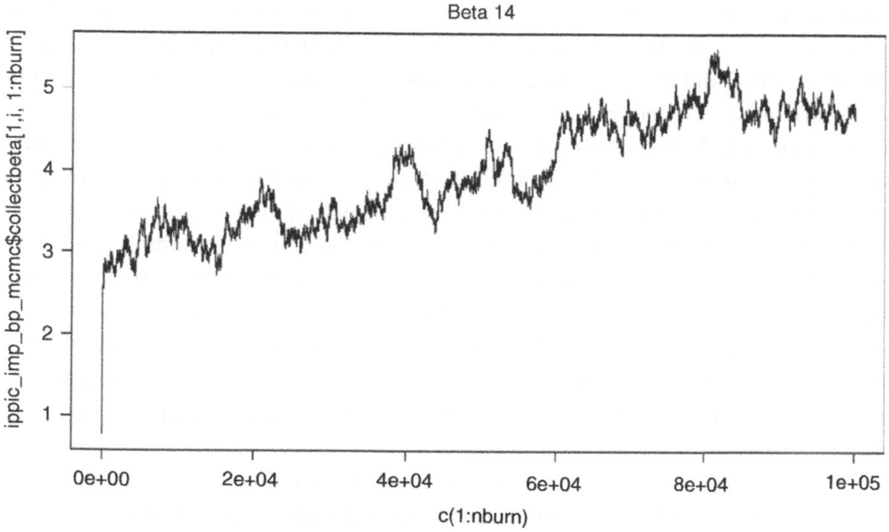

Figure 18.4 MCMC sampling chain for the beta corresponding to history of diabetes when using the multilevel joint modelling approach for imputation in the pre-eclampsia data, which provides concern that convergence has still not been achieved even after 100,000 iterations. *Source:* Kym Snell.

It is important to check the convergence of the multilevel joint model before sampling values from the posterior distribution for imputation of missing data. As part of the pre-eclampsia IPD meta-analysis project described in Section 18.2, Snell et al. used the multilevel joint modelling approach when developing a new pre-eclampsia risk prediction model.[318] When including some variables in the imputation, convergence of the imputation model was a concern even when using a large burn-in period. For example, Figure 18.4 shows the MCMC chain for the parameter corresponding to history of diabetes in the pre-eclampsia data and, even after 100,000 iterations, it remains questionable as to whether convergence was achieved and so whether subsequent results were reliable. Hence, such variables were removed from the imputation process. Other research has also identified concerns when checking imputations in an IPD meta-analysis setting.[343]

18.10.3 Multilevel Fully Conditional Specification

As discussed in Section 18.6.2, the FCS approach involves specifying a conditional distribution for each variable with missing values. For example, in a single study the method defines a linear regression model for a continuous variable, a logistic regression model for a binary variable, and so on. MCMC sampling is then used to estimate the parameters of these distributions and, after convergence, to generate imputations from the posterior distributions. The main analysis can then be applied to each imputed dataset, and the parameter estimates combined using Rubin's rules.

When using the FCS approach to deal with an IPD meta-analysis dataset, the specified conditional distributions must account for the clustering of participants within studies, and also potential between-study heterogeneity. This can be achieved by using either a one-stage or two-stage imputation approach. In the one-stage imputation approach, all the conditional models in FCS are allowed to have random study effects on the intercept and effects of explanatory covariates. For example, assume there are four variables (y_{ij}, x_{1ij}, x_{2ij}, and x_{3ij}). To impute missing values in an incomplete variable (y_j, say), a model of y_{ij} conditional on the other variables (covariates) x_{1ij}, x_{2ij}, and x_{3ij} is specified, with random study effects placed on the intercept and the effect of each of x_{1ij}, x_{2ij}, and x_{3ij}. Therefore, if y_{ij} is continuous a linear mixed effects regression model is specified, and if y_j is binary a logistic mixed effects regression model is specified, and so on. Each conditional imputation model may assume an unstructured between-study variance matrix to allow a unique variance for each random effect and a unique correlation for each pair of random effects. However, in practice, simplifications may be necessary to avoid estimation and convergence problems. It is, for instance, possible to specify random effects for a subset of explanatory variables, or to assume that the random effects are independent between studies. Further, when imputing continuous variables, heteroscedastic residual variances should be allowed, as discussed previously.[282] An MCMC procedure is used to estimate the parameters of the conditional models and, after convergence, draw missing values in each study, conditional on the study-specific random effects and residual variances.

In the two-stage approach, the first stage requires each conditional model to be specified separately per study. For example, a model for y_{ij} conditional on the other variables (covariates) x_{1ij}, x_{2ij}, and x_{3ij} is specified in each study separately, as described in Section 18.6.2. However, if a variable is systematically missing in a study then no conditional model is specified. For example, if y_{ij} is missing in study 1, then it is not possible to fit a model of y_{ij} conditional on the other variables (covariates) x_{1ij}, x_{2ij}, and x_{3ij}. Furthermore, in that study the conditional models for each of x_{1ij}, x_{2ij}, and x_{3ij} cannot include y_{ij} as a covariate. This means that the two-stage approach requires at least one study without systematically missing variables.

In the second stage, the parameter estimates of the conditional models are combined using a multivariate random-effects meta-analysis, separately for each variable. The imputation of missing values then distinguishes between two situations. When imputing systematically missing values, imputations are randomly generated from the pooled conditional models whilst allowing for the presence of between-study heterogeneity in their estimated parameters. When imputing sporadically missing values, imputations are randomly generated according to a Bayesian procedure that combines the pooled conditional models with the study-specific imputation models. This allows study-specific imputations whilst borrowing information across studies. Resche-Region and White provide full details of this method.[183]

The one-stage FCS approach is computationally intensive and slow to converge, particularly with binary variables. The two-stage approach is usually much faster to generate imputed datasets, especially when using analytic expressions (rather than iterative procedures) to derive and account for heterogeneity. However, Audigier et al. note that the two-stage approach tends to have a larger variance and is prone to (partial) separation problems when imputing binary variables in studies with few events.[282]

Returning to the IPD meta-analysis involving BNP, AFIB, LVEF and six other variables from the simulated GREAT data, we applied multilevel FCS to deal with sporadically and systematically missing variables, for each of the one-stage and two-stage approaches. For all conditional models, we placed random effects on the intercept term and the effect of BNP when included as explanatory covariate. When BNP was the response variable, we also allowed for random effects on the eight other variables included as covariates; this was done to improve compatibility of the conditional imputation models (Section 18.6.2). We subsequently generated 10 imputed datasets, and allowed for 20 imputation cycles. Results are shown in shown in Figure 18.3 (specifically consider the results labelled 'MMI-FCS'), and indicate that both one-stage and two-stage imputation methods lead to very similar summary estimates for AFIB and BNP, although standard errors and estimates of between-study heterogeneity do differ slightly. Importantly, both one-stage and two-stage FCS imputation approaches give larger estimate of between-study heterogeneity than both the complete-case and naive imputation method ignoring clustering. Also, the two-stage FCS imputation gives similar results to the multilevel joint modelling imputation with a heteroscedastic residual variance. For instance, both methods estimated the between-study standard deviation for BNP as 0.053.

18.11 Comparison of Methods and Recommendations

The pre-eclampsia and GREAT examples used throughout this chapter illustrate the imputation methods available for IPD meta-analysis; however, their results cannot be used to make general recommendations about which methods are best. Rather, guidance can be based on published simulation studies that compare the various methods.[281,282] These confirm that naive imputation methods which (largely) ignore the multilevel structure of the IPD meta-analysis dataset may subsequently underestimate between-study heterogeneity, as well as giving biased summary parameter estimates and too small standard errors. Therefore, our main recommendation is that researchers should use multilevel imputation methods to address missing values in an IPD meta-analysis, using either the FCS or joint modelling approaches described above, either based on within-study imputation or multilevel imputation. Also, results from simulation studies indicate that the best approach to deal with missing data in an IPD meta-analysis will be context specific,[281282] and so next we discuss some recommendations for when to use multilevel FCS or joint modelling approaches.

18.11.1 Multilevel FCS versus Joint Model Approaches

A summary of the advantages and limitations of the multilevel FCS and joint model imputation approaches is given in Table 18.6, based on the findings from simulation studies.[281,282] It is not possible to recommend one particular approach over the other, as their performance depends on the type of data that is being imputed, the number of studies in the IPD meta-analysis, the number of participants in each study, and the extent of between-study heterogeneity.[282]

The key advantage of the FCS approach is that it allows for greater flexibility in specifying conditional distributions for imputation of binary, count and other complex data types. However, a direct consequence of this flexibility is that the specified conditional distributions do not necessarily capture a well-defined joint distribution. Indeed, it has been demonstrated that a fully compatible model for systematically missing covariates may not exist,[281] and that the conditional distribution of multilevel models with a random slope is analytically intractable.[344] Nonetheless, simulations suggest that the use of incompatible imputation models rarely affects the validity of subsequent analyses.[184,311,345] Augidier et al. found that imputations from FCS were quite accurate for continuous variables, but less accurate for binary variables. Besides that, accurate parameter estimates (particularly with respect to the variance of the random effects) could only be obtained for IPD meta-analyses with a high (or moderate) number of studies.

Simulation studies also demonstrate that imputation using the joint model specification produces valid inferences,[281,282] even when data are not normally distributed. In fact, current implementations of joint modelling generally outperformed FCS when imputing binary variables. The Bayesian joint modelling approach proposed by Quartagno and Carpenter makes use of conjugate prior distributions,[184] such that sampling imputations from the posterior joint distribution does not require extensive use of MCMC methods. However, Audigier et al. argue that this joint modelling

Table 18.6 Key advantages and limitations of the multilevel joint modelling and fully conditional specification (FCS) approaches to dealing with both sporadically and systematically missing data in an IPD meta-analysis; recommendations are based on simulation studies.[281,282]

	Multilevel joint modelling multiple imputation	One-stage multilevel imputation by FCS	Two-stage multilevel imputation by FCS
Key areas for application			
IPD meta-analysis characteristics	Many and/or large studies	Small and/or few studies	Many and/or large studies
Imputation of continuous variables	Yes	Yes	Yes
Imputation of binary variables	Yes	No*	No*
Imputation of level-2 variables	Yes	Yes	Yes
Potential problems			
Summary effect estimates	Biased when the number of participants and/or studies is small	Biased when imputing sporadically missing data in binary variables.	Biased when the number of participants and/or studies is small. Biased when imputing sporadically missing data in binary variables.
Confidence intervals for summary effects	Too wide	Too narrow (when imputing continuous variables)	Too wide when imputing binary variables)
Between-study variance estimates	Too high when the number of participants and/or studies is small	Too low	Too high when the number of studies is small

* Fully conditional specification (FCS) one-stage is not tailored for imputing sporadically missing data in binary variables, and the two-stage estimator used in FCS two-stage is known to be biased when most studies in the IPD meta-analysis are small.
Source: Thomas Debray.

approach may lead to excessive standard errors when the proportion of missing values is very high and the variances of the random effects are low.[282]

Audigier et al. recommend the use of joint-modelling multiple imputation when the number of incomplete binary variables is large and when the number of studies is large.[282] Two-stage FCS approaches are advantageous when the number of studies with systematically missing variables is large, whereas one-stage FCS approaches appear beneficial when most studies are small. More generally,[281] when adopting (quasi-)Bayesian imputation methods in IPD meta-analysis with few participants or studies, the influence of prior distributions may become too influential. As such, 'default' prior distributions in statistical software (e.g. an inverse Wishart prior distribution for the between-study covariance matrix) should be used with caution, especially for variance components.

Although desirable, it is not always feasible to adopt the multilevel FCS or joint model imputation methods, for instance due to convergence issues or constraints on data sharing preventing the IPD to be housed in a single database (Chapter 4). For this reason, the within-study imputation approach of Section 18.8 may often be preferred for practical reasons, even though it does not allow imputation of systematically missing variables (and thus may require some studies to be excluded). For all imputation methods, it is helpful to include auxiliary variables in the imputation model in order to improve the accuracy of imputed values and make the MAR assumption more plausible. These variables are related to either the occurrence of missing data or the variables with missing data themselves, and are typically participant-level variables (as has been the focus in this chapter), but may represent study-level characteristics or even study means of the predictors.[183]

18.11.2 Sensitivity Analyses and Reporting

Regardless of the choice of imputation method, researchers should ideally explore the robustness of meta-analysis results under plausible departures from the MAR assumption. Sensitivity analyses may also be needed, for example to compare the impact of different prior distributions in the imputation modelling when the IPD meta-analysis has few or small studies. Clear reporting of the imputation process is also essential, to document the imputation method and its implementation, such as the inclusion of auxiliary variables, transformations, interactions, non-linear terms, and how clustering and between-study heterogeneity was accounted for. The implemented software package(s), the number of generated imputations, and the assessment of convergence should also be documented.

18.12 Software

Joint modelling multiple imputation is implemented in the R package *jomo*.[346] This allows for imputation of either continuous or discrete, participant-level or study-level, and systematically or sporadically missing data. A tutorial paper introducing the package has been published.[346] Additionally, *jomo* provides a function for substantive (main) model compatible imputation, which is the recommended method in the presence of non-linear effects or random slopes.[347] With continuous and participant-level data only, the R package *pan* uses a very similar algorithm, but has an advantage in terms of computational speed.[348] However, it does not allow for heteroscedasticity, as is recommended. Additionally, the R package *mitml* provides a user-friendly interface to *jomo* and *pan*, using the standard data-formula interface.[349]

Several options are available to perform multiple imputation using FCS. In particular, the R package *mice* offers the implementation of one-stage multilevel multiple imputation methods for handling systematically and sporadically missing data in clustered data, and has built-in functions for the imputation of continuous and binary variables. The functionalities of *mice* have been extended by the R package *micemd*, which offers the implementation of one-stage and two-stage multilevel imputation methods for continuous, binary and count variables. Other R packages are available for dealing with missing values in clustered data (e.g. *hmi* or *miceadds*), but they are generally not dedicated to handle systematically and sporadically missing data jointly.

18.13 Concluding Remarks

IPD meta-analysis projects often need to deal with missing participant values for key variables, including outcomes and covariates of interest. Novel methods for multiple imputation can be used in this situation, which account for clustering of participants within studies and potential between-study heterogeneity, by adopting either within-study imputation or multilevel imputation. Often the best approach to take is context specific, for example depending on the research question, the type of studies available, whether there are sporadically and systematically missing variables, and the assumptions being made about missing data (e.g. MAR). Software and methods for multilevel imputation are evolving, for example to deal with categorical data, interaction effects and non-linear terms,[350,351] and we will disseminate latest developments at www.ipdma.co.uk.

Part V References

1 Deeks JJ. Systematic reviews in health care: systematic reviews of evaluations of diagnostic and screening tests. *BMJ* 2001;323(7305):157–162.

2 Reitsma JB, Glas AS, Rutjes AW, et al. Bivariate analysis of sensitivity and specificity produces informative summary measures in diagnostic reviews. *J Clin Epidemiol* 2005;58(10):982–990.

3 Harbord RM, Deeks JJ, Egger M, et al. A unification of models for meta-analysis of diagnostic accuracy studies. *Biostatistics* 2007;8(2):239–251.

4 Chu H, Cole SR. Bivariate meta-analysis of sensitivity and specificity with sparse data: a generalized linear mixed model approach. *J Clin Epidemiol* 2006;59(12):1331–1332; author reply 32–33.

5 Leeflang MM, Deeks JJ, Rutjes AW, et al. Bivariate meta-analysis of predictive values of diagnostic tests can be an alternative to bivariate meta-analysis of sensitivity and specificity. *J Clin Epidemiol* 2012;65(10):1088–1097.

6 Harbord RM, Whiting P, Sterne JA, et al. An empirical comparison of methods for meta-analysis of diagnostic accuracy showed hierarchical models are necessary. *J Clin Epidemiol* 2008;61 (11):1095–1103.

7 Macaskill P, Gatsonis C, Deeks JJ, et al. Chapter 10: Analysing and presenting results. In: Deeks JJ, Bossuyt PM, Gatsonis C, eds. *Cochrane Handbook for Systematic Reviews of Diagnostic Test Accuracy* Version 10. The Cochrane Collaboration 2010. Available from: https://methodscochraneorg/sdt/resources-authors.

8 Rutter CM, Gatsonis CA. A hierarchical regression approach to meta-analysis of diagnostic test accuracy evaluations. *Stat Med* 2001;20(19):2865–2884.

9 Macaskill P. Empirical Bayes estimates generated in a hierarchical summary ROC analysis agreed closely with those of a full Bayesian analysis. *J Clin Epidemiol* 2004;57(9):925–932.

10 Phi XA, Houssami N, Obdeijn IM, et al. Magnetic resonance imaging improves breast screening sensitivity in BRCA mutation carriers age >/= 50 years: evidence from an individual patient data meta-analysis. *J Clin Oncol* 2015;33(4):349–356.

11 Dukic V, Gatsonis C. Meta-analysis of diagnostic test accuracy assessment studies with varying number of thresholds. *Biometrics* 2003;59(4):936–946.

12 Hamza TH, Arends LR, van Houwelingen HC, et al. Multivariate random effects meta-analysis of diagnostic tests with multiple thresholds. *BMC Med Res Methodol* 2009;9:73.

13 Kester AD, Buntinx F. Meta-analysis of ROC curves. *Med Decis Making* 2000;20(4):430–439.

14 Putter H, Fiocco M, Stijnen T. Meta-analysis of diagnostic test accuracy studies with multiple thresholds using survival methods. *Biom J* 2010;52(1):95–110.

15 Levis B, Benedetti A, Levis AW, et al. Selective cutoff reporting in studies of diagnostic test accuracy: a comparison of conventional and individual-patient-data meta-analyses of the Patient Health Questionnaire-9 depression screening tool. *Am J Epidemiol* 2017;185(10):954–964.

Individual Participant Data Meta-Analysis: A Handbook for Healthcare Research, First Edition.
Edited by Richard D. Riley, Jayne F. Tierney, and Lesley A. Stewart.

16 Levis B, Benedetti A, Thombs BD, et al. Accuracy of Patient Health Questionnaire-9 (PHQ-9) for screening to detect major depression: individual participant data meta-analysis. *BMJ* 2019;365:l1476.

17 Macaskill P, Walter SD, Irwig L, et al. Assessing the gain in diagnostic performance when combining two diagnostic tests. *Stat Med* 2002;21(17):2527–2546.

18 Tierney JF, Vale C, Riley R, et al. Individual participant data (IPD) meta-analyses of randomised controlled trials: guidance on their use. *PLoS Med* 2015;12(7):e1001855.

19 Debray TPA, Riley RD, Rovers MM, et al. Individual participant data (IPD) meta-analyses of diagnostic and prognostic modeling studies: guidance on their use. *PLoS Med* 2015;12(10):e1001886.

20 Ahmed I, Debray TP, Moons KG, et al. Developing and validating risk prediction models in an individual participant data meta-analysis. *BMC Med Res Methodol* 2014;14:3.

21 Abo-Zaid G, Sauerbrei W, Riley RD. Individual participant data meta-analysis of prognostic factor studies: state of the art? *BMC Med Res Methodol* 2012;12:56.

22 Riley RD, Lambert PC, Abo-Zaid G. Meta-analysis of individual participant data: rationale, conduct, and reporting. *BMJ* 2010;340:c221.

23 Craig JV, Lancaster GA, Taylor S, et al. Infrared ear thermometry compared with rectal thermometry in children: a systematic review. *Lancet* 2002;360(9333):603–609.

24 Dodd SR, Lancaster GA, Craig JV, et al. In a systematic review, infrared ear thermometry for fever diagnosis in children finds poor sensitivity. *J Clin Epidemiol* 2006;59(4):354–357.

25 Committee of Cincinnati Children's Hospital Medical Center. Evidence based clinical practice guideline for fever of uncertain source in children 2 to 36 months of age. Cincinatti Children's Hospital Medical Center (http://www.guidelines.gov) 2003.

26 Riley RD, Dodd SR, Craig JV, et al. Meta-analysis of diagnostic test studies using individual patient data and aggregate data. *Stat Med* 2008;27(29):6111–6136.

27 Bossuyt PM, Irwig L, Craig J, et al. Comparative accuracy: assessing new tests against existing diagnostic pathways. *BMJ* 2006;332(7549):1089–1092.

28 Shinkins B, Thompson M, Mallett S, et al. Diagnostic accuracy studies: how to report and analyse inconclusive test results. *BMJ* 2013;346:f2778.

29 Whiting PF, Rutjes AW, Westwood ME, et al. QUADAS-2: a revised tool for the quality assessment of diagnostic accuracy studies. *Ann Intern Med* 2011;155(8):529–536.

30 Leeflang MM, Deeks JJ, Takwoingi Y, et al. Cochrane diagnostic test accuracy reviews. *Syst Rev* 2013;2:82.

31 Haase R, Schlattmann P, Gueret P, et al. Diagnosis of obstructive coronary artery disease using computed tomography angiography in patients with stable chest pain depending on clinical probability and in clinically important subgroups: meta-analysis of individual patient data. *BMJ* 2019;365:l1945.

32 Schuetz GM, Schlattmann P, Achenbach S, et al. Individual patient data meta-analysis for the clinical assessment of coronary computed tomography angiography: protocol of the Collaborative Meta-Analysis of Cardiac CT (CoMe-CCT). *Syst Rev* 2013;2:13.

33 Stijnen T, Hamza TH, Özdemir P. Random effects meta-analysis of event outcome in the framework of the generalized linear mixed model with applications in sparse data. *Stat Med* 2010;29:3046–3067.

34 Hamza TH, van Houwelingen HC, Stijnen T. The binomial distribution of meta-analysis was preferred to model within-study variability. *J Clin Epidemiol* 2008;61(1):41–51.

35 Riley RD, Abrams KR, Sutton AJ, et al. Bivariate random-effects meta-analysis and the estimation of between-study correlation. *BMC Med Res Methodol* 2007;7(1):3.

36 Takwoingi Y, Guo B, Riley RD, et al. Performance of methods for meta-analysis of diagnostic test accuracy with few studies or sparse data. *Stat Methods Med Res* 2015;26(4):1896–1911.

37 Stata Statistical Software: Release 15 [program]: College Station, TX, 2017.

38 Pinheiro JC, Bates DM. Approximations to the log-likelihood function in the nonlinear mixed-effects model. *J Comput Graph Stat* 1995;4(1):12–35.
39 Bates D, Mächler M, Bolker B, et al. Fitting linear mixed-effects models using lme4. *J Stat Softw* 2015;67(1):1–48.
40 Zwinderman AH, Bossuyt PM. We should not pool diagnostic likelihood ratios in systematic reviews. *Stat Med* 2008;27(5):687–697.
41 Burke DL, Bujkiewicz S, Riley RD. Bayesian bivariate meta-analysis of correlated effects: impact of the prior distributions on the between-study correlation, borrowing of strength, and joint inferences. *Stat Methods Med Res* 2018;27(2):428–450.
42 Nikoloulopoulos AK. A mixed effect model for bivariate meta-analysis of diagnostic test accuracy studies using a copula representation of the random effects distribution. *Stat Med* 2015;34 (29):3842–3865.
43 Nikoloulopoulos AK. A vine copula mixed effect model for trivariate meta-analysis of diagnostic test accuracy studies accounting for disease prevalence. *Stat Methods Med Res* 2017;26(5):2270–2286.
44 Kuss O, Hoyer A, Solms A. Meta-analysis for diagnostic accuracy studies: a new statistical model using beta-binomial distributions and bivariate copulas. *Stat Med* 2014;33(1):17–30.
45 Riley RD, Ahmed I, Debray TP, et al. Summarising and validating test accuracy results across multiple studies for use in clinical practice. *Stat Med* 2015;34(13):2081–2103.
46 Higgins JP, Thompson SG, Spiegelhalter DJ. A re-evaluation of random-effects meta-analysis. *J Royal Stat Soc Series A* 2009;172:137–159.
47 Riley RD, Higgins JP, Deeks JJ. Interpretation of random effects meta-analyses. *BMJ* 2011;342:d549.
48 Jackson D, White IR. When should meta-analysis avoid making hidden normality assumptions? *Biom J* 2018;60(6):1040–1058.
49 Riley RD, Simmonds MC, Look MP. Evidence synthesis combining individual patient data and aggregate data: a systematic review identified current practice and possible methods. *J Clin Epidemiol* 2007;60(5):431–439.
50 Leeflang MM, Rutjes AW, Reitsma JB, et al. Variation of a test's sensitivity and specificity with disease prevalence. *CMAJ* 2013;185(11):E537–E544.
51 Leeflang MM, Bossuyt PM, Irwig L. Diagnostic test accuracy may vary with prevalence: implications for evidence-based diagnosis. *J Clin Epidemiol* 2009;62(1):5–12.
52 Chu H, Nie L, Cole SR, et al. Meta-analysis of diagnostic accuracy studies accounting for disease prevalence: alternative parameterizations and model selection. *Stat Med* 2009;28:2384–2399.
53 Debray TP, Moons KG, Ahmed I, et al. A framework for developing, implementing, and evaluating clinical prediction models in an individual participant data meta-analysis. *Stat Med* 2013;32 (18):3158–3180.
54 van Enst WA, Naaktgeboren CA, Ochodo EA, et al. Small-study effects and time trends in diagnostic test accuracy meta-analyses: a meta-epidemiological study. *Syst Rev* 2015;4:66.
55 Deeks JJ, Macaskill P, Irwig L. The performance of tests of publication bias and other sample size effects in systematic reviews of diagnostic test accuracy was assessed. *J Clin Epidemiol* 2005;58 (9):882–893.
56 McInnes MDF, Moher D, Thombs BD, et al. Preferred Reporting Items for a Systematic Review and Meta-analysis of Diagnostic Test Accuracy Studies: The PRISMA-DTA Statement. *JAMA* 2018;319 (4):388–396.
57 Bramwell R, West H, Salmon P. Health professionals' and service users' interpretation of screening test results: experimental study. *BMJ* 2006;333(7562):284.
58 Whiting PF, Davenport C, Jameson C, et al. How well do health professionals interpret diagnostic information? *A systematic review. BMJ Open* 2015;5(7):e008155.

59 Zhelev Z, Garside R, Hyde C. A qualitative study into the difficulties experienced by healthcare decision makers when reading a Cochrane diagnostic test accuracy review. *Syst Rev* 2013;2:32.

60 Deeks JJ, Bossuyt PM, Gatsonis C. *Cochrane Handbook for Systematic Reviews of Diagnostic Test Accuracy Version 1.0*. The Cochrane Collaboration 2010. Available from https://methods.cochrane.org/sdt/resources-authors.

61 Phillips B, Stewart LA, Sutton AJ. 'Cross hairs' plots for diagnostic meta-analysis. *Res Synth Methods* 2010;1(3–4):308–315.

62 Steinhauser S, Schumacher M, Rucker G. Modelling multiple thresholds in meta-analysis of diagnostic test accuracy studies. *BMC Med Res Methodol* 2016;16(1):97.

63 Riley RD, Takwoingi Y, Trikalinos T, et al. Meta-analysis of test accuracy studies with multiple and missing thresholds: a multivariate-normal model. *J Biomet Biostat* 2014;5:3.

64 Ensor J, Deeks JJ, Martin EC, et al. Meta-analysis of test accuracy studies using imputation for partial reporting of multiple thresholds. *Res Synth Methods* 2018;9(1):100–115.

65 Owen RK, Cooper NJ, Quinn TJ, et al. Network meta-analysis of diagnostic test accuracy studies identifies and ranks the optimal diagnostic tests and thresholds for health care policy and decision-making. *J Clin Epidemiol* 2018;99:64–74.

66 Hoyer A, Kuss O. Meta-analysis of full ROC curves: additional flexibility by using semiparametric distributions of diagnostic test values. *Res Synth Methods* 2019;10(4):528–538.

67 Hoyer A, Hirt S, Kuss O. Meta-analysis of full ROC curves using bivariate time-to-event models for interval-censored data. *Res Synth Methods* 2018;9(1):62–72.

68 Simoneau G, Levis B, Cuijpers P, et al. A comparison of bivariate, multivariate random-effects, and Poisson correlated gamma-frailty models to meta-analyze individual patient data of ordinal scale diagnostic tests. *Biom J* 2017;59(6):1317–1338.

69 Jones HE, Gatsonis CA, Trikalinos TA, et al. Quantifying how diagnostic test accuracy depends on threshold in a meta-analysis. *Stat Med* 2019;38(24):4789–4803.

70 Benedetti A, Levis B, Rücker G, et al. An empirical comparison of three methods for multiple cutoff diagnostic test meta-analysis of the Patient Health Questionnaire-9 (PHQ-9) depression screening tool using published data vs individual level data. *Res Synth Methods* 2020;11(6):833–848.

71 Localio A, Goodman S. Beyond the usual prediction accuracy metrics: reporting results for clinical decision making. *Ann Intern Med* 2012;157(4):294–295.

72 Vickers AJ, Van Calster B, Steyerberg EW. Net benefit approaches to the evaluation of prediction models, molecular markers, and diagnostic tests. *BMJ* 2016;352:i6.

73 Vickers AJ, Elkin EB. Decision curve analysis: a novel method for evaluating prediction models. *Med Decis Making* 2006;26(6):565–574.

74 Van Calster B, Wynants L, Verbeek JFM, et al. Reporting and interpreting decision curve analysis: a guide for investigators. *Eur Urol* 2018;74(6):796–804.

75 Kerr KF, Brown MD, Zhu K, et al. Assessing the clinical impact of risk prediction models with decision curves: guidance for correct interpretation and appropriate use. *J Clin Oncol* 2016;34(21):2534–2540.

76 Vickers AJ, Cronin AM, Elkin EB, et al. Extensions to decision curve analysis, a novel method for evaluating diagnostic tests, *prediction models and molecular markers. BMC Med Inform Decis Mak* 2008;8:53.

77 Steyerberg EW, Vickers AJ. Decision curve analysis: a discussion. *Med Decis Making* 2008;28(1):146–149.

78 Wynants L, Riley RD, Timmerman D, et al. Random-effects meta-analysis of the clinical utility of tests and prediction models. *Stat Med* 2018;37(12):2034–2052.

79 Takwoingi Y, Leeflang MM, Deeks JJ. Empirical evidence of the importance of comparative studies of diagnostic test accuracy. *Ann Intern Med* 2013;158(7):544–554.

80 Wang J, Bossuyt P, Geskus R, et al. Using individual patient data to adjust for indirectness did not successfully remove the bias in this case of comparative test accuracy. *J Clin Epidemiol* 2015;68 (3):290–298.

81 Ma X, Lian Q, Chu H, et al. A Bayesian hierarchical model for network meta-analysis of multiple diagnostic tests. *Biostatistics* 2018;19(1):87–102.

82 Nyaga VN, Aerts M, Arbyn M. ANOVA model for network meta-analysis of diagnostic test accuracy data. *Stat Methods Med Res* 2018;27(6):1766–1784.

83 Nyaga VN, Arbyn M, Aerts M. Beta-binomial analysis of variance model for network meta-analysis of diagnostic test accuracy data. *Stat Methods Med Res* 2018;27(8):2554–2566.

84 Trikalinos TA, Hoaglin DC, Small KM, et al. Methods for the joint meta-analysis of multiple tests. *Res Synth Methods* 2014;5(4):294–312.

85 Riley RD, van der Windt D, Croft P, et al., eds. *Prognosis Research in Healthcare: Concepts, Methods and Impact.* Oxford, UK: Oxford University Press 2019.

86 Hippisley-Cox J, Coupland C, Vinogradova Y, et al. Predicting cardiovascular risk in England and Wales: prospective derivation and validation of QRISK2. *BMJ* 2008;336(7659):1475–1482.

87 Schumacher M, Bastert G, Bojar H, et al. Randomized 2 x 2 trial evaluating hormonal treatment and the duration of chemotherapy in node-positive breast cancer patients. *German Breast Cancer Study Group. J Clin Oncol* 1994;12(10):2086–2093.

88 Riley RD, Hayden JA, Steyerberg EW, et al. Prognosis Research Strategy (PROGRESS) 2: prognostic factor research. *PLoS Med* 2013;10(2):e1001380.

89 Sutcliffe P, Hummel S, Simpson E, et al. Use of classical and novel biomarkers as prognostic risk factors for localised prostate cancer: a systematic review. *Health Technol Assess* 2009;13(5):iii, xi–xiii, 1–219.

90 Riley RD, Sauerbrei W, Altman DG. Prognostic markers in cancer: the evolution of evidence from single studies to meta-analysis, and beyond. *Br J Cancer* 2009;100(8):1219–1229.

91 Rifai N, Altman DG, Bossuyt PM. Reporting bias in diagnostic and prognostic studies: time for action. *Clin Chem* 2008;54(7):1101–1103.

92 Simon R. Evaluating prognostic factor studies. In: Gospodarowicz MK, O'Sullivan B, Sobin LH, eds. *Prognostic Factors in Cancer.* New York: Wiley-Liss 2001:49–56.

93 Sauerbrei W. Prognostic factors – confusion caused by bad quality of design, analysis and reporting of many studies. In: Bier H, ed. *Current Research in Head and Neck Cancer: Advances in Oto-Rhino-Laryngology. Basel*, Switzerland: Karger 2005:184–200.

94 Altman DG, Lyman GH. Methodological challenges in the evaluation of prognostic factors in breast cancer. *Breast Cancer Res Treat* 1998;52(1–3):289–303.

95 Simon R, Altman DG. Statistical aspects of prognostic factor studies in oncology. *Br J Cancer* 1994;69 (6):979–985.

96 Holländer N, Sauerbrei W. On statistical approaches for the multivariable analysis of prognostic marker studies. In: Auget J-L, Balakrishnan N, Mesbah M, et al., eds. *Advances in Statistical Methods for the Health Sciences.* Boston, MA: Birkhäuser 2007:19–38.

97 Altman DG, Lausen B, Sauerbrei W, et al. Dangers of using "optimal" cutpoints in the evaluation of prognostic factors. *J Natl Cancer Inst* 1994;86(11):829–835.

98 Riley RD, Abrams KR, Sutton AJ, et al. Reporting of prognostic markers: current problems and development of guidelines for evidence-based practice in the future. *Br J Cancer* 2003;88 (8):1191–1198.

99 Kyzas PA, Loizou KT, Ioannidis JP. Selective reporting biases in cancer prognostic factor studies. *J Natl Cancer Inst* 2005;97(14):1043–1055.

100 Sekula P, Mallett S, Altman DG, et al. Did the reporting of prognostic studies of tumour markers improve since the introduction of REMARK guideline? A comparison of reporting in published articles. *PLoS One* 2017;12(6):e0178531.

101 Schmitz-Dräger BJ, Goebell PJ, Ebert T, et al. p53 immunohistochemistry as a prognostic marker in bladder cancer. Playground for urology scientists? *Eur Urol* 2000;38 691–699.

102 Hemingway H, Riley RD, Altman DG. Ten steps towards improving prognosis research. *BMJ* 2009;339:b4184.

103 Kyzas PA, Denaxa-Kyza D, Ioannidis JP. Quality of reporting of cancer prognostic marker studies: association with reported prognostic effect. *J Natl Cancer Inst* 2007;99(3):236–243.

104 Parmar MK, Torri V, Stewart L. Extracting summary statistics to perform meta-analyses of the published literature for survival endpoints. *Stat Med* 1998;17(24):2815–2834.

105 Tierney JF, Stewart LA, Ghersi D, et al. Practical methods for incorporating summary time-to-event data into meta-analysis. *Trials* 2007;8:16.

106 Perneger TV. Estimating the relative hazard by the ratio of logarithms of event-free proportions. *Contemp Clin Trials* 2008;29:762–766.

107 Kyzas PA, Denaxa-Kyza D, Ioannidis JP. Almost all articles on cancer prognostic markers report statistically significant results. *Eur J Cancer* 2007;43(17):2559–2579.

108 Altman DG, Royston P. Statistics notes: the cost of dichotomising continuous variables. *BMJ* 2006;332:1080.

109 Royston P, Altman DG, Sauerbrei W. Dichotomizing continuous predictors in multiple regression: a bad idea. *Stat Med* 2006;25(1):127–141.

110 Cox DR. Note on grouping. *J Am Stat Assoc* 1957;52(280):543–547.

111 Altman DG. Systematic reviews of evaluations of prognostic variables. *BMJ* 2001;323(7306):224–228.

112 Riley RD, Moons KGM, Snell KIE, et al. A guide to systematic review and meta-analysis of prognostic factor studies. *BMJ* 2019;364:k4597.

113 Marmarou A, Lu J, Butcher I, et al. IMPACT database of traumatic brain injury: design and description. *J Neurotrauma* 2007;24(2):239–250.

114 McHugh GS, Engel DC, Butcher I, et al. Prognostic value of secondary insults in traumatic brain injury: results from the IMPACT study. *J Neurotrauma* 2007;24(2):287–293.

115 Trivella M, Pezzella F, Pastorino U, et al. Microvessel density as a prognostic factor in non-small-cell lung carcinoma: a meta-analysis of individual patient data. *Lancet Oncol* 2007;8(6):488–499.

116 Meert AP, Paesmans M, Martin B, et al. The role of microvessel density on the survival of patients with lung cancer: a systematic review of the literature with meta-analysis. *Br J Cancer* 2002;87 (7):694–701.

117 Thompson SG, Kaptoge S, White I, et al. Statistical methods for the time-to-event analysis of individual participant data from multiple epidemiological studies. *Int J Epidemiol* 2010;39 (5):1345–1359.

118 Crowther MJ, Riley RD, Staessen JA, et al. Individual patient data meta-analysis of survival data using Poisson regression models. *BMC Med Res Methodol* 2012;12:34.

119 Crowther MJ, Look MP, Riley RD. Multilevel mixed effects parametric survival models using adaptive Gauss-Hermite quadrature with application to recurrent events and individual participant data meta-analysis. *Stat Med* 2014;33(22):3844–3858.

120 Crowther MJ, Abrams KR, Lambert PC. Flexible parametric joint modelling of longitudinal and survival data. *Stat Med* 2012;31(30):4456–4471.

121 Berlin JA, Longnecker MP, Greenland S. Meta-analysis of epidemiologic dose-response data. *Epidemiology* 1993;4(3):218–228.

122 Greenland S, Longnecker MP. Methods for trend estimation from summarized dose-response data, with applications to meta-analysis. *Am J Epidemiol* 1992;135(11):1301–1309.

123 Hartemink N, Boshuizen HC, Nagelkerke NJ, et al. Combining risk estimates from observational studies with different exposure cutpoints: a meta-analysis on body mass index and diabetes type 2. *Am J Epidemiol* 2006;163(11):1042–1052.

124 Shi JQ, Copas JB. Meta-analysis for trend estimation. *Stat Med* 2004;23(1):3–19; discussion 159–162.

125 Orsini N, Li R, Wolk A, et al. Meta-analysis for linear and nonlinear dose-response relations: examples, an evaluation of approximations, *and software. Am J Epidemiol* 2012;175(1):66–73.

126 Gasparrini A, Armstrong B, Kenward MG. Multivariate meta-analysis for non-linear and other multi-parameter associations. *Stat Med* 2012;31:3821–3839.

127 Hemingway H, Croft P, Perel P, et al. Prognosis Research Strategy (PROGRESS) 1: a framework for researching clinical outcomes. *BMJ* 2013;346:e5595.

128 Moons KG, de Groot JA, Bouwmeester W, et al. Critical appraisal and data extraction for systematic reviews of prediction modelling studies: the CHARMS checklist. *PLoS Med* 2014;11(10):e1001744.

129 Debray TP, Damen JA, Snell KI, et al. A guide to systematic review and meta-analysis of prediction model performance. *BMJ* 2017;356:i6460.

130 Steyerberg EW, Moons KG, van der Windt DA, et al. Prognosis Research Strategy (PROGRESS) 3: prognostic model research. *PLoS Med* 2013;10(2):e1001381.

131 Perel P, Arango M, Clayton T, et al. Predicting outcome after traumatic brain injury: practical prognostic models based on large cohort of international patients. *BMJ* 2008;336(7641):425–429.

132 Steyerberg EW, Mushkudiani N, Perel P, et al. Predicting outcome after traumatic brain injury: development and international validation of prognostic scores based on admission characteristics. *PLoS Med* 2008;5(8):1251–1261.

133 Van Beek JGM, Mushkudiani NA, Steyerberg EW, et al. Prognostic value of admission laboratory parameters in traumatic brain injury: results from the IMPACT study. *J Neurotrauma* 2007;24 (2):315–328.

134 Green DJ, Lewis M, Mansell G, et al. Clinical course and prognostic factors across different musculoskeletal pain sites: a secondary analysis of individual patient data from randomised clinical trials. *Eur J Pain* 2018;22(6):1057–1070.

135 Ingui BJ, Rogers MA. Searching for clinical prediction rules in MEDLINE. *J Am Med Inform Assoc* 2001;8(4):391–397.

136 Geersing GJ, Bouwmeester W, Zuithoff P, et al. Search filters for finding prognostic and diagnostic prediction studies in Medline to enhance systematic reviews. *PLoS One* 2012;7(2):e32844.

137 Haynes RB, McKibbon KA, Wilczynski NL, et al. Optimal search strategies for retrieving scientifically strong studies of treatment from Medline: analytical survey. *BMJ* 2005;330(7501):1179.

138 Wong SS, Wilczynski NL, Haynes RB, et al. Developing optimal search strategies for detecting sound clinical prediction studies in MEDLINE. *AMIA Annu Symp Proc* 2003:728–732.

139 Riley RD, Burchill SA, Abrams KR, et al. A systematic review and evaluation of the use of tumour markers in paediatric oncology: Ewing's sarcoma and neuroblastoma. *Health Technol Assess* 2003;7 (5):1–162.

140 Hayden JA, van der Windt DA, Cartwright JL, et al. Assessing bias in studies of prognostic factors. *Ann Intern Med* 2013;158(4):280–286.

141 Wolff RF, Moons KGM, Riley RD, et al. PROBAST: a tool to assess the risk of bias and applicability of prediction model studies. *Ann Intern Med* 2019;170(1):51–58.

142 Moons KGM, Wolff RF, Riley RD, et al. PROBAST: a tool to assess risk of bias and applicability of prediction model studies: explanation and elaboration. *Ann Intern Med* 2019;170(1):W1–W33.

143 Sterne JA, Hernan MA, Reeves BC, et al. ROBINS-I: a tool for assessing risk of bias in non-randomised studies of interventions. *BMJ* 2016;355:i4919.

144 Wells GA, Shea B, O'Connell D, et al. The Newcastle-Ottawa Scale (NOS) for assessing the quality of nonrandomized studies in meta-analyses. *The Ottawa Hospital Research Institute* 2009. http://www.ohri.ca/programs/clinical_epidemiology/oxford.htm.

145 Altman DG, McShane LM, Sauerbrei W, et al. Reporting Recommendations for Tumor Marker Prognostic Studies (REMARK): explanation and elaboration. *PLoS Med* 2012;9(5):e1001216.

146 McShane LM, Altman DG, Sauerbrei W, et al. REporting recommendations for tumour MARKer prognostic studies (REMARK). *Br J Cancer* 2005;93(4):387–391.

147 Altman DG, Trivella M, Pezzella F, et al. Systematic review of multiple studies of prognosis: the feasibility of obtaining individual patient data. In: Auget J-L, Balakrishnan N, Mesbah M, et al., eds. *Advances in Statistical Methods for the Health Sciences.* Boston, MA: Birkhäuser 2006:3–18.

148 Hilsenbeck SG, Clark GM, McGuire WL. Why do so many prognostic factors fail to pan out? *Breast Cancer Res Treat* 1992;22(3):197–206.

149 Royston P, Sauerbrei W. *Multivariable Model-Building – A Pragmatic Approach to Regression Analysis Based on Fractional Polynomials for Modelling Continuous Variables.* Chichester, UK: Wiley 2008.

150 McShane LM, Altman DG, Sauerbrei W, et al. Reporting recommendations for tumor marker prognostic studies (REMARK). *J Natl Cancer Inst* 2005;97(16):1180–1184.

151 Groenwold RH, Moons KG, Pajouheshnia R, et al. Explicit inclusion of treatment in prognostic modeling was recommended in observational and randomized settings. *J Clin Epidemiol* 2016;78:90–100.

152 Rovers MM, Glasziou P, Appelman CL, et al. Predictors of pain and/or fever at 3 to 7 days for children with acute otitis media not treated initially with antibiotics: a meta-analysis of individual patient data. *Pediatrics* 2007;119(3):579–585.

153 Firth D. Bias reduction of maximum likelihood estimates. *Biometrika* 1993;80(1):27–38.

154 Thiébaut ACM, Bénichou J. Choice of time-scale in Cox's model analysis of epidemiologic cohort data: a simulation study. *Statistics in Medicine* 2004;23(24):3803–3820.

155 White IR, Kaptoge S, Royston P, et al. Meta-analysis of non-linear exposure-outcome relationships using individual participant data: a comparison of two methods. *Stat Med* 2019;38(3):326–338.

156 Gasparrini A, Armstrong B. Multivariate meta-analysis: a method to summarize non-linear associations. *Stat Med* 2011;30:2504–2506.

157 Sauerbrei W, Royston P. A new strategy for meta-analysis of continuous covariates in observational studies. *Stat Med* 2011;30(28):3341–3360.

158 Harrell FE, Jr. *Regression Modeling Strategies: With Applications to Linear Models, Logistic and Ordinal Regression, and Survival Analysis* (2nd edition). New York: Springer 2015.

159 Abo-Zaid G. Individual patient data meta-analysis of prognostic factor studies (PhD thesis). University of Birmingham, 2011.

160 Royston P, Sauerbrei W. A new approach to modelling interactions between treatment and continuous covariates in clinical trials by using fractional polynomials. *Stat Med* 2004;23 (16):2509–2525.

161 Royston P, Sauerbrei W. Interaction of treatment with a continuous variable: simulation study of power for several methods of analysis. *Stat Med* 2014;33(27):4695–4708.

162 Carroll RJ, Stefanski LA. Measurement error, instrumental variables and corrections for attenuation with applications to meta-analyses. *Stat Med* 1994;13(12):1265–1282.

163 Crowther MJ, Lambert PC, Abrams KR. Adjusting for measurement error in baseline prognostic biomarkers included in a time-to-event analysis: a joint modelling approach. *BMC Med Res Methodol* 2013;13:146.
164 Brakenhoff TB, van Smeden M, Visseren FLJ, et al. Random measurement error: Why worry? An example of cardiovascular risk factors. *PLoS One* 2018;13(2):e0192298.
165 White IR. Commentary: Dealing with measurement error: multiple imputation or regression calibration? *Int J Epidemiol* 2006;35(4):1081–1082.
166 Keogh RH, White IR. A toolkit for measurement error correction, with a focus on nutritional epidemiology. *Stat Med* 2014;33(12):2137–2155.
167 Guolo A. Robust techniques for measurement error correction: a review. *StatMethn Med Res* 2008;17 (6):555–580.
168 Carroll RJ, Ruppert D, Stefanski LA, et al. *Measurement Error in Nonlinear Models: A Modern Perspective* (2nd edition). Boca Raton, FL: CRC Press 2006.
169 Lawrence Gould A, Boye ME, Crowther MJ, et al. Joint modeling of survival and longitudinal non-survival data: current methods and issues. Report of the DIA Bayesian joint modeling working group. *Stat Med* 2015;34(14):2181–2195.
170 Emerging Risk Factors Collaboration. Collaborative meta-analysis of individual data on over 1 million participants in 96 prospective cohorts of lipid and inflammatory markers in cardiovascular diseases. *Eur J Epidemiol* 2007;22:839–869.
171 Burke DL, Ensor J, Riley RD. Meta-analysis using individual participant data: one-stage and two-stage approaches, and why they may differ. *Stat Med* 2017;36(5):855–875.
172 Hastie TJ, Tibshirani RJ. *Generalized Additive Models*. Boca Raton, FL: Chapman & Hall/CRC 1990.
173 Riley RD, Legha A, Jackson D, et al. One-stage individual participant data meta-analysis models for continuous and binary outcomes: comparison of treatment coding options and estimation methods. *Stat Med* 2020;39(1):2536–2555.
174 Riley RD, Steyerberg EW. Meta-analysis of a binary outcome using individual participant data and aggregate data. *Res Synth Meth* 2010;1:2–9.
175 van Smeden M, de Groot JA, Moons KG, et al. No rationale for 1 variable per 10 events criterion for binary logistic regression analysis. *BMC Med Res Methodol* 2016;16(1):163.
176 White IR. Multivariate meta-analysis. *Stata J* 2009;9:40–56.
177 White IR. Multivariate random-effects meta-regression: updates to mvmeta. *Stata J* 2011;11:255–270.
178 Sterne JA, White IR, Carlin JB, et al. Multiple imputation for missing data in epidemiological and clinical research: potential and pitfalls. *BMJ* 2009;338:b2393.
179 Little JA, Rubin DB. *Statistical Analysis with Missing Data*. New York: Wiley 2002.
180 Fibrinogen Studies Collaboration. Systematically missing confounders in individual participant data meta-analysis of observational cohort studies. *Stat Med* 2009;28(8):1218–1237.
181 Resche-Rigon M, White IR, Bartlett JW, et al. Multiple imputation for handling systematically missing confounders in meta-analysis of individual participant data. *Stat Med* 2013;32 (28):4890–4905.
182 Jolani S, Debray TP, Koffijberg H, et al. Imputation of systematically missing predictors in an individual participant data meta-analysis: a generalized approach using MICE. *Stat Med* 2015;34 (11):1841–1863.
183 Resche-Rigon M, White IR. Multiple imputation by chained equations for systematically and sporadically missing multilevel data. *Stat Methods Med Res* 2018;27(6):1634–1649.
184 Quartagno M, Carpenter JR. Multiple imputation for IPD meta-analysis: allowing for heterogeneity and studies with missing covariates. *Stat Med* 2016;35(17):2938–2954.

185 Siddique J, Reiter JP, Brincks A, et al. Multiple imputation for harmonizing longitudinal non-commensurate measures in individual participant data meta-analysis. *Stat Med* 2015;34 (26):3399–3414.

186 Rucker G, Schwarzer G, Carpenter JR, et al. Undue reliance on I(2) in assessing heterogeneity may mislead. *BMC Med Res Methodol* 2008;8:79.

187 Riley RD. Commentary: like it and lump it? Meta-analysis using individual participant data. *Int J Epidemiol* 2010;39(5):1359–1361.

188 Debray TPA, Moons KGM, Riley RD. Detecting small-study effects and funnel plot asymmetry in meta-analysis of survival data: A comparison of new and existing tests. *Res Synth Methods* 2018;9 (1):41–50.

189 Stroup DF, Berlin JA, Morton SC, et al. Meta-analysis of observational studies in epidemiology: a proposal for reporting. Meta-analysis Of Observational Studies in Epidemiology (MOOSE) group. *JAMA* 2000;283(15):2008–2012.

190 Stewart LA, Clarke M, Rovers M, et al. Preferred Reporting Items for Systematic Review and Meta-Analyses of individual participant data: the PRISMA-IPD statement. *JAMA* 2015;313 (16):1657–1665.

191 Huguet A, Hayden JA, Stinson J, et al. Judging the quality of evidence in reviews of prognostic factor research: adapting the GRADE framework. *Sys Rev* 2013;2:71.

192 Iorio A, Spencer FA, Falavigna M, et al. Use of GRADE for assessment of evidence about prognosis: rating confidence in estimates of event rates in broad categories of patients. *BMJ* 2015;350:h870.

193 Foroutan F, Guyatt G, Zuk V, et al. GRADE Guidelines 28: Use of GRADE for the assessment of evidence about prognostic factors: rating certainty in identification of groups of patients with different absolute risks. *J Clin Epidemiol* 2020;121:62–70.

194 Fisher DJ. Two-stage individual participant data meta-analysis and generalized forest plots. *Stata J* 2015;15(2):369–396.

195 Blettner M, Sauerbrei W, Schlehofer B, et al. Traditional reviews, meta-analyses and pooled analyses in epidemiology. *Int J Epidemiol* 1999;28(1):1–9.

196 Royston P. Explained variation for survival models. *Stata J* 2006;6:83–96.

197 Royston P, Sauerbrei W. A new measure of prognostic separation in survival data. *Stat Med* 2004;23 (5):723–748.

198 Pencina MJ, D'Agostino RB, Sr., D'Agostino RB, Jr., et al. Evaluating the added predictive ability of a new marker: from area under the ROC curve to reclassification and beyond. *Stat Med* 2008;27 (2):157–172.

199 Pennells L, Kaptoge S, White IR, et al. Assessing risk prediction models using individual participant data from multiple studies. *Am J Epidemiol* 2014;179(5):621–632.

200 Moons KG, Royston P, Vergouwe Y, et al. Prognosis and prognostic research: what, why, and how? *BMJ* 2009;338:b375.

201 Collins GS, Reitsma JB, Altman DG, et al. Transparent reporting of a multivariable prediction model for individual prognosis or diagnosis (TRIPOD): the TRIPOD statement. *Ann Intern Med* 2015;162:55–63.

202 Moons KG, Altman DG, Reitsma JB, et al. Transparent reporting of a multivariable prediction model for individual prognosis or Diagnosis (TRIPOD): explanation and elaboration. *Ann Intern Med* 2015;162(1):W1–W73.

203 Steyerberg EW. *Clinical Prediction Models: A Practical Approach to Development, Validation, and Updating*. New York: Springer 2009.

204 Anderson KM, Odell PM, Wilson PW, et al. Cardiovascular disease risk profiles. *Am Heart J* 1991;121(1 Pt 2):293–298.

205 Haybittle JL, Blamey RW, Elston CW, et al. A prognostic index in primary breast cancer. *Br J Cancer* 1982;45(3):361–366.

206 Galea MH, Blamey RW, Elston CE, et al. The Nottingham Prognostic Index in primary breast cancer. *Breast Cancer Res Treat* 1992;22(3):207–219.

207 Wells PS, Anderson DR, Rodger M, et al. Derivation of a simple clinical model to categorize patients probability of pulmonary embolism: increasing the models utility with the SimpliRED D-dimer. *Thromb Haemost* 2000;83(3):416–420.

208 Wells PS, Anderson DR, Bormanis J, et al. Value of assessment of pretest probability of deep-vein thrombosis in clinical management. *Lancet* 1997;350(9094):1795–1798.

209 Riley RD, Ensor J, Snell KI, et al. External validation of clinical prediction models using big datasets from e-health records or IPD meta-analysis: opportunities and challenges. *BMJ* 2016;353:i3140.

210 Royston P, Moons KGM, Altman DG, et al. Prognosis and prognostic research: developing a prognostic model. *Br Med J* 2009;338:b604.

211 Altman DG, Vergouwe Y, Royston P, et al. Prognosis and prognostic research: validating a prognostic model. *BMJ* 2009;338:b605.

212 Moons KG, Altman DG, Vergouwe Y, et al. Prognosis and prognostic research: application and impact of prognostic models in clinical practice. *BMJ* 2009;338:b606.

213 Hingorani AD, Windt DA, Riley RD, et al. Prognosis research strategy (PROGRESS) 4: stratified medicine research. *BMJ* 2013;346:e5793.

214 Pavlou M, Ambler G, Seaman SR, et al. How to develop a more accurate risk prediction model when there are few events. *BMJ* 2015;351:h3868.

215 Moons KG, Kengne AP, Woodward M, et al. Risk prediction models: I. Development, internal validation, and assessing the incremental value of a new (bio)marker. *Heart* 2012;98(9):683–690.

216 Bleeker SE, Moll HA, Steyerberg EW, et al. External validation is necessary in prediction research: A clinical example. *J Clin Epidemiol* 2003;56(9):826–832.

217 Debray TP, Vergouwe Y, Koffijberg H, et al. A new framework to enhance the interpretation of external validation studies of clinical prediction models. *J Clin Epidemiol* 2015;68(3):279–289.

218 Mallett S, Royston P, Waters R, et al. Reporting performance of prognostic models in cancer: a review. *BMC Med* 2010;8:21.

219 Reilly BM, Evans AT. Translating clinical research into clinical practice: impact of using prediction rules to make decisions. *Ann Intern Med* 2006;144(3):201–209.

220 Bouwmeester W, Zuithoff NP, Mallett S, et al. Reporting and methods in clinical prediction research: a systematic review. *PLoS Med* 2012;9(5):1–12.

221 Wyatt J, Altman DG. Commentary: Prognostic models: clinically useful or quickly forgotten? *BMJ* 1995;311:1539–1541.

222 Collins GS, Michaelsson K. Fracture risk assessment: state of the art, methodologically unsound, or poorly reported? *Curr Osteoporos Rep* 2012;10(3):199–207.

223 Geersing GJ, Zuithoff NP, Kearon C, et al. Exclusion of deep vein thrombosis using the Wells rule in clinically important subgroups: individual patient data meta-analysis. *BMJ* 2014;348:g1340.

224 Majed B, Tafflet M, Kee F, et al. External validation of the 2008 Framingham cardiovascular risk equation for CHD and stroke events in a European population of middle-aged men. The PRIME study. *Prev Med* 2013;57(1):49–54.

225 Den Ruijter HM, Peters SA, Anderson TJ, et al. Common carotid intima-media thickness measurements in cardiovascular risk prediction: a meta-analysis. *JAMA* 2012;308(8):796–803.

226 Kengne AP, Beulens JW, Peelen LM, et al. Non-invasive risk scores for prediction of type 2 diabetes (EPIC-InterAct): a validation of existing models. *Lancet Diabetes Endocrinol* 2014;2(1):19–29.

227 Debray TP, Koffijberg H, Nieboer D, et al. Meta-analysis and aggregation of multiple published prediction models. *Stat Med* 2014;33(14):2341–2362.

228 Debray TP, Koffijberg H, Vergouwe Y, et al. Aggregating published prediction models with individual participant data: a comparison of different approaches. *Stat Med* 2012;31(23):2697–2712.

229 Greving JP, Wermer MJ, Brown RD, Jr., et al. Development of the PHASES score for prediction of risk of rupture of intracranial aneurysms: a pooled analysis of six prospective cohort studies. *Lancet Neurol* 2014;13(1):59–66.

230 Janssen KJ, Moons KG, Kalkman CJ, et al. Updating methods improved the performance of a clinical prediction model in new patients. *J Clin Epidemiol* 2008;61(1):76–86.

231 Tzoulaki I, Liberopoulos G, Ioannidis JP. Assessment of claims of improved prediction beyond the Framingham risk score. *JAMA* 2009;302(21):2345–2352.

232 Cox DR, Snell EJ. *The Analysis of Binary Data* (2nd edition). London: Chapman & Hall 1989.

233 Nagelkerke N. A note on a general definition of the coefficient of determination. *Biometrika* 1991;78:691–692.

234 O'Quigley J, Xu R, Stare J. Explained randomness in proportional hazards models. *Stat Med* 2005;24 (3):479–489.

235 Brier GW. Verification of forecasts expressed in terms of probability. *Mon Weather Rev* 1950;78 (1):1–3.

236 Van Calster B, Nieboer D, Vergouwe Y, et al. A calibration hierarchy for risk models was defined: from utopia to empirical data. *J Clin Epidemiol* 2016; 74:167–176.

237 Royston P, Altman DG. External validation of a Cox prognostic model: principles and methods. *BMC Med Res Methodol* 2013;13:33.

238 Van Hoorde K, Van Huffel S, Timmerman D, et al. A spline-based tool to assess and visualize the calibration of multiclass risk predictions. *J Biomed Inform* 2015;54:283–293.

239 Austin PC, Steyerberg EW. The Integrated Calibration Index (ICI) and related metrics for quantifying the calibration of logistic regression models. *Statistics in Medicine* 2019;38 (21):4051–4065.

240 Hosmer DW, Lemeshow S. A goodness-of-fit test for the multiple logistic regression model. *Commun Stat* 1980;A10:1043–1069.

241 Harrell FE, Jr., Lee KL, Mark DB. Multivariable prognostic models: issues in developing models, evaluating assumptions and adequacy, and measuring and reducing errors. *Stat Med* 1996;15 (4):361–387.

242 Brentnall AR, Cuzick J. Use of the concordance index for predictors of censored survival data. *Stat Methods Med Res* 2018;27(8): 2359–2373.

243 Lambert J, Chevret S. Summary measure of discrimination in survival models based on cumulative/dynamic time-dependent ROC curves. *Stat Methods Med Res* 2016;25(5):2088–2102.

244 Yates JF. External correspondence: decompositions of the mean probability score. *Organization Behav Hum Perform* 1982;30:132–156.

245 Vergouwe Y, Steyerberg EW, Eijkemans MJ, et al. Substantial effective sample sizes were required for external validation studies of predictive logistic regression models. *J Clin Epidemiol* 2005;58 (5):475–483.

246 Collins GS, Ogundimu EO, Altman DG. Sample size considerations for the external validation of a multivariable prognostic model: a resampling study. *Stat Med* 2016;35(2):214–226.

247 Royston P, Parmar MKB, Sylvester R. Construction and validation of a prognostic model across several studies, with an application in superficial bladder cancer. *Stat Med* 2004;23:907–926.

248 Vergouwe Y, Moons KG, Steyerberg EW. External validity of risk models: use of benchmark values to disentangle a case-mix effect from incorrect coefficients. *Am J Epidemiol* 2010;172(8):971–980.

249 Mulherin SA, Miller WC. Spectrum bias or spectrum effect? Subgroup variation in diagnostic test evaluation. *Ann Intern Med* 2002;137(7):598–602.

250 Ransohoff DF, Feinstein AR. Problems of spectrum and bias in evaluating the efficacy of diagnostic tests. *N Engl J Med* 1978;299(17):926–930.

251 Steyerberg EW, Nieboer D, Debray TPA, et al. Assessment of heterogeneity in an individual participant data meta-analysis of prediction models: an overview and illustration. *Stat Med* 2019;38 (22):4290–4309.

252 Knottnerus JA. Between iatrotropic stimulus and interiatric referral: the domain of primary care research. *J Clin Epidemiol* 2002;55(12):1201–1206.

253 Oudega R, Hoes AW, Moons KG. The Wells rule does not adequately rule out deep venous thrombosis in primary care patients. *Ann Intern Med* 2005;143(2):100–107.

254 Pajouheshnia R, van Smeden M, Peelen LM, et al. How variation in predictor measurement affects the discriminative ability and transportability of a prediction model. *J Clin Epidemiol* 2019;105:136–141.

255 Luijken K, Groenwold RHH, Van Calster B, et al. Impact of predictor measurement heterogeneity across settings on the performance of prediction models: a measurement error perspective. *Stat Med* 2019;38(18):3444–3459.

256 van Klaveren D, Gonen M, Steyerberg EW, et al. A new concordance measure for risk prediction models in external validation settings. *Stat Med* 2016;35(23):4136–4152.

257 Snell KI, Ensor J, Debray TP, et al. Meta-analysis of prediction model performance across multiple studies: Which scale helps ensure between-study normality for the C-statistic and calibration measures? *Stat Methods Med Res* 2018;27(11):3505–3522.

258 Sidik K, Jonkman JN. A simple confidence interval for meta-analysis. *Stat Med* 2002;21 (21):3153–3159.

259 Hartung J, Knapp G. A refined method for the meta-analysis of controlled clinical trials with binary outcome. *Stat Med* 2001;20(24):3875–3889.

260 van Aert RCM, Jackson D. A new justification of the Hartung-Knapp method for random-effects meta-analysis based on weighted least squares regression. *Res Synths Methods* 2019;10 (4):515–527.

261 Higgins JP, Thompson SG, Deeks JJ, et al. Measuring inconsistency in meta-analyses. *BMJ* 2003;327 (7414):557–560.

262 Wang CC, Lee WC. A simple method to estimate prediction intervals and predictive distributions: summarizing meta-analyses beyond means and confidence intervals. *Res Synth Methods* 2019;10 (2):255–266.

263 Nagashima K, Noma H, Furukawa TA. Prediction intervals for random-effects meta-analysis: A confidence distribution approach. *Stat Methods Med Res* 2019;28(6):1689–1702.

264 Wynants L, Vergouwe Y, Van Huffel S, et al. Does ignoring clustering in multicenter data influence the performance of prediction models? A simulation study. *Stat Methods Med Res* 2018;27 (6):1723–1736.

265 Wynants L, Bouwmeester W, Moons KG, et al. A simulation study of sample size demonstrated the importance of the number of events per variable to develop prediction models in clustered data. *J Clin Epidemiol* 2015;68(12):1406–1414.

266 Falconieri N, Van Calster B, Timmerman D, et al. Developing risk models for multicenter data using standard logistic regression produced suboptimal predictions: a simulation study. *Biom J* 2020;62 (4):932–944.

267 Collins GS, Altman DG. An independent and external validation of QRISK2 cardiovascular disease risk score: a prospective open cohort study. *BMJ* 2010;340:c2442.

268 Wynants L, Kent DM, Timmerman D, et al. Untapped potential of multicenter studies: a review of cardiovascular risk prediction models revealed inappropriate analyses and wide variation in reporting. *Diagn Progn Res* 2019;3:6.

269 Li Y, Sperrin M, Martin GP, et al. Examining the impact of data quality and completeness of electronic health records on predictions of patients' risks of cardiovascular disease. *Int J Med Inform* 2020;133:104033.

270 Hippisley-Cox J, Coupland C, Brindle P. Development and validation of QRISK3 risk prediction algorithms to estimate future risk of cardiovascular disease: prospective cohort study. *BMJ* 2017;357:j2099.

271 Qin G, Hotilovac L. Comparison of non-parametric confidence intervals for the area under the ROC curve of a continuous-scale diagnostic test. *Stat Methods Med Res* 2008;17(2):207–221.

272 van Klaveren D, Steyerberg EW, Gonen M, et al. The calibrated model-based concordance improved assessment of discriminative ability in patient clusters of limited sample size. *Diagn Progn Res* 2019;3:11.

273 Steyerberg EW, Borsboom GJ, van Houwelingen HC, et al. Validation and updating of predictive logistic regression models: a study on sample size and shrinkage. *Stat Med* 2004;23 (16):2567–2586.

274 van Houwelingen HC, Thorogood J. Construction, validation and updating of a prognostic model for kidney graft survival. *Stat Med* 1995;14(18):1999–2008.

275 Schuetz P, Koller M, Christ-Crain M, et al. Predicting mortality with pneumonia severity scores: importance of model recalibration to local settings. *Epidemiol Infect* 2008;136(12):1628–1637.

276 Ensor J, Snell KIE, Debray TP, et al. Individual participant data meta-analysis for external validation, recalibration and updating of a flexible parametric prognostic model. *Stat Med* 2021 (in-press).

277 Snell KI, Hua H, Debray TP, et al. Multivariate meta-analysis of individual participant data helped externally validate the performance and implementation of a prediction model. *J Clin Epidemiol* 2016;69:40–50.

278 The R package 'mnormt': The multivariate normal and 't' distributions (version 1.5-1). http://azzalini.stat.unipd.it/SW/Pkg-mnormt [program], 2014.

279 Collins GS, Altman DG. Predicting the 10 year risk of cardiovascular disease in the United Kingdom: independent and external validation of an updated version of QRISK2. *BMJ* 2012;344:e4181.

280 Snell KIE, Allotey J, Smuk M, et al. External validation of prognostic models predicting pre-eclampsia: individual participant data meta-analysis. *BMC Med* 2020;18:302.

281 Kunkel D, Kaizar EE. A comparison of existing methods for multiple imputation in individual participant data meta-analysis. *Stat Med* 2017;36(22):3507–3532.

282 Audigier V, White IR, Jolani S, et al. Multiple imputation for multilevel data with continuous and binary variables. *Statist Sci* 2018;33(2):160–183.

283 Moons KG, de Groot JA, Linnet K, et al. Quantifying the added value of a diagnostic test or marker. *Clin Chem* 2012;58(10):1408–1417.

284 Riley RD, Snell KI, Ensor J, et al. Minimum sample size for developing a multivariable prediction model: Part II - binary and time-to-event outcomes. *Stat Med* 2019;38(7):1276–1296.

285 Riley RD, Snell KIE, Ensor J, et al. Minimum sample size for developing a multivariable prediction model: Part I - Continuous outcomes. *Stat Med* 2019;38(7):1262–1275.

286 Riley RD, Ensor J, Snell KIE, et al. Calculating the sample size required for developing a clinical prediction model. *BMJ* 2020;368:m441.

287 Collins GS, Ogundimu EO, Cook JA, et al. Quantifying the impact of different approaches for handling continuous predictors on the performance of a prognostic model. *Stat Med* 2016;35 (23):4124–4135.

288 Wolbers M, Blanche P, Koller MT, et al. Concordance for prognostic models with competing risks. *Biostatistics* 2014;15(3):526–539.

289 Wolbers M, Koller MT, Witteman JCM, et al. Prognostic models with competing risks: methods and application to coronary risk prediction. *Epidemiology* 2009;20:555–561.

290 Luijken K, Wynants L, van Smeden M, et al. Changing predictor measurement procedures affected the performance of prediction models in clinical examples. *J Clin Epidemiol* 2019;119:7–18.

291 Pavlou M, Ambler G, Seaman S, et al. A note on obtaining correct marginal predictions from a random intercepts model for binary outcomes. *BMC Med Res Methodol* 2015;15:59.

292 Westeneng H-J, Debray TPA, Visser AE, et al. Prognosis for patients with amyotrophic lateral sclerosis: development and validation of a personalised prediction model. *Lancet Neurol* 2018;17(5):423–433.

293 Royston P, Parmar MKB. Flexible parametric proportional-hazards and proportional-odds models for censored survival data, with application to prognostic modelling and estimation of treatment effects. *Stat Med* 2002;21:2175–2197.

294 Timmerman D, Van Calster B, Testa A, et al. Predicting the risk of malignancy in adnexal masses based on the Simple Rules from the International Ovarian Tumor Analysis group. *Am J Obstet Gynecol* 2016;214(4):424–437.

295 Van Calster B, Van Hoorde K, Valentin L, et al. Evaluating the risk of ovarian cancer before surgery using the ADNEX model to differentiate between benign, borderline, early and advanced stage invasive, and secondary metastatic tumours: prospective multicentre diagnostic study. *BMJ* 2014;349:g5920.

296 Wynants L, Timmerman D, Bourne T, et al. Screening for data clustering in multicenter studies: the residual intraclass correlation. *BMC Med Res Methodol* 2013;13:128.

297 Groll A, Tutz G. Variable selection for generalized linear mixed models by L1-penalized estimation. *Stat Comput* 2014;24(2):137–154.

298 Heinze G, Wallisch C, Dunkler D. Variable selection – a review and recommendations for the practicing statistician. *Biom J* 2018;60(3):431–449.

299 Steyerberg EW, Harrell FEJ, Borsboom GJ, et al. Internal validation of predictive models: efficiency of some procedures for logistic regression analysis. *J Clin Epidemiol* 2001;54:774–781.

300 van Smeden M, Moons KG, de Groot JA, et al. Sample size for binary logistic prediction models: beyond events per variable criteria. *Stat Methods Med Res* 2019;28(8):2455–2474.

301 Bouwmeester W, Moons KG, Kappen TH, et al. Internal validation of risk models in clustered data: a comparison of bootstrap schemes. *Am J Epidemiol* 2013;177(11):1209–1217.

302 Ensor J, Riley RD, Jowett S, et al. Prediction of risk of recurrence of venous thromboembolism following treatment for a first unprovoked venous thromboembolism: systematic review, prognostic model and clinical decision rule, and economic evaluation. *Health Technol Assess* 2016;20(12):i–xxxiii, 1–190.

303 Timmerman D, Testa AC, Bourne T, et al. Logistic regression model to distinguish between the benign and malignant adnexal mass before surgery: a multicenter study by the International Ovarian Tumor Analysis Group. *J Clin Oncol* 2005;23(34):8794–8801.

304 Testa A, Kaijser J, Wynants L, et al. Strategies to diagnose ovarian cancer: new evidence from phase 3 of the multicentre international IOTA study. *Br J Cancer* 2014;111(4):680–688.

305 Debray TPA, Collins GS, Riley RD, et al. Transparent reporting of multivariable prediction models developed or validated using clustered data: TRIPOD-Cluster. 2021 (submitted).

306 Roderick JAL. Regression with missing X's: a review. *J Am Stat Assoc* 1992;87(420):1227–1237.

307 Donders AR, van der Heijden GJ, Stijnen T, et al. Review: a gentle introduction to imputation of missing values. *J Clin Epidemiol* 2006;59(10):1087–1091.

308 Groenwold RH, Donders AR, Roes KC, et al. Dealing with missing outcome data in randomized trials and observational studies. *Am J Epidemiol* 2012;175(3):210–217.

309 Graham JW. *Missing Data: Analysis and Design*. New York: Springer 2012.

310 Carpenter JR, Kenward MG. *Multiple Imputation and Its Application*. Chichester, UK: Wiley 2013.

311 van Buuren S. *Flexible Imputation of Missing Data* (2nd Edition). Boca Raton, FL: Chapman & Hall/CRC 2018.

312 Groenwold RH, Moons KG, Vandenbroucke JP. Randomized trials with missing outcome data: how to analyze and what to report. *CMAJ* 2014;186(15):1153–1157.

313 Knol MJ, Janssen KJ, Donders AR, et al. Unpredictable bias when using the missing indicator method or complete case analysis for missing confounder values: an empirical example. *J Clin Epidemiol* 2010;63(7):728–736.

314 van der Heijden GJ, Donders AR, Stijnen T, et al. Imputation of missing values is superior to complete case analysis and the missing-indicator method in multivariable diagnostic research: a clinical example. *J Clin Epidemiol* 2006;59(10):1102–1109.

315 Groenwold RH, White IR, Donders AR, et al. Missing covariate data in clinical research: when and when not to use the missing-indicator method for analysis. *CMAJ* 2012;184(11):1265–1269.

316 Sullivan TR, White IR, Salter AB, et al. Should multiple imputation be the method of choice for handling missing data in randomized trials? *Stat Methods Med Res* 2018;27(9):2610–2626.

317 Allotey J, Snell KIE, Chan C, et al. External validation, update and development of prediction models for pre-eclampsia using an Individual Participant Data (IPD) meta-analysis: the International Prediction of Pregnancy Complication Network (IPPIC pre-eclampsia) protocol. *Diagnostic and Prognostic Research* 2017;1(1):16.

318 Allotey J, Snell KIE, Smuk M, Hooper R, Chan CL, Ahmed A, et al. Validation and development of models using clinical, biochemical and ultrasound markers for predicting pre-eclampsia: an individual participant data meta-analysis. *Health Technol Assess* 2020;24(72).

319 Crovetto F, Figueras F, Triunfo S, et al. First trimester screening for early and late preeclampsia based on maternal characteristics, biophysical parameters, and angiogenic factors. *Prenatal Diagnosis* 2015;35(2):183–191.

320 Leacy FP, Floyd S, Yates TA, et al. Analyses of sensitivity to the missing-at-random assumption using multiple imputation with delta adjustment: application to a tuberculosis/HIV prevalence survey with incomplete HIV-status data. *Am J Epidemiol* 2017;185(4):304–315.

321 Janssen KJ, Vergouwe Y, Donders AR, et al. Dealing with missing predictor values when applying clinical prediction models. *Clin Chem* 2009;55(5):994–1001.

322 Moons KG, Donders RA, Stijnen T, et al. Using the outcome for imputation of missing predictor values was preferred. *J Clin Epidemiol* 2006;59(10):1092–1101.

323 Tanner MA, Wong WH. The calculation of posterior distributions by data augmentation. *J Am Stat Assoc* 1987;82(398):528–540.

324 Goldstein H, Carpenter J, Kenward MG, et al. Multilevel models with multivariate mixed response types. *Stat Modelling* 2009;9(3):173–197.

325 Quartagno M, Carpenter JR. Multiple imputation for discrete data: evaluation of the joint latent normal model. *Biom J* 2019;61(4):1003–1019.

326 Vink G, Frank LE, Pannekoek J, et al. Predictive mean matching imputation of semicontinuous variables. *Statistica Neerlandica* 2014;68(1):61–90.

327 Hothorn T, Hornik K, Zeileis A. Unbiased recursive partitioning: a conditional inference framework. *J Comput Graph Stat* 2006;15(3):651–674.

328 Doove LL, Van Buuren S, Dusseldorp E. Recursive partitioning for missing data imputation in the presence of interaction effects. *Comput Stat Data Anal* 2014;72:92–104.

329 Shah AD, Bartlett JW, Carpenter J, et al. Comparison of random forest and parametric imputation models for imputing missing data using MICE: a CALIBER study. *Am J Epidemiol* 2014;179(6):764–774.

330 de Jong R, van Buuren S, Spiess M. Multiple imputation of predictor variables using generalized additive models. *Commun Stat - Simul Comput* 2016;45(3):968–985.

331 Chen HY. Compatibility of conditionally specified models. *Stat Probab Lett* 2010;80(7–8):670–677.

332 van Buuren S. Multiple imputation of discrete and continuous data by fully conditional specification. *Stat Methods Med Res* 2007;16(3):219–242.

333 White IR, Royston P, Wood AM. Multiple imputation using chained equations: issues and guidance for practice. *Stat Med* 2011;30(4):377–399.

334 Rubin DB. Inference and missing data. *Biometrika* 1976;63:581–592.

335 Meng X-L. Multiple-imputation inferences with uncongenial sources of input. *Statist Sci* 1994;9(4):538–558.

336 Burgess S, White IR, Resche-Rigon M, et al. Combining multiple imputation and meta-analysis with individual participant data. *Stat Med* 2013;32(26):4499–4514.

337 Marshall A, Altman DG, Holder RL, et al. Combining estimates of interest in prognostic modelling studies after multiple imputation: current practice and guidelines. *BMC MedRes Methodol* 2009;9(1):57.

338 Riley RD, Price MJ, Jackson D, et al. Multivariate meta-analysis using individual participant data. *Res Synth Method* 2015;6 157–174.

339 Andridge RR. Quantifying the impact of fixed effects modeling of clusters in multiple imputation for cluster randomized trials. *Biom J*2011;53(1):57–74.

340 GREAT Network. Managing acute heart failure in the ED – case studies from the Acute Heart Failure Academy (https://www.greatnetwork.org/p/2015/09/19/managing-acute-heart-failure-in-the-ed-case-studies-from-the-acute-heart-failure-academy/?lang=it) 2013.

341 Schafer JL, Yucel RM. Computational strategies for multivariate linear mixed-effects models with missing values. *J Comput Graph Stat* 2002;11(2):437–457.

342 Yucel RM. Random-covariances and mixed-effects models for imputing multivariate multilevel continuous data. *Stat Modelling* 2011;11(4):351–370.

343 Siddique J, de Chavez PJ, Howe G, et al. Limitations in using multiple imputation to harmonize individual participant data for meta-analysis. *Prev Sci* 2018;19(Suppl 1):95–108.

344 Grund S, Lüdtke O, Robitzsch A. Multiple imputation of missing covariate values in multilevel models with random slopes: a cautionary note. *Behav Res Methods* 2016;48(2):640–649.

345 Liu J, Gelman A, Hill J, et al. On the stationary distribution of iterative imputations. *Biometrika* 2013;101(1):155–173.

346 Quartagno M, Grund S, Carpenter J. jomo: A flexible package for two-level joint modelling multiple imputation. *R Journal* 2019;11(2):205–228.

347 Enders CK, Hayes T, Du H. A comparison of multilevel imputation schemes for random coefficient models: fully conditional specification and joint model imputation with random covariance matrices. *Multivariate Behav Res*2018;53(5):695–713.

348 Grund S, Lüdtke O, Robitzsch A. Multiple imputation of multilevel missing data: an introduction to the R package pan. *SAGE Open* 2016;6(4):1–17.

349 Grund S, Robitzsch A, Lüdtke O. mitml: Tools for multiple imputation in multilevel modeling (Version 0.3-7). 2019.

350 Enders CK, Keller BT, Levy R. A fully conditional specification approach to multilevel imputation of categorical and continuous variables. *Psychol Methods* 2018;23(2):298–317.

351 Enders CK, Du H, Keller BT. A model-based imputation procedure for multilevel regression models with random coefficients, interaction effects, and nonlinear terms. *Psychol Methods* 2020;25(1):88–112.

Index

Note: Page numbers in *italic* refer to figures and boxes, page numbers in **bold** refer to tables.

Individual Participant Data Meta-Analysis: A Handbook for Healthcare Research, First Edition.
Edited by Richard D. Riley, Jayne F. Tierney, and Lesley A. Stewart.

n

o

p

q

r

V

W

Printed and bound by CPI Group (UK) Ltd, Croydon, CR0 4YY
27/10/2024
14580360-0005